World Health Organization Classification of Tumours

WHO OMS

International Agency for Research on Cancer (IARC)

4th Edition

WHO Classification of Tumours of the Eye

Edited by

Hans E. Grossniklaus

Charles G. Eberhart

Tero T. Kivelä

International Agency for Research on Cancer

Lyon, 2018

World Health Organization Classification of Tumours

WHO Classification of Tumours of the Eye

Editors	Hans E. Grossniklaus, MD, MBA Charles G. Eberhart, MD, PhD Tero T. Kivelä, MD
IARC Editors	Ian A. Cree, MB ChB, PhD, FRCPath Valerie A. White, MD, MHSc, FRCPC Reiko Watanabe, MD, PhD
Project Assistant	Asiedua Asante
Assistants	Anne-Sophie Hameau Laura Brispot
Technical Editor	Jessica Cox
Database	Alberto Machado Delphine Nicolas
Layout	Meaghan Fortune
Printed by	Maestro Gestion D'Edition 69100 Villeurbanne, France Printed in Italy
Publisher	International Agency for Research on Cancer (IARC) 69372 Lyon Cedex 08, France

The WHO Classification of Tumours of the Eye presented in this book reflects the views of a Working Group that convened for a Consensus and Editorial Meeting at the International Agency for Research on Cancer, Lyon, 11–13 January 2018.

Members of the Working Group are indicated in the list of contributors on pages 185–188.

Published by the International Agency for Research on Cancer (IARC),
150 Cours Albert Thomas, 69372 Lyon Cedex 08, France

Distributed by
WHO Press, World Health Organization, 20 Avenue Appia, 1211 Geneva 27, Switzerland
Tel.: +41 22 791 3264; Fax: +41 22 791 4857; email: bookorders@who.int

Second print run (3000 copies)

Updated corrigenda can be found at
http://publications.iarc.fr/561

Format for bibliographic citations:
Grossniklaus HE, Eberhart CG, Kivelä TT, editors (2018).
WHO classification of tumours of the eye. 4th ed.
Lyon: IARC.

IARC Library Cataloguing-in-Publication Data

WHO classification of tumours of the eye / edited by Hans E. Grossniklaus, Charles G. Eberhart, Tero T. Kivelä. – 4th edition.

(World Health Organization classification of tumours)

1. Eye neoplasms – pathology 2. Eye neoplasms – genetics

I. Grossniklaus, Hans E. II. Series

ISBN 978-92-832-4497-4 (NLM Classification: WW 149)

Contents

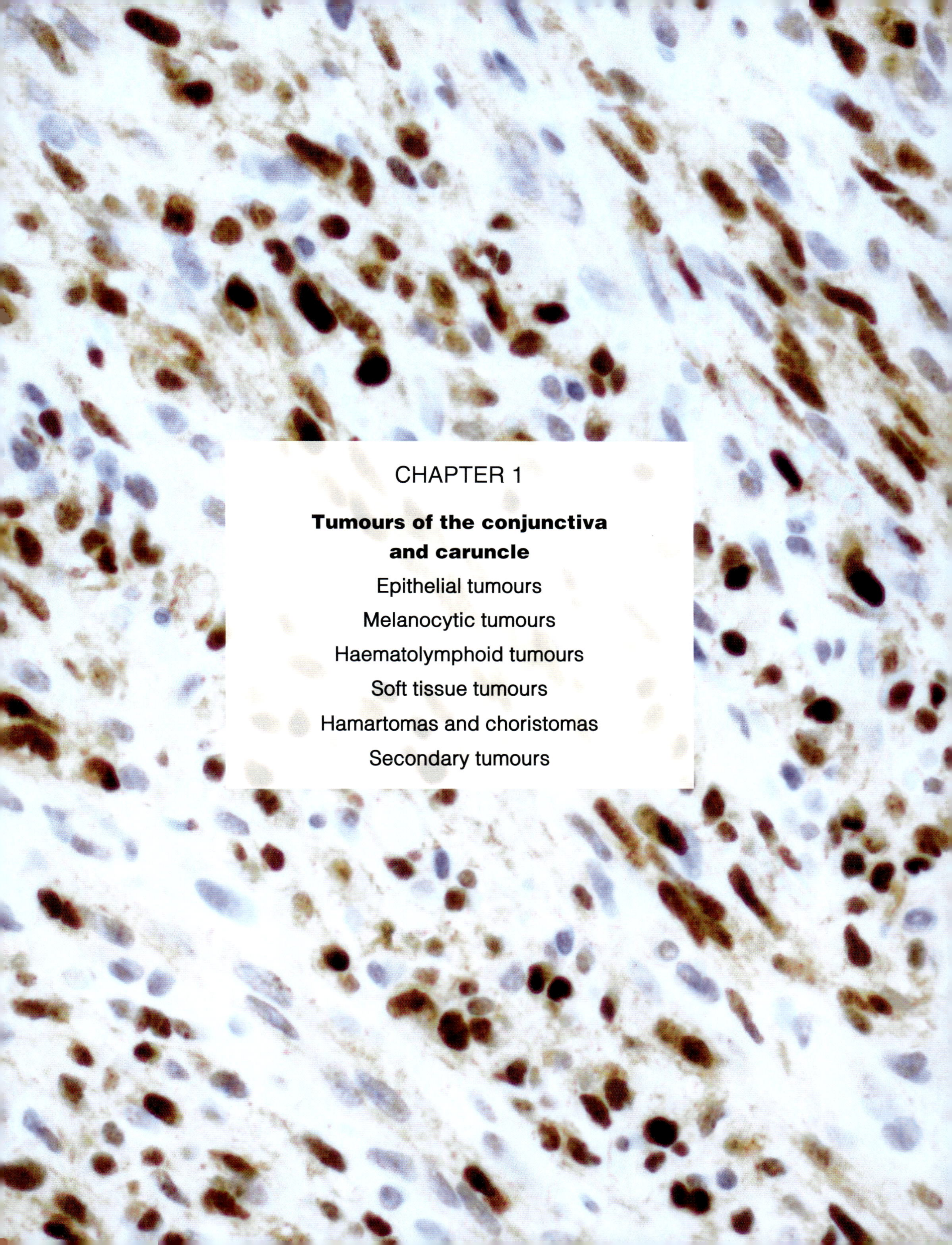

CHAPTER 1

Tumours of the conjunctiva and caruncle

WHO classification of tumours of the conjunctiva and carunder

Epithelial tumours	
Squamous cell carcinoma NOS	8070/3
Squamous cell carcinoma in situ with questionable stromal invasion	8076/2
Squamous cell carcinoma, keratinizing, NOS	8071/3
Basaloid squamous cell carcinoma	8083/3
Spindle cell carcinoma	8074/3
Mucoepidermoid carcinoma	8430/3
Adenosquamous carcinoma	8560/3
Keratoacanthoma	8071/3
Hereditary benign intraepithelial dyskeratosis	None
Conjunctival squamous intraepithelial neoplasia (conjunctival intraepithelial neoplasia and carcinoma in situ)	8077/2
Sebaceous carcinoma	8410/3
Oncocytoma	8290/0
Squamous papilloma	8052/0
Tumour-like lesions	
Cysts	None
Reactive epithelial hyperplasia	None
Pseudoglandular and pseudoepitheliomatous hyperplasia	None
Melanocytic tumours	
Melanoma NOS	8720/3
Nodular melanoma	8721/3
Melanoma in situ	8720/2
Junctional naevus	8740/0
Compound naevus	8760/0
Subepithelial (stromal) naevus	8750/0
Inflamed juvenile naevus	8770/0
Blue naevus	8780/0
Spitz naevus	8770/0
Benign epithelial melanoses	None
Haematolymphoid tumours	
Lymphoma	See note[a]
Papillary/follicular conjunctivitis	None
Reactive lymphoid hyperplasia	None
Soft tissue tumours	
Leiomyosarcoma	8890/3
Rhabdomyosarcoma NOS	8900/3
Embryonal rhabdomyosarcoma	8910/3
Spindle cell rhabdomyosarcoma	8912/3
Botryoid rhabdomyosarcoma	8910/3
Anaplastic rhabdomyosarcoma	8910/3
Alveolar rhabdomyosarcoma	8920/3
Pleomorphic rhabdomyosarcoma	8901/3
Kaposi sarcoma	9140/3
Angiosarcoma	9120/3
Benign fibrous histiocytoma	8830/0
Conjunctival stromal tumour	None
Myxoma	8840/0
Haemangioma	9120/0
Lymphangioma	9170/0
Neurofibroma	9540/0
Schwannoma	9560/0
Juvenile xanthogranuloma	None
Hamartomas and choristomas	
Epibulbar choristoma	None
Epibulbar osseous choristoma	None
Phakomatous choristoma	None
Secondary tumours	See note[b]

[a]Code primary and secondary conjunctival lymphomas according to the lymphoma subtype.

[b]Code secondary tumours according to the originating tumour type.

The morphology codes are from the International Classification of Diseases for Oncology (ICD-O) {381}. Behaviour is coded /0 for benign tumours; /1 for unspecified, borderline, or uncertain behaviour; /2 for carcinoma in situ and grade III intraepithelial neoplasia; and /3 for malignant tumours.

The classification is modified from the previous WHO classification, taking into account changes in our understanding of these lesions.

TNM classification of carcinoma of the conjunctiva

Carcinoma of Conjunctiva

(ICD-O-3 C69.0)

TNM Clinical Classification

T – Primary Tumour

TX	Primary tumour cannot be assessed
T0	No evidence of primary tumour
Tis	Carcinoma in situ
T1	Tumour 5 mm or less in greatest dimension invades through the conjunctival basement membrane
T2	Tumour more than 5 mm in greatest dimension, invades through the conjunctival basement membrane without invasion of adjacent structures*
T3	Tumour invades adjacent structures*
T4	Tumour invades the orbit or beyond
T4a	Tumour invades orbital soft tissues, without bone invasion
T4b	Tumour invades bone
T4c	Tumour invades adjacent paranasal sinuses
T4d	Tumour invades brain

Note

*Adjacent structures include: the cornea (3, 6, 9, or 12 clock hours), intraocular compartments, forniceal conjunctiva (lower and/or upper), palpebral conjunctiva (lower and/or upper), tarsal conjunctiva (lower and/or upper), lacrimal punctum and canaliculi (lower and/or upper), plica, caruncle, posterior eyelid lamella, anterior eyelid lamella and/or eyelid margin (lower and/or upper).

N – Regional Lymph Nodes

NX	Regional lymph nodes cannot be assessed
N0	No regional lymph node metastasis
N1	Regional lymph node metastasis

M – Distant Metastasis

M0	No distant metastasis
M1	Distant metastasis

pTNM Pathological Classification

The pT and pN categories correspond to the T and N categories.

pM – Distant Metastasis*

pM1	Distant metastasis microscopically confirmed

Note

*pM0 and pMX are not valid categories.

Stage

No stage is at present recommended.

The information presented here has been excerpted from the 8th edition of the *TNM classification of malignant tumours* (2017) {132}.
A help desk for specific questions about the TNM classification is available at http://www.uicc.org/resources/tnm/helpdesk.

TNM classification of skin carcinoma of the eyelid

Carcinoma of Skin of the Eyelid

(ICD-O C44.1)

TNM Clinical Classification

T – Primary Tumour

T0	No evidence of primary tumour	
Tis	Carcinoma in situ	
T1	Tumour 10 mm or less in greatest dimension	
	T1a	Not invading the tarsal plate or eyelid margin
	T1b	Invades tarsal plate or eyelid margin
	T1c	Involves full thickness of eyelid
T2	Tumour > 10 mm, but 20 mm or less in greatest dimension	
	T2a	Not invading the tarsal plate or eyelid margin
	T2b	Invades the tarsal plate or eyelid margin
	T2c	Involves full thickness of eyelid
T3	Tumour > 20 mm in greatest dimension	
	T3a	Not invading the tarsal plate or eyelid margin
	T3b	Invades tarsal plate or eyelid margin
	T3c	Involves full thickness of eyelid
T4	Any eyelid tumour that invades adjacent ocular, or orbital, or facial structures	
	T4a	Tumour invades ocular or intraorbital structures
	T4b	Tumour invades (or erodes through) the bony walls of orbit or extends to paranasal sinuses or invades the lacrimal sac/nasolacrimal duct or brain

N – Regional Lymph Nodes

NX	Regional lymph nodes cannot be assessed
N0	No evidence of lymph node involvement
N1	Metastasis in a single ipsilateral regional lymph node, 3 cm or less in greatest dimension
N2	Metastasis in a single ipsilateral lymph node more than 3 cm in greatest dimension or in bilateral or contralateral lymph nodes

M – Distant Metastasis

M0	No distant metastasis
M1	Distant metastasis

pTNM Pathological Classification

The pT and pN categories correspond to the T and N categories.

pM – Distant Metastasis*

pM1 Distant metastasis microscopically confirmed

Note

*pM0 and pMX are not valid categories.

Stage

Stage 0	Tis	N0	M0
Stage IA	T1	N0	M0
Stage IB	T2a	N0	M0
Stage IIA	T2b, T2c, T3	N0	M0
Stage IIB	T4	N0	M0
Stage IIIA	Any T	N1	M0
Stage IIIB	Any T	N2	M0
Stage IV	Any T	Any N	M1

The information presented here has been excerpted from the 8th edition of the *TNM classification of malignant tumours* (2017) {132}.
A help desk for specific questions about the TNM classification is available at http://www.uicc.org/resources/tnm/helpdesk.

TNM classification of melanoma of the conjunctiva

Malignant Melanoma of Conjunctiva

(ICD-O-3 C69.0)

TNM Clinical Classification

T – Primary Tumour

TX	Primary tumour cannot be assessed	
T0	No evidence of primary tumour	
Tis	Melanoma confined to the conjunctival epithelium (in situ)[a]	
T1	Melanoma of the bulbar conjunctiva	
	T1a	Tumour involves less than or equal to one quadrant[b]
	T1b	Tumour involves more than one but less than or equal to two quadrants
	T1c	Tumour involves more than two but less than or equal to three quadrants
	T1d	Tumour involves more than three quadrants
T2	Malignant conjunctival melanoma of the non-bulbar conjunctiva involving palpebral, forniceal, and/or caruncular conjunctiva	
	T2a	Non-caruncular tumour involves less than or equal to one quadrant
	T2b	Non-caruncular tumour involves more than one quadrant
	T2c	Caruncular tumour involves less than or equal to one quadrant of conjunctiva
	T2d	Caruncular tumour involves more than one quadrant of conjunctiva
T3	Tumour with local invasion into:	
	T3a	Globe
	T3b	Eyelid
	T3c	Orbit
	T3d	Paranasal sinus, nasolacrimal duct, and/or lacrimal gland
T4	Tumour invades central nervous system	

Notes

[a] Melanoma in situ (includes the term primary acquired melanosis) with atypia replacing greater than 75% of the normal epithelial thickness with cytological features of epithelial cells, including abundant cytoplasm, vesicular nuclei, or prominent nucleoli, and/or presence of intraepithelial nest of atypical cells.

[b] Quadrants are defined by clock hour, starting at the limbus (e.g. 6, 9, 12, 3) extending from the central cornea, to and beyond the eyelid margins. This will bisect the caruncle.

N – Regional Lymph Nodes

NX	Regional lymph nodes cannot be assessed
N0	No regional lymph node metastasis
N1	Regional lymph node metastasis

M – Distant Metastasis

M0	No distant metastasis
M1	Distant metastasis

pTNM Pathological Classification

pT – Primary Tumour

pTX	Primary tumour cannot be assessed	
pT0	No evidence of primary tumour	
pTis	Melanoma confined to the conjunctival epithelium (in situ)*	
pT1	Melanoma of the bulbar conjunctiva	
	T1a	Tumour 2.0 mm or less in thickness with invasion of the substantia propria
	T1b	Tumour more than 2.0 mm in thickness with invasion of the substantia propria
pT2	Melanoma of the palpebral, forniceal, or caruncular conjunctiva	
	T2a	Tumour 2.0 mm or less in thickness with invasion of the substantia propria
	T2b	Tumour more than 2.0 mm in thickness with invasion of the substantia propria
pT3	Melanoma invades the eye, eyelid, nasolacrimal system, or orbit	
	pT3a	Invades the globe
	pT3b	Invades the eyelid
	pT3c	Invades the orbit
	pT3d	Invades the paranasal sinus and/or nasolacrimal duct or lacrimal sac
pT4	Melanoma invades central nervous system	

pN – Regional Lymph Nodes

The pN categories correspond to the N categories.

pM – Distant Metastasis*

pM1 Distant metastasis microscopically confirmed

Note

*pM0 and pMX are not valid categories.

G – Histopathological Grading

Histological grade represents the origin of the primary tumour.

GX	Origin cannot be assessed
G0	Primary acquired melanosis without cellular atypia
G1	Conjunctival naevus
G2	Primary acquired melanosis with cellular atypia (epithelial disease only)
G3	Primary acquired melanosis with epithelial cellular atypia and invasive melanoma
G4	De novo malignant melanoma

Stage

No stage is at present recommended.

The information presented here has been excerpted from the 8th edition of the *TNM classification of malignant tumours* (2017) {132}.
A help desk for specific questions about the TNM classification is available at http://www.uicc.org/resources/tnm/helpdesk.

Tumours of the conjunctiva and caruncle: Introduction

Kivelä T.T.
Eberhart C.G.
Grossniklaus H.E.

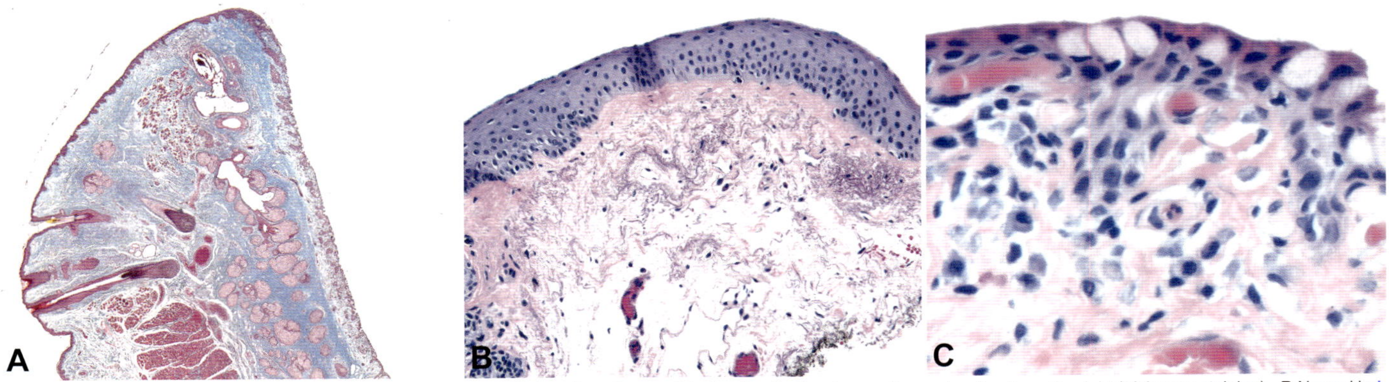

Fig. 1.01 Normal histology. **A** Normal eyelid; a low-power parasagittal section of an eyelid, showing the four layers; the conjunctiva is on the right (trichrome staining). **B** Normal bulbar conjunctiva shows stratified squamous epithelium; the underlying substantia propria is diaphanous, with small blood vessels and lymphatics; solar elastosis is present. **C** Normal tarsal conjunctiva shows thin stratified columnar epithelium containing numerous goblet cells.

The conjunctiva, together with the caruncle (its skin-like appendage located at the inner canthus of the eyelids), forms a protective sac that covers the anterior segment of the eye and the inner aspect of the eyelids. It consists of an epithelial layer and a stromal layer, and it is clinically divided into limbal, bulbar, forniceal, and palpebral parts. The epithelium is non-keratinizing and stratified columnar in type, and it harbours a population of basal melanocytes and superficial mucus-secreting goblet cells that are most abundant nasally and in crypt-like infoldings in the conjunctival fornices. It transitions to stratified squamous epithelium and abuts the corneal epithelium at the limbus, the epithelium of the lacrimal canaliculi at the lacrimal puncta, and the eyelid skin at the mucocutaneous junction (the so-called grey line) of the eyelid margin. The conjunctival stroma is fibrovascular and contains a population of melanocytes and inflammatory cells, including lymphocytes that can form follicles and germinal centres in the fornices; it also has lymphatics and contains accessory lacrimal glands. Lanugo hairs, sebaceous glands, sweat glands, and striated muscle are found only in the caruncle.

Most conjunctival masses encountered in primary care are degenerative or inflammatory, such as pingueculae, pterygia, and granulomas {12,32,35}. Tumours of the conjunctiva include choristomas – such as epibulbar dermoids, dermolipomas, and complex choristomas (occurring most commonly in children) – as well as epithelial tumours, such as papillomas; keratoacanthomas; intraepithelial neoplasia; and carcinomas of the squamous, spindle cell, and adenosquamous types (in particular towards the equatorial regions). Other tumours of the conjunctiva include various adnexal tumours and cysts; acquired melanosis and melanocytic tumours, including several types of naevi and conjunctival melanoma; various soft tissue tumours, including Kaposi sarcoma; vascular tumours, such as haemangioma and lymphangioma; and lymphoid tumours, in particular extranodal marginal zone lymphoma of mucosa-associated lymphoid tissue (MALT lymphoma) {1076,1425}. The conjunctiva can be secondarily involved by intraepithelial sebaceous cell carcinoma originating from sebaceous glands of the eyelids.

Conjunctival tumours can be readily biopsied, often by excisional biopsy. The conjunctiva and its tumours are also amenable to impression cytology before biopsy {83,573,593}, and sentinel lymph node biopsy is considered useful for a subset of conjunctival melanomas {214,1288}.

Epithelial tumours of the conjunctiva and caruncle

Conjunctival squamous cell carcinoma

Cherepanoff S.
Dubovy S.
Eberhart C.G.

Definition

Conjunctival squamous cell carcinoma (SCC) is an invasive epithelial neoplasm with evidence of squamous differentiation.

ICD-O codes

SCC NOS	8070/3
SCC in situ with questionable stromal invasion	8076/2
SCC, keratinizing, NOS	8071/3
Basaloid SCC	8083/3

Synonyms

Epidermoid carcinoma NOS; squamous carcinoma; squamous cell epithelioma; epidermoid carcinoma in situ with questionable stromal invasion; SCC, large cell, keratinizing; epidermoid carcinoma, keratinizing; basaloid SCC

Epidemiology

Conjunctival SCC is relatively rare; worldwide, the mean age-standardized incidence rate is 0.18 cases per 100 000 person-years among males and 0.08 cases per 100 000 person-years among females {404,851,1229,1393}. Two broad patterns of disease incidence are recognized. In immunocompetent populations in temperate countries, the incidence is higher in males and increases with age, sunlight exposure, and fairer skin {323,1229}. On the African continent, the incidence of conjunctival SCC is rising, and the disease mainly affects women, at a younger age; it is strongly associated with HIV infection and variably with HPV infection {404}, and it appears to have a more aggressive course {402}. The highest incidence of conjunctival SCC has been found at a latitude of 16° South {404}, where SCC is the most common primary conjunctival malignancy {404,691}. See Table 1.01 (p. 18) for a summary of the estimated age-standardized incidence rates of SCC of the eye by geographical region. The incidence rate has been found to decrease by 49% with each 10° increase in latitude {851}. Worldwide, a high incidence rate has been demonstrated among HIV-positive individuals {852,1034,1264} and in other immunosuppressed populations {434,1300}. A higher incidence is also seen in the setting of xeroderma pigmentosum {650}.

Etiology

The etiology of conjunctival SCC is not completely understood. It is unknown what proportion of cases arise from pre-existing epithelial dysplasia in flat lesions (conjunctival intraepithelial neoplasia) or papillomatous lesions versus cases that arise de novo. Ultraviolet (UV) radiation is the strongest etiological factor {851}, and it is the only risk factor for which a dose–response relationship has been established. UV radiation can directly damage DNA, causing mutations in the *TP53* gene {403}. Impaired immune surveillance clearly plays a role in the development of conjunctival SCC and links risk factors such as UV radiation (which suppresses cell-mediated immunity) and immunosuppression (e.g. due to HIV

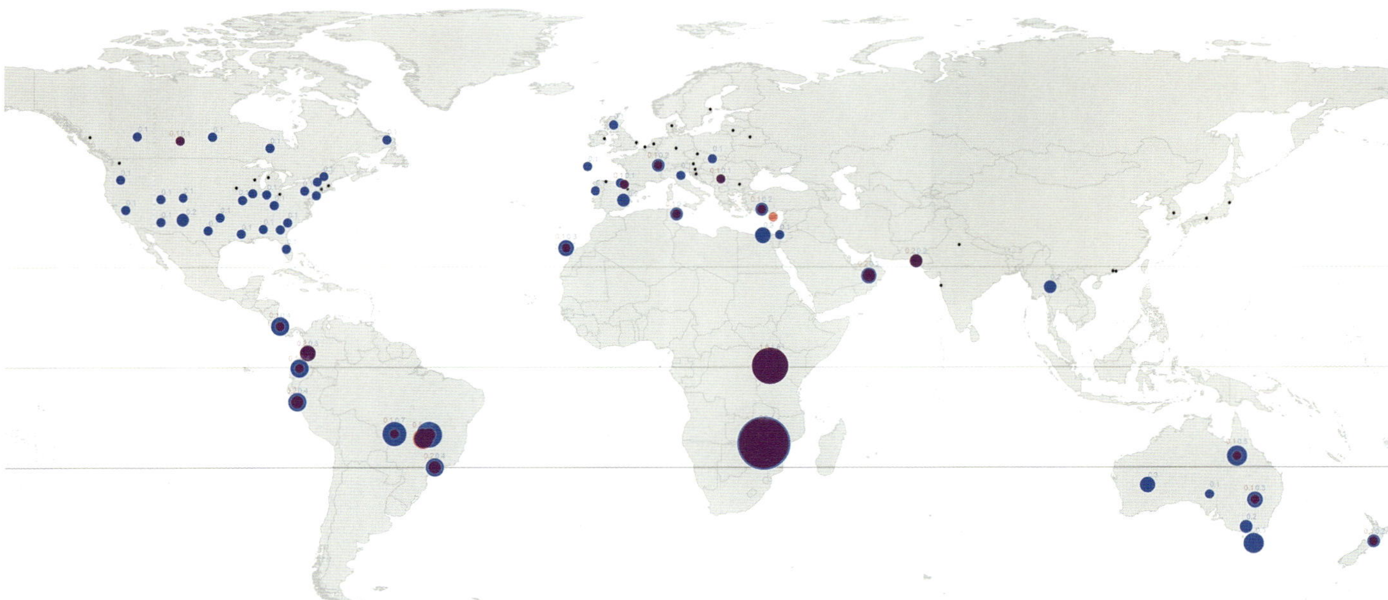

Fig. 1.02 Age-standardized incidence rates (per 100 000 person-years) of squamous cell carcinoma of the eye, by region. The data include all ocular squamous cell carcinoma cases, including those involving eyelid skin {239,404}. The dot size is directly proportional to incidence. Blue indicates rates among males and red indicates rates among females; overlaps between rates among males and females are shown in purple.

Table 1.01 Estimated age-standardized incidence rates of squamous cell carcinoma of the eye among males and females, by geographical region

Region	Mean number of cases per 100 000 person-years (95% CI)				*P* value
	Males		Females		
Africa	1.38	(−1.00 to 3.75)	1.18	(−1.08 to 3.43)	0.853
Central and South America	0.48	(0.33 to 0.62)	0.21	(0.10 to 0.33)	0.005
Oceania	0.28	(0.14 to 0.41)	0.05	(0.01 to 0.10)	0.002
North America	0.08	(0.06 to 0.10)	0.00	(0.00 to 0.01)	< 0.001
Asia	0.08	(0.01 to 0.14)	0.05	(0.00 to 0.09)	0.416
Europe	0.05	(0.02 to 0.08)	0.01	(0.00 to 0.03)	0.033
Southern Hemisphere	0.61	(0.14 to 1.09)	0.33	(−0.12 to 0.78)	0.355
Northern Hemisphere	0.10	(0.06 to 0.14)	0.05	(0.00 to 0.08)	0.045
Worldwide	**0.18**	**(0.09 to 0.26)**	**0.08**	**(0.01 to 0.15)**	**0.091**

CI, confidence interval.
The data include all ocular squamous cell carcinomas, including those involving eyelid skin {404}, and were extracted from *Cancer Incidence in Five Continents*, Vol. IX {239}.

infection or immunosuppressive therapy after organ transplantation). Reduced immunity also potentiates the effect of oncogenic viruses such as HPV {403}. In Africa, a confluence of low latitude, high prevalence of HIV infection, and high prevalence of HPV infection probably explains the high incidence of conjunctival SCC.

The relationship between HPV infection and conjunctival SCC in immunocompetent populations has been controversial because of small sample sizes and inconsistent detection methods {280}. Although the International Agency for Research on Cancer (IARC) did not find a strong causal association between HPV infection and conjunctival SCC when they evaluated the available data in 2007 {502}, other evidence suggests that the association may have been underestimated {9}.

The limbus (in particular the nasal limbus) is the most common site for conjunctival SCC. It has been hypothesized that limbal stem cells are particularly vulnerable to the oncogenic effects of UV radiation and viral infection {403} and that the conjunctival–corneal transition zone has vulnerabilities similar to those of the transition zone between the endocervix and ectocervix {9}.

Localization

Conjunctival SCC is most commonly located on the bulbar conjunctiva, within the sun-exposed interpalpebral fissure (including the caruncle), in particular at the limbus {777}. The tarsal and forniceal conjunctiva, the eyelid margin, and the cornea can be affected. Advanced tumours may also involve the surrounding tissues, including the orbit and intraocular structures.

Clinical features

Conjunctival SCCs are typically elevated and relatively well demarcated. Most are unilateral. They can be leukoplakic, gelatinous, or papilliform, and they are often associated with feeder blood vessels and intrinsic vasculature. They are pearly grey to pink in colour, depending on the vascularity. Pigmentation is variable, depending on the pigmentation of

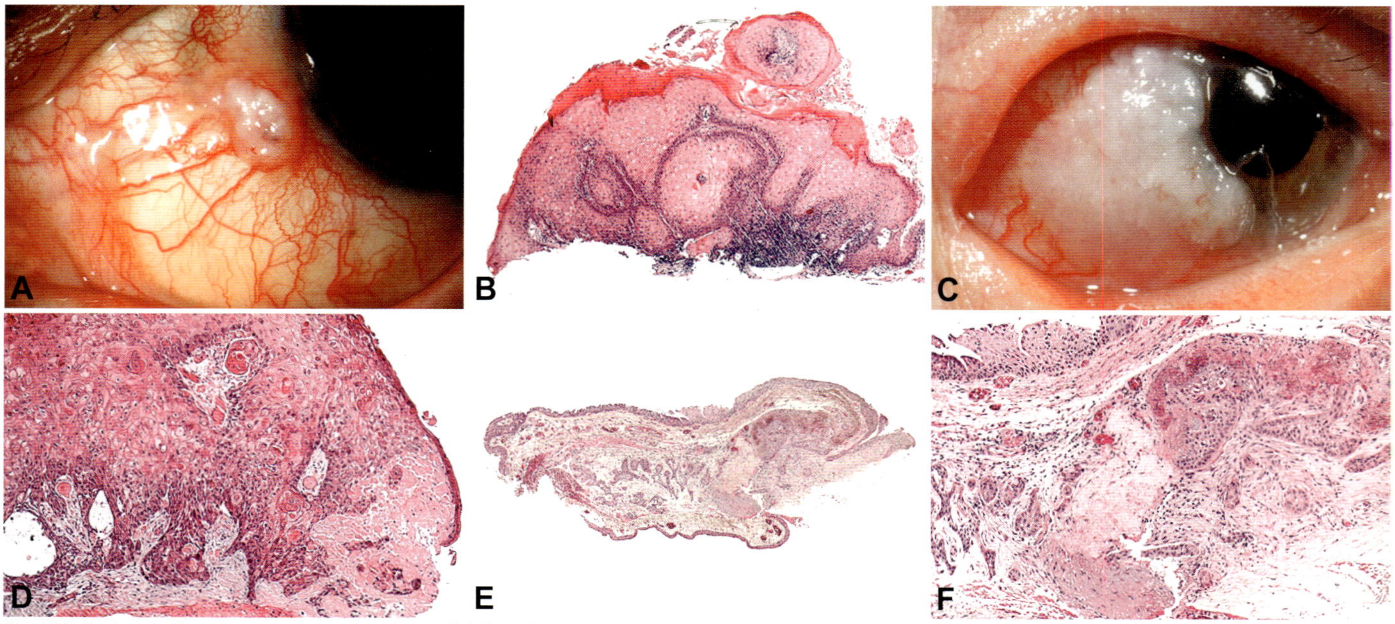

Fig. 1.03 Conjunctival invasive squamous cell carcinoma (SCC). **A** This keratotic nodule showed invasive SCC histologically. **B** The tumour has pushing, rather than infiltrative, deep borders; determining the degree of dysplasia and differentiating in situ from invasive disease can be clinically challenging. **C** The index of clinical suspicion for SCC is higher in larger lesions such as this one. **D** Histologically, this tumour has infiltrating borders. **E,F** Both in situ and invasive SCCs can occasionally involve pterygia.

the patient. Differentiating intraepithelial neoplasia from SCC is clinically challenging, and excisional biopsy is needed for definitive histopathological diagnosis.

Histopathology

Carcinoma in situ is a precursor lesion of conjunctival SCC. Invasive SCC breaches the epithelial basement membrane and extends into the subepithelial stroma. In some cases, the infiltration through the basement membrane is limited and superficial, and the designation "early stromal invasion" can be used. Grading of SCC is based on the degree of differentiation. Well-differentiated tumours produce keratin and have abundant eosinophilic cytoplasm, readily identifiable intercellular bridges, low mitotic counts, and minimal nuclear pleomorphism. Moderately differentiated SCCs show variable keratinization; compared with well-differentiated SCCs, they are more mitotically active and show more nuclear pleomorphism. Poorly differentiated SCCs can have a basaloid or spindled morphology. Basaloid SCCs have scant cytoplasm, and necrosis is often present. SCC can occasionally be present in pterygia.

Differential diagnosis

Immunohistochemical staining (for high-molecular-weight cytokeratins and p63) is typically required for the definitive diagnosis of poorly differentiated SCC, basaloid SCC, and spindle cell carcinoma (see *Conjunctival spindle cell carcinoma*, p. 19). The main differentials for basaloid SCC are basal cell carcinoma (usually a cutaneous primary secondarily involving the conjunctiva), poorly differentiated sebaceous carcinoma, and Merkel cell carcinoma. Adenosquamous carcinoma should be considered and excluded in older individuals because of its worse prognosis; the glandular component is usually found in the deeper aspect of the tumour. Adenosquamous carcinoma (see *Adenosquamous carcinoma of the conjunctiva and caruncle*, p. 20) can be readily distinguished from SCC using mucin staining. Adenosquamous carcinoma can be associated with adenosquamous carcinoma in situ or SCC in situ with mucinous differentiation.

Histogenesis

Conjunctival SCC is a malignant epithelial tumour of the conjunctival mucosa. The frequent limbal location suggests a vulnerability of limbal stem cells to oncogenic factors.

Genetic profile

UV radiation–induced mutations in the *TP53* gene are the only consistent genetic abnormality identified to date {403}.

Genetic susceptibility

There is an association with xeroderma pigmentosum. No other genetic susceptibilities have been demonstrated to date.

Prognosis and predictive factors

Conjunctival SCC has low metastatic potential but a high rate of local recurrence (12–40%) {1404}. The prognosis is generally favourable. Most lesions are treatable with local surgical excision and adjuvant cryotherapy and/or topical chemotherapy. Recurrence is most likely in cases with positive surgical margins {1236}. Orbital exenteration may be required for advanced-stage disease {802}. Recurrences can occur > 5 years after primary excision {802,1236}. The risk of metastasis and death is thought to be very low, but data are scarce. In a series of 38 T3 and T4 tumours, the reported rates of metastasis and death due to conjunctival SCC were 13% and 5%, respectively {802}. A mortality rate of 8% was found in a series of 26 cases {777}. Metastatic conjunctival SCC has been described in immunosuppressed patients, including patients with untreated HIV infection {258}.

Conjunctival spindle cell carcinoma

Alkatan H.
Syed N.

Definition

Conjunctival spindle cell carcinoma is a variant of conjunctival squamous cell carcinoma (SCC) characterized by predominant malignant spindle cells and/or pleomorphic cells {210,343,445}.

ICD-O code

Spindle cell carcinoma 8074/3

Synonyms

Metaplastic carcinoma; sarcomatoid carcinoma; pleomorphic carcinoma

Epidemiology

Conjunctival spindle cell carcinoma is rare. Of 2455 reported conjunctival lesions with histopathological diagnosis, only 4 cases of spindle cell carcinoma were found among 97 cases of SCC. In another large series, comprising 1643 conjunctival lesions including 219 epithelial tumours, no spindle cell carcinoma was found {428,1130}. More recently, 2 cases of spindle cell carcinoma were diagnosed in a series of 287 SCCs in 286 patients {168}. The peak incidence is in the fifth to seventh decades of life, with no sex preference {343,444}.

Localization

At this anatomical site, spindle cell carcinoma arises in the conjunctiva {168,210,428,1130}.

Clinical features

Clinically, spindle cell carcinomas can be a dome-shaped vascular pink mass arising from the limbus. They can appear pedunculated or they can present as a subconjunctival mass {210,212,1130}. A pterygium-like lesion has also been reported {1130}. Pain and tenderness have been described as symptoms {26,212}.

Histopathology

Spindle cell carcinoma consists of proliferating spindle-shaped, poorly differentiated, non-keratinizing squamous cells with pleomorphism, hyperchromatic nuclei, prominent nucleoli, and variable mitoses {26,210,1130}. The tumour invades the conjunctival stroma and may involve the adjacent cornea or underlying sclera {210,1130}. Immunohistochemical staining shows variable cytokeratin positivity, as well as positivity for other epithelial markers, such as epithelial membrane antigen, and p63 nuclear immunopositivity, which helps to differentiate spindle cell carcinoma from mesenchymal spindle cell tumours {26,210,294}. Staining for vimentin, SMA, and calponin highlights myoepithelial differentiation in spindle cell carcinoma {210}.

Differential diagnosis

Spindle cell carcinoma can easily be misdiagnosed. Desmoplastic melanoma is the main differential. Some reported cases have initially been misdiagnosed as SCC, malignant fibrous histiocytoma (now termed undifferentiated pleomorphic sarcoma), schwannoma, and

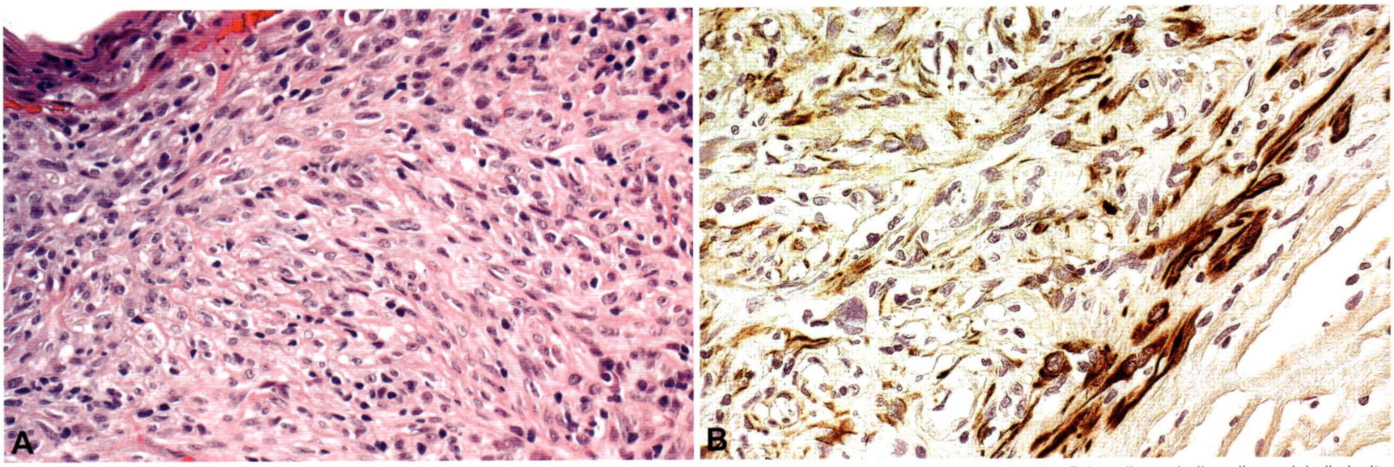

Fig. 1.04 Spindle cell carcinoma. **A** A superficial area of the tumour showing poorly differentiated squamous and spindle-shaped cells. **B** Invading spindle cells are labelled with antibodies to cytokeratin.

malignant schwannoma {212,343,1130}. In addition to spindle cell carcinoma's immunopositivity for p63, electron microscopy can also be used to support the histopathological diagnosis: ultrastructurally, spindle cell carcinoma cells show tonofilament-associated desmosomes and keratohyalin granules {445,855}. Anterior segment optical coherence tomography and ultrasound biomicroscopy are useful additional clinical diagnostic tools {549,1130}.

Histogenesis

Limbal epithelial stem cells may play a role in the histogenesis {810}. It has been postulated that spindle cell carcinoma cells result from epithelial–mesenchymal transition of classic SCC {444}.

Prognosis and predictive factors

Spindle cell carcinoma has an unfavourable prognosis, possibly because of its rarity, tumour-related factors (i.e. local aggressiveness), and the lack of standardized treatment {26,212,343,428}. Patient age, primary tumour location, and American Joint Committee on Cancer (AJCC) staging have been found to be independent prognostic indicators for spindle cell carcinomas located elsewhere {343}. Recurrence, which is common after incomplete excision, tends to be associated with intraocular invasion, resulting in exenteration in some cases; in one reported case, there was bilateral pulmonary metastasis 3 years after surgery, followed by death 3 months later {26,212,855}.

Adenosquamous carcinoma of the conjunctiva and caruncle

Mudhar H.S.
Edward D.P.
Chan A.S.Y.

Definition

Adenosquamous carcinoma of the conjunctiva and caruncle is a carcinoma composed of a variable combination of squamous (epidermoid) cells and mucous cells, arranged in invasive sheets, cords, and ducts.

ICD-O code

Mucoepidermoid carcinoma	8430/3
Adenosquamous carcinoma	8560/3

Synonyms

Mucoepidermoid carcinoma; squamous cell carcinoma with glandular differentiation

Epidemiology

This tumour is rare. The mean patient age at presentation is 64 years, and there is a male predilection {163,818,953}.

Localization

At this anatomical site, the most common location is the limbus, but adenosquamous carcinoma can also occur in the bulbar or palpebral conjunctiva {163,556}.

Clinical features

Patients present with mild irritation, with a limbal or bulbar conjunctival mass of short duration (usually several weeks to < 6 months) {982}. Palpebral conjunctival involvement is rare. The neoplasm may present as a nodular, leukoplakic, infiltrative, ulcerative, or papillomatous lesion and may mimic an inflamed pterygium {818}.

Histopathology

In the salivary and lacrimal glands, mucoepidermoid carcinoma is composed of three cell types (squamous, intermediate and mucous). The literature also refers to so-called mucoepidermoid carcinomas of the conjunctiva, but these tumours are composed of only two cell types (squamous and mucous), and they may include an in situ component; therefore, "mucoepidermoid carcinoma" is considered an incorrect term for tumours at this location. A conjunctival carcinoma with squamous and mucous elements is best designated as an adenosquamous carcinoma.
The ratio of squamous to mucous cells varies from case to case. The squamous cells, which are atypical and have eosinophilic polygonal cytoplasm, are arranged in sheets or cords. The mucous cells are often smaller and have intracytoplasmic cystic spaces that contain mucin. Intercellular spaces containing mucin may also be seen {953,1056}. Ductular structures are sometimes present {480}. The intercellular cysts are often accompanied by individual cells with well-defined intracytoplasmic vacuoles, resembling signet-ring cells. The cysts and intracellular vacuoles are positive for mucin by mucicarmine, Alcian blue, and periodic acid–Schiff (PAS) with diastase staining {550}. Occasionally, the mucous component

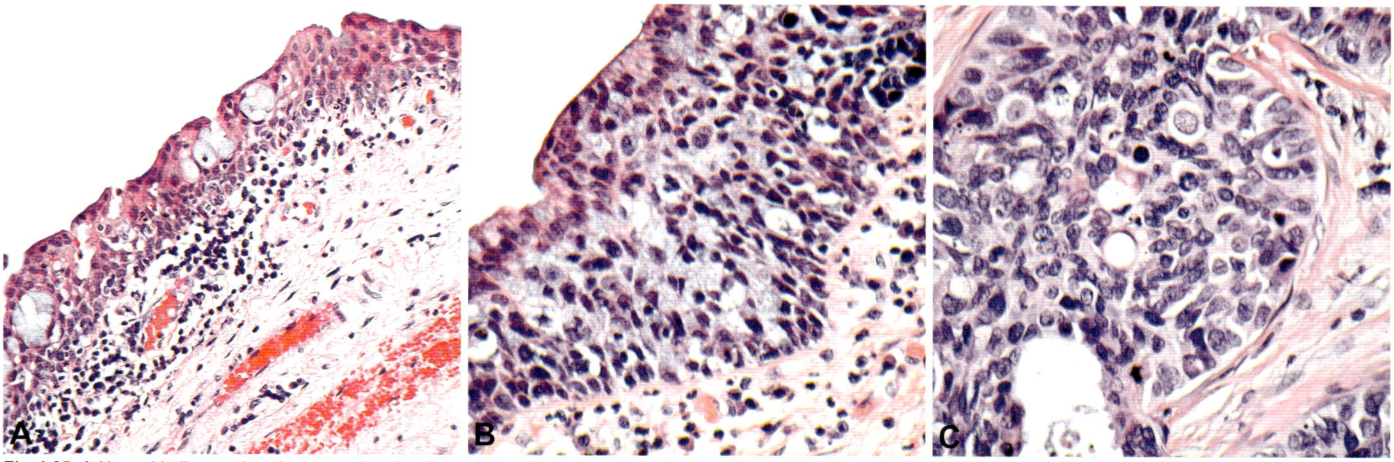

Fig. 1.05 **A** Normal bulbar conjunctiva; a section showing goblet cell clusters. **B** Conjunctival intraepithelial neoplasia with adenosquamous (mucoepidermoid) differentiation; note the atypical, hyperchromatic nuclei and the prominent light-blue intracellular mucin. **C** Invasive conjunctival adenosquamous carcinoma; a lobule of invasive tumour composed of squamous cells, with a cystic space at the bottom and occasional signet-ring–like intracytoplasmic circular vacuoles containing mucin.

is more prominent when the tumour invades the globe {140,439}. Conjunctival squamous intraepithelial neoplasia with mucous differentiation may sometimes be seen adjacent to an invasive tumour {556}. Immunohistochemistry can show positivity for high-molecular-weight cytokeratins, epithelial membrane antigen, and CEA {550}.

Differential diagnosis
The differentia diagnosis includes squamous cell carcinoma and pseudoglandular hyperplasia {757}. Squamous cell carcinoma does not feature mucous cells, and pseudoglandular hyperplasia does not show cytological atypia or true invasion.

Histogenesis
Adenosquamcus carcinoma arises from conjunctival squamous cell carcinoma in situ or conjunctival squamous intraepithelial neoplasia with mucous differentiation {556,755}.

Prognosis and predictive factors
The clinical course is aggressive, with extensive local recurrence that can involve the orbit and the globe after local (or even wider) resection {163,818,982}. Local control may require enucleation or exenteration. Lymph node metastasis is uncommon. Mortality from this tumour has rarely been reported. A rare low-grade variant has been reported {818}.

Keratoacanthoma of the conjunctiva and caruncle

Auw-Haedrich C.
Dubovy S.
Iacob C.E.
Grossniklaus H.E.

Definition
Keratoacanthoma of the conjunctiva and caruncle is a common, rapidly growing squamoproliferative tumour that may spontaneously regress. It is histologically indistinguishable from (and considered to be a variant of) well-differentiated cutaneous invasive squamous cell carcinoma, with distinct clinical behaviour {673}.

ICD-O code
Keratoacanthoma 8071/3

Epidemiology
Compared with its cutaneous counterpart, conjunctival keratoacanthoma occurs in younger patients, who are typically aged 26–65 years {229,1044}, although a case has also been reported in an 82-year-old patient {870}. It occurs most often in men, and most patients are White {377,870,1000}.

Etiology
The etiology is most likely related to ultraviolet (UV) radiation {1044}.

Localization
The most common location is the limbal and perilimbal conjunctiva {229,834, 870,1044}. One keratoacanthoma in the caruncle has been described {562}.

Clinical features
Patients present with a rapidly growing whitish tumour that markedly enlarges within a few weeks {870}. In most cases, the tumour is solitary and presents as a crater-like lesion.

Histopathology
Acanthotic epithelium with an intact basal cell layer, keratinization, and mild to marked cytological dysplasia is accompanied by numerous mitoses (including atypical ones) and a central crater filled with keratin. Eosinophils are common, but plasma cells are rare. Perineural invasion may occur {1044}.

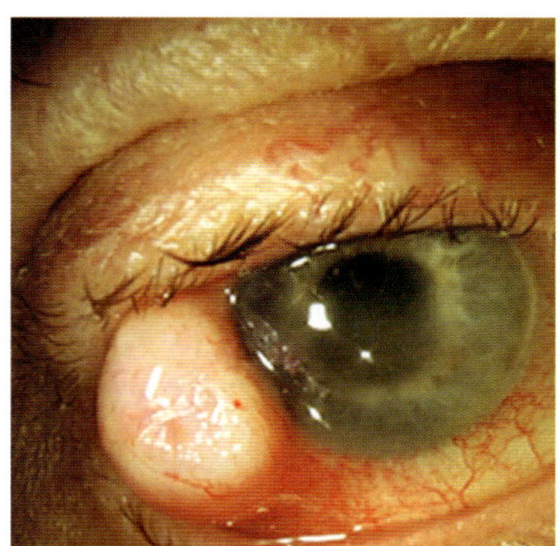

Fig. 1.06 Conjunctival keratoacanthoma. A leukoplakic tumour on the bulbar conjunctiva at the time of presentation situated at the temporal limbus, with surrounding dilated and tortuous vessels {870}.

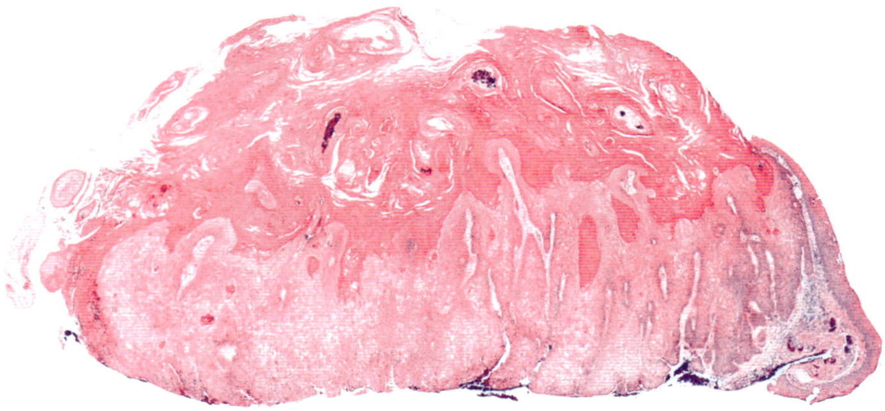

Fig. 1.07 Conjunctival keratoacanthoma. This lesion, which is buttressed by normal epithelium, is composed of a somewhat crater-like centre filled with keratin and keratin debris.

Differential diagnosis
The differential diagnosis includes squamous cell carcinoma, papilloma, and amelanotic melanoma. Keratoacanthoma is now considered to be a form of well-differentiated squamous cell carcinoma.

Histogenesis
Conjunctival keratoacanthoma arises from the conjunctival epithelium.

Genetic profile
The genetic profile is unknown, but cases associated with hereditary multiple self-healing palmoplantar carcinoma (MIM number: 615225) have been described {745}. Multiple self-healing palmoplantar carcinoma is associated with mutations in *NLRP1* on chromosome 17, leading to inflammasome activation {1416}.

Prognosis and predictive factors
Theoretically, conjunctival keratoacanthomas have the potential for spontaneous resolution, but no such case has been described to date. The lesion has not been reported to recur after 4–24 months of follow-up, except for an isolated case with keratoacanthoma features and intraocular invasion of a recurrence 1 month after primary excision {430}.

Hereditary benign intraepithelial dyskeratosis of the conjunctiva

Iacob C.E.
Eberhart C.G.

Definition
Hereditary benign intraepithelial dyskeratosis (HBID) is a non-neoplastic hyperkeratotic and dyskeratotic epithelial disorder of the conjunctiva and oral mucosa.

ICD-O code
None

Synonym
Witkop–von Sallmann syndrome

Epidemiology
This is a very rare condition that is almost exclusively encountered in the indigenous Haliwa-Saponi tribe native to the US state of North Carolina. This triracial isolate group is called Haliwa because its ancestral homelands are located in the counties of Halifax and Warren. There have also been isolated reports of cases in families with no relation to this tribe {146}.

Etiology
HBID is an autosomal dominant disease (MIM number: 127600).

Localization
HBID presents with semilunar limbal conjunctival lesions, frequently accompanied by similar hyperkeratotic patches in the oral mucosa.

Clinical features
HBID appears as a raised, leukoplakic, generously vascularized, and usually inflamed plaque. The lesions are frequently bilateral and change shape over time. The severity ranges from mild (erythematous limbal spots only) to moderate (elevated leukoplakic plaques limited to the conjunctiva) to severe (with some corneal involvement). Seasonal variability has been noted, with exacerbation during spring and summer followed by partial remission in autumn {238}.

Histopathology
The lesions are sharply demarcated from the surrounding conjunctiva, and they show marked acanthosis with substantial multilayered parakeratosis displaying copious cytoplasmic dyskeratotic material and pyknotic nuclei. No intervening granular layer is seen. Accompanying features include chronic inflammation and capillary telangiectasias in the lamina propria. The basement membrane remains intact. Malignant transformation has never been observed {449}.

Differential diagnosis
HBID must be distinguished from conjunctival intraepithelial neoplasia and squamous cell carcinoma. The bilateral presentation, lack of nuclear pleomorphism, and lack of atypical mitoses can facilitate this. Other ocular surface lesions to be ruled out include pterygium, limbal vernal nodule, and conjunctival papillomas. Multiple self-healing palmoplantar carcinoma is characterized by recurrent keratoacanthomas in palmoplantar skin, as well as in conjunctival and corneal epithelia, where they may appear histopathologically similar to HBID {745,1416}. The skin lesions and mutated *NLRP1* gene on chromosome 17 establish the diagnosis of multiple self-healing palmoplantar carcinoma {1202}.

Genetic profile
HBID has been mapped to chromosome 4q35, where copy-number variation (duplication) and three alleles have been described {30,70}. No protein-coding

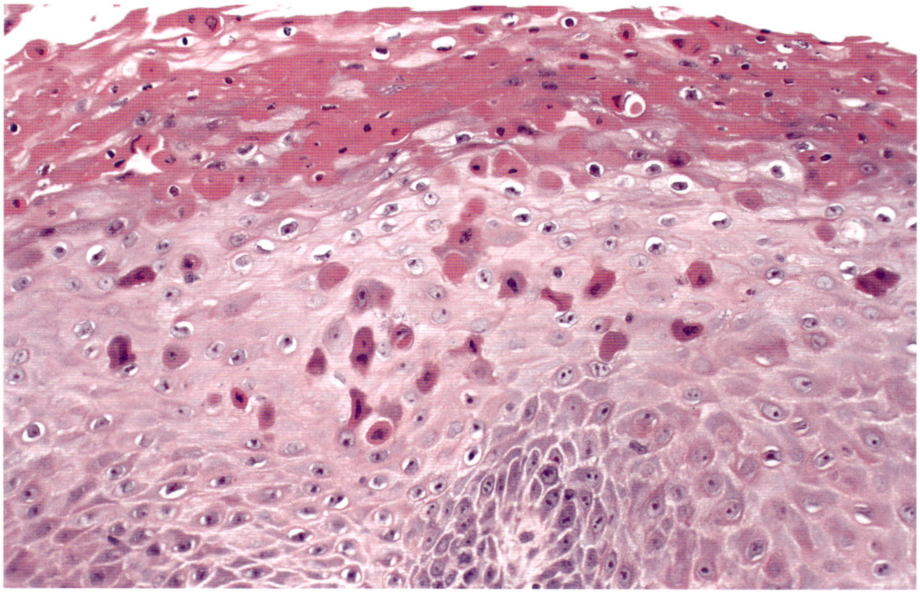

Fig. 1.08 Hereditary benign intraepithelial dyskeratosis. An example showing bright eosinophilic dyskeratotic squamous cells.

genes are known to occur in this location {146}.

Genetic susceptibility

HBID is often found in multiple generations of an affected family.

Prognosis and predictive factors

The lesions of HBID are self-limiting and do not require treatment.

Conjunctival squamous intraepithelial neoplasia

Alkatan H.
Auw-Haedrich C.
Croxatto J.O.
Dubovy S.
Eberhart C.G.
Iacob C.E.
Li B.
Loeffler K.U.
Vemuganti G.

Definition

Conjunctival squamous intraepithelial neoplasia constitutes a spectrum of disease involving the epithelium to a varying extent. Superficial maturation is still present in conjunctival squamous intraepithelial neoplasia, whereas dysplasia encompassing essentially the full epithelial thickness is designated conjunctival carcinoma in situ (cCIS). None of these dysplastic proliferations of the ocular surface squamous epithelium breach the basement membrane {600}. The clinical term "ocular surface squamous neoplasia" encompasses the entire spectrum of epithelial dysplasia and neoplasia, including squamous cell carcinoma {1108}.

ICD-O code

Conjunctival squamous intraepithelial neoplasia (conjunctival intraepithelial neoplasia and carcinoma in situ) 8077/2

Synonyms

Intraepithelial neoplasia of the conjunctiva; ocular surface squamous neoplasia; conjunctival squamous dysplasia; conjunctival epithelial dyskeratosis; Bowen disease

Epidemiology

Conjunctival squamous intraepithelial neoplasia is the most common conjunctival malignancy in the USA, and the third most common ocular tumour in the adult population {584}. The estimated incidence is 17–20 cases per 1 million person-years {690}.

Etiology

Conjunctival squamous intraepithelial neoplasia is an acquired condition linked to chronic ultraviolet B (UVB) radiation exposure and seen predominantly in older adults. The risk is increased in individuals with immunosuppression or autoimmune disease and in those with a history of HIV, hepatitis B or C, or HPV infection {397,1079}. Additional risk factors include heavy cigarette smoking, exposure to petroleum products or chemicals, ocular surface injury, and xeroderma pigmentosum. HIV testing should be considered for patients with conjunctival squamous intraepithelial neoplasia who are aged < 40 years and have no other risk factors {451}.

Localization

Conjunctival squamous dysplasias generally occur on the conjunctival surface in sun-exposed regions of the eye. The most common location is the limbus, either nasally or temporally, and lesions can spread onto the cornea {846,1109}. The forniceal or palpebral conjunctiva is occasionally involved {1108}.

Clinical features

Conjunctival squamous intraepithelial neoplasia and cCIS generally present as fleshy, sessile or minimally elevated lesions. Clinically, conjunctival squamous intraepithelial neoplasia most commonly appears as a gelatinous lesion with tufts of blood vessels and a pearly grey appearance. However, some have a leukoplakic appearance secondary to hyperkeratosis. They can show papillary features or spread onto the cornea, and they may show associated pigmentation in individuals with racial pigmentation of the conjunctiva {1108}. These intraepithelial lesions move freely over the underlying episclera; this is in contrast to invasive carcinoma, which is fixed to the underlying tissue {401,846}.

Histopathology

Conjunctival squamous intraepithelial neoplasia is composed of dysplastic cells that originate from the basal cell layer and extend towards the surface, with increased cell proliferation, abnormalities in maturation, and irregularity of individual epithelial cells. The lesions can contain large squamous cells, small epithelial cells, or spindle-shaped epithelial cells. In more-advanced lesions, suprabasal mitotic figures can be seen. Generally, conjunctival squamous intraepithelial neoplasia and cCIS are sharply demarcated from the normal conjunctival epithelium at their peripheral edges. The epithelium is often thickened, sometimes with associated sessile papillomatous

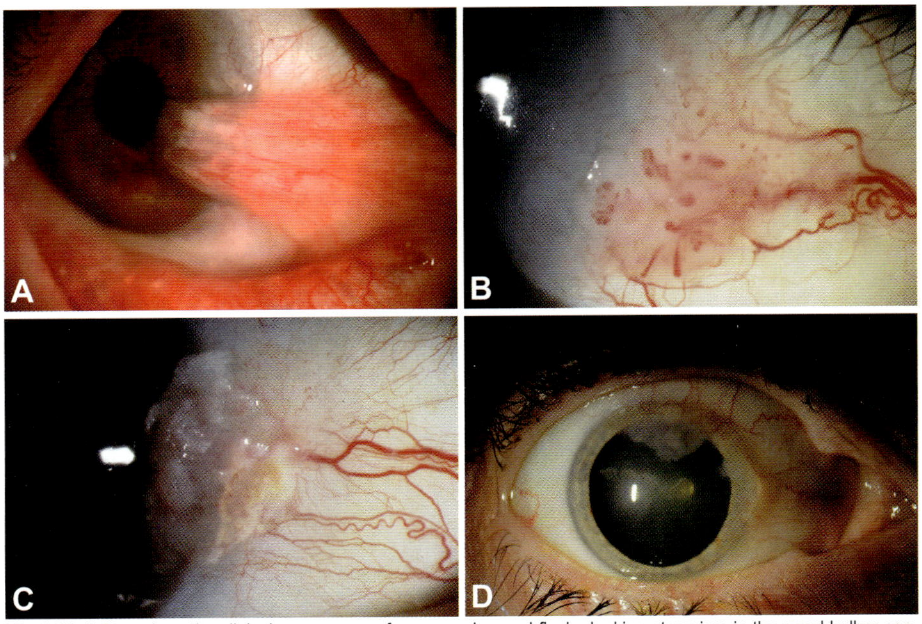

Fig. 1.09 **A** Pterygium; the clinical appearance of a more advanced fleshy-looking pterygium in the nasal bulbar conjunctiva, with advanced corneal involvement. **B** Severe conjunctival dysplasia, papillary pattern; clinically, there is a papillary tumour present near the limbus that contains corkscrew-like blood vessels. **C** Conjunctival carcinoma in situ; this example presents as a fleshy, gelatinous conjunctival mass near the limbus. **D** Corneal epithelial dysplasia; islands of dysplastic epithelium form plaques on the corneal surface.

changes, but atrophic forms of dysplasia can occasionally occur.

Conjunctival squamous intraepithelial neoplasia is classified as mild, moderate, or severe depending on the extent of the epithelial involvement and the degree of cellular atypia. Mild dysplasia is confined to the lower third of the conjunctival epithelial thickness, moderate dysplasia extends into the middle third, and severe dysplasia spreads to the upper third but retains substantial surface differentiation {451,553}. cCIS exhibits full-thickness replacement of the surface epithelium with dysplastic epithelial cells {1108}.

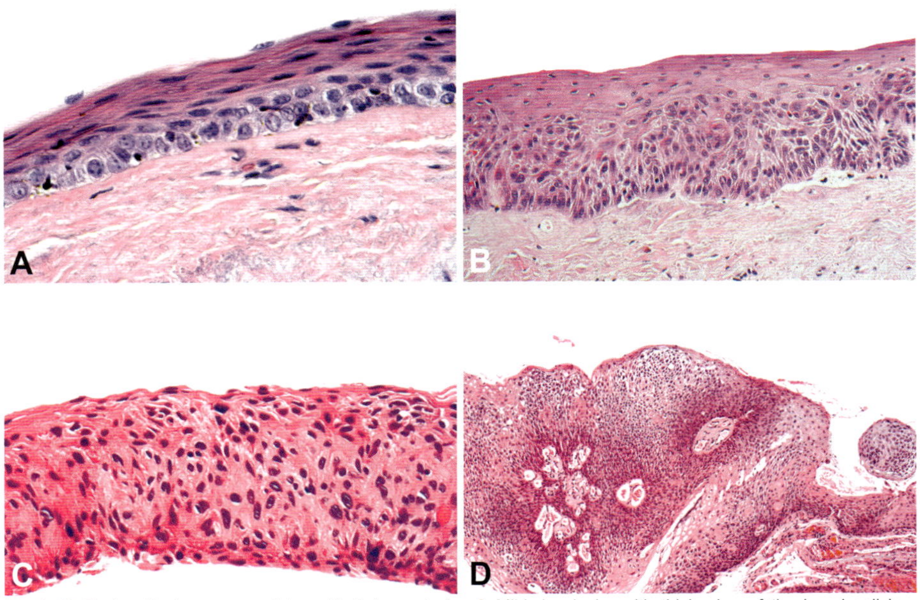

Fig. 1.10 Conjunctival squamous intraepithelial neoplasia. **A** Mild dysplasia, with thickening of the basal cell layer. **B** Moderate dysplasia, with thickening of the basal cell layer extending into the middle third of the conjunctival epithelial thickness. **C** Corneal epithelial dysplasia; the corneal epithelium peels off in a sheet and is replaced by dysplastic keratinocytes. **D** Severe conjunctival dysplasia, papillary pattern; there is acanthotic epithelium overlying central vascular cores present in this corneal dysplasia.

Differential diagnosis

The differential diagnosis includes invasive squamous cell carcinoma, intraepithelial sebaceous carcinoma, amelanotic conjunctival naevus or melanoma, lymphoproliferative or histiocytic diseases, hereditary benign intraepithelial dyskeratosis, and papilloma {138,248}. Most cases of conjunctival squamous intraepithelial neoplasia and cCIS can be distinguished from these other lesions on the basis of appearance alone; when necessary, immunohistochemical stains for sebaceous, melanocytic, lymphoid, or histiocytic markers can also be used.

Conjunctival squamous intraepithelial neoplasia and cCIS can occasionally develop in other common ocular lesions associated with sunlight/ultraviolet (UV) radiation exposure, including pinguecula and pterygium.

Pingueculae are common degenerative tumour-like lesions that arise most commonly at the 9 o'clock or 3 o'clock position on the limbal conjunctiva and can be bilateral. Clinically, they appear whitish-yellow, with a smooth, elevated, sometimes slightly leukoplakic surface. Microscopically, the surface is covered by goblet cell–containing conjunctival epithelium with various degrees of keratinizing metaplasia. The subepithelial connective tissue shows actinic elastosis and sometimes contains spheroid bodies.

Pterygia (from the Greek word "*pterygos*", meaning "wing") are thin triangular conjunctival proliferations that invade over the corneal surface {173,594,984}. Bilateral presentation is common. The pooled prevalence is 10%, with a higher prevalence among men, in the elderly, and at lower latitudes {720}. Multifactorial pathogenesis has been reported, with associated factors including UV radiation, environmental factors (microtrauma caused by wind and dust), chronic inflammation, dry eyes, residence in rural or tropical regions, and adenovirus and HPV infection {173,594,939}. Pterygia are characterized histopathologically by stromal pseudoelastotic degeneration of collagen, with fragmented curly fibres in the substantia propria and fibrovascular proliferation with variable chronic inflammatory cell infiltration. The overlying epithelium may show reactive changes (thinning, hyperplasia, and/or metaplasia) or (more rarely) dysplasia; dysplasia can sometimes occur at the advancing head of a pterygium and resemble actinic keratosis of the skin, with associated epithelial acanthosis, hyperkeratosis, and parakeratosis {1108}.

Histogenesis
Conjunctival squamous intraepithelial neoplasia arises from conjunctival epithelial cells that originate from the ocular surface ectoderm {1289}. Their preferred limbal location suggests that most cases may arise from limbal epithelial stem cells.

Genetic profile
Somatic *TP53* mutations have been reported {1266}, along with chromosomal alterations involving loci encoding DNA repair genes {59}. Conjunctival dysplasia has been linked to overexpression of telomerase due to *TERT* promoter mutations consistent with UV radiation–induced damage {1049}.

Genetic susceptibility
Deficiency of DNA repair in some hereditary diseases (e.g. xeroderma pigmentosum) confers an increased risk of carcinoma of the conjunctiva and of rarer conjunctival lesions such as atypical fibroxanthoma {1067}.

Prognosis and predictive factors
Conjunctival squamous intraepithelial neoplasia is considered to be a low-grade malignancy, but it can progress to invasive squamous cell carcinoma {901}. The risk of recurrence depends on the involvement of the surgical margins, as well as on the histological grade, corneal location, and size. After surgery, carcinoma in situ may recur in > 50% of patients, even years later {977}. Lower recurrence rates are reported after topical chemotherapy.

Sebaceous carcinoma of the conjunctiva and caruncle

Dubovy S.
Eberhart C.G.
Vemuganti G.

Definition
Sebaceous carcinoma of the conjunctiva and caruncle is a malignant tumour arising from sebaceous glands of the ocular adnexa (including the Meibomian glands and the glands of Zeis) and sebaceous glands of the eyelid and caruncle.

ICD-O code
Sebaceous carcinoma 8410/3

Synonyms
Sebaceous adenocarcinoma; Meibomian gland carcinoma; sebaceous gland carcinoma

Epidemiology
Sebaceous carcinoma of the ocular adnexa is generally considered to be the second most common neoplasm of this anatomical region, after basal cell carcinoma {1125}. It accounts for about 5% of all malignant eyelid tumours. Risk factors include advanced age, Asian race, and female sex {249}. The mean patient age at diagnosis is 57–72 years {1150}.

Etiology
Sebaceous carcinoma is acquired. Several cases have occurred within an irradiated field.

Localization
Sebaceous carcinoma usually originates from the tarsus of the upper eyelid or (less commonly) the lower eyelid, the glands of Zeis, or the sebaceous glands of the caruncle. In addition to large masses in the eyelid stroma, secondary involvement of the conjunctival or squamous epithelium by pagetoid invasion is common {586}. Cases of sebaceous carcinoma confined to the conjunctival epithelium without involvement of the tarsus or dermis have also been reported {490,1125}.

Clinical features
These tumours often present as solitary ulcerated nodules or more-diffuse eyelid thickening, sometimes yellow in colour. They can be confused clinically with chalazion. More rarely, diffuse intraepithelial sebaceous carcinoma with associated tarsoconjunctival inflammation can masquerade as chronic blepharoconjunctivitis {756,758}. Abnormal vascular patterns and loss of eyelashes are distinguishing features.

Histopathology
Lobules of epithelial or basaloid cells with distinct cell borders and variably vacuolated cytoplasm form in the tarsal plate and dermis, with larger ones often featuring central necrosis in a comedonecrosis pattern. Other variants include the solid and papillary patterns. Peripheral palisading and clefting of the type seen in basal cell carcinoma are absent. Mitotic figures and apoptotic bodies are common. Cellular nuclei are amphophilic. Most periocular sebaceous carcinomas are relatively poorly differentiated, and cytoplasmic vacuolization can be limited or focal. Oil Red O staining for sectioning of frozen or fixed unprocessed tissue (or adipophilin immunostaining) can be helpful in confirming sebaceous differentiation {805,1047}. Intraepithelial spread of sebaceous carcinoma is relatively common; it can be bowenoid, pagetoid, or papillary {954}. Bowenoid spread is characterized by replacement of the epithelium by large pleomorphic cells, pagetoid spread by scattered individual or clustered tumour cells. The rarer papillary pattern exhibits papillary projections with areas of confluent tumour cells. Sebaceous carcinoma can extend (in a pagetoid fashion) great distances from the main tumour mass; immunostaining for adipophilin, p53, p16, androgen

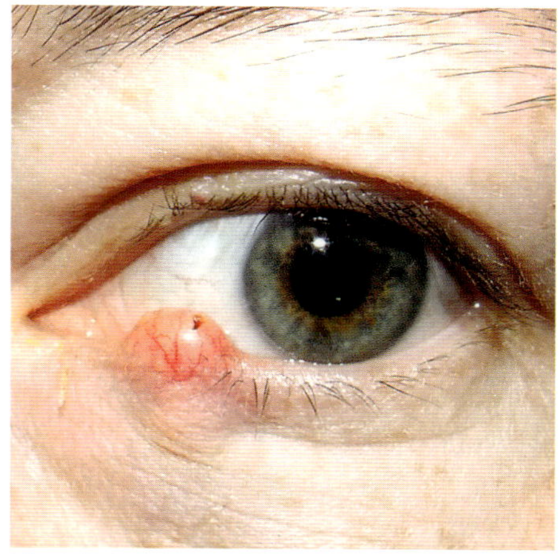

Fig. 1.11 Sebaceous carcinoma of the eyelid. The left lower eyelid contains a nodular, yellowish mass, with associated loss of eyelashes.

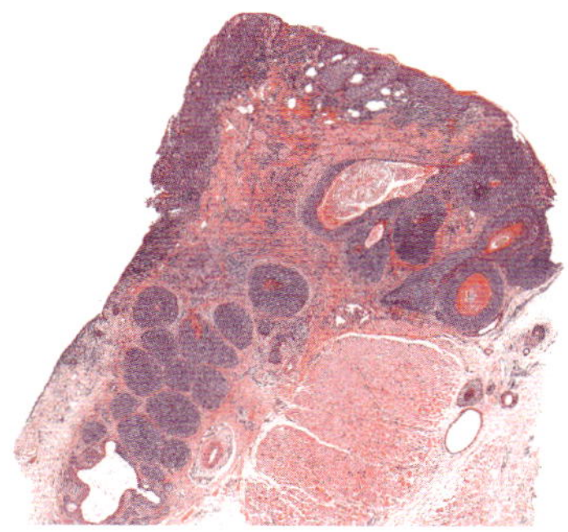

Fig. 1.12 Sebaceous carcinoma of the eyelid. The tumour involves the Meibomian glands, the glands of Zeis, and the epithelium of the conjunctiva and eyelid margin; the cells are amphophilic, with pleomorphic nuclei and cytoplasmic vacuolation.

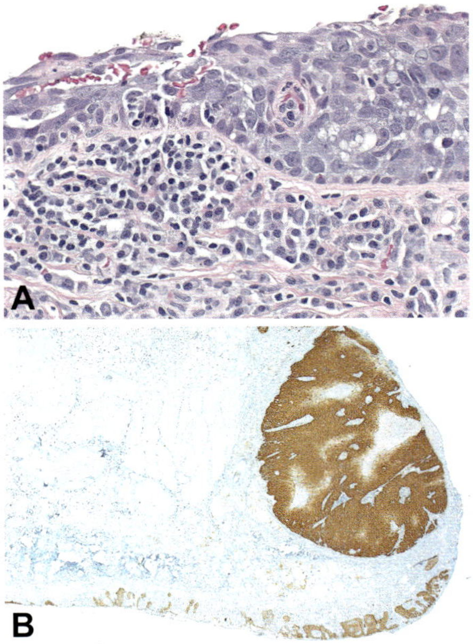

Fig. 1.13 A Intraepithelial sebaceous carcinoma; vacuolated tumour cells with atypical nuclei fill the conjunctival epithelium. B Sebaceous carcinoma; in this full thickness eyelid section, p16 immunostaining highlights both the main tumour nodules and the intraepithelial spread through conjunctiva (at the bottom of the image).

receptor, and perforin has been used to distinguish small numbers of intraepithelial carcinoma cells from reactive epithelial changes {92,805,814,1047}.

Differential diagnosis
The differential diagnosis includes histiocytic lesions, as well as squamous cell, basal cell, and adnexal cancers showing clear cell changes.

Histogenesis
Sebaceous carcinoma originates from sebaceous glands. Primary conjunctival intraepithelial sebaceous carcinoma may arise de novo {490}.

Genetic profile
Sebaceous carcinoma has been associated with dysregulation of several pathways, namely, the MAPK and JAK/STAT {665}, NF-κB, PTEN, and TGF-β {1251} pathways. Ultraviolet (UV) radiation–independent *TP53* mutations have been found in a high proportion of sebaceous carcinomas {504}. Immunochemical positivity for ERBB2 (HER2) has been found in as many as 82% of cases, with 75% of these cases showing *ERBB2* amplification by FISH {918}.

Genetic susceptibility
Sebaceous carcinoma associated with Muir–Torre syndrome (MIM number: 158320) shows microsatellite instability and loss of expression of the DNA mismatch repair genes *MLH1*, *MSH2*, and *MSH6*; these findings are not usually seen in sporadic sebaceous carcinoma {632,1213}.

Prognosis and predictive factors
Sebaceous carcinomas with large size, pagetoid invasion of the overlying epithelia, poor differentiation, and multifocal origin have worse prognosis {954,1239}.

Oncocytoma of the conjunctiva and caruncle

van der Valk P.
Grossniklaus H.E.
Iacob C.E.

Definition
Oncocytoma of the conjunctiva and caruncle is a benign epithelial tumour composed largely of oncocytic cells with abundant light, eosinophilic, granular cytoplasm.

ICD-O code
Oncocytoma 8290/0

Synonyms
Oxyphilic adenoma; oncocytic adenoma; eosinophilic cystadenoma

Epidemiology
Oncocytomas are rare in all locations.

Localization
Oncocytomas occur in two main locations in the periocular region: (1) the lacrimal gland and sac and (2) the conjunctiva, where they have a preference for the caruncle, although they may also occur in other conjunctival areas {879}. Oncocytomas of the lacrimal sac seem to occur preferentially in elderly women; no other sex preference is noted. These tumours are predominantly seen in the elderly, although exceptional cases in young patients have been reported.

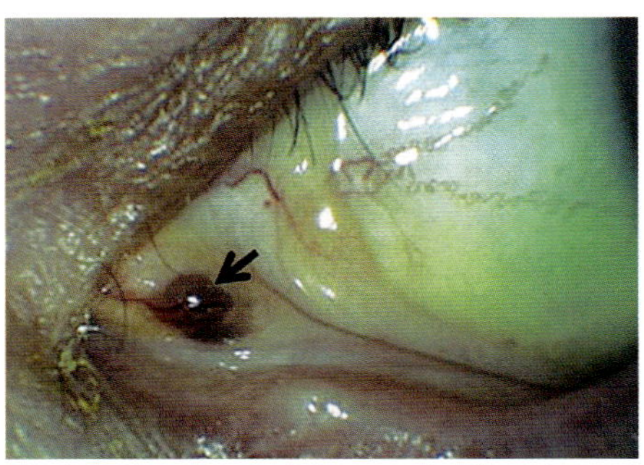

Fig. 1.14 Oncocytoma of the caruncle. There is a red nodular lesion (arrow) present in the caruncle.

Clinical features
The signs and symptoms depend on the location. Lacrimal gland oncocytomas cause swelling and proptosis, whereas those in the conjunctiva cause a visible tumour. Imaging of lacrimal gland oncocytoma reveals a tumour in the lacrimal gland area.

Histopathology
Classically, larger specimens are sharply demarcated lobular tumours that are reddish-brown on macroscopic examination, apparently because of the high content of cytochrome in the tumour cells. This appearance is similar to that of oncocytomas in other locations.

Microscopically, oncocytomas are glandular in appearance or composed of solid cell nests or cords. The cells have abundant cytoplasm that is slightly eosinophilic and distinctly granular because of the presence of large numbers of mitochondria. The nuclei are small to medium-sized and often show a fairly prominent nucleolus. The N:C ratio is low {152,1319}.

These tumours have no specific immunohistochemical profile. They are cytokeratin-positive, with reactivity for both low- and high-molecular-weight keratins. Not surprisingly, markers for mitochondria are strongly positive {879}. The abundant mitochondria can also be clearly seen ultrastructurally.

Histogenesis
The abnormal mitochondrial numbers seem to be related to truncating mutations in complex I of the respiratory chain (also seen in other oncocytic tumours). Such mutations impair cellular respiration, which may contribute to maintaining the tumour cells in a low-proliferative state {925}.

Genetic profile
No studies on genetic abnormalities in oncocytomas from the ocular adnexa have been reported.

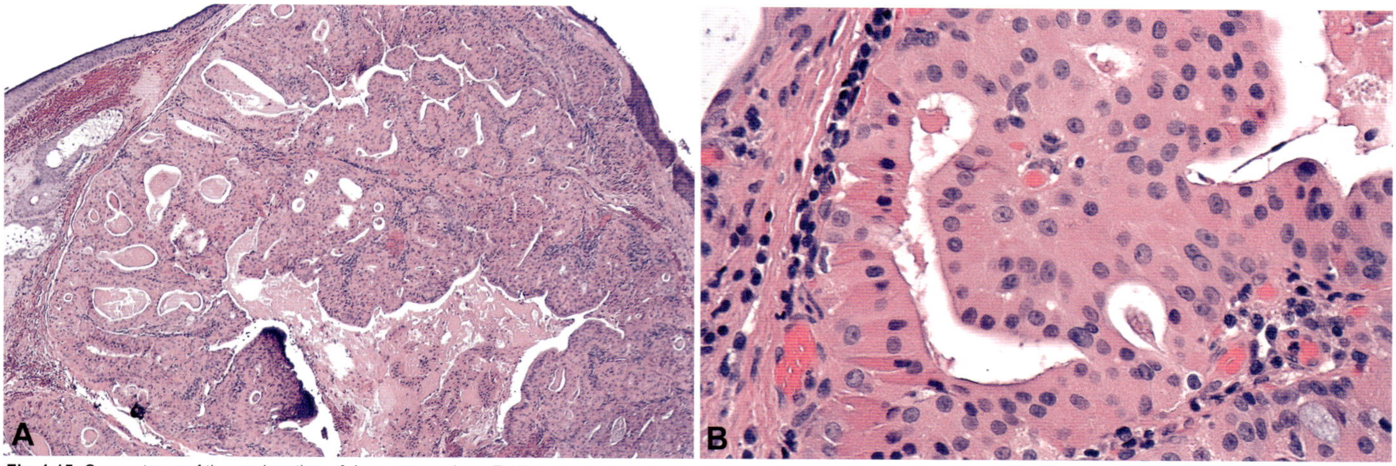

Fig. 1.15 Oncocytoma of the conjunctiva. **A** Low-power view. **B** High-power view showing large columnar cells with strongly eosinophilic cytoplasm and regular nuclei.

Prognosis and predictive factors
Oncocytomas are benign tumours; excision is curative.

Conjunctival squamous papilloma

Auw-Haedrich C.
Iacob C.E.
Loeffler K.U.

Definition
Conjunctival squamous papilloma is a benign papillomatous neoplasm generally composec of non-keratinizing epithelium, including goblet cells.

ICD-O code
Squamous papilloma 8052/0

Synonyms
Conjunctival papilloma; caruncular papilloma

Epidemiology
Children and adults can be affected {565,1108}, adults most often in the third and fourth decades of life {817,1194}. A male preponderance has been reported {56,776,1194}.

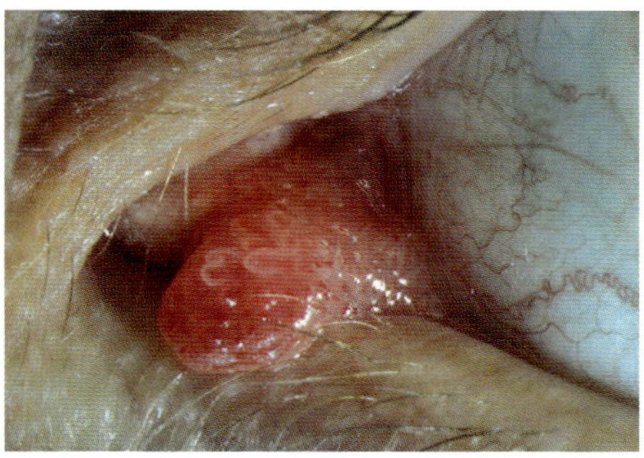

Fig. 1.16 Squamous papilloma. A caruncle papilloma (in a 39-year-old man) showing the characteristic vascularized papillomatous architecture.

Etiology
Most cases (60–90%) are positive for HPV6 or HPV11 (alpha papillomavirus genus strains of HPV) {817,1323}, and a minority are positive for HPV9, HPV12, HPV20, HPV21, HPV22, or HPV24 (beta papillomavirus genus strains) {817}. Some cases are positive for the high-risk HPV16 {1017,1195}.

Localization
Squamous papilloma is most common in the non-limbal conjunctiva; cases in this location are strongly associated with HPV6 and HPV11 positivity {817}. Squamous papilloma can also occur in the medial and inferior limbal and caruncular conjunctiva {1194}.

Clinical features
Patients present with a papillomatous, vascularized pink tumour, sometimes with keratinized areas. The tumour is either sessile or pedunculated with a fibrovascular peduncle. Squamous papilloma can be solitary (the most common presentation in adults), with extension over the cornea, or multiple (the most common presentation in children), located in the lower conjunctival fornix {1108}.

Histopathology
There is papillomatous hyperplastic thickening of either non-keratinizing or (rarely)

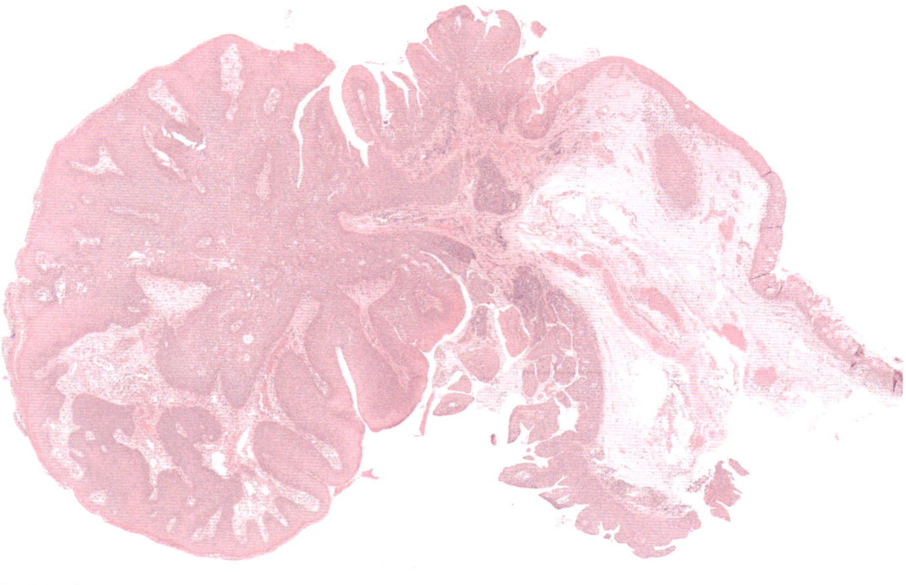

Fig. 1.17 Squamous papilloma. Histological aspect of the caruncle papilloma in fibrovascularized fronds covered by papillomatous epithelial hyperplasia with non-keratinizing epithelium and areas containing metaplasia towards keratinizing epithelium, including goblet cells without any dysplasia.

keratinizing epithelium with intermingled goblet cells; in some cases (6–20%), there is mild dysplasia {817,1194}. There is subepithelial fibrous vascularized tissue, either flat or pedunculated, usually with a scattered intraepithelial neutrophilic infiltrate.

Differential diagnosis
The differential diagnosis of squamous cell carcinoma is especially important for cases that are widespread or show corneal involvement.

Histogenesis
Squamous papillomas originate from the conjunctival epithelium.

Prognosis and predictive factors
In one large study, conjunctival papillomas in younger patients (aged ≤ 20 years) were significantly larger and more numerous, less likely to contain feeder vessels, more likely to recur, and more likely to require repeated treatment than conjunctival papillomas in patients aged > 20 years {565}. One case with conversion from HPV-negative to HPV16-positive and progression to squamous cell carcinoma has been described {131}.

Tumour-like lesions of the conjunctiva and caruncle

Auw-Haedrich C.
Eberhart C.G.
Grossniklaus H.E.
Iacob C.E.
Margo C.

Cysts of the conjunctiva and caruncle

Definition
Cysts of the conjunctiva and caruncle are cysts lined by conjunctival epithelium.

ICD-O code
None

Synonym
Epithelial inclusion cysts

Epidemiology
Conjunctival epithelial cysts can occur at any age. They show no sex predisposition.

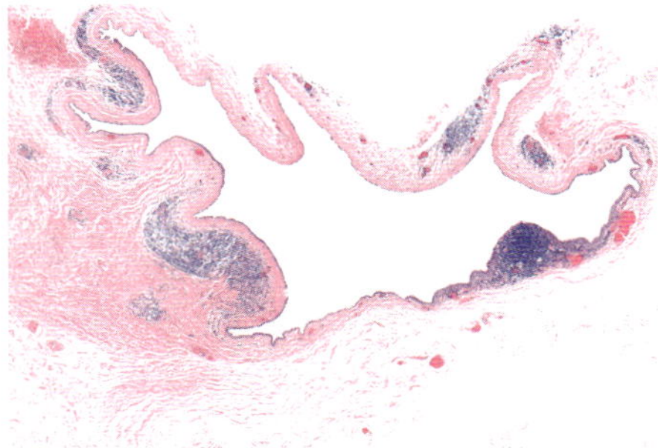

Fig. 1.18 Conjunctival epithelial cyst. An epithelium-lined cyst with mild fibrous and inflammatory reaction.

Etiology
These cysts generally originate from epithelial implantation, and they can be related to previous surgery on the ocular surface, enucleation {559}, or eye injury. They can arise years after the initiating event {678}.

Localization
Most conjunctival epithelial cysts are located under the bulbar conjunctiva away from the limbus, in areas where the conjunctiva or extraocular muscles have been surgically manipulated. Deeper epithelial cysts in the orbit have also been described with intraconal or extraconal expansion related to previous injury or enucleation {559,1410}, but some are not associated with prior injury {436}. Another classic location of conjunctival cysts is the caruncle.

Clinical features
The cyst can be more or less elevated above the surface of the eye depending on its size, and it is usually freely movable, translucent, and compressible. Intraorbital epithelial cysts can cause prominent proptosis and compression of the optic nerve and other orbital structures, ultimately resulting in visual impairment.

Histopathology
Conjunctival epithelial cysts are lined by flattened stratified non-keratinizing epithelium with rare goblet cells. The contents of the cysts are mostly proteinaceous and sometimes lightly mucinous. They can elicit a mild surrounding fibrous or inflammatory reaction. Periodic acid–Schiff (PAS) staining can be useful in highlighting goblet cells and cyst contents.

Differential diagnosis
In the anatomically diverse, skin-like caruncle, the differential diagnosis includes epidermal inclusion cyst, infundibular cyst, steatocystoma, hidrocystoma, and cystic oncocytoma {735,1118}.

Histogenesis
Normal conjunctival epithelium can undergo cystic proliferation in the lamina propria or orbit as a result of implantation after surgery or injury.

Prognosis and predictive factors
Complete excision is curative for epithelial cysts of the bulbar conjunctiva or caruncle. Complete resection of orbital epithelial cysts can be technically problematic, and recurrences can occur from epithelial residues.

Reactive epithelial hyperplasia of the conjunctiva and caruncle

Definition
Reactive epithelial hyperplasia of the conjunctiva and caruncle is a non-neoplastic epithelial proliferation.

ICD-O code
None

Epidemiology
Reactive epithelial changes are relatively common at this site, but their precise incidence is difficult to estimate.

Etiology
Infection, injury, allergy, autoimmune disease, and drug reaction have been associated with reactive epithelial hyperplasia {236,396,926}.

Localization
The bulbar, forniceal, and palpebral conjunctiva, as well as the caruncle, can be involved.

Clinical features
The affected conjunctival area is generally slightly elevated; in some cases it can be pedunculated. It lacks true papillomatous features and vascularized fronds. Leukoplakia, with its typical whitish appearance, is often present.

Histopathology

In most cases the epithelium is thickened, with accompanying metaplasia towards keratinizing epithelium. The maturation of the cells is normal, but hyperkeratosis and parakeratosis may be present. Dysplasia is not a feature, although reactive atypia can sometimes be found. Goblet cell hyperplasia is unusual, but it has been reported in some cases {871}.

Differential diagnosis

The main differential diagnoses are actinic degeneration (with or without dysplasia), hereditary benign intraepithelial dyskeratosis, and papillomas, as well as malignancies such as squamous cell carcinoma and sebaceous carcinoma.

Histogenesis

Reactive epithelial hyperplasia occurs as the result of a proliferation of conjunctival epithelium in the setting of dry eye and lagophthalmos, and as a reaction to local friction caused by other pathological processes (e.g. foreign bodies, space-occupying lesions, and tumours in the lamina propria).

Prognosis and predictive factors

These lesions can recur, but they do not become malignant.

Pseudoglandular and pseudoepitheliomatous hyperplasia of the conjunctiva and caruncle

Definition

Pseudoglandular hyperplasia of the conjunctiva and caruncle is a proliferation of the conjunctival epithelium (featuring prominent glandular elements) in response to irritating stimuli. Pseudoepitheliomatous hyperplasia of the conjunctival epithelium is a proliferation of the squamous epithelium alone.

ICD-O code

None

Synonyms

Pseudoglandular hyperplasia:
pseudoadenomatous hyperplasia

Pseudoepitheliomatous hyperplasia:
pseudocarcinomatous hyperplasia

Epidemiology

These lesions are reported in children and adults of both sexes.

Etiology

These lesions have been associated with granular cell myoblastoma, blastomycosis, thermal burns, and previous surgery, but no antecedent etiology is known in most instances {341,347,753,757,1379}.

Localization

Pseudoglandular hyperplasia affects the tarsal conjunctiva, the conjunctival fornix, or both. Pseudoepitheliomatous hyperplasia may affect the bulbar conjunctiva, including the limbus.

Clinical features

Pseudoglandular hyperplasia appears as a fleshy, poorly defined mass {757}. Pseudoepitheliomatous hyperplasia may appear as a fleshy to white (leukoplakic) mass that is minimally raised or thickened {341}.

Histopathology

Pseudoglandular hyperplasia is composed of prominent pseudoglands of Henle, which are lined by stratified squamous epithelium and goblet cells that may be numerous. Mucin often fills the lumina of the pseudoglands. Pseudoepitheliomatous hyperplasia is composed of acanthotic epithelium in which the keratinocytes display normal maturation. Squamous metaplasia may be present, including keratohyalin granules in the cytoplasm of superficial cells and surface keratinization.

Differential diagnosis

The main differential diagnosis for pseudoglandular hyperplasia is well-differentiated adenosquamous carcinoma of the conjunctiva, which is more cellular than pseudoglandular hyperplasia and shows nuclear atypia in the keratinocytes lining the glandular structures. The mitotic activity in dysplasia and adenosquamous carcinoma differentiates them from their benign counterparts. The main differential diagnoses for pseudoepitheliomatous hyperplasia include papilloma, inverted papilloma, and conjunctival squamous epithelial dysplasia. Normal maturation of keratinocytes is lost in epithelial dysplasia, and the keratinocytes display pleomorphic nuclei with variable amounts of cytoplasm.

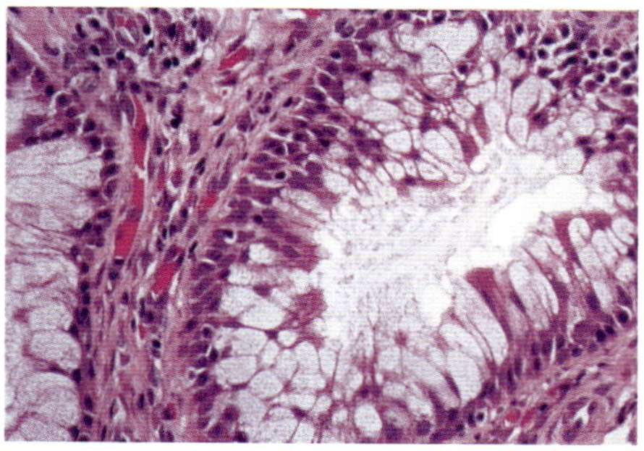

Fig. 1.19 Pseudoglandular hyperplasia. This reactive process contains prominent hyperplastic pseudoglands of Henle with relatively consistent N:C ratios.

Histogenesis

These proliferations are often idiopathic in nature, although they may be associated with antecedent inflammatory, infectious, or subepithelial processes that result in invagination or entrapment of epithelium with goblet cells (in the case of pseudoglandular hyperplasia) or overlying hyperplasia (in the case of pseudoepitheliomatous hyperplasia).

Prognosis and predictive factors

These are benign reactive processes with a good prognosis. Overtreatment may occur because of misdiagnosis of these lesions as carcinomas.

Melanocytic tumours of the conjunctiva and caruncle

Conjunctival melanoma

Margo C.
Coupland S.E.
Moulin A.
Roberts F.

Definition

Conjunctival melanoma is an invasive tumour arising from conjunctival melanocytes.

ICD-O codes

Melanoma NOS	8720/3
Nodular melanoma	8721/3

Synonym

Ocular melanoma (discouraged because uveal melanoma is also ocular)

Epidemiology

Conjunctival melanomas account for 5% of all ocular melanomas. The annual incidence is 0.1–0.7 cases per 1 million person-years {497,812,1064,1272}. Geographical variations reflect the racial compositions of populations in different parts of the world. Increasing incidence rates have been observed in several populations over the past 50 years {682,1287,1406}. About 10% of conjunctival melanomas arise in or involve the caruncle {1338}. The average patient age at diagnosis is in the late 50s {684,864}. These tumours are rare in children and show no sex predilection {243,244,498,1287}.

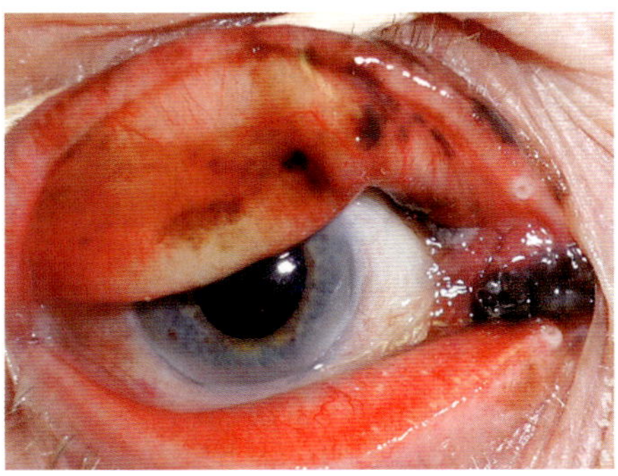

Fig. 1.20 Melanoma of the caruncle. A brown, multinodular mass has effaced the right caruncle; there is patchy brown discolouration of the upper tarsal conjunctiva; most of the tarsal pigmentation is flat, but some areas have discernible thickening.

Etiology

Evidence linking chronic ultraviolet (UV) radiation exposure to conjunctival melanoma is accumulating, but is less robust than for cutaneous melanoma {978,1272}. No other environmental cause has been established.

Localization

Most melanomas of the conjunctiva and caruncle arise on the bulbar surface of the conjunctiva within the interpalpebral fissure. Most are contiguous with the limbus {36,244,1096}.

Clinical features

Conjunctival melanomas range from solitary symmetrical domes to irregularly shaped plaques and nodules. Their colour, which can be uniform or patchy, varies from pale tan to dark brown, with as many as 20% of cases reported as non-pigmented {244,1096}. Tumours arising from underlying intraepithelial disease (i.e. conjunctival melanocytic intraepithelial neoplasia or primary acquired melanosis with atypia) are surrounded by flat conjunctiva displaying various shades of brown. Melanomas arising in the fornix or tarsal conjunctiva can be mistaken for primary eyelid tumours.

Conjunctival melanomas can invade contiguous tissues. They metastasize via lymphatics and blood vessels to regional lymph nodes and distant sites {1096}. The utility of sentinel lymph node examination is unclear {329,911,1288}.

Histopathology

Conjunctival melanomas consist of various combinations of atypical spindle cells, polyhedral cells, and epithelioid cells. Large epithelioid cells can assume bizarre shapes, and their nuclei contain conspicuous nucleoli. In contrast, smaller polyhedral cells can often be difficult to distinguish from naevus cells. Spindle-shaped melanoma cells tend to be less pigmented than polyhedral and epithelioid cells. Spindle melanoma cells may occasionally induce a desmoplastic reaction. Clusters of so-called balloon cells with clear or vacuolated cytoplasm are occasionally encountered.

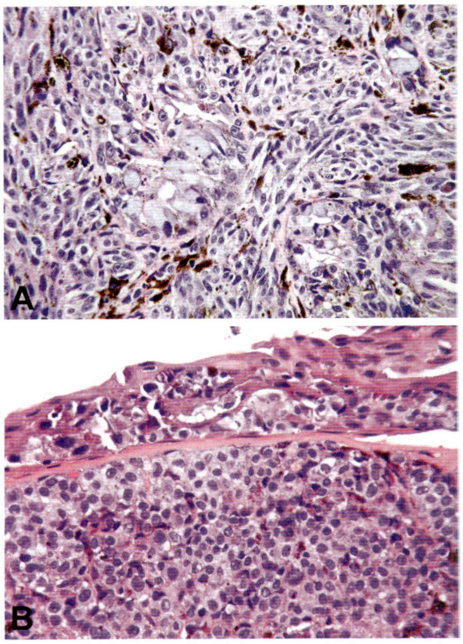

Fig. 1.21 Melanoma. **A** Melanoma of the caruncle; a biopsy specimen of the caruncle shown in Fig. 1.20 shows moderately pleomorphic spindle-shaped cells with various amounts of melanin; many of the nuclei contain centrally clumped chromatin. **B** Conjunctival melanoma arising in primary acquired melanosis; biopsy shows that most of the epithelium has been replaced with markedly atypical melanocytes; the substantia propria is filled with epithelioid melanoma cells.

Differential diagnosis

Early conjunctival melanoma must be distinguished from atypical melanocytic naevus, combined naevus, and inflamed juvenile conjunctival naevus. Naevi occurring in childhood or adolescence and recurrent naevi after excision can exhibit considerable cellular pleomorphism. Helpful distinguishing features of melanoma include the absence of maturation from top to bottom, strong HMB45 staining at the base {1069}, an elevated Ki-67 proliferation index (> 5%), and necrosis {523,525}.

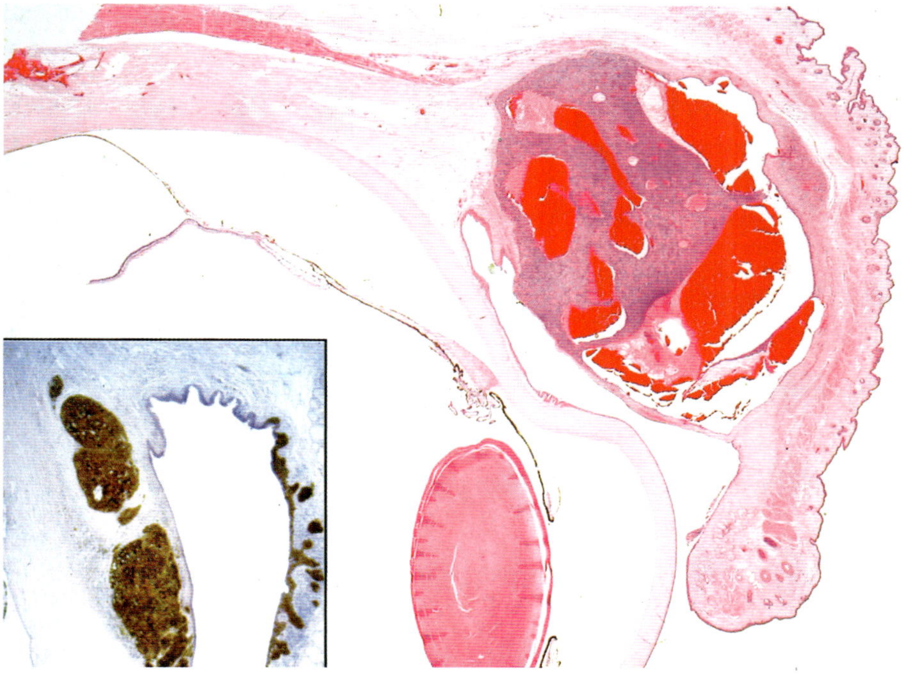

Fig. 1.22 Conjunctival melanoma. This large tumour arising in the upper palpebral conjunctiva contains spaces filled with blood; the tumour was mistaken clinically for a primary eyelid tumour. **Inset**: A deeper section with immunohistochemical staining for S100 protein shows melanoma in the bulbar conjunctiva; melanoma in situ of the palpebral conjunctiva is evident in the areas of positive staining.

Histogenesis
About 65% of conjunctival melanomas arise from melanocytic intraepithelial neoplasia; others may arise from a pre-existing naevus or de novo {243,360}.

Genetic profile
About 30–50% of conjunctival melanomas have *BRAF* mutations, and nearly 20% have *NRAS* mutations; these proportions are similar to those observed in cutaneous melanoma {682,684,1338}. Other (less common) mutations involve *TERT* and *KIT* {88,421,422,677}.

Prognosis and predictive factors
The 10-year melanoma-related mortality rate is 25–30% {329,892,1096}. Tumour-related death has been associated with de novo origin, non-limbal location, large tumour size, orbital invasion, nodular growth, and multicentric origin {36,892,1096}. Non-limbal location and thickness > 2 mm have been proposed as indicators that sentinel lymph node biopsy should be considered {1288}. *BRAF* mutations may be associated with greater risk of distant metastasis, but these mutations are less common in melanomas occurring in extrabulbar locations {684}. Incisional biopsy and excision without adjuvant therapy have also been correlated with poor outcome {244,684,1338}.

Conjunctival melanocytic intraepithelial neoplasia

Eberhart C.G.
Coupland S.E.
Folberg R.
Margo C.
Rao N.

Definition
Conjunctival melanocytic intraepithelial neoplasia represents a spectrum of neoplastic changes ranging from melanocytic hyperplasia through degrees of atypia to melanoma in situ.

Various terminologies have been used to classify these lesions. "Primary acquired melanosis (PAM) with and without atypia" and "conjunctival melanocytic intraepithelial neoplasia (C-MIN)" are terms used to describe the morphological changes associated with conjunctival and caruncular intraepithelial melanocytic neoplasia, often associated with hyperpigmentation, and to denote the estimated risk of progression to melanoma (see Table 1.02, p. 32).

ICD-O code
Melanoma in situ 8720/2

Synonyms
"C-MIN" and "PAM with atypia" are synonymous terms for describing melanocytic neoplasia at this site. Older terms include "precancerous melanosis" and "premalignant melanosis". More recently, the term "intraepithelial melanocytic proliferation with atypia" has been proposed {522}.

Epidemiology
All of these lesions are most common in middle-aged and elderly White people, but they can occasionally occur in individuals with darker pigmentation, and even in teenagers or young adults. The precise incidence of pigmented conjunctival lesions is difficult to estimate. In a North American analysis of 311 eyes with PAM, 96% of the cases were in White individuals and 4% in African-Americans, Hispanics, or Asians, with a patient age range of 15–90 years (mean: 56 years) {1163}. Males and females are affected in equal numbers.

Etiology
No environmental cause has been clearly established, but atypical conjunctival melanocytic proliferations develop most frequently in the interpalpebral zone, suggesting an association with ultraviolet (UV) radiation {1406}.

Localization
These lesions are generally unilateral but often multifocal; they vary in size, involving a mean of 3 clock hours of the conjunctiva {683,1163}. In decreasing frequency, they involve the bulbar, limbal, forniceal, and palpebral conjunctiva; they can also extend to the cornea and occur in the caruncle {1163}.

Clinical features
C-MIN/PAM lesions appear as flat, irregular brown discolourations of the conjunctiva. The distribution of pigment and thus the size of the lesion may change over time. The pigmentation is mobile over the substantia propria and episclera. In rare cases, C-MIN/PAM with atypia can be amelanotic, making it difficult to recognize clinically.

Histopathology
PAM without atypia: In PAM without atypia, the density of melanocytic cells is only modestly increased, and the melanocytes remain cytologically bland and

Table 1.02 Neoplastic conjunctival melanocytic lesions

PAM system modified to include melanoma in situ	C-MIN scoring system[a]	Proposed simplified WHO terminology with low- and high-grade stratification[b]
PAM without atypia	C-MIN score = 1	Low-grade conjunctival melanocytic intraepithelial lesion
PAM with mild atypia	C-MIN score = 2	
PAM with moderate atypia	C-MIN score = 3	High-grade conjunctival melanocytic intraepithelial lesion
PAM with severe atypia (≤ 75% of epithelium)	C-MIN score = 4–5	
Melanoma in situ	C-MIN score > 5	Melanoma in situ
Invasive melanoma	Invasive melanoma	Invasive melanoma

PAM, primary acquired melanosis; C-MIN, conjunctival melanocytic intraepithelial neoplasia.
[a]The highest possible total score of the C-MIN scoring system = 10, based on the extent of horizontal and vertical epithelial involvement, as well as the degree of melanocytic cytological atypia; based on proposals from {243}, {595}, and {522}. [b]Modification of proposals from {1225} and Raymond Barnhill, unpublished presentation at the 28th Congress of the European Society of Pathology, Cologne, 25–29 September 2016.

restricted to the basal layer. The presence of rare suprabasal dendritic melanocytes can also be compatible with this diagnosis. Increased melanin is almost always noted within the conjunctival epithelium, generally involving multiple layers of keratinocytes {360,522,595}. These features correspond with a score of 1 in the C-MIN scoring system {595}; however, because it is not clear that these bland lesions truly constitute clonal neoplasms, they may be better designated as proliferations rather than neoplasms.

PAM with atypia: Melanocytic neoplasia with higher degrees of atypia (C-MIN score 2–5) is a synonymous designation for conjunctival intraepithelial proliferations of atypical melanocytes with the presumed potential for progression to melanoma in situ and, ultimately, invasive conjunctival melanoma. PAM with atypia features melanocytic proliferation with various degrees of cytological atypia and abnormal patterns of spread within the epithelium {360,522,595}. Mitotic activity, nesting, pagetoid spread, cellular enlargement, epithelioid appearance, hyperchromatic nuclei, and prominent nucleoli are all associated with increasing atypia. Atypia is generally graded as mild, moderate, or severe. In one study, cells with mild cytological atypia were found to deviate only slightly from normal melanocytes. Moderately atypical cells showed nuclear enlargement and often prominent nucleoli or epithelioid changes, and severe atypia was associated with bizarre nuclear shapes {360}. Substantial melanocytic proliferation not limited to the epithelial base has been associated with increased melanoma risk. Numerical scores for melanocytic hyperplasia, nesting, pagetoid spread, cytological atypia, and Ki-67 proliferation index have been used to stratify mild, moderate, and severe atypia, with good correlation with recurrence and progression {744}. It has also been proposed that PAM with atypia be divided into low-risk and high-risk groups {1225}.

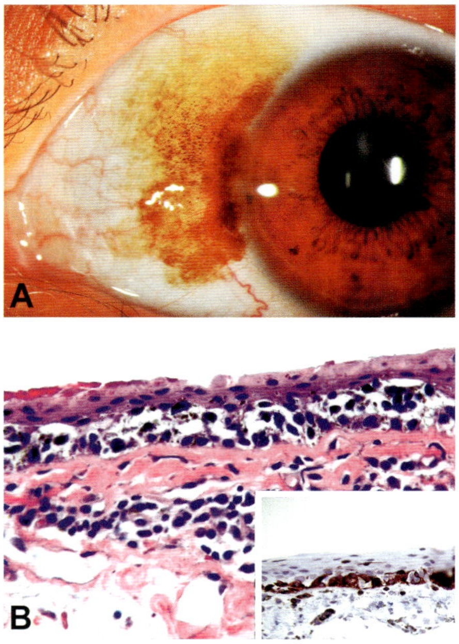

Fig. 1.23 Primary acquired melanosis with atypia. **A** An example presenting as a flat, variably pigmented lesion in the bulbar conjunctiva and limbus. **B** A lentiginous proliferation of melanocytes highlighted by melan-A immunostaining (**inset**).

C-MIN scoring: This suggested scoring system uses a scale of 1–10 based on the extent of horizontal and vertical epithelial involvement, as well as the degree of melanocytic cytological atypia {245}. With respect to horizontal growth, basal cells are scored 1 point, scattered pagetoid cells 2, isolated nests 3, and confluent nests 4. Vertical spread (suprabasilar extension) is scored as 1 (1–50% involvement), 2 (50–90%), or 3 (> 90%). With respect to cytological atypia, three characteristics are evaluated, each scored 1 point if present: melanocytic nuclei of equal or greater size than those of the basal epithelial cells, melanocytic cytoplasm of equal or greater size than that of the basal epithelial cells, and nucleoli and/or mitotic figures. A total score of 1 equates to PAM without atypia, 2–3 to PAM with mild or moderate atypia, 4–5 to PAM with severe atypia, and 5–10 to melanoma in situ {595}. Although this scoring system provides a potentially helpful quantitative approach, its use is not obligatory for diagnosis. The designation "PAM with severe atypia" has been used by many instead of "melanoma in situ", and use of the latter term in the conjunctiva has been somewhat controversial. In the current TNM staging guidelines {132}, melanoma in situ is defined by > 75% of the normal conjunctival epithelial thickness being replaced by atypical melanocytes.

Atypical melanocytic lesions of the conjunctiva are immunoreactive for S100 protein, MITF, melan-A, and SOX10. HMB45 staining is typically positive, and proliferation is highlighted by Ki-67 staining {964}. Extension of C-MIN/PAM or melanoma in situ into conjunctival epithelial invaginations in the underlying lamina propria (pseudoglands of Henle) should not be misdiagnosed as invasive melanoma.

Differential diagnosis

Potential mimics of C-MIN/PAM with atypia include conjunctival naevi, in particular those with junctional activity. Pure junctional naevi are generally found in children or young adults. In middle-aged or older patients, a basal melanocytic proliferation lacking a subepithelial component is much more likely to be C-MIN/PAM than a naevus. Pigmented ocular surface squamous neoplasia can clinically mimic C-MIN/PAM with atypia {1095}.

Pigmented conjunctival lesions characterized by increased melanin production by cytologically normal-looking melanocytes, with no increase in melanocyte number, are discussed in the section *Benign epithelial melanoses of the conjunctiva* (p. 38).

Histogenesis

C-MIN/PAM with atypia arises from basal conjunctival melanocytes {522}.

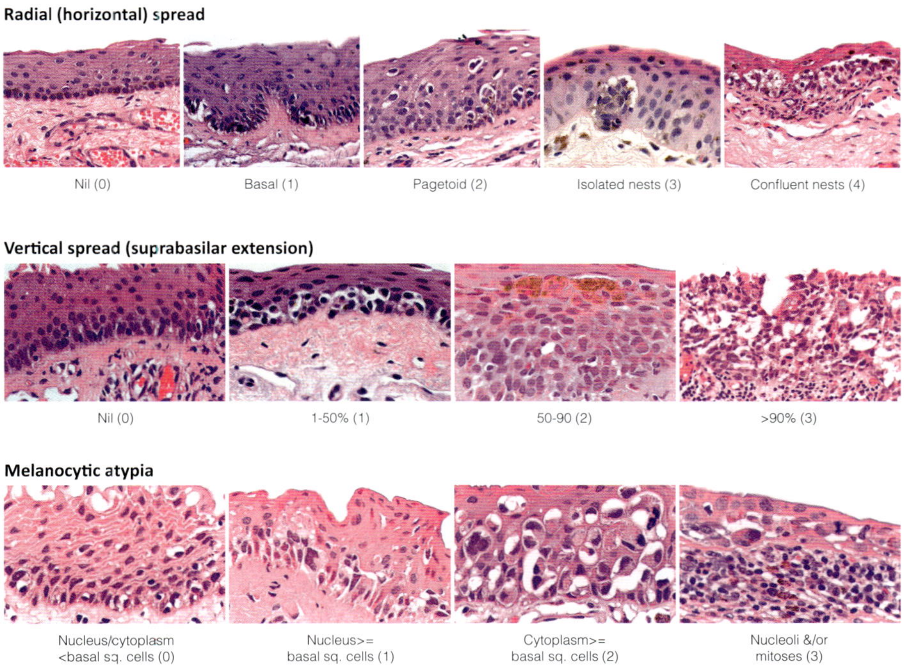

Fig. 1.24 Conjunctival melanocytic intraepithelial neoplasia (C-MIN) scoring. C-MIN is scored out of 10 based on the extent of horizontal (radial) spread and vertical spread (suprabasilar extension) of melanocytes, as well as the degree of atypia. sq., squamous.

Genetic profile

Little is known about the genetic alterations in C-MIN/PAM. BRAF p.V600E alterations occur in approximately 40% of conjunctival melanomas, but some studies suggest that these cases arise from naevi with mutations rather than from PAM {158,684}. *TERT* promoter mutations were found in 2 of 25 cases of PAM with atypia {646}. *GNAQ* and *GNA11* mutations are not present in intraepithelial or invasive conjunctival melanoma {297}.

Genetic susceptibility

PAM with atypia has been reported in patients with neurofibromatosis type 1, but this association may be coincidental {1211}.

Prognosis and predictive factors

As many as 70% of conjunctival melanomas arise from C-MIN/PAM with atypia {595}. PAM without atypia has not been associated with a significantly increased risk of progression to melanoma {360,744,1163}. The risk of melanoma depends on the severity of the C-MIN/PAM with atypia. In one early study, the presence of epithelioid cells was associated with a 75% chance of melanoma development {360}. A single-institution retrospective study of 29 cases of PAM with atypia stratified on the basis of microscopic criteria into low-risk and high-risk groups found that 15% and 94% of cases, respectively, progressed to melanoma {1225}. Atypical cytological features, including epithelioid cells, hyperchromatic nuclei, and prominent nucleoli, have been found to have greater prognostic value than do architectural alterations (e.g. the extent of pagetoid spread) {1411}. A larger study including 112 eyes with biopsy-confirmed PAM found recurrence in 11% of the cases without atypia, 26% of those with mild atypia, and 50% of those with severe atypia; 13% of the cases with severe atypia (but none with mild or no atypia) progressed to melanoma {1163}. Extensive lesions are also thought to have a greater risk of progression.

Conjunctival junctional, compound, and subepithelial naevi

Pe'er J.
Milman T.
Rašić D.M.

Definition

Conjunctival junctional, compound, and subepithelial naevi are benign melanocytic neoplasms composed of naevocellular naevus cells located within the conjunctival epithelium and its invaginations at the epithelial–subepithelial junction. Pure junctional naevus and predominantly junctional naevus show no or only minimal (respectively) subepithelial colonization in the conjunctival stroma; compound naevus shows subepithelial colonization both at the epithelial–subepithelial junction and in the stroma; and subepithelial naevus shows subepithelial colonization entirely in the stroma, with no junctional component at all {359,669,1411}.

ICD-O codes

Junctional naevus	8740/0
Compound naevus	8760/0
Subepithelial (stromal) naevus	8750/0

Synonym

Melanocytic naevi

Epidemiology

Junctional naevi account for 3–6% of biopsied conjunctival naevi {24,398,1082}; the male-to-female ratio is 2:1 {398}, and cases are typically diagnosed in childhood or adolescence {398,1082,1411}. Compound naevi account for 70–78% of biopsied conjunctival naevi and are diagnosed at a median patient age of 22 years (range: 5–74 years) {359,398,1082}. Subepithelial naevi account for 15–24% of biopsied conjunctival naevi and are diagnosed at a mean age of 46 years (range: 12–87 years) {24,398,1082}. Compound and subepithelial naevi occur with equal frequency in males and females and are more common in White populations.

Etiology

Conjunctival naevi are considered to be a subtype of acquired melanocytic naevus. Analogous to its dermal counterpart, conjunctival junctional naevus is thought to be the first stage of the conjunctival naevocellular naevus ontology {359,669,1411}. Compound naevus constitutes an intermediate stage characterized by the migration of intraepithelial naevus cells into the conjunctival stroma (substantia propria), and subepithelial naevus corresponds to the final stage, after the disappearance of the junctional component {359}.

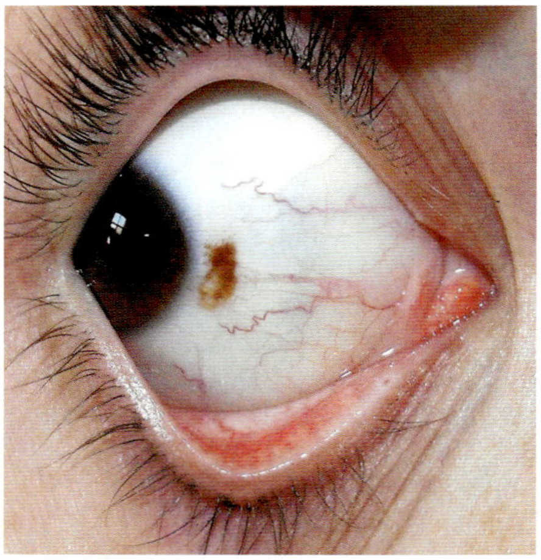

Fig. 1.25 Conjunctival junctional naevus. A juxtalimbal focal, flat, well-circumscribed, moderately pigmented conjunctival lesion with amelanotic foci.

Localization

Junctional naevi are found almost exclusively in the juxtalimbal bulbar conjunctiva and are very rare in other conjunctival sites {1082}. Most compound and subepithelial naevi (98%) are located in the bulbar (commonly juxtalimbal) conjunctiva, caruncle, and plica semilunaris; they are very rare in the palpebral conjunctiva and the fornix {359,398,602,1082}. Corneal involvement is characteristically absent {1411}.

Clinical features

Conjunctival naevi are well-circumscribed brown to tan (or rarely, amelanotic) lesions that can be freely moved over the scleral surface. Junctional naevi are usually focal and flat {24,1082,1411}. Feeder or intrinsic vessels are typically absent {24,1082,1411}, and epithelial inclusion cysts are uncommon {24,1082,1411}. Compound naevi are usually elevated, and epithelial cysts are common (occurring in 70% of cases). Subepithelial naevi are also elevated, with an average thickness of < 1 mm. Both compound and subepithelial naevi harbour epithelial cysts and often intrinsic vessels {359,1082}, but feeder vessels are typically absent.

Histopathology

Junctional naevi appear as an intraepithelial proliferation of type A (round to oval, plump, epithelioid) naevocytes and/or type B (oval to cuboidal, intermediate, or lymphocyte-like) naevocytes {359,1411}. The naevocytes may form single, confluent, or irregular nests, and they sometimes form lentiginous proliferations along the epithelial–subepithelial junction anterior to the epithelial basement membrane, which is typically intact {359,1411}. Some nests may protrude superficially into the substantia propria {359}. The epithelium overlying the nests is commonly reduced to a thin rim. No notable pagetoid scatter is present. Sporadic nuclear pleomorphism and small squamous whorls can be seen {359}. The nucleoli are small, basophilic, sometimes prominent, and without atypia. Mitotic activity is very low {359,1411}. Lymphocytic infiltrate may be present in the substantia propria.

Compound naevi contain naevus cells both within the epithelium and in the substantia propria, with maturation towards the deeper layers. Type A cells are seen in the junctional nests and superficial substantia propria, and type B cells in the deeper layers of the subepithelial compartment. In older patients, the deepest cells may display spindle-like neuroid differentiation (type C). Solid and cystic epithelial rests are common; the cysts are lined by conjunctival epithelium and occasional goblet cells. Polyhedral balloon cells and spindle cells can also be found. Multinucleated cells and pleomorphism can be seen but do not imply malignancy. Mitotic activity, if present, appears in the superficial layer {359,1411}.

Subepithelial naevi typically appear as symmetrically arranged intrastromal

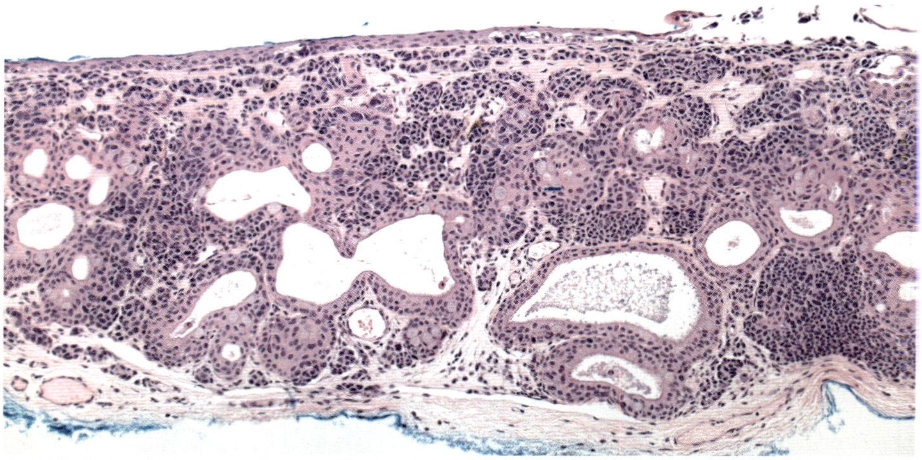

Fig. 1.26 Conjunctival compound naevus. Prominent induction of conjunctival cysts is common in conjunctival naevi.

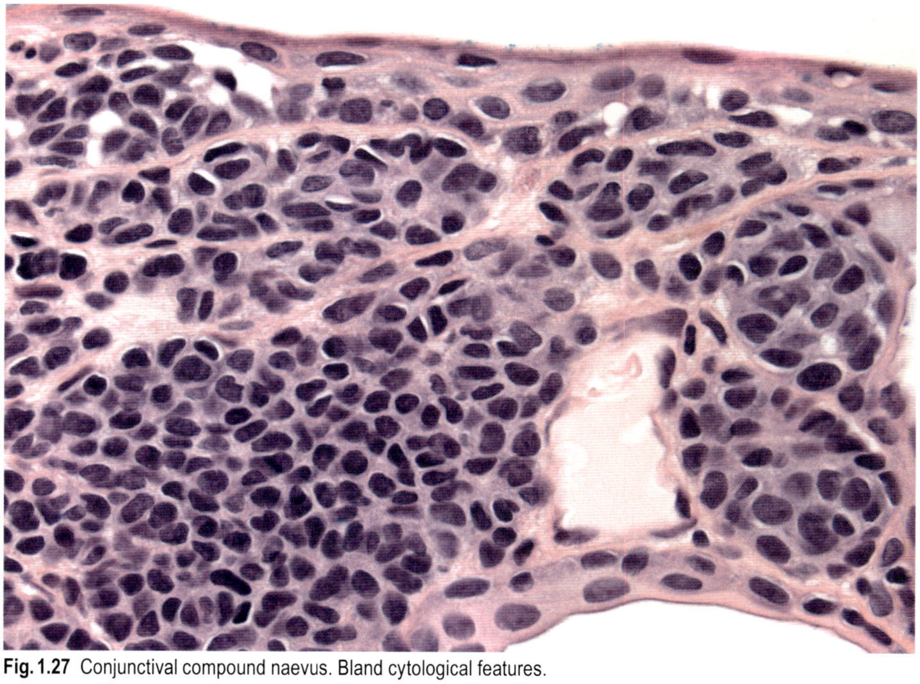

Fig. 1.27 Conjunctival compound naevus. Bland cytological features.

proliferations of predominantly type B cells, with occasional intranuclear vacuoles, often organized in large nests. Although maturation is not as pronounced in conjunctival subepithelial naevi as in their dermal counterparts, the superficial naevus cells tend to be larger and more polygonal (type A), whereas the deep naevus cells may display neuroid differentiation (type C) {359,523}. Naevus giant cells and sporadic pleomorphism can be seen. Mitotic figures are generally absent {523}. Cystic and solid rests of conjunctival epithelium entrapped within the melanocytic proliferation are seen microscopically in about half of these lesions {523,1082}. Compared with junctional and compound naevi, subepithelial naevi are more likely to be amelanotic or minimally pigmented, and they are rarely associated with lymphocytic infiltrate {523}.

Conjunctival naevi stain positively for S100 protein, melan-A, and (more weakly) HMB45 antigen {523,964,1069}. HMB45 antigen is characteristically found in the junctional component. The Ki-67 proliferation index is low (~2%), with Ki-67 staining usually limited to the junctional component of junctional and compound naevi and generally limited to rare superficial stromal melanocytes in subepithelial naevi {523,964,1069}.

Differential diagnosis

Both clinically and histopathologically, conjunctival junctional naevi may mimic conjunctival melanocytic intraepithelial neoplasia/primary acquired melanosis. Any junctional melanocytic lesion in an adult should be assumed to be conjunctival melanocytic intraepithelial neoplasia until proved otherwise {359,1411}. Clinically, compound naevi and subepithelial naevi should be differentiated from other elevated pigmented conjunctival lesions, in particular conjunctival melanoma and extraocular extension of uveal melanoma, both of which may be adherent to the globe and typically show no epithelial cysts. Histologically, melanoma cells tend to be larger than naevus cells; they also demonstrate higher grades of nuclear atypia and mitotic activity, and epithelial rests are absent or rare {359}. Immunohistochemically, conjunctival melanoma is more likely to be diffusely positive for HMB45 antigen and to have a high mean Ki-67 proliferation index {523,526,964,1069}.

Histogenesis

Conjunctival junctional, compound, and subepithelial naevi arise from neural crest–derived melanocytes {359}.

Genetic profile

Data on the genetic profile of naevocellular conjunctival naevi are limited. *BRAF* c.1799T>A (p.V600E) mutation has been found in as many as half of the acquired naevocellular conjunctival naevi evaluated {410,683}. *GNAQ* and *GNA11* mutations were not detected in conjunctival naevi {297}.

Genetic susceptibility

Dysplastic naevus syndrome and a family history of cutaneous melanoma have been rarely described in patients with acquired naevocellular conjunctival naevi {359,669,1082}.

Prognosis and predictive factors

Rarely, a junctional or compound naevus of the conjunctiva can give rise to conjunctival melanoma {359,669,1082}. Subepithelial naevus cells are predominantly postmitotic, and they are believed to have an extremely low risk of progression to melanoma {359}.

Inflamed juvenile conjunctival naevus

Pe'er J.
Chévez-Barrios P.
Kivelä T.T.

Definition

Inflamed juvenile conjunctival naevus (IJCN) is a compound naevus that appears in children and adolescents and shows inflammatory features {359,1256, 1408}.

ICD-O code

Inflamed juvenile naevus 8770/0

Synonym

Inflamed naevus of puberty and young adulthood

Epidemiology

IJCN affects children and adolescents at a mean age of 11–13 years and occurs with equal frequency in males and females. It is usually accompanied by asymptomatic or symptomatic allergic conjunctivitis {703,744,1256,1408}.

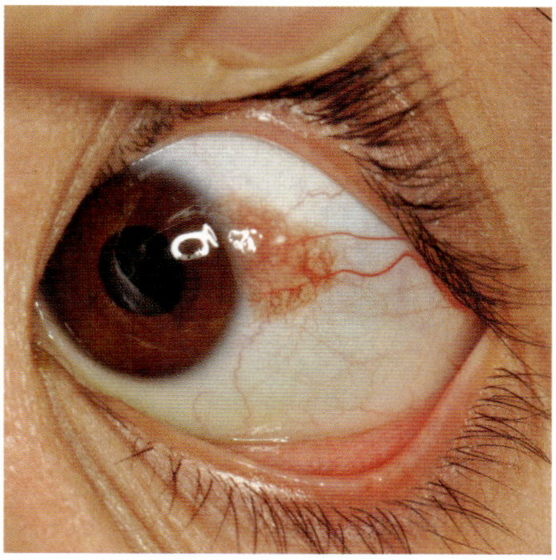

Fig. 1.28 Inflamed juvenile conjunctival naevus. An amelanotic conjunctival lesion adjacent to the temporal limbus, with prominent cysts, feeder vessels, and intrinsic vascularity.

Etiology

IJCN is a subtype of compound naevus associated with chronic conjunctival inflammation, the triggering factors of which are unknown. The inflammatory reaction might induce the growth of the naevi at an early age. Alternatively, this process might constitute a direct immune response induced by the naevus itself {703}.

Localization

IJCNs are perilimbal and may also involve the limbus itself {1408}.

Clinical features

IJCN is an elevated, well-circumscribed nodule. An amelanotic inflamed naevus is more common than a pigmented one, although changes in the degree of pigmentation may occur during growth. The naevus usually shows cystic structures and is freely movable, except when it involves the limbus. IJCNs frequently cause undue concern, because they can grow rapidly, they appear vascularized, and they can have congested feeding vessels {744,1256,1408}.

Histopathology

IJCN shares features with conjunctival compound naevus, including cystic and solid epithelial rests in most cases. The cystic component often contains goblet cells, and periodic acid–Schiff (PAS) staining highlights this component {204}. Prominent lymphocytic inflammation is

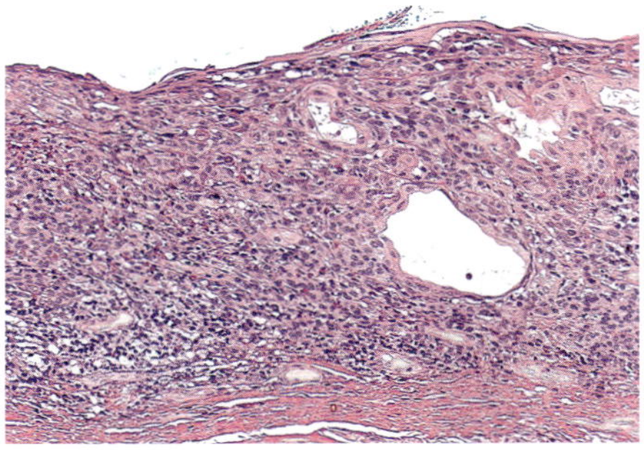

Fig. 1.29 Inflamed juvenile conjunctival naevus. A compound naevus of the conjunctiva involving the junctional area and the substantia propria, with cystic epithelial rests; the naevus is infiltrated and surrounded by inflammatory cells, including lymphocytes, with a remarkable number of eosinophils.

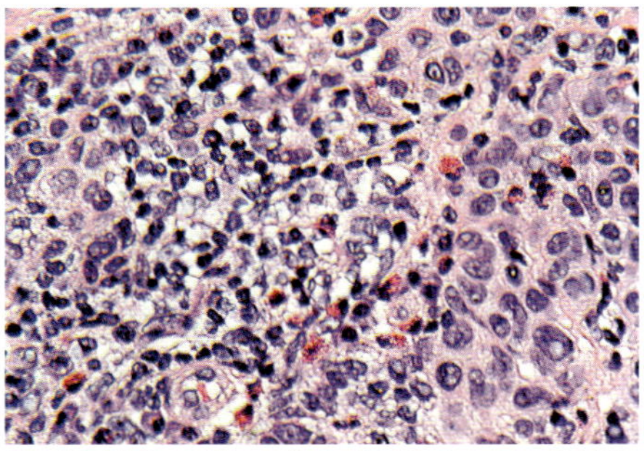

Fig. 1.30 Inflamed juvenile conjunctival naevus. A high-power view showing naevus cells to the right and inflammation, which is rich in eosinophils and lymphoid cells, to the left.

characteristic. Well-defined germinal centres may be present. Plasma cells and eosinophils are seen in about three quarters of IJCNs. Periods of rapid growth result from inflammatory infiltration and cystic enlargement by mucin production and accumulation {204,359,710,1408}. IJCNs show apparent disordered growth, such as prominent confluent junctional nests and lack of (or incomplete) maturation or paradoxical so-called reverse maturation, in which the nuclear and cytoplasmic size of the naevus cells is greater in the subepithelial component than in the junctional region. This may lead to misdiagnosis as a premalignant or malignant melanocytic lesion. The junctional component often extends horizontally beyond the subepithelial component {744,1256,1411}. Mitotic figures are rarely seen, and the Ki-67 proliferation index is low. IJCN is positive for HMB45 antigen in the superficial layer only. Immunostaining for leukocyte common antigen, CD3, and CD20 reveals a mixed population of B cells and T cells {204,744,1256}.

Differential diagnosis

The clinical appearance and rapid growth of IJCN often raise concern for malignancy, such as conjunctival melanoma, which is very rare in children and adolescents. The histological patterns may also raise suspicion for melanoma. The patient's young age and the cystic nature of a typical IJCN are indicators of a benign lesion. Amelanotic IJCN should also be differentiated from the so-called salmon patch of conjunctival lymphoproliferative lesions, including conjunctival lymphoma {204,359,1408,1411}. Plasma cells may be abundant and some are IgG4-positive, but they do not meet the full diagnostic criteria for IgG4-related disease {204}.

Histogenesis

IJCN arises from neural crest–derived melanocytes accompanied by an inflammatory infiltrate, usually of presumed allergic type {703}.

Genetic profile

BRAF c.1799T>A mutation was identified in 1 of 4 IJCNs {410}.

Genetic susceptibility

There is no known genetic susceptibility. Dysplastic naevus syndrome or a family history of cutaneous melanoma has not been described in patients with IJCN {1256,1408}.

Prognosis and predictive factors

IJCN rarely recurs if excised, and it is rarely the source of conjunctival melanoma {1256,1408}.

Blue naevus of the conjunctiva

Milman T.
Mihic-Probst D.
Rao N.

Definition

Blue naevus of the conjunctiva is a benign melanocytic neoplasm composed of dendritic and spindle-shaped melanocytes in the subepithelial connective tissue {96}.

ICD-O code

Blue naevus 8780/0

Epidemiology

Blue naevi account for < 4% of conjunctival and caruncular naevi, occur with equal frequency in males and females, and are more common in White populations {24,398,1082}. Most blue naevi are diagnosed between the third and fifth decades of life {24,96,398,1082}.

Localization

Distribution is relatively even throughout the bulbar, forniceal, and palpebral

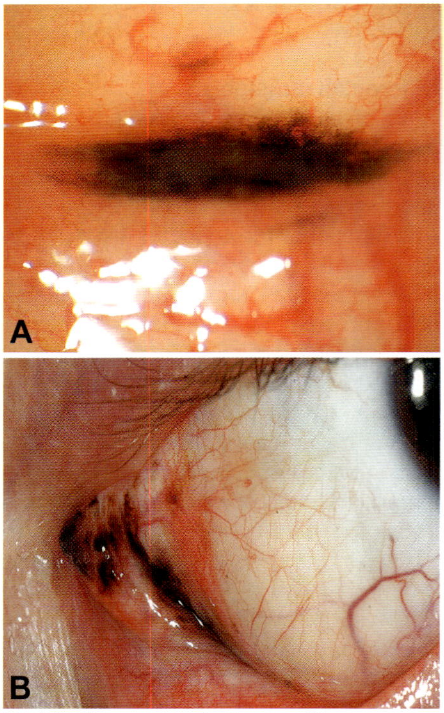

Fig. 1.31 Blue naevus. **A** Common blue naevus; a well-circumscribed, darkly pigmented lesion involves the forniceal conjunctiva. **B** Cellular blue naevus; a multifocal, darkly pigmented lesion involves the caruncle, plica semilunaris, and forniceal conjunctiva.

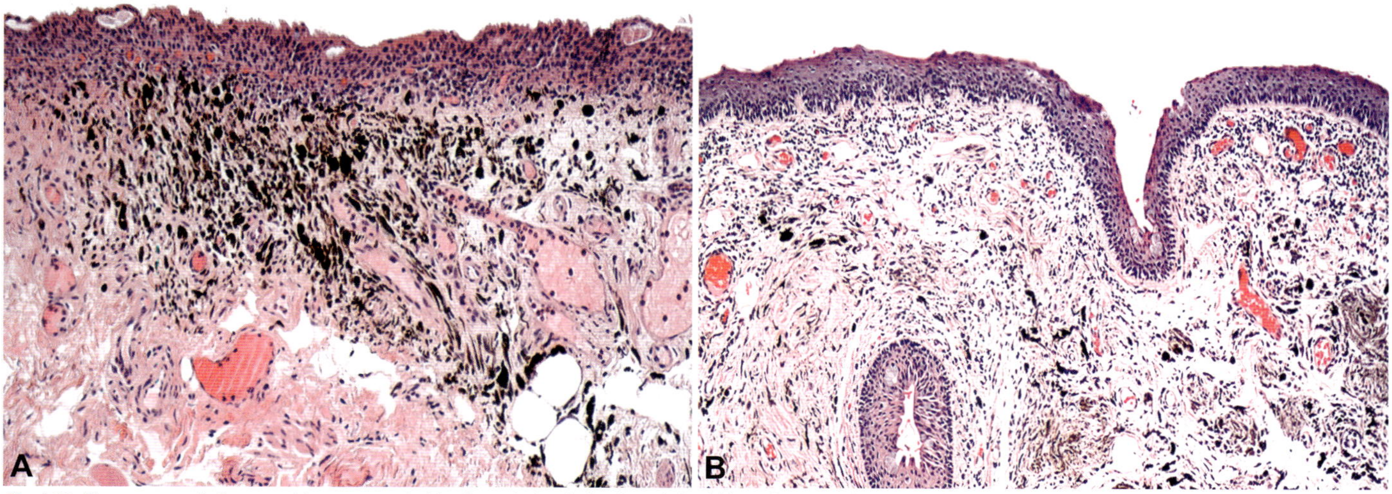

Fig. 1.32 Blue naevus. A Common blue naevus; darkly pigmented, spindle-shaped dendritic melanocytes interspersed with melanophages are present in the substantia propria. B Cellular blue naevus; several dense aggregates of lightly pigmented melanocytes are present in a background of common blue naevus.

conjunctiva and the caruncle {24,96,533, 1082}.

Clinical features

Blue naevi present as dark-brown to black, sharply demarcated, unifocal or multifocal, slightly elevated conjunctival masses, with a thickness of approximately 2 mm {96}. Unlike the common acquired naevocellular conjunctival naevi, blue naevi lack epithelial cysts and infrequently contain intrinsic or feeder vessels {96,1082}.

Histopathology

Blue naevi are characterized by proliferation of dendritic and/or fusiform melanocytes in the subepithelial connective tissues {96,319,359,525}. There is no associated junctional melanocytic proliferation or entrapped epithelial cysts, except in combined or collision lesions such as combined naevus, which shows features of both naevocellular and blue naevi {234,602}. Common blue naevi are characterized by the presence of variably pigmented, spindle-shaped dendritic melanocytes, which show slender, branching networks of dendritic processes in the substantia propria. Melanophages and stromal fibrosis are frequently associated {96,319,359}. Cellular blue naevi contain dense aggregates of cytologically bland spindle and/or epithelioid amelanotic melanocytes, frequently set in a background of common blue naevus {112,272,359}. In all benign blue naevus variants, mitotic figures are characteristically absent {359}. Immunohistochemically, the dendritic cells are positive for S100 protein, melan-A, and SOX10, and they can be positive for HMB45 antigen. There is neither necrosis nor proliferation {533,542,602}.

Differential diagnosis

The differential diagnosis includes conjunctival melanoma, malignant blue naevus, uveal melanoma with extrascleral extension, and pigmented epithelioid melanocytoma {107,359}. Melanomas are more pleomorphic and they demonstrate mitotic activity. Unlike malignant blue naevus, conjunctival melanoma usually has an intraepithelial component {207,523,964}. Cutaneous melanomas associated with or mimicking blue naevi frequently demonstrate loss of nuclear BAP1 immunohistochemical expression {223}.

Histogenesis

Blue naevus is believed to arise as the result of an arrest in migration of neural crest–derived melanocytes in the subepithelial connective tissue {991}.

Genetic profile

The genetic profile of conjunctival blue naevi remains unclear. Cutaneous blue naevi have been shown to harbour mutations in *GNA11* and *GNAQ* {991,1305,1399}.

Prognosis and predictive factors

Cellular blue naevi can rarely evolve into melanoma {272}.

Spitz naevus of the conjunctiva

Van Ginderdeuren R.
Mihic-Probst D.
Milman T.

Definition

Spitz naevus of the conjunctiva is a neoplasm consisting of a proliferation of large spindle-shaped or epithelioid melanocytes with distinctive architectural features.

ICD-O code

Spitz naevus	8770/0

Synonym

Spindle and/or epithelioid cell naevus

Epidemiology

Because of its extreme rarity (< 10 cases reported) the incidence of conjunctival Spitz naevus is unknown {542,576,1325, 1341}.

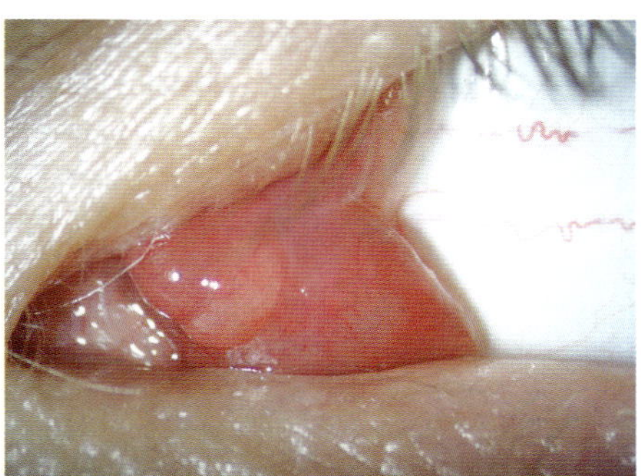

Fig. 1.33 Caruncular Spitz naevus. An example in a 28-year-old man.

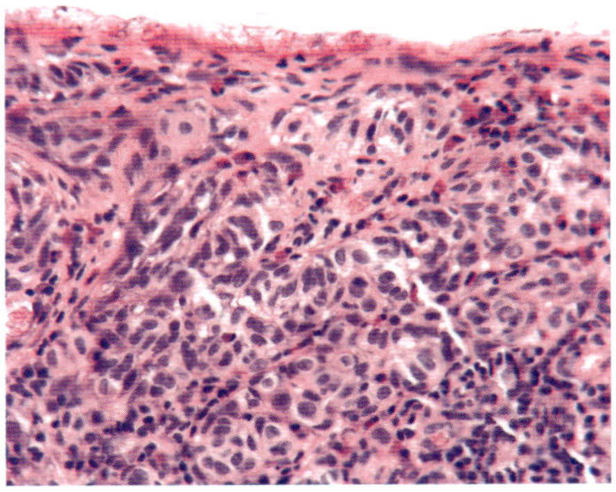

Fig. 1.34 Conjunctival Spitz naevus. Clusters of large eosinophilic epithelioid non-pigmented melanocytes; there is an obvious nucleolus, as well as multiple eosinophilic granulocytes between the naevus cells.

Localization
At this anatomical site, Spitz naevus occurs in the bulbar and caruncular conjunctiva {215,542,576,1325}.

Clinical features
The clinical presentation is nonspecific: a rapidly growing, pinkish-red, vascularized, solitary lesion seen mostly in young patients {1119}. Spitz naevi involving the bulbar conjunctiva are freely movable over the sclera, whereas naevi in the caruncle are immobile {359,1119}. A rapid growth phase is typical, followed by a stable period.

Histopathology
The lesion resembles the dermal variant of Spitz naevus. These non-pigmented compound melanocytic neoplasms are well circumscribed, with symmetrical borders. A benign lymphoplasmacytic infiltrate is present around the tumour, with multiple epithelial invaginations or cysts with goblet cells. The neoplastic cells are distributed in circumscribed nests and fascicles, oriented perpendicular to the surface. The eosinophilic cells are large and epithelioid or spindle-shaped, with medium to large nuclei. Mitoses can be found in the superficial layers. The cytomorphology of the cells is uniform throughout the entire lesion. High-grade atypia must be absent. Maturation of the tumour cells can be observed. Immunohistochemically, the cells stain for melan-A and S100 protein. Junctional cells are HMB45-positive. Ki-67 staining can be positive in the superficial layers {215,988,1325}.

Differential diagnosis
Common conjunctival naevus, inflamed conjunctival naevus, and conjunctival melanoma are differentiated on the basis of strict regularity and symmetry; the deeper parts of Spitz naevi lack atypia and mitoses.

Prognosis and predictive factors
Spitz naevi are benign lesions {542,576,1325,1341}.

Benign epithelial melanoses of the conjunctiva

Edward D.P.
Mihic-Probst D.
Kivelä T.T.
Chan A.S.Y.

Definition
Benign epithelial melanoses of the conjunctiva are a group of clinical entities characterized by increased production of melanin without proliferation of conjunctival melanocytes; the melanocytes remain normal in size and location and may transfer melanin into adjacent keratinocytes {243}.

ICD-O code
None

Synonyms
Racial melanoses; constitutional melanoses; complexion-associated melanoses; non-proliferative melanocytic pigmentary patches; ephelides; freckles {243,522}

Epidemiology
Benign epithelial melanoses are common. They are more frequent in people with darker pigmentation, occurring with decreasing frequency in African, Asian, and White populations {243}.

Etiology
Benign epithelial melanoses are a biological trait. People whose ancestors lived closer to the equator for many generations have melanocytes that produce larger quantities of melanin to protect them from ionizing ultraviolet (UV) radiation.

Localization
Benign epithelial melanoses are usually bilateral; they are most common in the perilimbal region, but they can also occur in the bulbar conjunctiva and extend to the palpebral conjunctiva {458}.

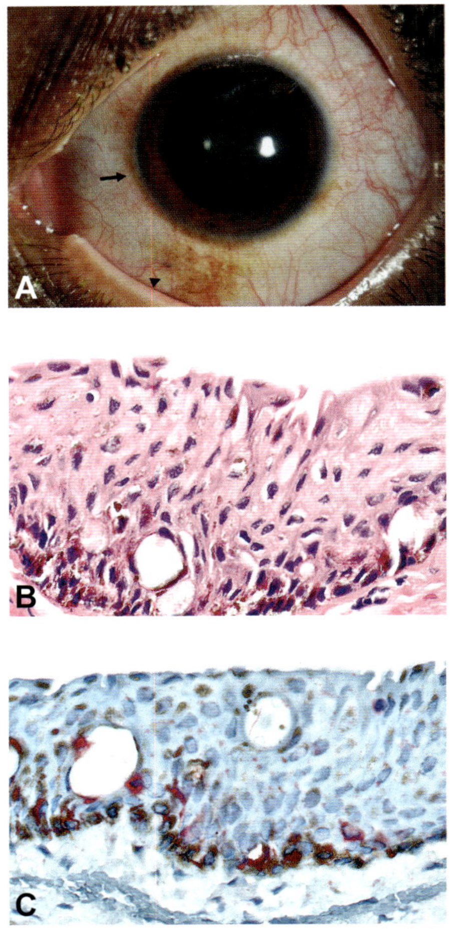

Fig. 1.35 Congenital conjunctival hypermelanosis. **A** An anterior segment photo showing patchy brown pigmentation at the limbus (arrow) and extending over the inferior bulbar conjunctiva (arrowhead); note the superficial nature of the pigmentation, which can be seen overlying the episcleral vessels. **B** Increased melanin pigmentation within melanocytes and adjacent keratinocytes; note the melanin cap over the nucleus. **C** HMB45 immunostaining highlights the normal number of melanocytes present.

Clinical features
Congenital conjunctival hypermelanosis may be visible from birth as mottled or patchy intraepithelial pigmented lesions that are not fixed to the sclera. The pigmentation may extend into the corneal epithelium. The lesions darken and may increase in size during childhood and adolescence {990}. The melanin granules in the recipient epithelial cells accumulate over the nuclei to diminish the chance of harmful mutations caused by UV radiation.

Histopathology

Normal conjunctival melanocytes are dendritic and are located within the basal epithelium. Congenital conjunctival hypermelanosis appears microscopically as increased melanin pigmentation within these melanocytes, which are normal in number. Features such as nuclear enlargement, prominent nucleoli, and mitoses are not present {243}. Melanocytes transfer melanin granules to keratinocytes to such an extent that the pigmented keratinocytes typically outnumber the melanocytes, as determined with antibodies against the two cell types. The cells are HMB45-positive.

Differential diagnosis

The differential diagnosis includes conjunctival melanocytic intraepithelial neoplasia/primary acquired melanosis with atypia and secondary conjunctival melanosis {243,458,522}.

Histogenesis

Benign epithelial melanoses arise from normally developed melanocytes with abundant melanin.

Prognosis and predictive factors

Benign epithelial melanoses are benign non-neoplastic lesions; the malignant potential of their cells is no higher than that of any other melanocyte {458}. Malignant transformation into conjunctival melanocytic intraepithelial neoplasia/primary acquired melanosis with atypia and conjunctival melanoma is exceedingly rare, especially in people with dark pigmentation.

Haematolymphoid tumours of the conjunctiva and caruncle

Lymphomas of the conjunctiva and caruncle

Coupland S.E.
Heegaard S.
Loeffler K.U.
van der Valk P.
Bermúdez Magner A.

Definition

Primary conjunctival lymphomas are primary monoclonal proliferations of atypical lymphocytes arising in the conjunctiva. Secondary conjunctival lymphomas are manifestations of systemic lymphoma in the conjunctiva {233}.

ICD-O codes

Code according to the lymphoma subtype.

Synonym

Conjunctival non-Hodgkin lymphomas

Epidemiology

Primary conjunctival lymphomas account for 25–30% of all ocular adnexal lymphomas, which in turn constitute 2% of all extranodal lymphomas {231}. They occur more commonly in middle-aged and elderly individuals, although they can also occur in young adults. Low-grade primary conjunctival lymphomas tend to occur in the sixth decade of life, whereas high-grade tumours affect people aged > 70 years {231,350,614,831,1192}. Women are affected slightly more commonly than men. The incidence of conjunctival non-Hodgkin lymphoma increased as much as 3% per year from 1980 to 2005 {1192}.

Etiology

One of the proposed risk factors for conjunctival lymphoma development is autoimmune disease; others include *Chlamydia psittaci*, *Helicobacter pylori*, and HIV infection {185,231,350,831,1192}.

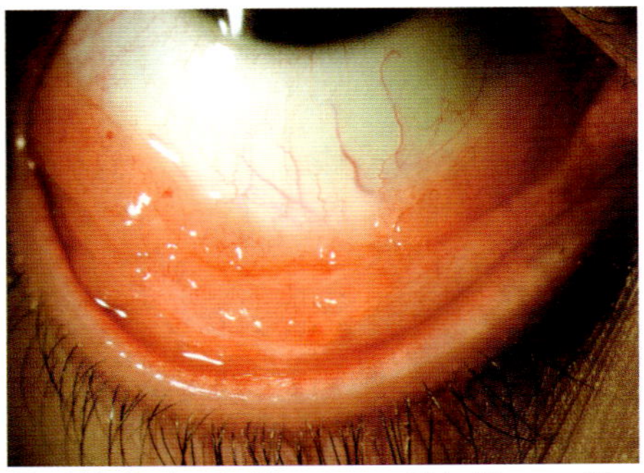

Fig. 1.36 Conjunctival lymphoma. Clinical image of the right lower eyelid of a 53-year-old man who presented with a slow-growing, painless, pink swelling of the conjunctiva.

Localization

The palpebral conjunctiva and forniceal conjunctiva are most commonly affected. As many as 90% of patients have unilateral disease {231,350}.

Clinical features

These tumours present as a slow-growing, painless, salmon-pink, fleshy patch or swelling. Primary conjunctival non-Hodgkin lymphoma presents as limited disease, defined as stage IE by the Ann Arbor staging system and T1 by the TNM staging system {233}. Secondary conjunctival non-Hodgkin lymphoma tends to appear more rapidly and as part of widely spread disease {831,960}. Recurrence or disease progression is observed in about 40% of patients with primary conjunctival lymphomas, with subsequent relapses frequently occurring at extraocular sites {231,350,1192,1260}.

Histopathology

Most primary conjunctival lymphomas (98%) are non-Hodgkin lymphomas of B-cell type, whereas T-cell non-Hodgkin lymphomas are rare (accounting for only 2% of cases) {614}. The three most common primary conjunctival non-Hodgkin lymphoma types are extranodal marginal zone lymphoma of mucosa-associated lymphoid tissue (MALT lymphoma), accounting for 60% of cases; follicular lymphoma, accounting for 10%; and

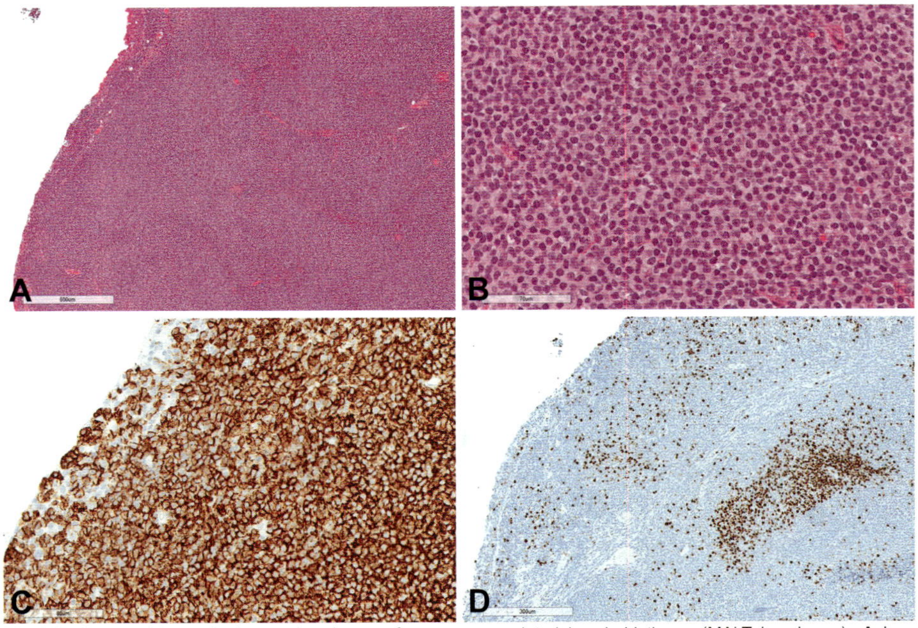

Fig. 1.37 Extranodal marginal zone lymphoma of mucosa-associated lymphoid tissue (MALT lymphoma). **A** Low power shows monotonous sheets of small lymphoid cells with a vaguely nodular pattern. **B** Higher power shows that the cells resemble normal small lymphocytes with slightly irregular nuclei and tiny nucleoli. **C** CD20 staining highlights the lymphoma cells within the substantia propria, as well as those that infiltrate the epithelium. **D** There is a low Ki-67 proliferation index in the majority of the lymphoma; the clusters of positively staining cells highlight a germinal centre infiltrated by lymphoma cells.

diffuse large B-cell lymphoma (DLBCL), accounting for 9%.
Hodgkin lymphoma occurs as a secondary manifestation and is exceptionally rare. The most common secondary conjunctival non-Hodgkin lymphomas are mantle cell lymphomas, plasmacytomas, and T-cell lymphomas. The morphological, immunophenotypic, and genomic features of each of these tumours have been reviewed elsewhere {231,350,1192,1260}.

Differential diagnosis
The differential diagnosis includes reactive lymphoid hyperplasia, chronic (allergic) conjunctivitis, and granulomatous conjunctival inflammation.

Histogenesis
The histogenesis depends on the B-cell lymphoma subtype and its associated neoplastic clone in the B-cell differentiation pathway {1231}.

Genetic profile
Conjunctival MALT lymphomas are characterized by the following translocations: t(11;18)(q21;q21), t(1;14)(p22;q32), t(14;18)(q32;q21), and t(3;14)(p13;q32), resulting in uncontrolled activation of the NF-κB signalling pathway {1231}. The *TNFAIP3* (*A20*) gene (located at 6q23.3) is frequently down-regulated by gene deletion, mutation, and hypermethylation in these tumours {184}.
Conjunctival follicular lymphoma shows the pathognomonic translocation t(14;18)(q32;q21), involving *BCL2* gene rearrangement, resulting in apoptosis arrest in the neoplastic B cells {961}.
Most conjunctival DLBCLs demonstrate immunophenotypic and molecular features of the activated B-cell–like subtype {831,1231}. Multiple oncogenic alterations and dysregulating signal transduction pathways have been documented in DLBCL, including mutations of *MYD88*. A recurrent target of genetic lesions is NF-κB, particularly in the less curable activated B-cell–like subtype {156,896}.

Prognosis and predictive factors
Treatment, which depends on the tumour stage and subtype, includes surgical resection, cryotherapy, radiotherapy, and systemic chemotherapy – usually including targeted anti–B-cell therapy (i.e. rituximab) {1397}.
The prognosis of conjunctival and caruncular lymphomas depends on the lymphoma subtype (i.e. MALT vs non-MALT) and the clinical stage of disease (i.e. stage IE vs > IIE and < T2 vs ≥ T3). Patients with stage IE conjunctival MALT lymphoma and follicular lymphoma have a favourable prognosis, with reported 5-year lymphoma-related survival rates of 82% and 72%, respectively, whereas patients with DLBCL and mantle cell lymphoma have a poor prognosis, with reported rates of 33% and 8%, respectively {831,960}.
Patient age and sex are reliable predictors of disease-specific survival for MALT lymphoma and follicular lymphoma, as are the Ann Arbor and TNM stages of disease for MALT lymphoma, follicular lymphoma, and DLBCL {231,962}. The growth fraction (Ki-67 proliferation index) of the tumour cells is also postulated to be prognostic {231}. Conjunctival T-cell non-Hodgkin lymphoma is associated with a poor prognosis, with 50% of cases progressing or recurring within the first year after diagnosis {614}.

Papillary/follicular conjunctivitis

Coupland S.E.
Heegaard S.
Loeffler K.U.
van der Valk P.
Bermúdez Magner A.

Definition
Conjunctivitis is categorized as either papillary or follicular according to the macroscopic and microscopic appearances. Papillary conjunctivitis shows a cobblestone arrangement of flattened nodules with a central vascular core. Follicular conjunctivitis is characterized by hyperaemia and small, dome-shaped nodules without a prominent central vessel.

ICD-O code
None

Synonyms
Atopic conjunctivitis; allergic conjunctivitis

Epidemiology
The exact incidence is difficult to determine. The proportion of individuals with allergic conjunctival diseases diagnosed by ophthalmologists is about 12% among children and 15% among adults. The incidence of atopic keratoconjunctivitis is increasing, particularly among children {219,514,699,700,1259}.

Etiology
Neither papillary nor follicular conjunctivitis is pathognomonic for any particular disease entity. Papillary conjunctivitis is most commonly associated with an allergic immune response (as is the case in vernal and atopic keratoconjunctivitis), or it is a response to a foreign body (e.g. a contact lens or an ocular prosthesis). Follicular conjunctivitis has a variety of causes, such as microorganisms (e.g. viruses and atypical bacteria) and toxins (including topical medications). A common infectious cause of follicular conjunctivitis is *Chlamydia trachomatis* (serotypes D–K); *Chlamydophila felis*, *Chlamydia psittaci*, and *Chlamydophila pneumoniae* are less frequent causes {219,699,1248,1259}.

Localization
In papillary conjunctivitis, papillae coat the tarsal surface of the upper eyelid. Cases in which these papillae reach large sizes (≥ 1 mm in diameter) are termed giant papillary conjunctivitis. Perilimbal Horner–Trantas dots, which may occur in vernal keratoconjunctivitis, are focal white limbal dots consisting of degenerated epithelial cells and eosinophils {143}. The follicles in follicular conjunctivitis are typically most prominent in the inferior palpebral and forniceal conjunctiva.

Clinical features
The main subjective symptoms in both conjunctivitis types are ocular itching, hyperaemia, eye discharge, and a foreign body sensation. In advanced cases of atopic keratoconjunctivitis with giant papillae, a secondary so-called shield ulcer of the (mostly superior) cornea can occur {699}.

Histopathology
Histological examination of papillary conjunctivitis shows closely packed, flat-topped projections, with numerous eosinophils, lymphocytes, plasma cells, and mast cells in the stroma surrounding a central vascular channel. The morphology is the same regardless of the cause. In follicular conjunctivitis, lymphoid

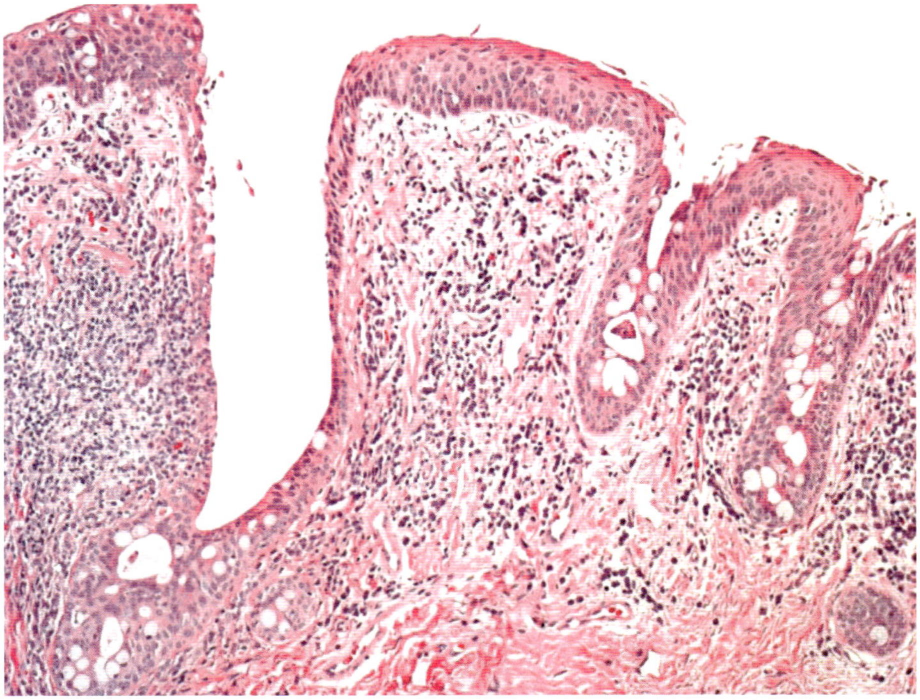

Fig. 1.38 Papillary conjunctivitis. Low-power magnification demonstrating the so-called flat top of the conjunctival papillae, which occur as a result of the chronic inflammation in papillary conjunctivitis.

follicles are situated in the subepithelial region; these follicles consist of a germinal centre (containing immature, proliferating lymphocytes) and a surrounding corona (containing mature lymphocytes and plasma cells).

Differential diagnosis
The differential diagnosis includes numerous other causes of red eye, including dry eye disease and infections.

Histogenesis
Papillary and follicular conjunctivitis arises as a result of complex reactive inflammation, involving hypersensitivity and T-cell–mediated inflammation mechanisms {390,793}. Giant papillary conjunctivitis shows features of both an immediate (type I) IgE-mediated hypersensitivity reaction and a delayed (type IV) reaction {390}. IL-6sR, IL-11, CCL24 (eotaxin-2), MIP-1δ, and TIMP2 are elevated in giant papillary conjunctivitis {1172}.

Genetic susceptibility
The genetic susceptibility is generally unknown, but there is an increased risk in the setting of hyper-IgE syndrome {463}.

Prognosis and predictive factors
The treatment of papillary/follicular conjunctivitis depends on the underlying etiology; it includes topical and systemic steroids, antiallergic medication, and lubricants, which usually resolve the disease {68,835}. Vernal keratoconjunctivitis tends to be self-resolving during puberty, whereas atopic conjunctivitis is seasonally chronic.

Reactive lymphoid hyperplasia of the conjunctiva and caruncle

Coupland S.E.
Heegaard S.
Loeffler K.U.
van der Valk P.
Bermúdez Magner A.

Definition
Reactive lymphoid hyperplasia (RLH) of the conjunctiva and caruncle is a polyclonal proliferation of lymphoid tissue that typically occurs in young adults {43}.

ICD-O code
None

Synonyms
Benign lymphoid hyperplasia; conjunctival lymphoid hyperplasia

Epidemiology
This lesion is typically found in young adults and occasionally in children, but it can occur at any age {17,43,231,1079, 1119}. There is a higher incidence in males. RLH seems to be increasing in frequency, but this may be due to increased recognition. There is no race predilection {43}.

Etiology
The etiology is unknown, but RLH is probably caused by chronic antigen stimulation (by either exogenous or endogenous antigens) leading to chronic conjunctivitis and ultimately RLH. Implicated exogenous antigens include antigens associated with *Chlamydia psittaci, Chlamydophila pneumoniae*, *Chlamydia trachomatis*, *Helicobacter pylori*, EBV, and HTLV-1 {43}. Implicated endogenous antigens include those occurring in autoimmune diseases.

Localization
The medial conjunctiva is affected most commonly, but this lesion also occurs commonly in the fornices {481,1079,1119}. The caruncle is involved in about 30% of cases {43}.

Clinical features
This lesion usually (i.e. in 70% of cases) presents as a unilateral, red or orange, painless swelling {481,1079,1119}. It is clinically and radiologically indistinguishable from low-grade non-Hodgkin lymphoma, so tissue biopsy is required in all cases {224}. There is no evidence of underlying systemic lymphoma.

Histopathology
The diagnosis is made by exclusion, requiring histopathological evaluation, immunophenotyping, and molecular studies (e.g. IGH PCR). RLH shows a diffuse infiltrate of mature lymphocytes within the substantia propria, as well as scattered irregular secondary lymphoid follicles with regular germinal centres and narrow marginal and mantle zones. The infiltrate comprises a mixture of B cells and T cells arranged physiologically. The germinal centres are immunoreactive for BCL6 and CD10 but negative for BCL2, with a normal Ki-67 proliferation index. IGH PCR shows a polyclonal or oligoclonal amplification product {231}.

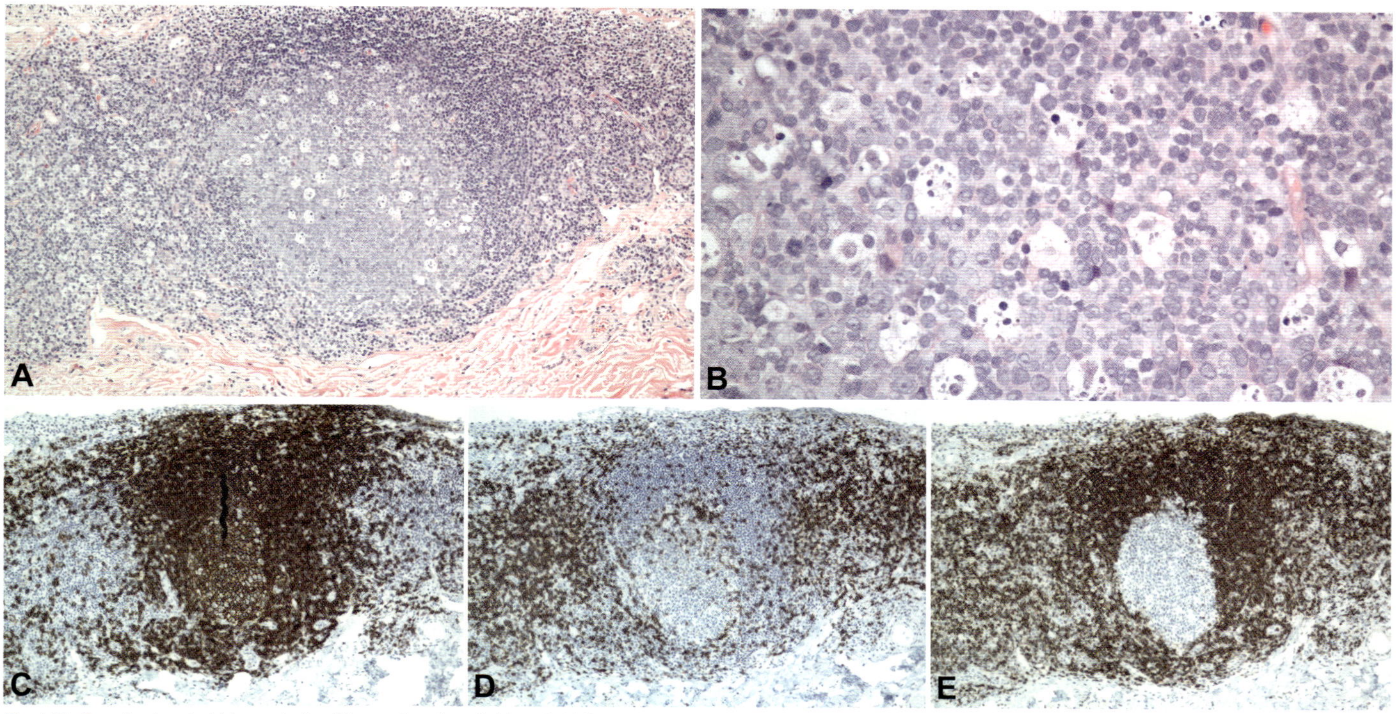

Fig. 1.39 Reactive lymphoid hyperplasia of the conjunctiva. **A** A lymphoid follicle with a large reactive germinal centre. **B** A high-power image of the germinal centre, showing numerous tingible body macrophages. **C** The follicle (including the germinal centre and the mantle zone) stains uniformly for CD20. **D** The interfollicular zone stains for CD3. **E** There is no staining for BCL2 in this benign follicle, although the surrounding reactive lymphocytes are positive.

Differential diagnosis

The differential diagnosis includes chronic allergic conjunctivitis, contact lens intolerance, idiopathic cicatricial disease, oculocutaneous pemphigoid, conjunctival granulomas, and sarcoidosis {481}, as well as extranodal marginal zone lymphoma of mucosa-associated lymphoid tissue (MALT lymphoma) and follicular lymphoma {43,1079}.

Histogenesis

Chronic antigen stimulation leads to polyclonal expansion of B cells and T cells {510}.

Prognosis and predictive factors

RLH can be treated medically (e.g. with topical steroids), by surgical excision with or without additional cryotherapy, and/or with low-dose external beam radiation therapy. Most cases have a favourable outcome, but recurrence and malignant transformation with time can rarely occur {231,350}.

Soft tissue tumours of the conjunctiva and caruncle

Leiomyosarcoma

Vemuganti G.
Bermúdez Magner A.

Definition
Leiomyosarcoma is a sarcoma with smooth muscle differentiation.

ICD-O code

Leiomyosarcoma	8890/3

Epidemiology
There are < 10 cases reported in the literature as conjunctival leiomyosarcomas; most occurred in the seventh decade of life {435,792,820,838,1366}.

Localization
Leiomyosarcoma occurs in the conjunctival stroma.

Clinical features
Patients present with an elevated, fleshy, pale, vascularized conjunctival mass that may extend into the cornea.

Histopathology
The elongated spindle-shaped tumour cells are arranged in fascicles and sheets. The cells have indistinct borders; moderate amounts of eosinophilic cytoplasm; and elongated, oval, centrally located, blunt-ended and cigar-shaped nuclei with coarse chromatin and prominent nucleoli. Leiomyosarcoma may exhibit variable nuclear pleomorphism, tumour giant cells, and mitotic figures with a fibrotic stroma. The tumour cells are immunoreactive for SMA and vimentin, and the reported cases have been negative for cytokeratins, desmin, MYOD1, myogenin, S100 protein, and CD34 {820,838}. Ultrastructurally, they show irregular grooved nuclei with prominent nucleoli, numerous well-oriented myofilaments and dense bodies, immature cell junctions, and discontinuous basal laminar material along the cell surface {435}.

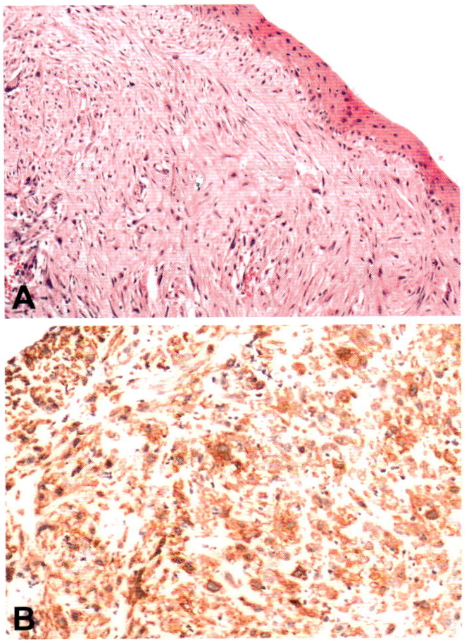

Fig. 1.40 Leiomyosarcoma of the conjunctiva. **A** Stratified squamous epithelium of the conjunctiva and spindle and ovoid tumour cells are arranged in narrow cords with hyalinized stroma below; these cells show vesicular nuclei with nucleoli and a rim of fibrillary cytoplasm. **B** The spindle cells exhibit strong cytoplasmic positivity for SMA.

Differential diagnosis
The differential diagnosis includes myofibrosarcoma and fibrosarcoma.

Histogenesis
Leiomyosarcoma originates from vascular smooth muscle or primitive mesenchymal cells of soft tissue.

Genetic susceptibility
Leiomyosarcoma is associated with Gardner syndrome, neurofibromatosis, and hereditary syndromes associated with genomic instability (e.g. Li–Fraumeni syndrome and Werner syndrome) {416,1293A}.

Prognosis and predictive factors
Complete resection by exenteration is associated with a favourable life prognosis. The 1-year survival in case reports is 80%. Soft tissue sarcomas in the conjunctiva tend to be < 5 cm in largest dimension; according to the TNM classification system, they are T1a if superficial and T1b if deep {132}. Recurrent lesions may warrant radiotherapy and chemotherapy {838,1247}.

Rhabdomyosarcoma of the conjunctiva and caruncle

Saornil M.A.
van der Valk P.
Bermúdez Magner A.

Definition
Rhabdomyosarcoma of the conjunctiva and caruncle is a malignant mesenchymal tumour with skeletal muscle differentiation.

ICD-O codes

Rhabdomyosarcoma NOS	8900/3
Embryonal rhabdomyosarcoma	8910/3
Spindle cell rhabdomyosarcoma	8912/3
Botryoid rhabdomyosarcoma	8910/3
Anaplastic rhabdomyosarcoma	8910/3
Alveolar rhabdomyosarcoma	8920/3
Pleomorphic rhabdomyosarcoma	8901/3

Synonyms
Rhabdosarcoma; myosarcoma; malignant rhabdomyoma

Epidemiology
Primary conjunctival rhabdomyosarcoma is rare, with few case reports in the literature; it accounts for 12% of ocular rhabdomyosarcomas {1114}. The embryonal type is most frequently seen in the first decade of life, accounting for > 90% of published cases of conjunctival origin. Alveolar rhabdomyosarcoma is observed in adolescents and young adults. Pleomorphic rhabdomyosarcoma occurs almost exclusively in adults, and no cases of conjunctival origin have been described.

Localization
The most common location is the bulbar and forniceal conjunctiva, but the tumour

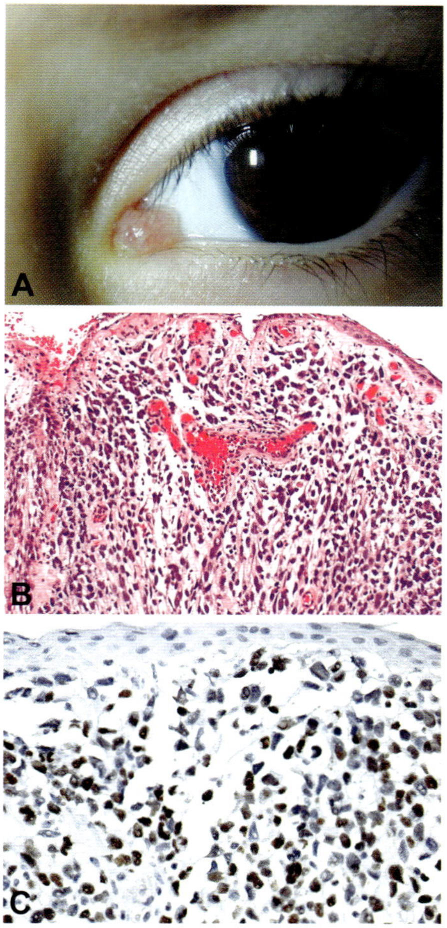

Fig. 1.41 Embryonal rhabdomyosarcoma (botryoid type). **A** An example in the caruncle of a 4-year-old boy with a 1-month history of a fast-growing papillomatous lesion in the left eye. **B** A polypoid lesion with intact conjunctival epithelium and subepithelial proliferation of loosely cohesive spindle cells with small hyperchromatic nuclei; the cells tend to condense into a dense layer (a so-called cambium layer) beneath the epithelium. **C** The nuclei stain positively for MYOD1.

may also occur in the plica semilunaris and the caruncle.

Clinical features

The characteristic presentation is a rapidly growing fleshy pink or reddish mass or papillomatous conjunctival lesion.

Histopathology

Almost all reported conjunctival cases are embryonal {1114}. The tumour cells, which appear in the substantia propria beneath the epithelium, are loosely spindle-shaped cells with hyperchromatic nuclei with indistinct tapered cytoplasmic processes, some with long ribbons of eosinophilic cytoplasm (tadpole cells), with variable degrees of pleomorphism and proliferative rates. The botryoid type contains linear condensations of tumour cells underneath the epithelial layer (a so-called cambium layer) and polypoid nodules with abundant, loose, myxoid stroma; this type originates just beneath a mucous membrane, with a predominance of spindle cells or with striking anaplasia. Alveolar rhabdomyosarcoma is a small round blue cell neoplasm, with a worse prognosis. The term "alveolar" refers to a growth pattern in nests with central discohesion, separated by fibrovascular septa. The pleomorphic variant has not been described in the periocular region {368,942}.

The presence of specific immunohistochemical markers for muscle correlates with the degree of tumour cell differentiation. Desmin and actin are expressed by developing rhabdomyoblasts. Myoglobin, myosin, and creatine kinase correspond to terminal differentiation. Immunostaining for MYOD1 and myogenin (MYF4) is sensitive and specific for rhabdomyosarcoma {942,1319}.

Differential diagnosis

In young patients, the differential diagnosis includes other rapidly growing reddish conjunctival tumours, as well as other small round blue cell and spindle cell tumours, including pyogenic granuloma, lymphangioma, lymphoma, myeloid sarcoma, leukaemia, metastatic neuroblastoma, and Langerhans cell histiocytosis.

Histogenesis

Rhabdomyosarcoma arises from undifferentiated pluripotent mesenchymal cells with a predilection to differentiate into skeletal muscle cells. Rhabdomyoblasts are diagnostic.

Genetic profile

Embryonal rhabdomyosarcoma is characterized by loss of heterozygosity on the short arm of chromosome 11 (11p15.5), suggesting inactivation of a tumour suppressor gene. In contrast, the majority of alveolar rhabdomyosarcomas have the reciprocal chromosomal translocation t(2;13)(q35;q14) or t(1;13)(p36;q14). The translocation t(2;13)(q35;q14), found in about 70% of cases, results in a chimeric fusion gene involving *PAX3* on chromosome 2 and a member of the forkhead box family (*FOXO1*) on chromosome 13 {313,389}.

Prognosis and predictive factors

Rhabdomyosarcoma is one of the few life-threatening conditions that the ophthalmologist is typically first to face; recognition resulting in prompt investigation and treatment may be lifesaving {952}. Poor prognostic factors in adults include advanced age, pleomorphic histological subtype, and more-advanced disease at presentation {1227}. The embryonal type has a better prognosis. Of the published cases of primary conjunctival rhabdomyosarcoma, only one case presented with metastasis.

Kaposi sarcoma of the conjunctiva and caruncle

Bermúdez Magner A.
Grossniklaus H.E.
van der Valk P.

Definition

Kaposi sarcoma of the conjunctiva and caruncle is an HHV8-associated vascular proliferation. Whether it qualifies as a true sarcoma is still a matter of debate {301}. In immunocompromised individuals, HHV8 infection induces vascular proliferation characterized by disorganized endothelial cell growth, resulting in the formation of erythrocyte-containing clefts, organized neovascularization, and an associated inflammatory infiltrate {182}.

ICD-O code

Kaposi sarcoma	9140/3

Epidemiology

There are four clinical forms of Kaposi sarcoma {1358}.

Classic Kaposi sarcoma occurs predominantly in elderly men of Mediterranean and eastern European descent. It is indolent and slowly progressive, and it tends to involve the distal extremities, in particular the legs and feet.

African (endemic) Kaposi sarcoma occurs predominantly in HIV-negative children and middle-aged adults in equatorial Africa. A rapidly fatal lymphadenopathic form can occur in children.

Iatrogenic Kaposi sarcoma occurs in solid organ transplant recipients and patients who are on immunosuppressive regimens for other diseases.

AIDS-associated Kaposi sarcoma is an aggressive form with frequent extracutaneous involvement. It occurs especially frequently in men who have sex with men.

The majority of periocular and ocular Kaposi sarcoma cases are iatrogenic or AIDS-associated, but conjunctival Kaposi sarcoma is also rarely reported in immunocompetent patients {799}.

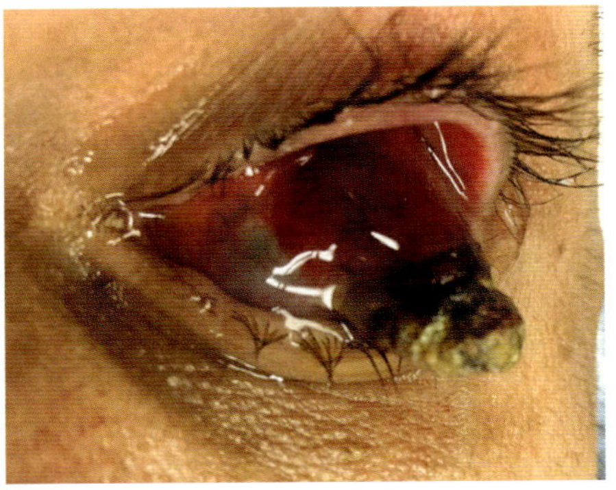

Fig. 1.42 Kaposi sarcoma of the conjunctiva. The tumour is a red mass with surface necrosis.

Etiology

The causative agent in all clinical forms is HHV8 infection of endothelial cells {462,1323}. The exact mode of transformation of the infected cells is unknown.

Localization

Ocular Kaposi sarcoma is uncommon {889}, but during the early period of the AIDS epidemic, it was reported that 20% of patients had periocular lesions {1174}. In the ocular region, the most commonly affected site is the skin of the eyelids, but the conjunctival surfaces may also be involved. Orbital and intraocular (e.g. choroidal) localizations have been reported but are very rare; they are mostly seen in the setting of widely disseminated Kaposi sarcoma {889}.

Clinical features

The predominant feature in ocular Kaposi sarcoma is skin lesions, which can appear as red macules in the beginning of the disease; as purple, bluish, or dark-brown patches or plaques; or as violaceous nodules, which can ulcerate when the disease is more established {799,970,1249,1358}. The medical history is very important, and biopsy is usually also necessary. Intraocular signs and symptoms are rare. The orbital signs are those of a mass lesion in the orbit (e.g. proptosis and double vision).

Histopathology

The morphology of Kaposi sarcoma is variable {470,945,1358}. Very early lesions are diagnostically treacherous, because the changes are very subtle. There is often a vascular proliferation around vessels and adnexae, as well as small bundles of spindle cells, but these features are easily overlooked. Immunohistochemistry is very helpful in such cases, but a high index of suspicion is very important. In later stages, the lesion is easily recognized. It is a predominantly spindle cell neoplasm, often with extravasated erythrocytes between the spindle cells and with hyaline globules. The tumour cells are only mildly atypical, but mitotic figures can usually be found. This spindle cell morphology is also seen in other sites, and makes diagnosis fairly easy. Because this is an endothelial neoplasm, markers for endothelial differentiation (i.e. CD31, CD34, and ERG) can be used {470}. Positivity for these markers in combination with morphology is diagnostic, but demonstration of HHV8 infection using an antibody {462} to latency-associated nuclear antigen (LANA) is highly specific and distinguishes Kaposi sarcoma from other vascular neoplasms.

Differential diagnosis

The differential diagnosis includes other spindle cell neoplasms, in particular angiosarcoma.

Histogenesis

This tumour derives from transformed vascular endothelial cells.

Genetic profile

A variety of genetic abnormalities have been reported in a small numbers of cases, but a consistent genetic landscape has yet to emerge. Genes from the FGF family are attractive potential targets. Molecular studies do not play a role in diagnosis.

Genetic susceptibility

The genetic susceptibility is unknown.

Prognosis and predictive factors

With the rise of antiretroviral therapy, Kaposi sarcoma is on the decline and is becoming more difficult to predict. Because most ocular cases are AIDS-associated, the prognosis is predominantly

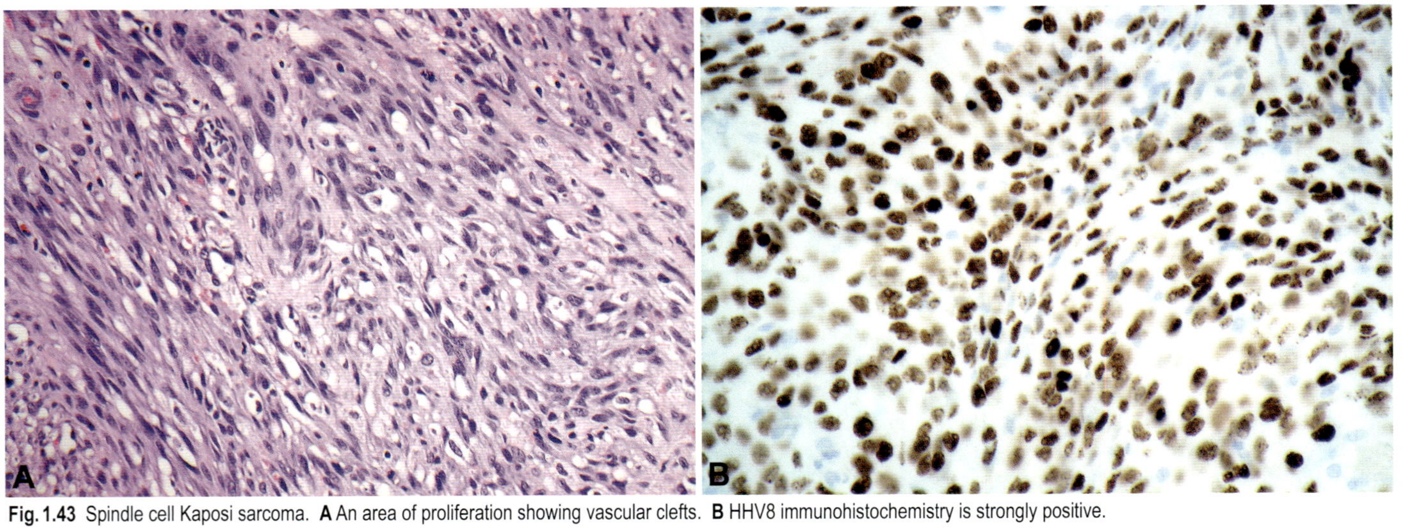

Fig. 1.43 Spindle cell Kaposi sarcoma. **A** An area of proliferation showing vascular clefts. **B** HHV8 immunohistochemistry is strongly positive.

dependent on swift treatment. Not surprisingly, wide dissemination at diagnosis is a prognostically unfavourable sign.

Angiosarcoma of the conjunctiva and caruncle

Bermúdez Magner A.
Grossniklaus H.E.
van der Valk P.

Definition
Angiosarcoma of the conjunctiva and caruncle is a highly malignant neoplasm with endothelial differentiation.

ICD-O code
Angiosarcoma 9120/3

Synonyms
Lymphangiosarcoma; haemangiosarcoma; malignant (haemangio)endothelioma

Epidemiology
Angiosarcoma is a rare tumour with unknown incidence in the conjunctiva. In the periocular region, it is mostly found in the skin and more rarely in the orbit, where it accounts for no more than 3% of all periocular angiosarcomas {1319}.

Localization
At this anatomical site, angiosarcoma arises in the conjunctiva.

Clinical features
Patients present with a poorly defined reddish or bluish plaque, somewhat resembling a bruise {470,1377}. The tumour usually extends far beyond the visible lesion, which makes complete excision very difficult; identifying the edge can be virtually impossible. Local recurrence is therefore extremely common. Metastasis is also common and can occur late in the course of the disease {267,1358}.

Histopathology
The cutaneous form of angiosarcoma is usually a recognizable vascular lesion in which the vessels are lined by cytologically atypical endothelium. The degree of atypia varies. However, some degree of nuclear enlargement and either hyperchromasia or hypochromasia are always present. Nucleoli are sometimes also present, in particular in the epithelioid variant. The tumour infiltrates between pre-existing collagen fibres; because of the varying atypia, its recognition in resection margins can be difficult {470,605,1358,1377}. Given this fact and the unpredictable pattern of spread, resection is often non-radical, and recurrence is frequent. In the epithelioid variant, plump tumour cells fill the vascular spaces, creating an epithelial appearance {1358}. Mitotic figures are often found.

Orbital tumours can be less differentiated, with a more spindle cell morphology. The formation of vessels is less pronounced than in cutaneous lesions. Features suggesting the endothelial origin of such tumours are the presence of erythrocytes between tumour cells and the formation of intracellular lumina, sometimes containing an erythrocyte {1177,1358}.

The tumour expresses markers of endothelial differentiation, such as CD31, CD34, ERG, and factor VIII–related antigen, but any of these can also be negative, so it is prudent not to rely on any single marker. HHV8 is usually negative {267,470,890,1358}.

Ultrastructurally, the endothelial tumour cells are characterized by the presence of Weibel–Palade bodies {1358}. However, the use of electron microscopy in the diagnosis of angiosarcoma has been almost completely superseded by the use of immunohistochemistry.

Differential diagnosis
Distinguishing the cutaneous form from non-neoplastic vessels is problematic. For the orbital form, the differential diagnosis includes other sarcomas and spindle cell tumours.

Genetic profile
Angiosarcoma shows no characteristic molecular abnormalities. Many cases show complex cytogenetic aberrations, involving a variety of loci, but a diagnostically useful marker has not yet been identified {470}.

Prognosis and predictive factors
Angiosarcomas are high-grade sarcomas with a poor prognosis. The growth rate is variable, but recurrence and metastasis are common. Surgery, despite its limitations, is the mainstay of therapy, and additional therapeutic modalities are sometimes used with some success {256,1358}.

Fibrous histiocytoma of the conjunctiva and caruncle

Alkatan H.
Loeffler K.U.
Grossniklaus H.E.
Lazar A.J.

Definition
Fibrous histiocytoma of the conjunctiva and caruncle is a benign mesenchymal tumour that consists of spindled to polymorphic cells of uncertain derivation, with various proportions of fibroblastic, myofibroblastic, and histiocytic differentiation {55,1007}.

ICD-O code
Benign fibrous histiocytoma 8830/0

Synonym
Fibrous histiocytoma involving the skin is called dermatofibroma.

Epidemiology
The age of onset ranges from infancy to the eighth decade of life (mean age: 37 years), and there is no sex predilection {603}. Fibrous histiocytoma is rare, accounting for only 0.2% of all conjunctival tumours {1080}.

Localization
At this anatomical site, fibrous histiocytoma occurs in the bulbar conjunctiva {577,603}.

Clinical features
Patients present with an acquired, painless, tan-coloured, dome-shaped mass, often of recent onset. Unlike amelanotic melanoma, fibrous histiocytoma lacks a feeder vessel at the base, but it sometimes has visible vascularization over the surface {55,603,633}. The mass can be yellowish in colour because of the presence of admixed foamy macrophages {489}.

Histopathology
The lesions are composed of spindled to polymorphous cells and often show a conspicuous storiform to vaguely spindled architecture and variably prominent collagenous or fibrous background {529,633}. Immunohistochemically, there are no specific markers for fibrous histiocytoma {1210}. The tumour cells usually show strong positivity for vimentin

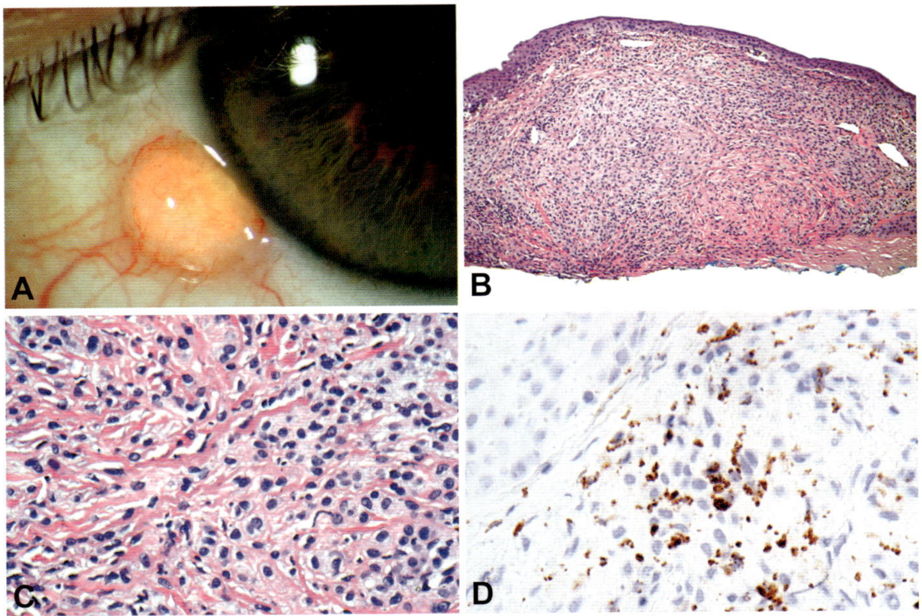

Fig. 1.44 Fibrous histiocytoma of the limbal conjunctiva. A nodular tumour (**A**) with expansion of the stroma (**B**) by plump spindle cells (**C**), which are immunoreactive for factor XIII (**D**).

and often for CD68; positivity has also been reported for α_1-antitrypsin, factor XIIIa, and CD163 {113,165,529,1205}. Ultrastructural studies may reveal prominent rough endoplasmic reticulum with granular material and lipid vacuoles {515,904}.

Differential diagnosis

Nodular episcleritis, juvenile xanthogranuloma, spindle cell carcinoma, and solitary fibrous tumour can be ruled out by a lack of immunohistochemical expression of HMB45 antigen, S100 protein, diffuse CD34 or STAT6, and cytokeratins {113,165,904}. Atypical fibroxanthoma is uncommon at this site, but has been reported in association with xeroderma pigmentosum {529,1067}.

Histogenesis

The cell of origin is unknown, but it is likely to be mesenchymal {679}.

Genetic profile

Gene fusions between protein kinase C isoforms (e.g. *PRKCB* and *PRKCD*) and a variety of partner genes (including *PDPN*, *CD63*, and *LAMTOR1*) have been seen in various types of cutaneous benign fibrous histiocytoma {887,916,1348}, although no such fusions have been documented in conjunctival lesions.

Prognosis and predictive factors

Complete excision is usually curative, with no recurrence {529,577,603,1205}. The tumour previously termed malignant fibrous histiocytoma (now designated undifferentiated pleomorphic sarcoma) has no histogenic connection to benign fibrous histiocytoma. Conjunctival sarcoma is exceedingly rare {1080}.

Conjunctival stromal tumour

Herwig-Carl M.C.
Grossniklaus H.E.
Auw-Haedrich C.

Definition

Conjunctival stromal tumour is a benign stromal tumour of the bulbar conjunctiva, composed of myxoid/collagenous stroma, spindle-shaped cells with pseudonuclear inclusions, and multinuclear cells.

ICD-O code

None

Epidemiology

The few described cases of conjunctival stromal tumour (7 published and 1 unpublished) have occurred in middle-aged White men (median age: 47 years) {483,1295}.

Etiology

The etiology is unknown, but conjunctival stromal tumour appears to be reactive in nature.

Localization

The typical location is the bulbar conjunctiva. Involvement of the cornea is possible in lesions adjacent to the limbus.

Clinical features

The tumours are whitish, yellowish, or reddish in colour and typically soft. A cystoid or gelatinous appearance has been described. Patients may report a foreign body sensation and mild ocular injection.

Histopathology

Conjunctival stromal tumour is a stromal lesion composed of varying proportions of myxoid and collagenous fibrovascular tissues infiltrated by loosely arranged spindle-shaped cells. Some cells exhibit pseudonuclear inclusions or are multinucleated, occasionally in a floret-like configuration. There are typically no mitotic figures. Scattered aggregates of lymphocytes and histiocytes may be present. Immunohistochemical staining for CD34 and vimentin is typically positive. The stroma may stain positively with Alcian blue/colloidal iron.

Differential diagnosis

The clinical differential diagnosis includes benign and malignant lesions of the conjunctival stroma. The histological differential diagnosis includes conjunctival myxoma, giant cell angiofibroma, and rhabdomyosarcoma. Myxoma (the

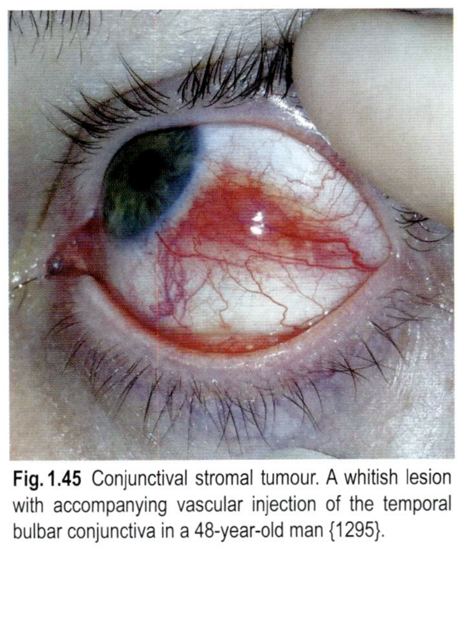

Fig. 1.45 Conjunctival stromal tumour. A whitish lesion with accompanying vascular injection of the temporal bulbar conjunctiva in a 48-year-old man {1295}.

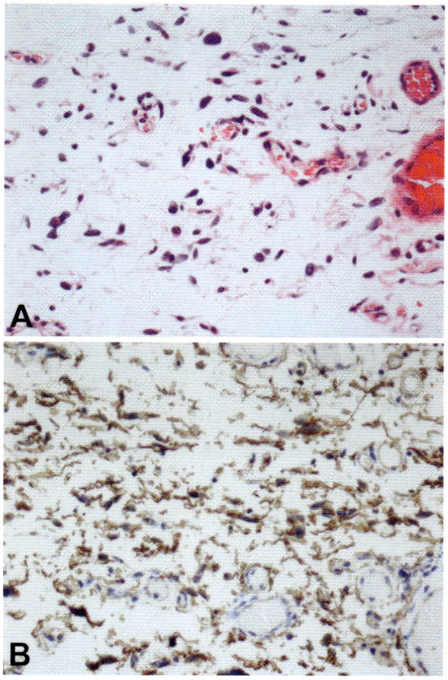

Fig. 1.46 Conjunctival stromal tumour. **A** There are loosely arranged spindle-shaped cells with pseudonuclear inclusions in the stroma. **B** CD34 is positive in the cells and the stroma.

most common differential diagnosis) can be excluded by the presence of CD34-positive stromal cells.

Histogenesis
Conjunctival stromal tumour is of mesenchymal derivation.

Prognosis and predictive factors
There are no reported cases of malignant change or metastasis. Recurrence was described in one case after incomplete excision in an 11-year-old boy {1295}.

Myxoma of the conjunctiva and caruncle

Laver N.
Alkatan H.
Loeffler K.U.

Definition
Myxoma of the conjunctiva and caruncle is a benign lesion composed mostly of myxoid material, showing sparse cellularity and variable vascularization.

ICD-O code
Myxoma 8840/0

Epidemiology
The incidence is about 2 cases per 1 million person-years, with no sex predilection {1386}.

Etiology
Myxoma can occur as an isolated process or can be a presenting component of Carney complex type 1 (MIM number: 160980), an autosomal dominant disease characterized by myxomas, skin pigmentation, and endocrine overactivity {162}. The precise origin is unknown.

Localization
Myxoma commonly occurs in the temporal bulbar conjunctiva, and it may involve the caruncle and the limbus of the cornea {428,681}.

Clinical features
Patients present with a soft, freely movable, pinkish-white lesion that may resemble a cyst; myxoma is usually unilateral {902}.

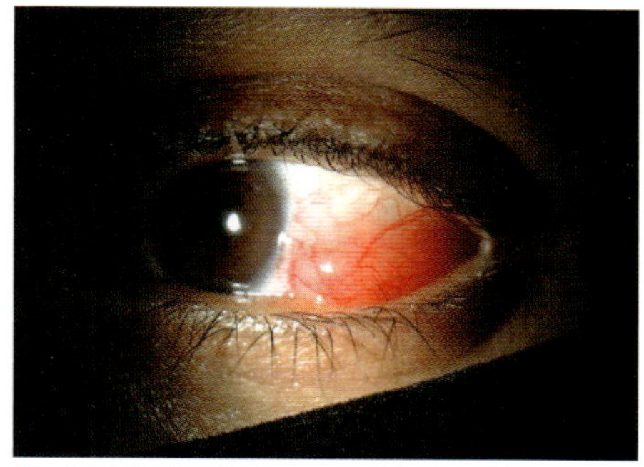

Fig. 1.47 Conjunctival myxoma. A lesion of the temporal bulbar conjunctiva, present for 3 years.

Histopathology
Myxoma is a paucicellular lesion composed of sparse stellate and spindle-shaped mesenchymal cells interspersed in a myxoid stroma. Macrophages, lymphocytes, and mast cells can rarely be

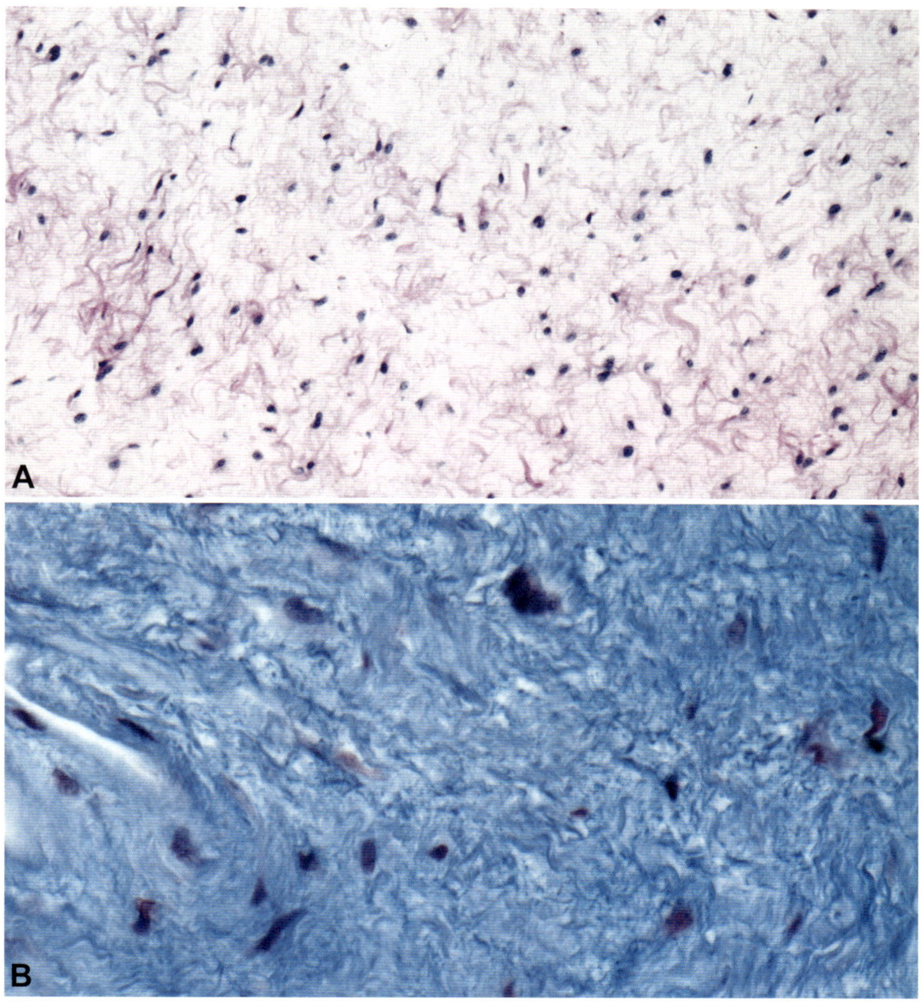

Fig. 1.48 Conjunctival myxoma. **A** There are a few stellate and spindle-shaped cells in a loose, myxoid stroma. **B** Alcian blue staining of the myxoid stroma.

found. Cytoplasmic vacuoles, focal mild pleomorphism, and pseudonuclear inclusions might be present; mitoses are absent. Alcian blue stains the myxoid material between the cells; it can be dissolved with hyaluronidase, demonstrating the mucopolysaccharide nature of the material {482,1070}. Mucicarmine and colloidal iron also stain the cells, and myxomas are immunoreactive for vimentin and SMA (focally) {1070,1386}. The Ki-67 proliferation index is < 1%.

Differential diagnosis

Other lesions with myxoid stroma include fibromyxoma, lipomyxoma, myxomatous degeneration of tissue, conjunctival stromal tumour {483}, spindle cell lipoma, amelanotic naevus, myxoid neurofibroma, myxoid liposarcoma, rhabdomyosarcoma, myxoid solitary fibrous tumour, and nodular fasciitis. Myxomas lack substantial cellularity; mitotic figures and cellular pleomorphism are helpful in distinguishing myxoma from other soft tissue tumours.

Genetic profile

Inactivation of the gene *PRKAR1A* (at 17q24.2) is found in myxomas associated with Carney complex {493}.

Prognosis and predictive factors

If the lesion is removed by complete surgical excision {14}, recurrence is uncommon. Conjunctival myxoma in a younger patient should prompt evaluation to rule out Carney complex {270,428}.

Haemangioma of the conjunctiva and caruncle

Alkatan H.
Harocopos G.

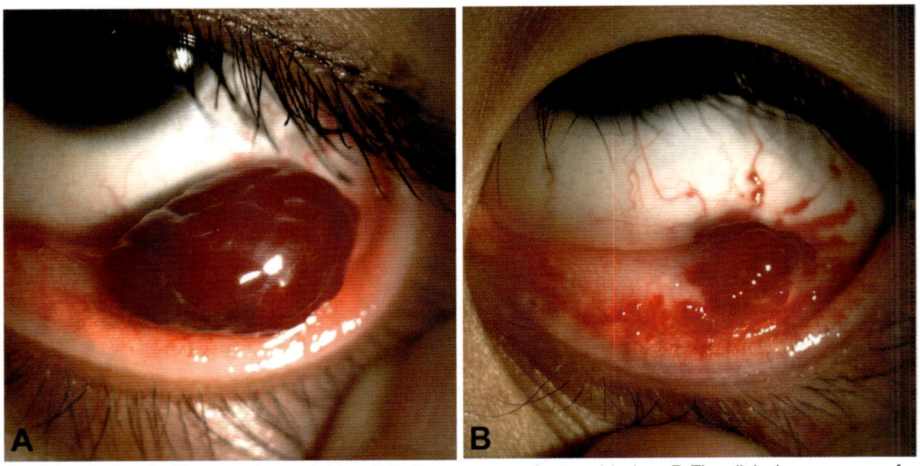

Fig. 1.49 Conjunctival haemangioma. **A** The clinical appearance of a tarsal lesion. **B** The clinical appearance of a lesion deep in the fornix.

Definition

Haemangioma of the conjunctiva and caruncle is a benign neoplasm/hamartoma of vascular phenotype.

ICD-O code

Haemangioma 9120/0

Synonyms

Racemose haemangioma: arteriovenous malformation; arteriovenous communication

Epidemiology

In a series of 140 vascular lesions of the conjunctiva (including lymphangioma, pyogenic granuloma, varix, glomus tumour, and Kaposi sarcoma), capillary haemangiomas accounted for 14% of the lesions, acquired sessile haemangiomas for 7%, racemose haemangiomas for 5%, and cavernous haemangiomas for 2% {1143}. Except for infantile capillary haemangioma, these vascular tumours typically occur in adults (median age: 41 years) {1143}. De novo acquired capillary haemangioma has been reported in older children and adults {346,406}. Haemangiomas are generally sporadic, but capillary haemangiomas can occasionally be familial, with an autosomal dominant pattern of inheritance (MIM number: 602089) {111,601}.

Etiology

Haemangiomas are typically regarded as congenital, hamartomatous lesions. Cell-autonomous defects and a developmental origin underlying haemangiogenesis in these lesions have been described, as have etiologies related to growth factors, hormones, and stromal cells {94,751}.

Localization

These lesions are typically unilateral. In the series of 140 vascular lesions of the conjunctiva mentioned above, the following conjunctival locations were reported: bulbar (extralimbal in 57% of cases and limbal in 14%), tarsal (in 17%), forniceal (in 17%), and (least commonly) caruncular {1143}.

Clinical features

Haemangiomas are generally solitary lesions, although multiple close lesions may occur in capillary haemangioma {95}. Capillary haemangiomas generally present in infancy {1143}, but de novo presentation or growth is rarely reported in older children and young adults {346,406}. Other types of haemangiomas may present at any age. Capillary haemangioma is circumscribed or diffuse, flat or elevated, and pinkish in colour {489,1143}. Cavernous haemangioma is multiloculated, reddish-blue, and located deep in the stroma {489,1143}. Clinically, racemose haemangioma has been described as showing an afferent deeper blood vessel forming a loop, then continuing as a more superficial efferent vessel. It may be associated with Wyburn–Mason syndrome {489,1143}. Acquired sessile haemangioma is a rarely reported conjunctival vascular tumour {1141,1143} that appears as a flat lesion of tortuous intertwining blood vessels without systemic association {734,1141}.

Histopathology

Capillary haemangioma consists of capillaries with numerous intervening proliferating endothelial cells {1143}. Cavernous haemangioma is composed of dilated, blood-filled venous spaces separated by fibroconnective tissue septa of varying thickness {1141}. Racemose haemangioma consists of loops of dilated communicating arteries and veins that have an irregular muscular layer and thin walls, and that do not pass through a bed of capillaries {489,540,1143}. Sessile haemangioma consists of multiple layers of

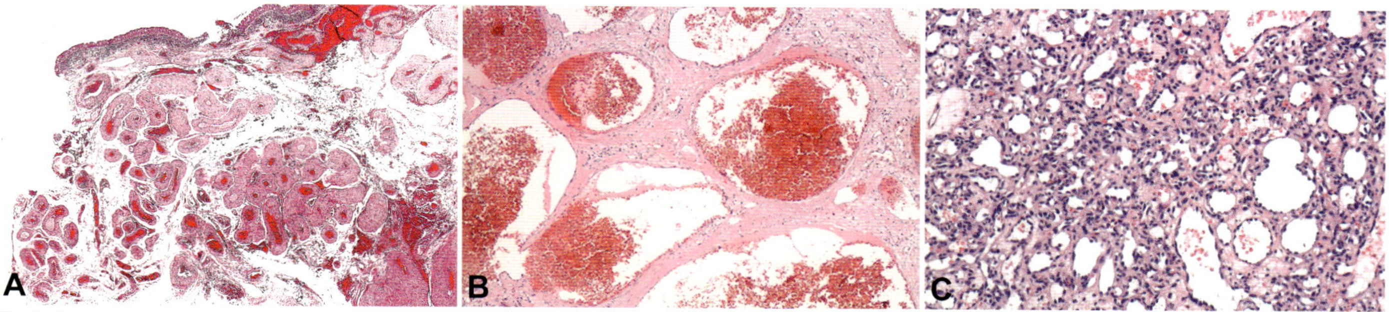

Fig. 1.50 Haemangioma. **A** Sessile haemangioma with congested dilated blood vessels in layers. **B** Cavernous haemangioma of the conjunctiva showing large, endothelial-lined, blood-filled vascular spaces with intervening septations. **C** Capillary haemangioma of the conjunctiva showing numerous capillary-like blood vessels with proliferating endothelial cells.

congested, dilated blood vessels that are histologically unremarkable {1141}. In all haemangiomas, the positive immunohistochemical staining of endothelial cells for CD31 and CD34 indicates vascular origin {540}.

Differential diagnosis

The differential diagnosis includes Kaposi sarcoma, pyogenic granuloma (also known as lobular capillary haemangioma), haemorrhagic lymphangioma, varix, and glomus tumour {489}.

Histogenesis

The endothelial cells composing capillary haemangioma have been found to be clonal in origin, suggesting development from a common precursor cell {126}. The angiogenesis inhibitor endostatin, which inhibits migration of normal endothelial cells, has been shown to stimulate migration of capillary haemangioma endothelial cells {126}. In mice, the release of stromal cell factors, which results in an angiogenic response, was blocked by neutralizing anti-VEGF IgG {94}.

Genetic profile

Loss of heterozygosity of chromosome 5q, initially described in familial cases of capillary haemangioma, has also been found in sporadic cases, with *FGFR4*, *PDGFRB*, and *FLT4* (*VEGFR3*) identified as possible candidate genes. This finding suggests that most cases (i.e. sporadic cases) of capillary haemangioma may result from somatic mutation events {95,1345}. Somatic mutation in the *KDR* (*VEGFR2*, *FLK1*) gene on chromosome 4 has also been reported in capillary haemangioma; therefore, it has been proposed that all of these mutations may result in alteration of the VEGF signalling pathway in endothelial and/or pericytic cells {1346}.

Genetic susceptibility

Hereditary mutations in chromosomes 2p (*ANTXR1*), 4q (*KDR*), and 5q may result in an autosomal dominant predisposition to developing capillary haemangioma, but the vast majority of cases of capillary haemangioma are sporadic, associated with somatic mutations in these lesions {95,1345}.

Prognosis and predictive factors

Capillary haemangioma is benign, showing an early rapid proliferation phase within the first year of life followed by slow spontaneous regression (the involution phase) by 4–7 years of age, but it can be treated earlier (e.g. with beta blockers) if it causes amblyopia or strabismus {180,751}. The other types of haemangiomas are also benign; they can be observed or surgically excised for cosmetic reasons or if symptomatic {489,540}.

Lymphangioma of the conjunctiva and caruncle

Alkatan H.
Harocopos G.

Definition

Lymphangioma of the conjunctiva and caruncle is a hamartomatous mass of dilated lymphatic channels.

ICD-O code

Lymphangioma 9170/0

Synonyms

Lymphatic malformation; lymphatic venous malformation

Epidemiology

Isolated conjunctival lymphangioma is rare {1057}. In a series of 140 cases of conjunctival vascular lesions, lymphangiomas accounted for 20% of the cases {1143}.

Etiology

Lymphangioma is a vascular hamartoma of lymphatic or venolymphatic origin {551}. One case report suggested a possible association with tuberous sclerosis {378}.

Localization

Conjunctival lymphangioma is unilateral, and most often constitutes the superficial component of an orbital lymphangioma, but lymphangioma can occasionally be isolated to the conjunctiva {551,1057,1143}.

Clinical features

Patients present with a diffuse or circumscribed, soft, red, painless conjunctival lesion with focal or diffuse haemorrhage, which often enlarges during upper respiratory tract infections. Recurrent haemorrhage is common; over time, blood may become multiloculated, leading to the formation of a so-called chocolate cyst within the lesion {1057,1143}.

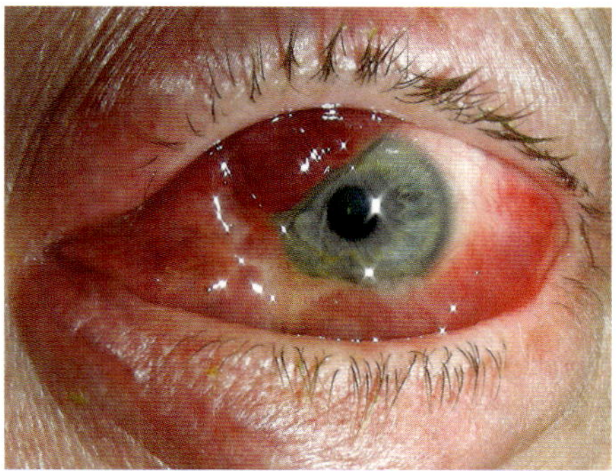

Fig. 1.51 Lymphangioma. The clinical appearance of an extensive conjunctival lymphangioma with bleeding.

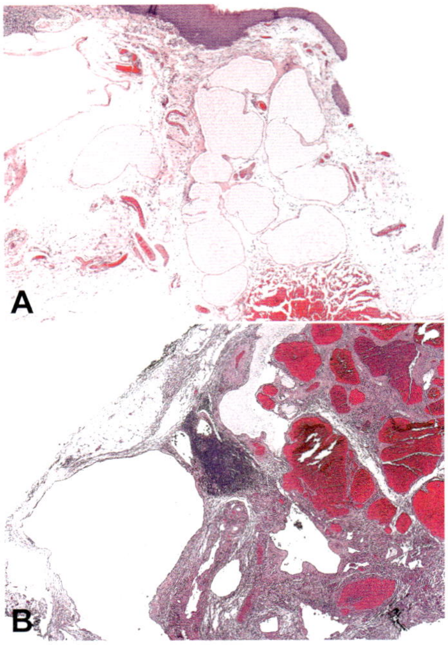

Fig. 1.52 Lymphangioma. **A** Endothelial-lined channels filled with lymph. **B** An example showing a combination of pure lymphatic channels and channels filled with blood in addition to an aggregate of lymphocytes.

Histopathology
An unencapsulated irregular mass of endothelial-lined channels of various sizes is separated by fibroconnective tissue septa that lack smooth muscle, unlike in cavernous haemangioma. The connective tissue may show aggregates of small mature lymphocytes, which often form lymphoid follicles. The channels may contain clear fluid, blood, or both, hence the alternative term "lymphatic venous malformation". Vascular endothelial cells in general are highlighted by CD31 staining {104,883,1190}. More-specific immunohistochemistry for lymphatic endothelium includes staining for podoplanin {240,241} and LYVE1 {104,241,876,919}; the D2-40 podoplanin antibody is often used {104,540,1190}.

Differential diagnosis
The differential diagnosis includes cavernous haemangioma, varix, cystic compound melanocytic naevus, and conjunctival lymphangiectasis (constituting dilation of existing lymphatic channels) {1151}.

Histogenesis
Lymphangiomas are regarded as hamartomatous in origin.

Genetic profile
The genetic profile of lymphangioma has not been confirmed. There has been one report of presumed conjunctival lymphangioma (diagnosed clinically) in a patient with tuberous sclerosis, which is associated with the *TSC1* gene (encoding hamartin) {378}.

Genetic susceptibility
These hamartomas are sporadic, with no known genetic susceptibility. It is unknown whether tuberous sclerosis (i.e. mutations in the TSC genes) may confer increased susceptibility.

Prognosis and predictive factors
Lymphangioma is a benign lesion with no reported tendency for malignancy. The clinical course is variable, ranging from spontaneous regression to gradual progression. Very rarely, conjunctival or orbital lymphangioma may be associated with systemic generalized lymphangiomatosis {335,1143}.

Neurofibroma of the conjunctiva and caruncle

Cummings T.
Stemmer-Rachamimov A.O.
Verdijk R.M.

Definition
Neurofibroma of the conjunctiva and caruncle is a benign peripheral nerve sheath tumour composed of Schwann cells, with intermixed perineurial cells, fibroblasts, mast cells, and axons in a variably myxoid to collagenous extracellular matrix.

ICD-O code
Neurofibroma 9540/0

Synonyms
Solitary conjunctival neurofibroma; plexiform conjunctival neurofibroma

Epidemiology
Solitary conjunctival neurofibromas are very rare. In one large series of 1643 conjunctival tumours, only one neurofibroma was found {1080}. Plexiform neurofibromas of the eyelid and orbit, which are typically associated with neurofibromatosis type 1 (MIM number: 162200), may extend to involve the conjunctiva {141}.

Etiology
Neurofibroma results from allelic loss and inactivation of the *NF1* gene region located on chromosome 17q {110}.

Localization
Neurofibroma occurs in the conjunctival stroma.

Clinical features
Neurofibromas of the conjunctiva may be of the solitary, diffuse, or plexiform type {570}.

Histopathology
Neurofibroma is characterized by a haphazard proliferation of Schwann cells and fibroblasts {570}. Mast cells are often present as well. Tactile-like structures (pseudo-Meissner corpuscles) may be seen. Degenerative nuclear atypia may occur. A gelatinous or myxomatous extracellular matrix is often present. Neurofibroma shows patchy, variable immunoreactivity for S100 protein. Axons permeate the lesion and are highlighted by immunohistochemical staining for NFP.

Differential diagnosis
The differential diagnosis includes traumatic neuroma, circumscribed solitary neuroma, schwannoma, low-grade malignant peripheral nerve sheath tumour, perineurioma, and myxoma {189}.

Histogenesis
Neurofibroma is composed of a mixture of endoneurial-derived fibroblastic cells, Schwann cells, and axons.

Genetic profile
Plexiform neurofibromas occur mainly in the context of neurofibromatosis type 1, in association with inactivation and allelic loss of both copies of the *NF1* gene on chromosome 17q {217}.

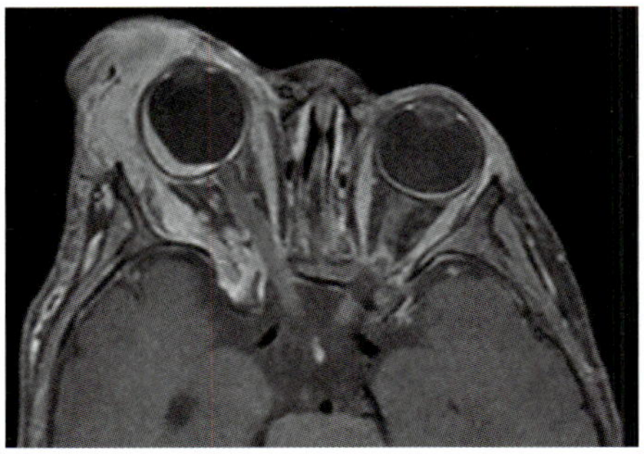

Fig. 1.53 Neurofibroma. T1-weighted MRI showing a plexiform tumour involving the orbit, eyelid, and conjunctiva.

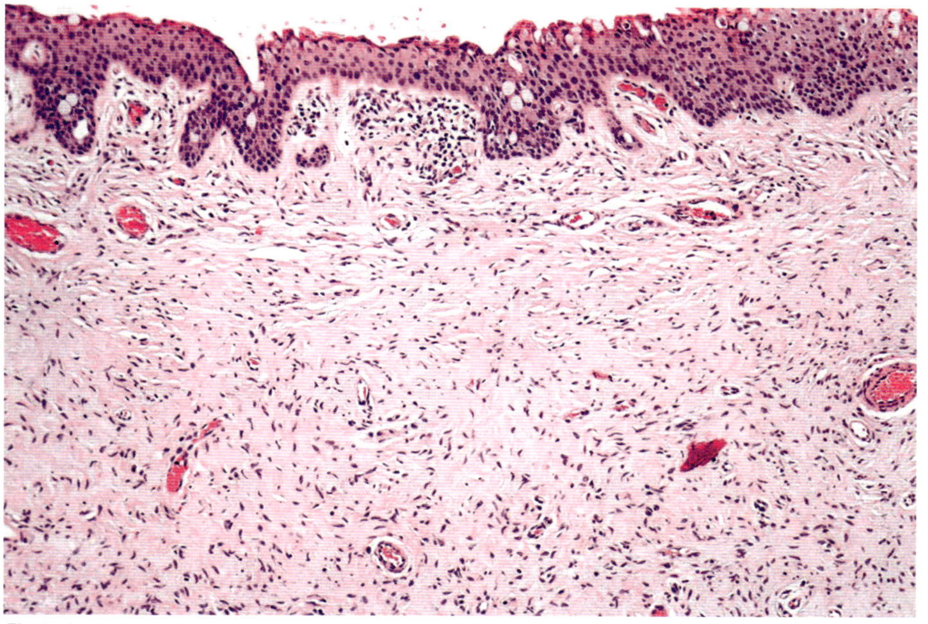

Fig. 1.54 Neurofibroma of the conjunctiva. Conjunctival epithelium with goblet cells is visible at the top of the field.

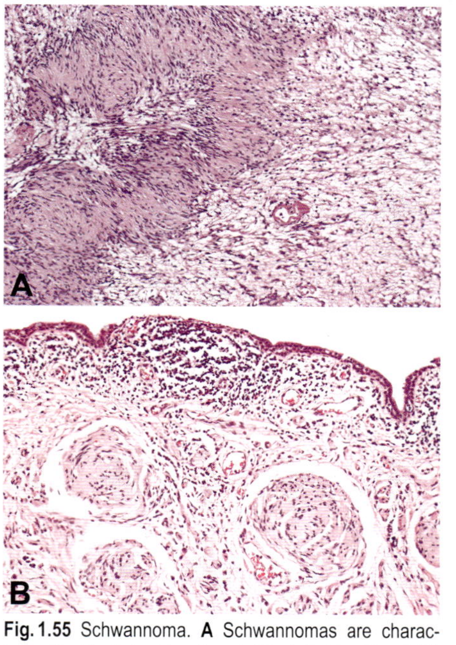

Fig. 1.55 Schwannoma. **A** Schwannomas are characterized by the Antoni A pattern (at the left side of the field) and the looser Antoni B pattern (at the right side of the field). **B** Conjunctiva with subepithelial schwannoma.

Genetic susceptibility
There is an association with neurofibromatosis type 1 {141}.

Prognosis and predictive factors
Solitary lesions can be excised. Plexiform lesions are difficult to remove, and scarring and recurrences may occur. Malignant transformation is rare.

Schwannoma of the conjunctiva and caruncle

Cummings T.
Biswas J.
Stemmer-Rachamimov A.O.
Verdijk R.M.

Definition
Schwannoma of the conjunctiva and caruncle is a benign peripheral nerve sheath tumour derived from Schwann cells.

ICD-O code
Schwannoma 9560/0

Synonym
Neurilemmoma

Epidemiology
Schwannomas isolated to the conjunctiva are rare. Orbital schwannomas may occur in 10% of patients with neurofibromatosis type 1 (MIM number: 162200).

Etiology
The etiology of sporadic conjunctival schwannoma is unknown.

Localization
Schwannomas are typically localized to the bulbar or tarsal conjunctival stroma {189,428}. The caruncle is rarely involved {972}.

Clinical features
Conjunctival schwannoma usually presents as a yellowish-pink elevated mass.

Histopathology
Schwannoma is characterized by a nodular (solitary), diffuse, or plexiform proliferation of Schwann cells with spindled and tapered nuclei. Two patterns of growth, known as the Antoni A and Antoni B patterns, are typically seen. The Antoni A areas show cells arranged in wavy, interlacing, or whorled bundles. The elongated nuclei may be arranged in palisades called Verocay bodies. Antoni B areas have a loose myxoid appearance with microcysts and foamy macrophages. Blood vessels are thickened, and haemosiderin pigment is often present. Nuclear atypia with hyperchromatic pleomorphic nuclei is observed in ancient schwannoma. Malignant change of schwannoma is exceptionally rare. Schwannomas are immunopositive for S100 protein. Perineurium positive for epithelial membrane antigen may be present. Rare histological variants include cellular, plexiform, microcystic, reticular, and melanotic schwannomas {189}.

Differential diagnosis
The differential diagnosis includes schwannomatous neurofibroma, cellular neurofibroma, and fibromatosis.

Histogenesis
Schwannomas are derived from Schwann cells.

Genetic profile
Schwannomas may exhibit complete or partial loss of chromosome 22, resulting in the loss of the protein merlin (also known as NF2 and schwannomin) {1215}.

Genetic susceptibility
Multiple schwannomas may be seen in neurofibromatosis type 2 and schwannomatosis {110}.

Prognosis and predictive factors
Surgical resection is often recommended. Recurrences are rare.

Juvenile xanthogranuloma of the conjunctiva and caruncle

Iacob C.E.
Alkatan H.
Bermúdez Magner A.

Definition
Juvenile xanthogranuloma of the conjunctiva and caruncle is a benign, self-healing proliferation of macrophages with a variable degree of lipidization, in the absence of a metabolic disorder. The adult form is better termed xanthogranuloma or adult-onset xanthogranuloma of the conjunctiva and caruncle.

ICD-O code
None

Synonyms
Xanthogranuloma; solitary xanthogranuloma; naevoxanthoendothelioma

Epidemiology
Juvenile xanthogranuloma and adult-onset xanthogranuloma are similar (if not identical) rare entities with a slight male predominance and a relatively wide age range (mean patient age: 36 years), but xanthogranuloma is more common in infancy and childhood. Limbal and conjunctival lesions are estimated to account for 13–18% of all juvenile xanthogranuloma lesions arising in the second decade of life {461,575}.

Localization
At this anatomical site, juvenile xanthogranuloma occurs at periocular preseptal locations in the eyelid and conjunctiva, including the caruncle and (most frequently) the limbus {644}.

Clinical features
Juvenile xanthogranuloma presents as dome-shaped soft yellow masses with smooth borders and a steady growth rate over several years. Concomitant skin lesions, ranging from small papules and nodules to larger tumours, can sometimes be found, typically in the upper parts of the body. Juvenile xanthogranuloma has been reported in association with neurofibromatosis and lymphoproliferative conditions. No systemic associations are typically seen with the adult-onset type {643}, although one case was reported in association with multiple endocrine neoplasia type 1 {27}.

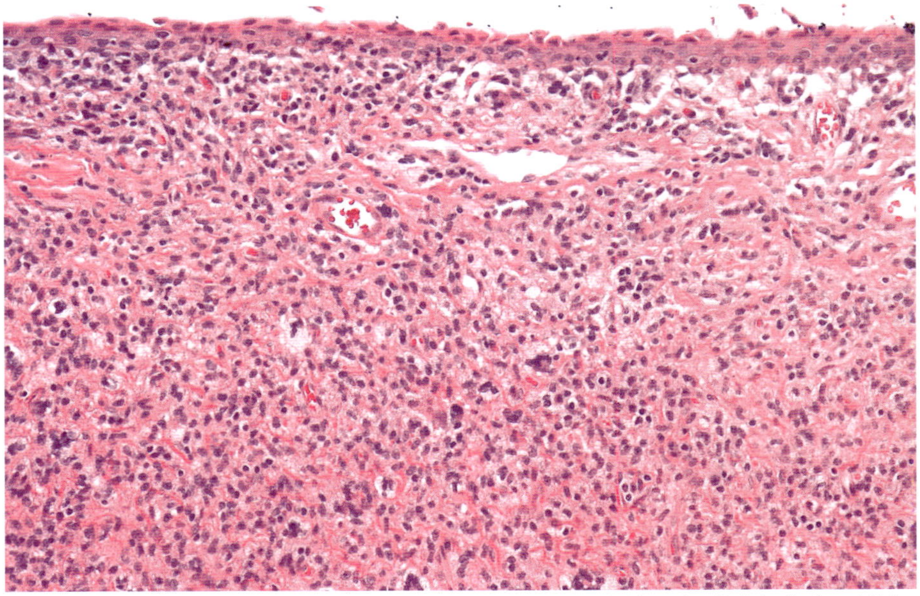

Fig. 1.56 Juvenile xanthogranuloma. Thin conjunctival epithelium with an underlying subepithelial collection of histiocytes and a few Touton-type multinucleated giant cells typical of this entity.

Histopathology
Xanthogranuloma shows well-delineated, unencapsulated nodules consistent with granulomatous chronic inflammation with macrophages in a lymphocyte-rich background, accompanied by few eosinophils, plasma cells, neutrophils, and mast cells. Macrophages vary in morphology from mononuclear small oval/spindle cells with eosinophilic cytoplasm in early lesions to progressively larger and lipid-laden cells resulting in frankly foamy macrophages in late lesions. Characteristic Touton-type giant histiocytes with peripheral foamy cytoplasm and a ring-like central distribution of nuclei are almost always present. Fibrosis increases with time. Histiocytes in these lesions stain positively with CD11c, CD68, CD163, HAM56, and lysozyme antibodies but are negative for CD1a and S100 protein {608,860}.

Differential diagnosis
The differential diagnosis includes Langerhans cell histiocytosis, lymphoproliferative processes, mesenchymal nodular lesions, systemic histiocytosis (Erdheim–Chester disease), and necrobiotic xanthogranuloma.

Genetic profile
Non-recurrent somatic mutations have been reported in 3 cases of cutaneous juvenile xanthogranuloma, including *PIK3CD* mutations (identified in multiple skin specimens in one case {28,172}), suggesting a pathogenetic role of ERK pathway activation {28}.

Genetic susceptibility
An association between juvenile xanthogranuloma, neurofibromatosis type 1 and type 2, and juvenile myelomonocytic leukaemia has been documented in approximately 20 cases {547}.

Prognosis and predictive factors
Complete surgical excision is usually curative.

Hamartomas and choristomas of the conjunctiva and carunce

Epibulbar choristoma

Herwig-Carl M.C.
Moulin A.
Verdijk R.M.

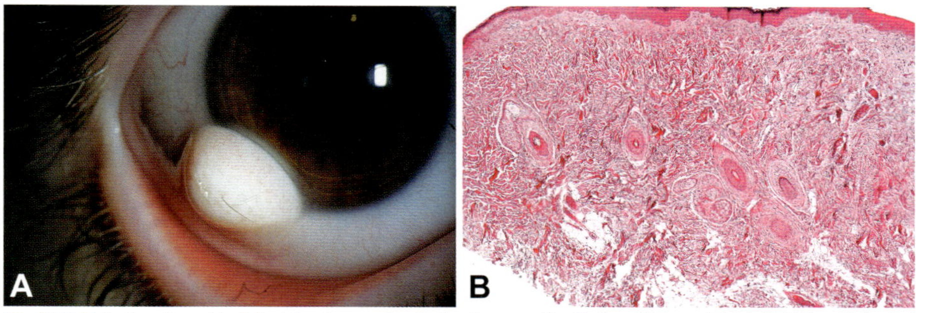

Fig. 1.57 Epibulbar dermoid. **A** An inferotemporal epibulbar tumour with cilia in a 12-year-old girl. **B** Histopathological analysis of the excised lesion shows a tumour covered by keratinized squamous epithelium; the tumour is composed of wiry collagen fibres; hair follicles with adjacent sebaceous glands are present.

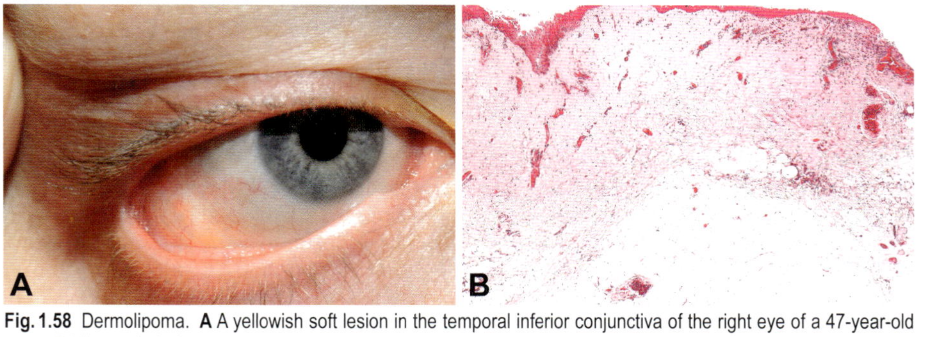

Fig. 1.58 Dermolipoma. **A** A yellowish soft lesion in the temporal inferior conjunctiva of the right eye of a 47-year-old man. **B** Histopathologically, a tumour covered by non-keratinized squamous epithelium is seen; the tumour is composed of wiry collagen fibres and a large amount of adipose tissue.

Definition

Epibulbar choristoma is a benign congenital developmental lesion of histologically mature tissue in an abnormal location. Epibulbar dermoid is an epibulbar choristoma composed of dermal and epidermal elements. Dermolipoma additionally contains large amounts of adipose tissue. Complex choristoma contains two or more ectopic tissues normally absent from the conjunctiva and caruncle.

ICD-O code

None

Synonyms

Epibulbar dermoid: limbal dermoid; dermoid tumour
Dermolipoma: lipodermoid
Complex choristoma: mixed dermoid

Epidemiology

As congenital lesions, epibulbar dermoids and dermolipomas are predominantly (in 60–70% of cases) diagnosed during childhood; they have a higher incidence in females and in White populations {1076,1119}. The incidence of complex choristomas is unknown, but they may be slightly more frequent in males than in females. Together, these choristomatous lesions account for approximately 8% of all epibulbar tumours in children {1076,1119}; in adults, this relative proportion is substantially lower (< 1%) {1076}. All three types of epibulbar choristoma are frequently observed in patients with Goldenhar syndrome and linear naevus sebaceous syndrome (MIM number: 163200; also known as organoid naevus syndrome, Schimmelpenning syndrome, and naevus sebaceus of Jadassohn), in which as many as 50% of patients are affected by ocular anomalies, most commonly epibulbar choristomas {592,599,849,921}. Epibulbar choristomas may be part of other syndromes as well {84}.

Etiology

The occurrence of complex choristoma has been partially attributed to early fetal altered migration of the palpebral portion of the lacrimal gland {1368}.

Localization

Epibulbar dermoids are typically located close to the inferotemporal limbus beneath the conjunctiva {1076}. If extensive, they can occupy the entire temporal quadrant. Dermoids are usually unilateral but can occur bilaterally in syndromic cases {1344}. Dermolipomas are typically located in the superotemporal quadrant {934}. If extensive, they can also occupy the entire temporal quadrant, including the upper and lower fornix. They are rarely observed in the lower eyelid {1275}. Both types may also involve parts of the cornea. Complex choristomas commonly extend from the superior temporal conjunctiva to the cornea. They may involve the entire temporal conjunctiva or, more rarely, the inferotemporal {300} or superior nasal conjunctiva {1156}. Occurrences in the caruncle {67} and bilaterality {300} are exceptional.

Clinical features

Epibulbar dermoids are whitish, firm lesions with cilia {489}. They are not movable because they are attached to the underlying sclera, hampering complete removal. Dermolipomas are yellowish, soft, non-mobile lesions that can also contain cilia {489}. The appearance of complex choristomas depends on their composition: they appear yellowish if they contain adipose tissue and pinkish with gelatinous elevations if they contain lacrimal gland {921}. The mass can also appear whitish, harbour cilia, and display fine superficial vasculature.

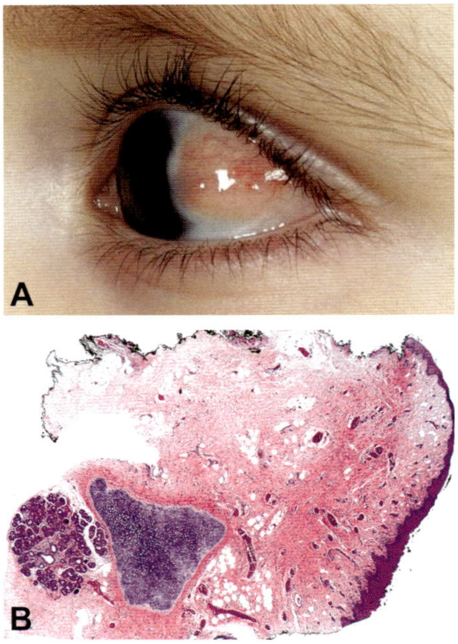

Fig. 1.59 Complex choristoma. **A** A temporal, pinkish, finely vascularized mass. **B** The lesion contains ectopic lacrimal gland, cartilage, adipose tissue, and fibrous tissue.

Histopathology
Epibulbar dermoids are composed of interweaving collagen bundles and covered by squamous epithelium (keratinized or non-keratinized, with or without goblet cells). Dermal appendages, in particular cilia with associated sebaceous glands and sweat glands, are generally present, in varying numbers and combinations. Variable amounts of fat can be found. Dermolipomas contain a large amount of adipose tissue and collagen bundles. Skin appendages can be present, but are less common and less numerous than in epibulbar dermoids. Cartilage and lacrimal gland tissue have been described in dermolipoma, but their occurrence formally denotes complex choristoma {425,921,1031,1368}. Other possible components of complex choristoma include smooth muscle {300,749} and nerve fascicles {300}, as well as (more rarely) myxomatous tissue {1276}, bone {478}, striated muscle {749}, and immature tooth and brain {322}.

Differential diagnosis
The differential diagnosis includes epibulbar xanthogranuloma and herniated orbital fat.

Histogenesis
Epibulbar choristoma arises from tissues of dermal and mesenchymal origin.

Genetic susceptibility
Epibulbar choristoma is associated with linear naevus sebaceous syndrome.

Prognosis and predictive factors
Malignant transformation has not been described. Documented growth, possibly due to local reactive changes, has exceptionally been reported {921,1276}. Excision is sometimes necessary to mitigate the risk of amblyopia associated with corneal lesions or for cosmetic reasons {1218}. The lesion can be partly removed (debulking) to avoid complications {609}.

Epibulbar osseous choristoma

Moulin A.
Herwig-Carl M.C.
Verdijk R.M.

Definition
Epibulbar osseous choristoma is a choristoma composed of mature bone.

ICD-O code
None

Synonyms
Episcleral osseous choristoma; osteoma

Epidemiology
The incidence of epibulbar osseous choristoma is unknown. These choristomas

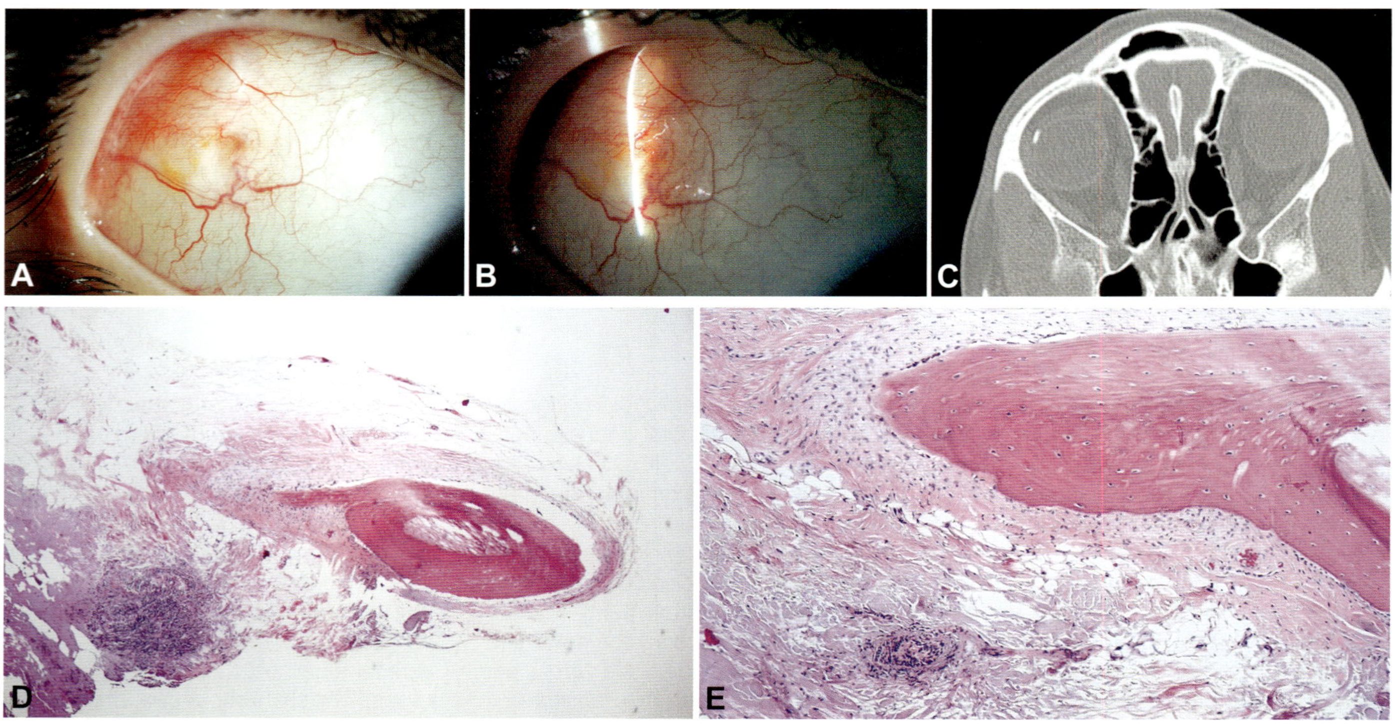

Fig. 1.60 Epibulbar osseous choristoma. **A,B** A multinodular whitish and firm mass can be seen in the superotemporal conjunctiva. **C** Transverse CT showing bone in the temporal anterior episclera of the right eye. **D** The lesion is composed of bone surrounded by fibrous and adipose tissue. **E** Normal compact lamellar bone with adjacent periosteum.

frequently present in patients aged < 20 years {395,1296}, but they can also be discovered later in life {1280}. They seem to be more frequent in females {395,1104}. A few cases have been reported in African-American patients {121,1104}.

Etiology

Epibulbar osseous choristoma is by definition a choristoma (a benign congenital lesion of histologically mature tissue in an abnormal location).

Localization

Epibulbar osseous choristomas are typically unilateral and located in the superotemporal conjunctiva {121,395,1104,1296}. They can also occur temporally {121} and (exceptionally) in the inferotemporal conjunctiva {878}.

Clinical features

Epibulbar osseous choristoma presents as a yellow, orange, pink, or white subconjunctival mass that may be multinodular and more or less adherent to the sclera. The mass usually extends from the equator to the superotemporal fornix. Epibulbar osseous choristomas are firm, and calcifications can be seen using CT.

Histopathology

Epibulbar osseous choristomas are composed of compact lamellar bone with normal osteocytes. Haversian canals can be found. Haematopoietic bone marrow is usually absent but has been rarely reported {349,395,878}. The bone is surrounded by dense fibrous tissue (periosteum), and an internal osteogenic layer can sometimes be observed {121}.

Differential diagnosis

The differential diagnosis includes dermolipoma and ectopic lacrimal gland (typically occurring in the same region), as well as a foreign body or an inflammatory process.

Histogenesis

Epibulbar osseous choristoma arises from cortical bone.

Prognosis and predictive factors

Epibulbar osseous choristomas are benign, and malignant transformation has not been described. It is believed that these lesions do not grow, although slight enlargement has been reported {121,878,1296}.

Phakomatous choristoma

Eagle R.C. Jr
Syed N.
Thaung C.

Definition

Phakomatous choristoma is a congenital choristomatous lesion of lenticular anlage, composed of extraocular crystalline lens tissue {1423}.

ICD-O code

None

Synonym

Zimmerman's tumour

Epidemiology

Phakomatous choristoma is very rare. The male-to-female ratio is 2:1.

Etiology

This is a developmental abnormality thought to be related to faulty separation of embryonic lens vesicle from the surface ectoderm.

Localization

The lesion occurs in the inferonasal eyelid or anterior orbit {1063}.

Clinical features

Patients present with a firm subcutaneous mass in the lower eyelid, present at birth.

Histopathology

There are nests, lobules, tubules, cords, and islands of cytologically bland cells resembling those of the crystalline lens, within dense fibrocollagenous stroma {1423}. The ectopic lens material comprises linear arrays of cuboidal lens epithelial cells, as well as cellular debris, granular amorphous material, and cells with copious eosinophilic cytoplasm that resemble the Wedl cells of posterior subcapsular cataract. The foci of ectopic lens cells are surrounded by, or aligned along, segments of basement membrane analogous to lens capsule, which give a positive periodic acid–Schiff (PAS) reaction. Focal calcification resembling psammoma bodies may be present {1274}. The ectopic lens material is immunoreactive for S100 protein, vimentin, and lens crystalline proteins {320,572} and negative for cytokeratins. Electron microscopy reveals 10 nm whorled cytoplasmic microfilaments within degenerating epithelial cells {782,995}.

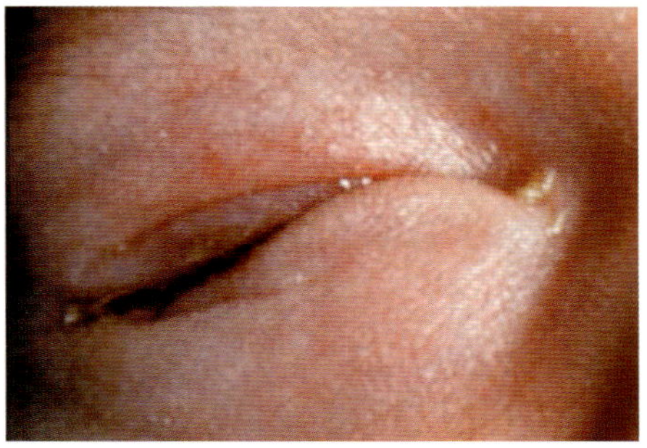

Fig. 1.61 Phakomatous choristoma. A congenital mass involving the medial lower eyelid.

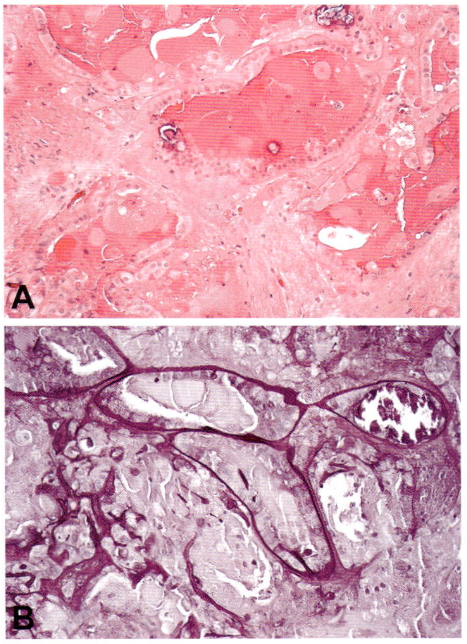

Fig. 1.62 Phakomatous choristoma. **A** Linear arrays of lens epithelial cells envelop lens material, including cells resembling the Wedl cells of posterior subcapsular cataract. **B** Periodic acid–Schiff (PAS) staining highlights prominent basement membrane (analogous to lens capsule) surrounding ectopic lens material.

Differential diagnosis

The differential diagnosis includes cystic dermoid and adnexal neoplasms.

Histogenesis

Pathogenic theories include faulty separation of the embryonic lens vesicle from the surface ectoderm or migration of putative lens tissue through the closing optic fissure.

Prognosis and predictive factors

Phakomatous choristoma is benign. The ipsilateral eye is usually normal, but a myopic eye with a colobomatous hypoplastic optic disc and staphyloma has been reported {1253}.

Secondary tumours of the conjunctiva

Mudhar H.S.
Coupland S.E.

Definition

Secondary tumours of the conjunctiva are tumours that originate elsewhere and involve the conjunctiva by metastasis or by direct spread from adjacent anatomical structures.

ICD-O codes

Code according to the originating tumour type.

Epidemiology

Metastases to the conjunctiva account for < 1% of all conjunctival tumours {428,612,1076,1080}; the female-to-male ratio is 1.2:1, and the average patient age is 54 years {1076,1080}. Direct tumour spread from adjacent sites accounts for 3% of all conjunctival tumours; the female-to-male ratio is about 1.4:1, and the average patient age is 64 years {1076,1080}.

Clinical features

Patients with conjunctival metastases can present with a discrete mass, red eye, foreign body sensation, or tearing {612}. Metastases are fast-growing, usually unifocal, and commonly present on the bulbar conjunctiva; they manifest after the primary tumour (at a mean of 44 months later; range: 8–130 months) {612}. Metastases can be yellow, red, or brown, depending on the nature of the primary tumour. Most patients with conjunctival metastasis also have concurrent metastases to adjacent ocular sites (uvea and orbit) and non-ocular sites {612,1080}.

Tumours involving the conjunctiva by direct spread present in one of two main ways: as a discrete ovoid mass involving the extralimbal conjunctiva or with a diffuse distribution. Extraocular extension of uveal melanoma commonly presents as a discrete mass {1076,1080}, whereas sebaceous carcinoma from the eyelid skin is commonly diffuse {954}. Secondary lymphomas and leukaemias present as either diffuse or nodular pink painless masses.

Histopathology

Metastatic tumours occur in the substantia propria and are often separated from the epithelium by a thin rim of stromal collagen. The tumour deposits may be unifocal or multifocal and associated with lymphatic/blood vessel dissemination. The epithelium shows no evidence of intraepithelial neoplasia.

The histopathology of metastatic tumours depends on the nature of the primary. Metastases from the breast are often ductal or lobular tumours {612}. Metastatic carcinomas from the lung are usually non-small cell lung carcinoma {612}. Metastatic melanomas from the skin tend to be amelanotic and composed of mitotically active epithelioid and/or spindle cells {353,1080}; some cases can show pigmented melanoma cells in lymphatic vessels.

Uveal melanoma spreading directly to the conjunctiva is composed of variably pigmented spindle and/or epithelioid cells. Sebaceous carcinoma spreading to the conjunctiva shows a distinctive intraepithelial pagetoid spread pattern, which often spares the basal layer of the conjunctival epithelium. The cells contain bubbly cytoplasm due to intracytoplasmic lipid, which often indents the nucleus.

The histological and immunohistochemical features seen in secondary involvement of the conjunctiva by lymphoma or leukaemia depend on the lymphoma/leukaemia subtype (see *Lymphomas of the conjunctiva and caruncle*, p. 40) {1231}.

Immunohistochemistry is very useful in distinguishing between various metastatic tumours. Some of the most commonly used immunohistochemical markers are shown in Table 2.01 (p. 103) in Chapter 2.

Histogenesis

Primary origin of tumours metastasizing to the conjunctiva

Carcinoma: The primary sites that most commonly give rise to conjunctival metastases are the breast and lung {612,1080}. Other sites that give rise to conjunctival metastases include the stomach, urinary

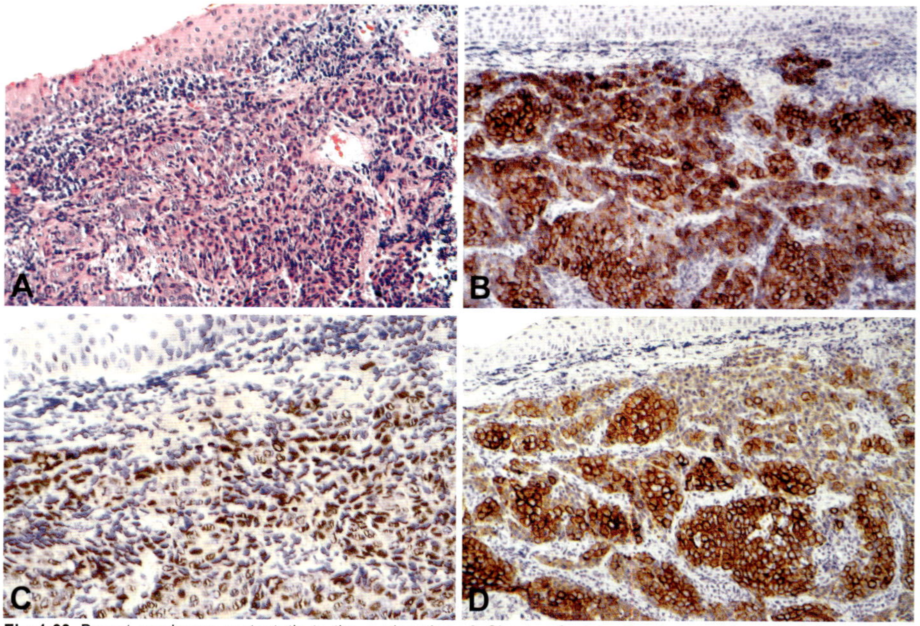

Fig. 1.63 Breast carcinoma metastatic to the conjunctiva. **A** Sheets of minimally pleomorphic epithelial cells in the substantia propria are surrounded by a lymphocytic infiltrate. The infiltrating carcinoma is highlighted by immunohistochemical staining for cytokeratin (**B**), estrogen receptor (**C**), and GCDFP-15 (**D**).

bladder, kidney, colon, cervix, thyroid, and larynx.

Melanoma: The primary site that most commonly gives rise to conjunctival metastases is the truncal skin {353}.

Lymphoma and leukaemia: Secondary involvement of the conjunctiva by lymphoma or leukaemia is relatively rare, but the precise frequency varies considerably depending on the lymphoma/leukaemia subtype and its associated aggressiveness {614,960}. The B-cell lymphoma that most commonly affects the conjunctiva secondarily is mantle cell lymphoma, followed by diffuse large B-cell lymphoma and follicular lymphoma {231,614,960}. The T-cell lymphomas that most commonly affect the conjunctiva secondarily are peripheral T-cell lymphoma NOS, adult T-cell leukaemia/lymphoma, anaplastic large cell lymphoma, and mycosis fungoides {614}. Chronic lymphocytic leukaemia is the most common secondary leukaemia subtype in adults {231}, but with the advent of allogeneic bone marrow transplantation, there has been an increased frequency of acute leukaemias in both adults and children {1072}.

Other tumour types: One case of metastatic testicular seminoma {391A}, one case of metastatic neuroendocrine tumour (carcinoid) of uncertain origin {612}, and one case of metastatic pleural mesothelioma have been documented {209}.

Primary origin of tumours directly spreading to the conjunctiva

Extraocular extension of uveal melanoma and pagetoid spread of sebaceous carcinoma of the eyelid to the conjunctiva are well documented {954,1076,1080}. Extraocular spread of uveal melanoma is found in 13% of enucleated eyes {8,1066}. Pagetoid spread of sebaceous carcinoma to the conjunctiva is reported to occur in 40–80% of cases {185A,954,1076}. Eyelid basal cell carcinoma and lacrimal gland tumours rarely involve the conjunctiva {1076,1080}.
Lymphomas can also spread directly to the conjunctiva from adjacent anatomical sites. Reported examples include extraocular extension of primary choroidal lymphoma {488}, as well as involvement of the conjunctiva by mycosis fungoides of the outer eyelid and (rarely) by extranodal NK/T-cell lymphomas of nasal type infiltrating from the nasal mucosa {231}.

Genetic profile

A tumour's genetic profile may be helpful in distinguishing metastatic skin melanoma from direct spread of uveal melanoma. Cutaneous melanomas commonly harbour *BRAF* and *NRAS* mutations, which are not usually present in uveal melanomas (excluding iris melanomas, which can show *BRAF* mutations in some cases {475A,1304}). Uveal melanomas show mutations in *GNAQ* and *GNA11* {875A,1306} and loss of chromosome 3 {979}, whereas skin melanomas usually do not.
ALK and *EGFR* mutations occur in non-small cell lung carcinoma, and ERBB2 (HER2) status may be positive in breast carcinoma. Sebaceous carcinomas can show mutations in the DNA mismatch repair genes and can be associated with Muir–Torre syndrome {908}.
The molecular genetic features seen in secondary involvement of the conjunctiva by lymphoma or leukaemia depend on the lymphoma/leukaemia subtype (see *Lymphomas of the conjunctiva and caruncle*, p. 40) {1231}.

Prognosis and predictive factors

Conjunctival metastases manifest at an advanced stage, with a mean survival of 9 months after diagnosis {612}; death occurs as a result of widespread metastases. In the largest series reported to date, patients were offered localized radiotherapy, excision, and chemotherapy to control the conjunctival disease {612}.
Extraocular spread of uveal melanoma correlates with orbital tumour recurrence, development of metastases, and tumour-related death {93,225A}.
Sebaceous carcinoma with conjunctival pagetoid spread is more likely to be exenterated than tumours without pagetoid spread, but there is no difference in terms of tumour-related metastases {185A}.
The prognosis in secondary involvement of the conjunctiva by lymphoma or leukaemia depends on the lymphoma/leukaemia subtype {1231}.

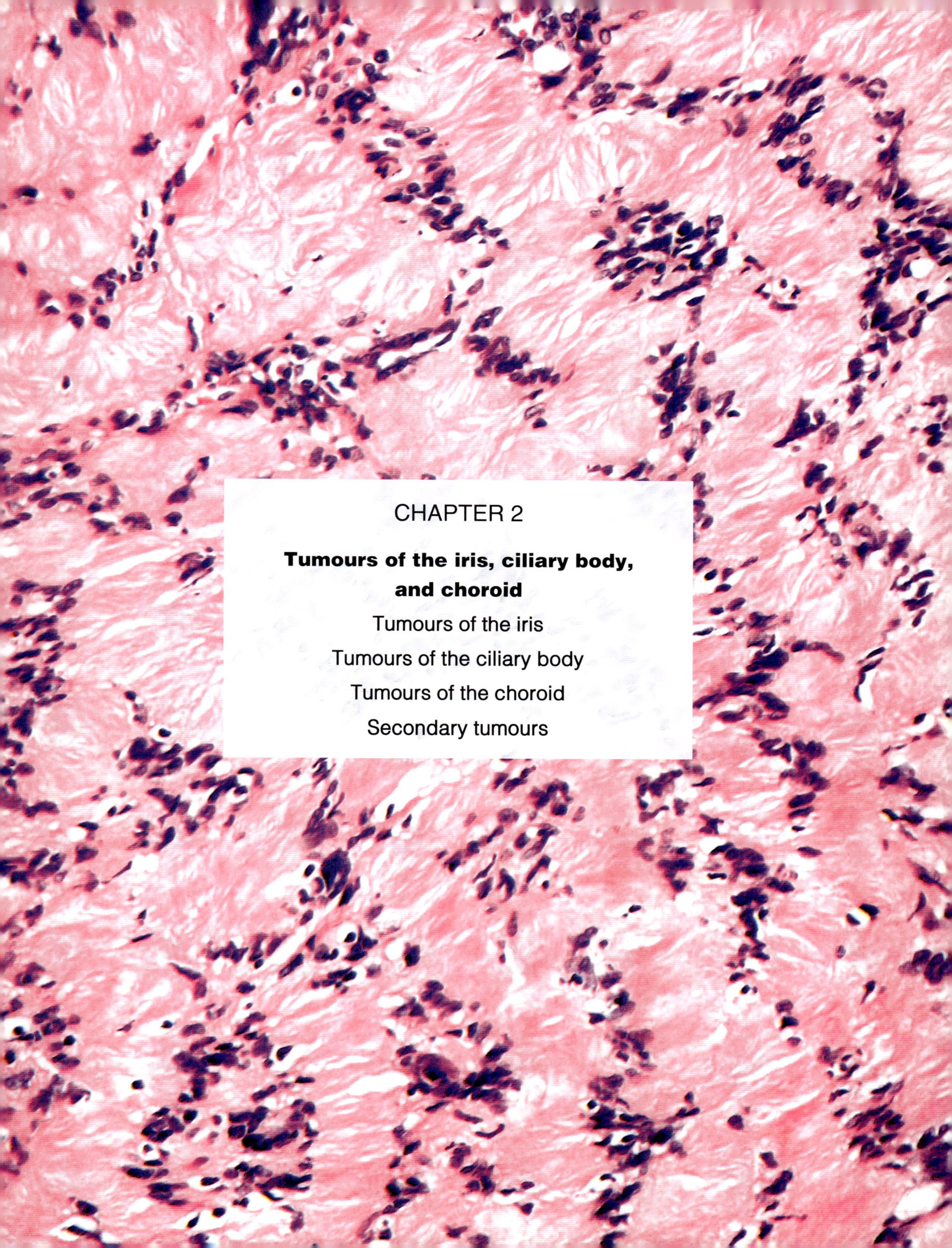

CHAPTER 2

Tumours of the iris, ciliary body, and choroid

Tumours of the iris

Tumours of the ciliary body

Tumours of the choroid

Secondary tumours

WHO classification of tumours of the iris, ciliary body, and choroid

Tumours of the iris	
Uveal melanoma	8720/3
Iris melanoma	8720/3
Iris naevus	8720/0
Ocular melanocytosis	None
Lisch nodule	None
Pigmented epithelial cyst	None
Implantation cyst	None
Ectopic lacrimal gland	None
Histiocytic tumours	
Juvenile xanthogranuloma	None
Rosai–Dorfman disease	None
Langerhans cell histiocytosis	9751/1
Erdheim–Chester disease	9749/3
Tumours of the ciliary body	
Melanocytoma (of the ciliary body, iris, and choroid)	8726/0
Ciliary body adenocarcinoma	8140/3
Ciliary body adenoma	8140/0
Adenomatous hyperplasia	None
Reactive epithelial hyperplasia	None
Medulloepithelioma, benign	9501/0
Medulloepithelioma, malignant	9501/3
Teratoid medulloepithelioma, benign	9502/0
Teratoid medulloepithelioma, malignant	9502/3
Leiomyoma	8890/0
Schwannoma	9560/0
Glioneuroma	9490/0
Tumours of the choroid	
Mixed epithelioid and spindle cell uveal melanoma	8770/3
Epithelioid cell uveal melanoma	8771/3
Spindle cell uveal melanoma NOS	8772/3
Spindle cell uveal melanoma, type A	8773/3
Spindle cell uveal melanoma, type B	8774/3
Uveal naevus	8720/0
Bilateral diffuse uveal melanocytic hyperplasia	None
Neurofibroma	9540/0
Ganglioneuroma	9490/0
Schwannoma	9560/0
Haemangioma	9120/0
Osteoma	9180/0
Primary choroidal lymphoma	9699/3
Secondary lymphomatous infiltration of the choroid	See note[a]
Leukaemic infiltration of the choroid	See note[a]
Secondary tumours	See note[b]

[a]Code secondary lymphomatous and leukaemic infiltration of the choroid according to the lymphoma/leukaemia subtype.

[b]Code secondary tumours according to the originating tumour type.

The morphology codes are from the International Classification of Diseases for Oncology (ICD-O) {381}. Behaviour is coded /0 for benign tumours; /1 for unspecified, borderline, or uncertain behaviour; /2 for carcinoma in situ and grade III intraepithelial neoplasia; and /3 for malignant tumours.

The classification is modified from the previous WHO classification, taking into account changes in our understanding of these lesions.

TNM classification of melanoma of the uvea

Malignant Melanoma of Uvea

(ICD-O C69.3,4)

TNM Clinical Classification

T – Primary Tumour

TX Primary tumour cannot be assessed
T0 No evidence of primary tumour

Iris*

T1 Tumour limited to iris
- T1a not more than 3 clock hours in size
- T1b more than 3 clock hours in size
- T1c with secondary glaucoma

T2 Tumour confluent with or extending into the ciliary body, choroid, or both
- T2a Tumour confluent with or extending into the ciliary body without secondary glaucoma
- T2b Tumour confluent with or extending into the choroid without secondary glaucoma
- T2c Tumour confluent with or extending into the ciliary body and/or choroid with secondary glaucoma

T3 Tumour confluent with or extending into the ciliary body, choroid, or both, with scleral extension

T4 Tumour with extrascleral extension
- T4a less than or equal to 5 mm in diameter
- T4b more than 5 mm in diameter

Note
*Iris melanomas originate from, and are predominantly located in, this region of the uvea. If less than half of the tumour volume is located within the iris, the tumour may have originated in the ciliary body and consideration should be given to classifying it accordingly.

Ciliary Body and Choroid

Primary ciliary body and choroidal melanomas are classified according to the four tumour size categories listed in Fig. 2.01.[a,b]

Thickness (mm)

Thickness (mm)	≤ 3.0	3.1–6.0	6.1–9.0	9.1–12.0	12.1–15.0	15.1–18.0	>18
>15					4	4	4
12.1–15.0				3	3	4	4
9.1–12.0		3	3	3	3	3	4
6.1–9.0	2	2	2	2	3	3	4
3.1–6.0	1	1	1	2	2	3	4
≤ 3.0	1	1	1	1	2	2	4

Largest basal diameter (mm)

Fig. 2.01 Classification for ciliary body and choroid uveal melanoma based on thickness and diameter.

T1 Tumour size category 1
- T1a without ciliary body involvement and extraocular extension
- T1b with ciliary body involvement
- T1c without ciliary body involvement but with extraocular extension less than or equal to 5 mm in diameter
- T1d with ciliary body involvement and extraocular extension less than or equal to 5 mm in diameter

T2 Tumour size category 2
- T2a without ciliary body involvement and extraocular extension
- T2b with ciliary body involvement
- T2c without ciliary body involvement but with extraocular extension less than or equal to 5 mm in diameter
- T2d with ciliary body involvement and extraocular extension less than or equal to 5 mm in diameter

T3 Tumour size category 3
- T3a without ciliary body involvement and extraocular extension
- T3b with ciliary body involvement
- T3c without ciliary body involvement but with extraocular extension less than or equal to 5 mm in diameter
- T3d with ciliary body involvement and extraocular extension less than or equal to 5 mm in diameter

T4 Tumour size category 4

(Continued on next page)

Malignant Melanoma of Uvea

(Continued)

T4 Tumour size category 4
- T4a without ciliary body involvement and extraocular extension
- T4b with ciliary body involvement
- T4c without ciliary body involvement but with extraocular extension less than or equal to 5 mm in diameter
- T4d with ciliary body involvement and extraocular extension less than or equal to 5 mm in diameter
- T4e Any tumour size category with extraocular extension more than 5 mm in diameter

Notes

[a] In clinical practice, the largest tumour basal diameter may be estimated in optic disc diameters (dd, average: 1 dd = 1.5 mm). Tumour thickness may be estimated in dioptres (average: 2.5 dioptres = 1 mm). However, techniques such as ultrasonography and fundus photography are used to provide more accurate measurements. Ciliary body involvement can be evaluated by the slit-lamp, ophthalmoscopy, gonioscopy, and transillumination. However, high-frequency ultrasonography (ultrasound biomicroscopy) is used for more accurate assessment. Extension through the sclera is evaluated visually before and during surgery, and with ultrasonography, computed tomography, or magnetic resonance imaging.

[b] When histopathological measurements are recorded after fixation, tumour diameter and thickness may be underestimated because of tissue shrinkage.

N – Regional Lymph Nodes

NX Regional lymph nodes cannot be assessed
N0 No regional lymph node metastasis
N1 Regional lymph node metastasis

M – Distant Metastasis

M0 No distant metastasis
M1 Distant metastasis
- M1a Largest metastasis 3 cm or less in greatest dimension
- M1b Largest metastasis is larger than 3 cm in greatest dimension but not larger than 8 cm
- M1c Largest metastasis is larger than 8 cm in greatest dimension

pTNM Pathological Classification

The pT and pN categories correspond to the T and N categories.

pM – Distant Metastasis*

pM1 Distant metastasis microscopically confirmed

Note
*pM0 and pMX are not valid categories.

Stage*

Stage I	T1a	N0	M0
Stage IIA	T1b–d, T2a	N0	M0
Stage IIB	T2b, T3a	N0	M0
Stage IIIA	T2c–d	N0	M0
	T3b–c	N0	M0
	T4a	N0	M0
Stage IIIB	T3d	N0	M0
	T4b–c	N0	M0
Stage IIIC	T4d–e	N0	M0
Stage IV	Any T	N1	M0
	Any T	Any N	M1

Note
*The stage groups are for malignant melanoma of the choroid and ciliary body but not of the iris.

The information presented here has been excerpted from the 8th edition of the *TNM classification of malignant tumours* (2017) {132}.
A help desk for specific questions about the TNM classification is available at http://www.uicc.org/resources/tnm/helpdesk.

Tumours of the iris, ciliary body, and choroid: Introduction

Grossniklaus H.E.
Eberhart C.G.
Kivelä T.T.

The uveal tract occupies the middle coat of the eye and consists of the iris, ciliary body, and choroid. The iris has five layers, from anterior to posterior: the anterior border layer, the stroma, the muscular layer (the dilator and sphincter muscles), the anterior pigment epithelium, and the posterior pigment epithelium. The ciliary body comprises (from outermost to innermost within the eye) the supraciliary space, the muscular layer (longitudinal, radial, and circular fibres), the stroma, the pigmented epithelium, and the non-pigmented epithelium. The choroid comprises (from outermost to innermost within the eye) the lamina fusca, Haller's layer, Sattler's layer, and the choriocapillaris. These tissues contain melanocytes, fibrocytes, smooth muscle, vascular channels, and nerves; they can be infiltrated by lymphocytes, histiocytes, and other cells of haematopoietic origin. The tumours that arise from these tissues include naevi and melanomas (from melanocytes), schwannomas and neurofibromas (from nerves and nerve sheaths), adenomas and adenocarcinomas (from the pigmented and non-pigmented epithelia), and lymphoma (from lymphocytes).

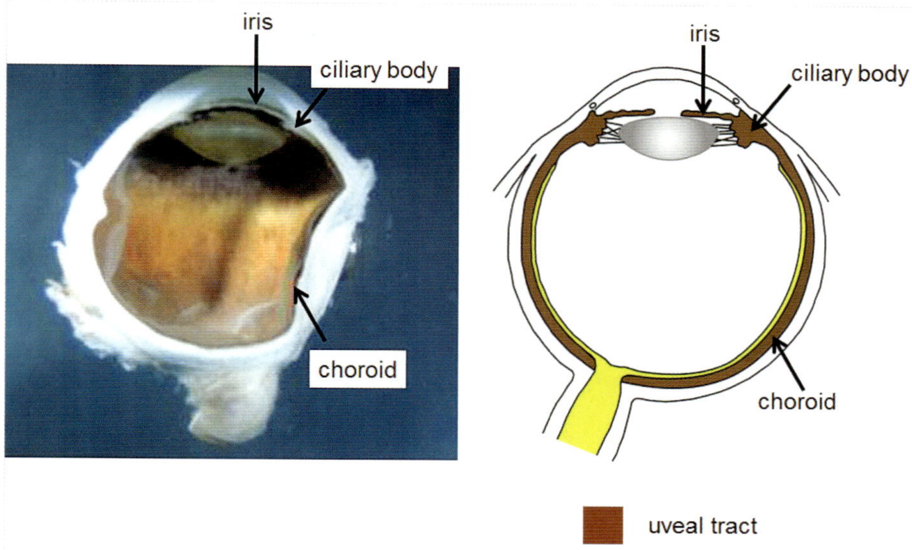

Fig. 2.02 Anatomy of the uveal tract. The uveal tract is the middle coat of the eye, lying between the outer coat (the cornea and sclera) and the inner coat (the ciliary epithelium and retina); the uvea consists of the iris, ciliary body, and choroid.

For gross and microscopic examination of tumours of the uveal tract, it is advisable to section the eye such that the centre of the tumour is in the same plane as the centre of the pupil and the centre of the optic nerve (resulting in a specimen called a P-O section). This can be accomplished by transilluminating the eye, outlining the transillumination blockage corresponding to the uveal tumour, and sectioning the eye accordingly. First, a calotte (a small cap) is removed from one side. The eye is then examined under a dissecting microscope and its gross features described. A second calotte is then removed from the opposite side of the eye to create a P-O section, from which slides are then prepared and examined, and the tumour is described in terms of its size, shape, location, cellular characteristics, and effects on surrounding tissue. Along with the uveal tract tumour itself, the surrounding tissue and the eye as a whole are also examined microscopically.

The primary uveal tract malignancy most commonly examined in the pathology laboratory is melanoma; metastases to the uveal tract are more common clinically, but they are less frequently examined microscopically. Similarly, naevi are far more common than melanomas, but they are much less frequently sampled by fine-needle aspiration biopsy. The advent of molecular diagnostic techniques, such as gene expression profiling and FISH analysis for chromosome 3 aneuploidy, has enabled small amounts of tumour to be sampled and genetically examined. In general, these molecular techniques improve the description of a tumour, but they do not replace careful histological and/or cytological examination.

Clinicopathological correlation is essential for the investigation of uveal tract tumours. For example, a cystic lesion on the posterior surface of the iris seen on ultrasound biomicroscopy is probably a cyst of the iris pigment epithelium; when pigmented epithelial cysts of the iris are excised, they often collapse, revealing essentially normal, redundant iris pigment epithelium. That appearance in combination with the ultrasound biomicroscopy findings leads to the correct diagnosis. Another example is a ciliary body tumour that does not block light on

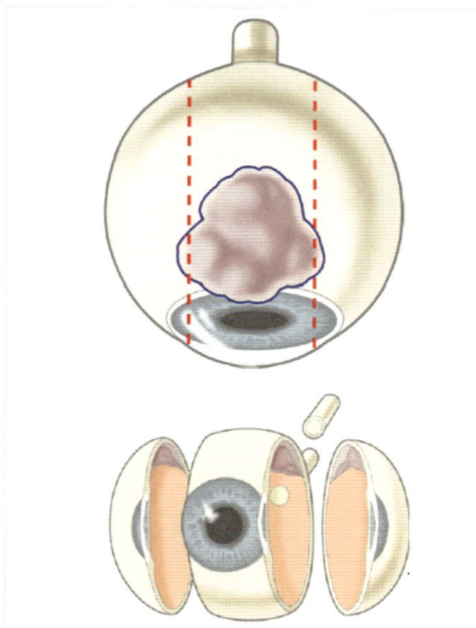

Fig. 2.03 Sectioning of an eye with uveal melanoma. The eye is sectioned such that the centre of the tumour is in the same plane that contains the centre of the pupil and the centre of the optic nerve (resulting in a specimen called a P-O section).

transillumination, presenting in a young woman; these characteristics are clinically suggestive of a leiomyoma (or mesectodermal leiomyoma), and this should be taken into consideration when evaluating fine-needle aspiration biopsy or excision specimens from the lesion. Adenomas of the ciliary epithelium appear clinically as multilobulated lesions, whereas melanomas generally have a smooth surface. Examining pathologists should be familiar with the clinical characteristics of the uveal tract tumour being investigated, and they should take these characteristics into consideration when examining the tumour microscopically.

Within this volume, some of the rarer entities that can arise throughout the uveal tract are discussed only in their most common site; for example, bilateral diffuse uveal melanocytic hyperplasia is grouped with tumours of the choroid, and ocular melanocytosis is grouped with tumours of the iris.

Tumours of the iris

Iris melanoma

Bechrakis N.E.
Grossniklaus H.E.
Schoenfield L.

Definition

Iris melanoma is a tumour that arises from the melanocytes of the iris stroma.

ICD-O codes

Uveal melanoma	8720/3
Iris melanoma	8720/3

Synonyms

Uveal melanoma (less specific, because this includes ciliary body and choroidal tumours); ocular melanoma (imprecise, discouraged)

Epidemiology

Iris melanomas account for 5% of all uveal melanomas.

Etiology

A possible association with ultraviolet (UV) radiation has been proposed, because most iris melanomas are located in the inferior half of the iris (most commonly at the inferior temporal quadrant), where UV irradiation due to sun exposure is most prominent {1090}.

Localization

Iris melanomas can occur anywhere on the iris, but most (an estimated 80% of cases) are located in the inferior half of the iris (most commonly at the inferior temporal quadrant) {1090}. Iris melanomas may invade into the ciliary body, and they may seed the anterior chamber, trabecular meshwork, and associated aqueous outflow channels.

Clinical features

Iris melanomas can have heterogeneous pigmentation, with the tumours ranging from almost translucent and amelanotic to deeply pigmented. They are usually associated with deformation and irregularity of the pupillary margin, as well as ectropion uveae, although these characteristics are not pathognomonic of malignancy. Their margins can be distinct or poorly defined. Iris melanomas can be nodular and well circumscribed; multinodular; or diffuse with infiltration of tumour cells and nests over the entire iris surface, lens surface, and trabecular meshwork. They can also infiltrate into the ciliary body, either in a circumscribed fashion or over the entire circumference of the trabecular meshwork and ciliary body, producing a so-called ring melanoma. Ring melanomas are associated with elevated intraocular pressure (secondary glaucoma) that does not respond to conventional glaucoma medication. The vascularity of the lesions can be visualized with fluorescein angiography of the anterior segment of the eye.

Non-pigmented iris melanomas with multiple tumour nodules over the entire iris surface have been called tapioca melanomas. When iris melanomas infiltrate posteriorly, they can touch the lens, producing a sectorial cataract and/or astigmatism resulting in vision deterioration, which in some cases might be the first symptom a patient notices.

Diffuse iris melanoma may result in heterochromia and secondary glaucoma. Patients with these symptoms may present late as a result of diagnostic delay and confusion with iridocorneal endothelial syndrome and/or pigmentary glaucoma.

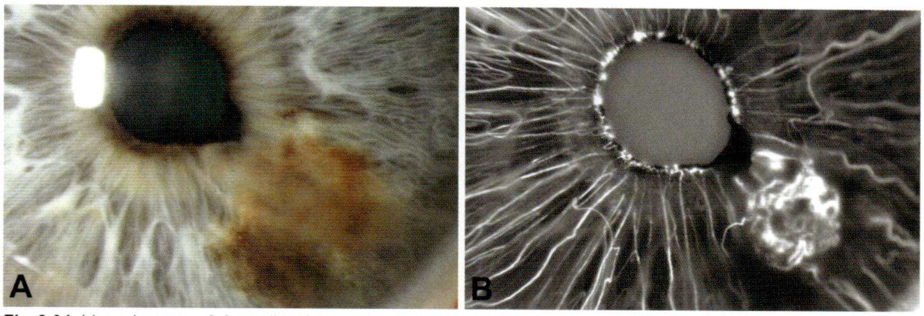

Fig. 2.04 Iris melanoma. **A** A small melanoma located at the inferior temporal quadrant, with heterogeneous pigmentation and ectropion uveae. **B** Fluorescein angiography shows the prominent vascularity of this small melanocytic lesion.

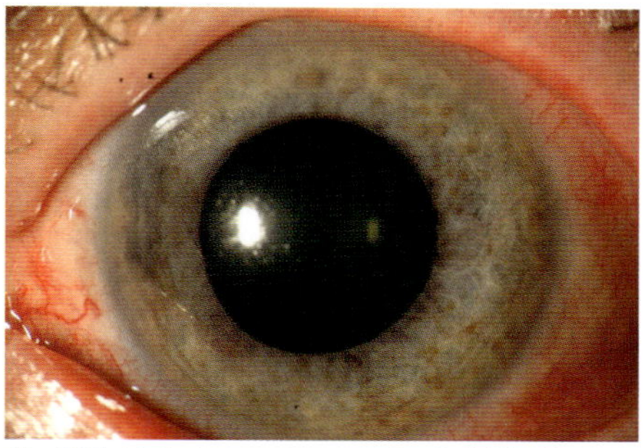

Fig. 2.05 Iris tapioca melanoma. Small, lightly pigmented nodules scattered diffusely over the surface of the iris.

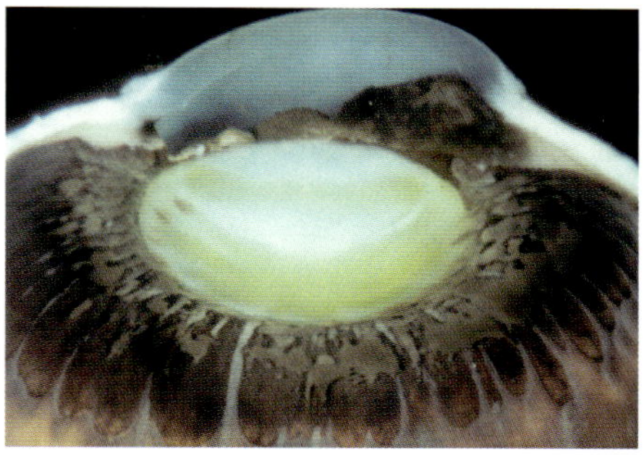

Fig. 2.06 Iris melanoma. A macroscopic view of a diffusely infiltrating iris ring melanoma, with posterior extension into the ciliary body and around the equator of the lens.

Histopathology

Iris melanomas can have very heterogeneous pigmentation, varying from completely amelanotic to densely pigmented. They may have blander morphology than do choroidal and ciliary body melanomas.

Cytopathologically, iris melanomas can display the full spectrum of melanocytic differentiation, from spindle cells to epithelioid cells. Spindle cell nuclei can have fine linear interdigitation of their nuclear membrane, usually referred to

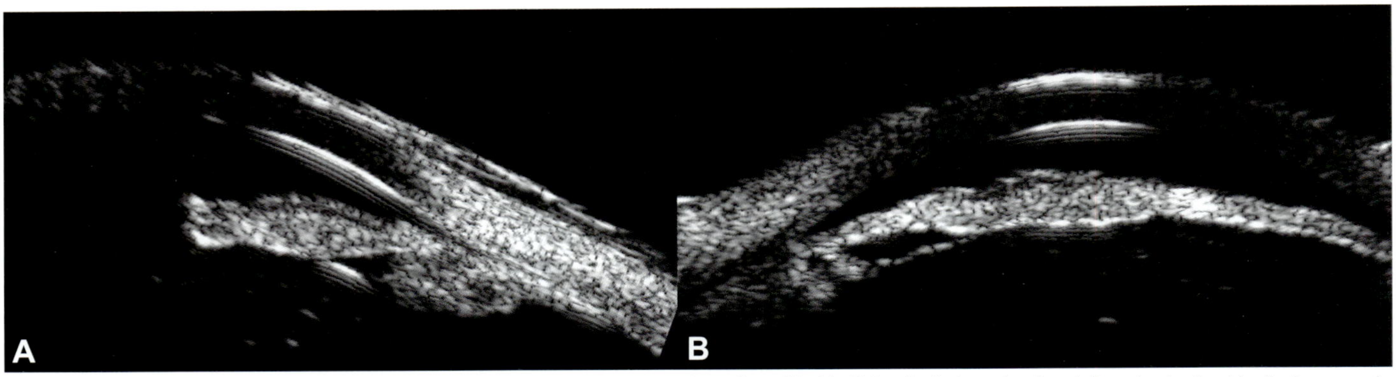

Fig. 2.07 Iris melanoma. Ultrasound biomicroscopy (20 MHz) reveals spread on the anterior surface of the iris (**A**; longitudinal scan) and posterior extension touching the lens capsule (**B**; transversal scan).

as a chromatin strip, with small nucleoli (spindle B cells) or without small nucleoli (spindle A cells). At the other end of the differentiation spectrum, iris melanomas can be composed of epithelioid cells, which are usually less pigmented than spindle cells (or even amelanotic). Epithelioid cells may be seen at the base (ciliary body side) of iris melanomas. The parts of iris melanomas located on the surface of the iris and protruding towards the anterior chamber are cytologically more loosely and non-coherently arranged, which increases the risk of dispersion of cells within the anterior chamber upon surgical manipulation. Iris melanomas that are biopsied for diagnostic purposes usually have a smaller spindle cell, well-differentiated melanocytic morphology, with small or even absent nucleoli, probably because they are captured (clinically and histopathologically) at an early stage of their dedifferentiation process. On immunohistochemistry, iris melanomas exhibit the same features as choroidal and ciliary body melanomas, namely, positivity for S100 protein, HMB45 antigen, and melan-A. In one study, 189 lesions originally diagnosed as iris melanomas were retrospectively reclassified; 87% were reassigned to one of six categories of naevi and 13% were classified as melanomas {532}.

Melanoma cells on the iris surface can undergo aqueous humour modification and appear smaller (with a naevoid appearance) than the larger melanoma cells in the stroma beneath {828A}. These modified surface cells have a lower proliferation rate and express pro-differentiation proteins {828A}.

Differential diagnosis

The differential diagnosis includes naevi and melanocytomas, metastatic lesions to the iris, leiomyoma of the iris stroma, non-neoplastic granulomatous lesions, and infectious infiltrates.

Histogenesis

Iris melanomas arise from neural crest–derived melanocytes, which are normally scattered within the iris stroma. There is a reported tendency for cytological dedifferentiation from normal melanocytes to the spindle cell variant, and further to the epithelioid phenotype, during the natural evolution of these lesions {89}.

Genetic profile

Iris melanomas show chromosomal aberrations similar to those seen in choroidal melanomas. Cytogenetically, most iris melanomas have a low-metastatic-risk profile, reflecting their relatively benign clinical course {657,1105}. The mutations found in iris melanoma, which are similar to those found in choroidal and ciliary body melanomas, include mutations of *GNAQ*, *GNA11*, *EIF1AX*, and *SF3B1* {1048,1304}, as well as *BAP1* {442,1304}. In one study, iris melanomas were found to show mutations similar to those seen in cutaneous melanoma, namely, mutations in *NRAS*, *BRAF*, *PTEN*, *KIT*, and *TP53* {1304}. However, these findings contrast

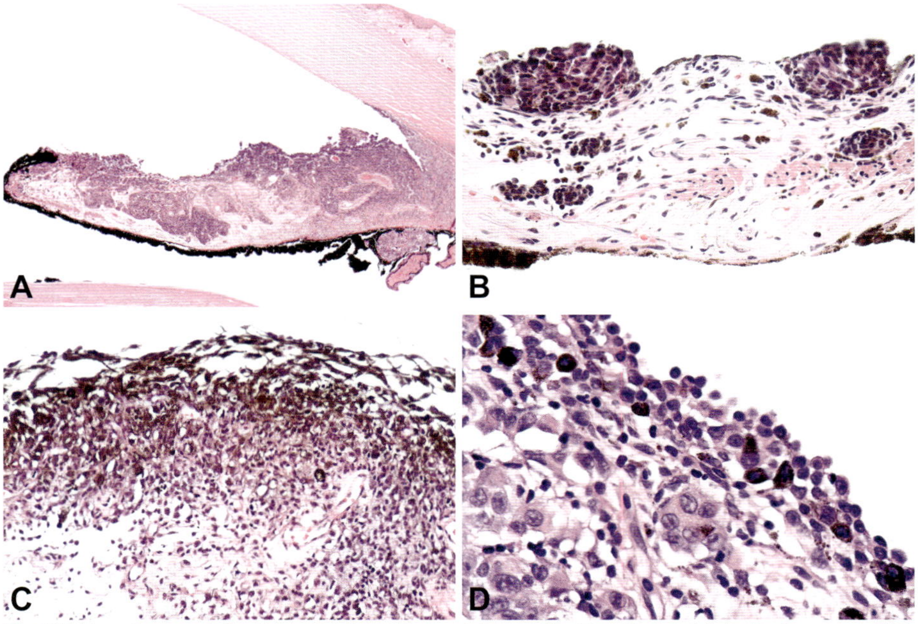

Fig. 2.08 Iris melanoma. **A** A melanoma on the surface and stroma of the iris, with associated ectropion uveae. **B** Iris tapioca melanoma; a microscopic image of the melanoma shown in Fig. 2.05 shows clusters of well-differentiated melanocytic cells with prominent nucleoli, both on the iris surface and within the iris stroma. **C** An iris melanoma with heterogeneous pigmentation; the tumour is moderately vascularized and exhibits a loose connectivity on the surface towards the anterior chamber. **D** Iris surface melanoma cells much smaller than stromal melanoma cells, secondary to aqueous modification.

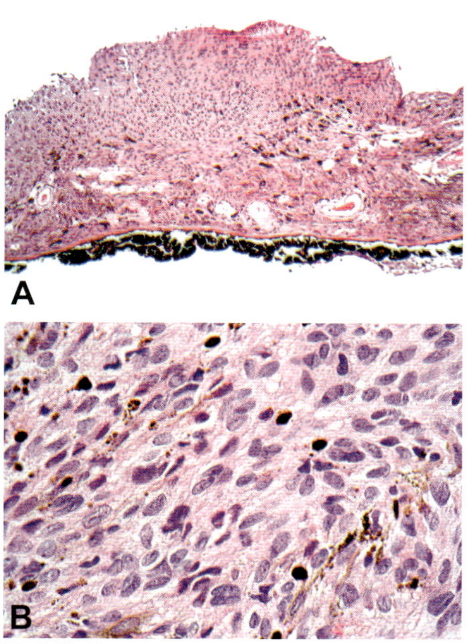

Fig. 2.09 Iris melanoma. **A** Melanoma present on the iris surface. **B** This example contains spindle B cells.

with those of other studies, in which no *BRAF* mutations were detected in any of the examined iris melanoma cases {657}.

Genetic susceptibility
The familial *BAP1* tumour predisposition syndrome is associated with uveal melanomas.

Prognosis and predictive factors
The prognosis of iris melanoma is good, because most lesions are treated at an early stage. According to a Kaplan–Meier life table analysis, metastasis occurs in 3% of patients by 5 years after diagnosis, 5% by 10 years, and 10% by 20 years. Clinical factors at the time of initial evaluation that are prognostic of eventual metastasis from iris melanoma include older patient age, elevated intraocular pressure, posterior tumour margin at the angle or iris root (vs the midzone), extraocular extension, and prior surgical treatment of the tumour before referral (vs observation). The method of management (i.e. resection, radiation therapy, or enucleation) does not affect the risk of metastasis {1116}.

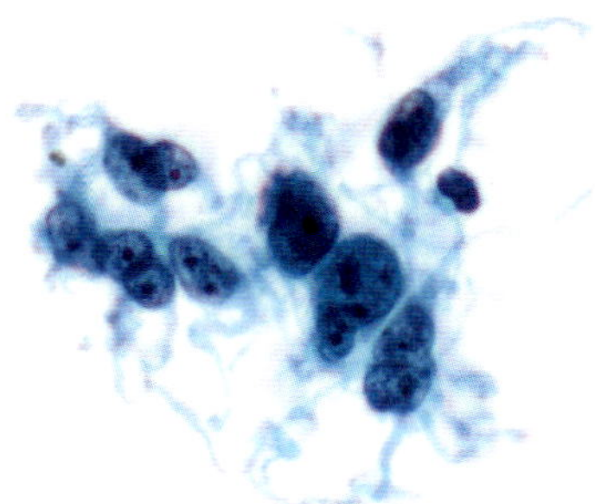

Fig. 2.10 Iris melanoma. A fine-needle aspiration biopsy specimen shows melanoma cells with atypia and prominent nucleoli.

Melanocytic naevus of the iris

Schoenfield L.
Grossniklaus H.E.
Pe'er J.

Definition
Melanocytic naevus of the iris is a benign proliferation of melanocytes, usually pigmented.

ICD-O code
Iris naevus 8720/0

Synonyms
Naevus; melanocytoma (which is a specific type of naevus)

Epidemiology
Iris naevi, which are more common in light-coloured irides than in dark-coloured irides, occur in approximately 4% of the population overall. This incidence rate is much lower than that of iris freckles (which occur in 60% of the population) or choroidal naevi (in 17%) {454,1053}. Iris naevi account for 60% of solid melanocytic iris tumours {1092}.

Etiology
Sunlight exposure may play an etiological role similar to its role in the formation of iris freckles {1051}. The etiology of melanocytic naevi may be multifactorial. Their development may be related to the migration and maturation of melanoblasts during embryogenesis {1052,1053,1258}. Choroidal naevi have been found to be associated with body mass index and other systemic factors {941}.

Localization
Most are located in the inferior half of the iris {1053,1307}.

Clinical features
The majority (> 90%) of iris naevi are pigmented, but some are amelanotic {1145}. They alter the iris stroma (unlike iris freckles), and there may be an associated cyst. The lesions can be flat or elevated, and they can be circumscribed or diffuse. Iris naevi have been classified as sectoral, incomplete sectoral, or solitary {1053}.

Histopathology
The naevus cells are bland, usually pigmented, spindle cells with small fusiform nuclei, dispersed chromatin, and indistinct nucleoli. The nuclei may show a longitudinal fold (chromatin stripe) or pseudonuclear inclusions. The naevus cells may have elongated cellular processes (dendritic cells), a more epithelioid appearance, or vacuolated cytoplasm (balloon cells). One classification system categorizes iris naevi as melanocytomas, spindle cell naevi with surface plaque, spindle cell naevi with a stromal component, and epithelioid cell naevi {532}.

Differential diagnosis
The differential diagnosis includes melanoma, metastasis, cysts, and non-melanocytic lesions (e.g. xanthogranuloma, neurofibroma, and leiomyoma) {1092}.

Genetic profile
GNA11 or *GNAQ* mutations, found in 83% of uveal melanomas, are also present in a smaller proportion of cutaneous blue naevi and naevi of Ota, but not in

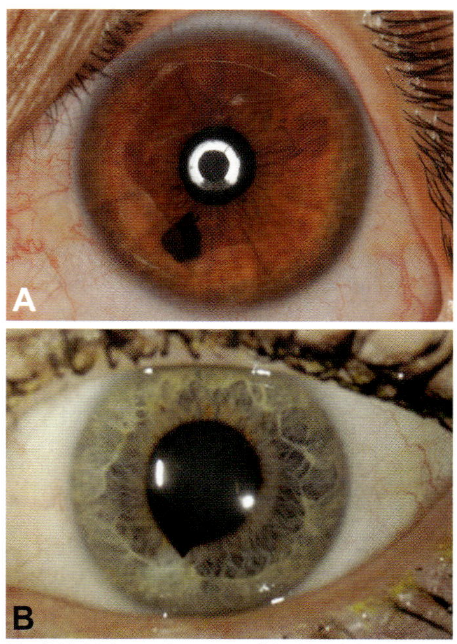

Fig. 2.11 Melanocytic naevus of the iris. **A** A pigmented naevus at the 7 o'clock position. **B** An amelanotic naevus at the 7 o'clock position.

common naevi {1306}. Recent genetic studies of iris naevi have identified mutations in *EIF1AX*, *NRAS*, *PTEN*, *KIT*, and *TP53* as well as *GNAQ* and *GNA11* {1048,1304}. Some iris naevi harbour *BAP1* mutations; these cases have been designated iris melanocytic tumours of uncertain malignant potential {1304}.

Prognosis and predictive factors
Most naevi are stable. Periodic examinations with photographic documentation and ultrasound are recommended to monitor for increasing lesion size and other features suggestive of progression to melanoma {200}.

Ocular melanocytosis

Singh A.
Kivelä T.T.

Definition
Ocular melanocytosis is a congenitally increased population of non-proliferating hyperpigmented melanocytes.

ICD-O code
None

Synonyms
Ocular melanocytosis: melanosis oculi
When occurring together with adjacent cutaneous melanocytosis: oculodermal melanocytosis; naevus of Ota; naevus fusco-caeruleus ophthalmo-maxillaris
When occurring together with naevus flammeus: phakomatosis pigmentovascularis

Epidemiology
Ocular and oculodermal melanocytoses combined occur in approximately 0.04% of White people, in 1.4–2.7% of all patients with uveal melanoma, and in 3.1–4.3% of young patients with uveal melanoma {15,164,412,1088}. These disorders are believed to be more common among Asians, but prevalence data are not available.

Etiology
This is a congenital hamartoma-like disorder.

Localization
Ocular melanocytosis is usually unilateral. It can involve, in a diffuse or sectoral pattern, any or all of the following: the sclera, iris, ciliary body, choroid, and orbit. Ocular melanocytosis associated with adjacent cutaneous pigmentation is called oculodermal melanocytosis.

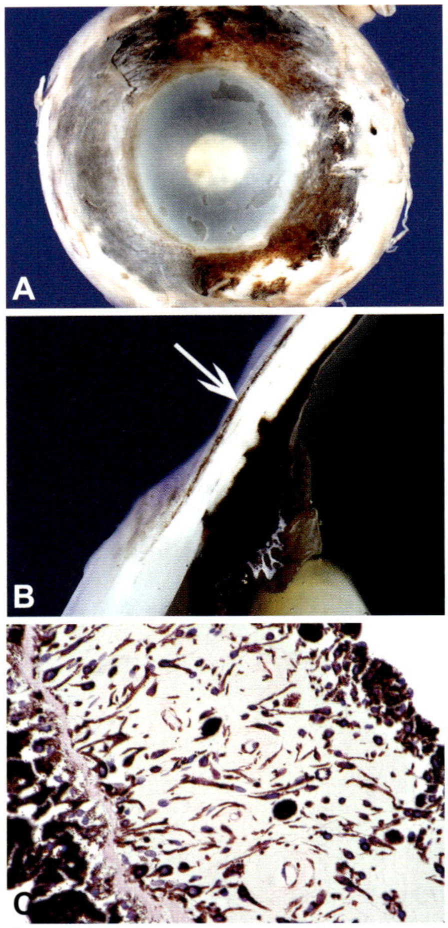

Fig. 2.12 Oculodermal melanocytosis. **A** A macroscopic image showing episcleral pigmentation of the globe. **B** A macroscopic image showing the episcleral brown pigment on cut surface (arrow). **C** Heavily pigmented melanocytes on the iris surface and in the stroma.

Clinical features
Patients present with hyperchromic heterochromia that gives the iris a velvety or mammillated appearance, which is especially striking if the fellow (uninvolved) eye is blue. There is slate-grey, patchy pigmentation of the sclera, as well as dark-brown choroid. In oculodermal melanocytosis, there is cutaneous hyperpigmentation in the trigeminal distribution (V1 or V2); adjacent orbital tissues may also be involved.

Histopathology
The iris and choroid are heavily pigmented and slightly thickened because of increased numbers of heavily pigmented melanocytes; there is some resemblance to melanocytoma {1394}. Similar melanocytes are abundant in the ciliary body and between scleral lamellae. Mitoses are not seen. Thickened areas should be carefully examined to exclude an embedded early uveal melanoma.

Differential diagnosis
The differential diagnosis includes diffuse uveal melanoma and conjunctival melanosis.

Histogenesis
The histogenesis of ocular melanocytosis is similar to that of cellular blue naevus and Mongolian spot; it involves abnormal migration of neural crest–derived melanocytes to the eye and dermis rather than to the dermoepidermal junction {293}.

Genetic profile
Somatic activating mutations of *GNA11* or *GNAQ* have been found in some cases associated with cutaneous melanocytosis, as well as in phakomatosis pigmentovascularis {1257}.

Prognosis and predictive factors
Ocular melanocytosis in itself is innocuous; however, it is associated with an increased risk of glaucoma {917}. It is also an important predisposing factor for uveal melanoma, associated with a lifetime risk of 1 in 400 {1180}. In atypical cases of uveal melanoma, such as multifocal, bilateral, and paediatric cases, as well as in orbital and leptomeningeal melanomas, underlying melanocytosis should be suspected. Melanocytosis-associated uveal melanomas may have a higher risk of metastasis {15,763,1091}. The association with uveal melanoma may be due to a shared predisposing mutation in *GNAQ* {1305}.

Lisch nodule

Schoenfield L.
Cummings T.
Stemmer-Rachamimov A.O.

Definition
A Lisch nodule is an iris hamartoma consisting of a proliferation of melanocytes (a naevus) occurring in the setting of neurofibromatosis type 1 (NF1). Lisch nodules are one of the seven National Institutes of Health (NIH) criteria for the diagnosis of

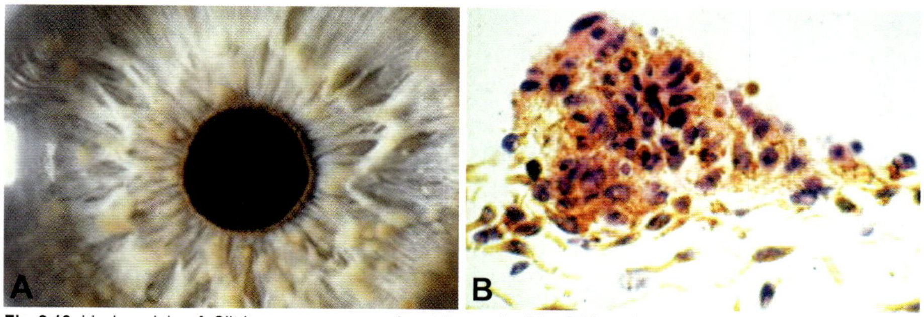

Fig. 2.13 Lisch nodule. **A** Slit-lamp appearance of nodules on the iris. **B** There is a proliferation of melanocytes with benign cytological features on the surface of the iris.

NF1 {848}, and they are the most common ocular manifestation of the disorder.

ICD-O code
None

Synonyms
Sakurai–Lisch nodule; iris hamartoma; melanocytic hamartoma
The term "benign tumour of the iris" has been proposed because of the possible role of ultraviolet (UV) radiation (presumably via DNA damage) in Lisch nodules' development {115}.

Epidemiology
NF1 is an autosomal dominant disorder (phakomatosis); it is the most common of the three types of neurofibromatosis (the other types being neurofibromatosis type 2 and schwannomatosis). NF1 has an estimated birth prevalence of 1 case per 3000 live births, with no predilection for race, sex, ethnicity, or geographical location {380}. Lisch nodules have been found in 95% of all patients with NF1 and in 100% of those aged ≥ 16 years {503}.

Etiology
The etiological factors include *NF1* mutation with other genetic factors, iris colour, and possibly UV radiation exposure modifiers {115}.

Localization
Lisch nodules occur in the iris, usually in the inferior hemifield {115}.

Clinical features
Lisch nodules appear in early childhood, first arising in children aged about 2 years. The lesions present as dome-shaped or confluent nodules, sometimes with ragged borders. They may be creamy white in dark-coloured irides or brown in light-coloured irides {3}.

Histopathology
There is a spindle-type naevus on the anterior surface of the iris.

Differential diagnosis
The differential diagnosis includes naevi, primary melanoma, and (in particular in the absence of NF1) metastases.

Histogenesis
The histogenesis is related to *NF1* mutation and possibly UV radiation–induced DNA damage {115}.

Genetic profile
NF1 is caused by heterozygous loss of function mutations in the tumour suppressor gene *NF1* (chromosome 17q11.2) {80}, which encodes neurofibromin (NF1), a negative regulator of RAS signalling. Disease penetrance is 100%, but the phenotypic expressivity varies. De novo (spontaneous) mutations occur in approximately 50% of affected individuals {554}.

Genetic susceptibility
Genetic susceptibility is associated with *NF1* gene mutations, which show variable expressivity, even within families; this variability is attributed to genetic and possibly environmental modifiers {115, 307,1235}.

Prognosis and predictive factors
Lisch nodules do not interfere with vision. Patients with NF1 have other ocular abnormalities, such as plexiform neurofibromas, optic pathway gliomas, and choroidal naevi, as well as cutaneous neurofibromas. There is an 8–16% lifetime risk of developing malignant peripheral nerve sheath tumour, generally from a pre-existing plexiform neurofibroma {332,1294}. A reported 50–80% of children with NF1 have neurocognitive deficits {1294}.

Pigmented epithelial cyst of the iris

Bechrakis N.E.
Eagle R.C. Jr
Kivelä T.T.

Definition
Pigmented epithelial cyst of the iris is a cystic lesion arising from the iris pigment epithelium at the posterior iris surface.

ICD-O code
None

Synonym
Iris flocculi (multiple pigmented epithelial cysts at the pupillary margin)

Epidemiology
Cysts of the iris pigment epithelium are detected most often in young adults; 34% of cases are diagnosed in the third or fourth decade of life {1152}.

Etiology
In most cases the etiology is unknown. Rare cases can be inherited in an autosomal dominant pattern with variable penetrance. There have been reports of pigmented epithelial cysts developing secondary to chronic topical use of miotics (e.g. pilocarpine) or prostaglandin $F_{2\alpha}$ analogues (e.g. latanoprost) {728,1142,1152,1162,1361}.

Localization
Primary cysts of the iris pigment epithelium can be peripheral (63% of cases), mid-zonal (28%), central at the pupillary margin (7%), or dislodged/free-floating in either the anterior chamber or the vitreous cavity (2%) {1152}.

Clinical features
Iris pigmented epithelial cysts can be singular or multiple, and some are bilateral. They are dark-brown matte lesions that vary in size and can bulge the iris stroma forwards towards the anterior chamber. The cysts are easier to see after pupillary dilatation, and they can roll anteriorly over the pupillary margin. Iris pigmented epithelial cysts can collapse spontaneously or after laser treatment (which is rarely necessary).
Iris pigmented epithelial cysts can induce an anterior shift of the iris stroma, mimicking solid neoplasia. Epithelial cysts can

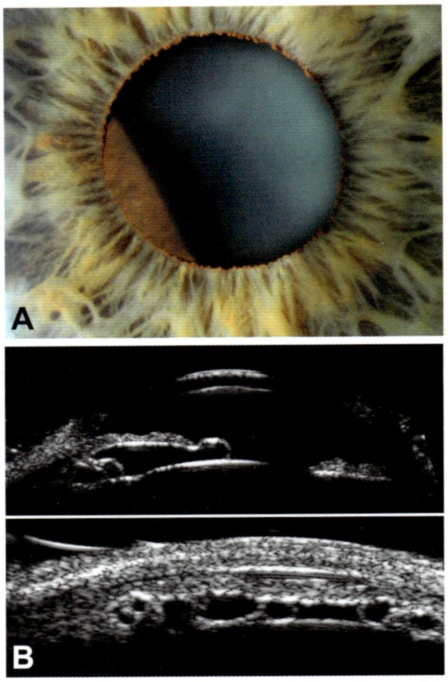

Fig. 2.14 Iris/ciliary body pigmented epithelial cyst. **A** A cyst is visible at the pupillary margin. **B** Longitudinal and transversal ultrasound biomicroscopy sections revealed multiple cysts in this patient.

also arise from the epithelial layers of the ciliary body; cysts that arise from the outer layer are pigmented, whereas cysts that arise from the inner layer are non-pigmented and have the same presentation as cysts arising from the pigmented double epithelial layers of the iris.

Histopathology
Iris pigmented epithelial cysts contain clear fluid or keratin flocculi in their lumen, surrounded by a monolayer of pigmented epithelial cells.

Differential diagnosis
The differential diagnosis includes primary iris stromal cyst, iris melanoma, iris melanocytoma, ciliary body melanoma, ciliary body melanocytoma, adenoma of the iris pigment epithelium, and medulloepithelioma.

Genetic susceptibility
Most iris pigmented epithelial cysts are sporadic, but there have been a few reports of an autosomal dominant pattern of inheritance (with variable penetrance) in multiple and bilateral cases.

Prognosis and predictive factors
The prognosis is excellent. Treatment is usually unnecessary for asymptomatic cases, but cysts may be excised or decompressed if necessary. Iris flocculi may be associated with dissecting aortic aneurysm; therefore, patients with this condition should have their aorta imaged {1142}.

Implantation cyst of the iris

Bechrakis N.E.
Eagle R.C. Jr
Kivelä T.T.

Definition
Implantation cyst of the iris is a squamous epithelium–lined cyst.

ICD-O code
None

Synonyms
Primary iris stromal cyst; acquired epithelial implantation cyst

Etiology
Iris stromal cysts are defined as primary if there is no recognizable cause and secondary if they are induced by penetrating anterior chamber injury. Epithelial, mesenchymal, and/or conjunctival goblet cells can be introduced into the anterior chamber as a result of trauma, giving rise to a secondary implantation cyst {159,1003}.

Localization
Iris stromal cysts can arise anywhere on or in the iris, but they occur most commonly in the mid-periphery and the inferior or superonasal quadrant {729}.

Clinical features
Iris stromal cysts have a thin, slightly translucent anterior wall, allowing visualization of the iris pigment epithelium through the (usually atrophic) underlying iris stroma. The cysts contain a clear or slightly opaque fluid and can be septated by thin translucent membranes. They tend to enlarge towards the chamber angle and optical axis, inducing secondary glaucoma, corneal oedema, and amblyopia {159,729,1003}.

Histopathology
Primary iris stromal cysts are lined by multilayered stratified squamous epithelium, with or without goblet cells. Keratinization has been found in some cases, and corneal endothelial cells covering the cyst wall have also been described.

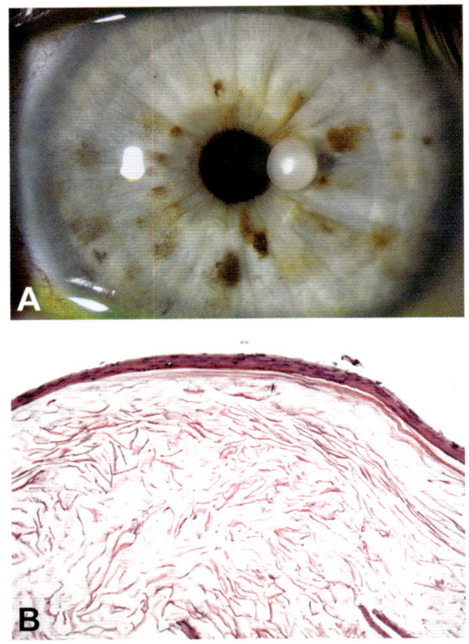

Fig. 2.15 Implantation cyst on the iris stroma. **A** A cyst with opaque content close to the pupillary margin, after cataract extraction and corneal lamellar surgery. **B** Microscopic examination of the cyst reveals an epithelial implantation cyst lined by stratified keratinized epithelium, containing keratin within the lumen.

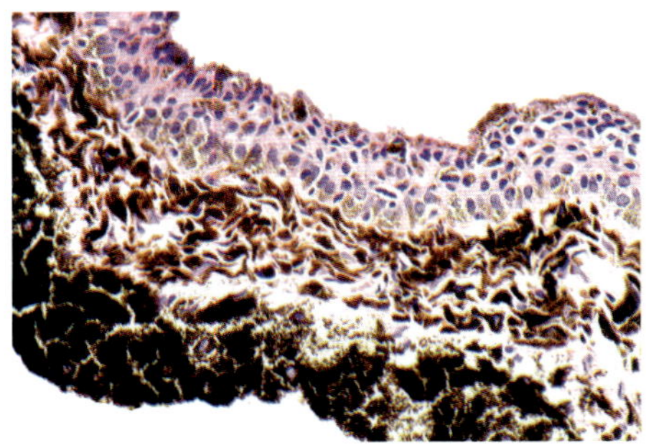

Fig. 2.16 Congenital iris stromal cyst. The cyst is lined by non-keratinized stratified squamous epithelium; its histological appearance is similar to that of an implantation cyst.

Differential diagnosis
The differential diagnosis includes pigmented and non-pigmented tumours of the iris such as melanoma, melanocytoma, iris metastases, leiomyoma, juvenile xanthogranuloma, and various types of inflammatory and autoimmune-associated granulomas of the iris surface and stroma {407}.

Histogenesis
Iris stromal cysts probably originate as a result of the implantation of cells from

the eye surface into the anterior chamber, iris surface, or iris stroma; this may occur at various points during prenatal development or after birth. Some cases have been associated with penetrating trauma, including inadvertent penetration of the anterior chamber during amniocentesis.

Prognosis and predictive factors

Surgical excision or drainage may be necessary, because of the high probability of progressive enlargement of the cyst with involvement of the visual axis and the development of complications such as secondary glaucoma and cataract {638}.

Ectopic lacrimal gland in the iris

Cherepanoff S.
Kivelä T.T.

Definition

Ectopic lacrimal gland in the iris is a choristoma composed of lacrimal gland tissue.

ICD-O code

None

Synonym

Heterotopic lacrimal gland

Epidemiology

The incidence in unknown. Fewer than 20 case reports of ectopic lacrimal gland in the iris have been published, with most of the reported cases occurring in an infant or young child {1134,1140}. Most lacrimal ectopias are found in extraocular sites (such as the orbit and conjunctiva) {910,921}.

Etiology

Possible etiologies include displacement of lacrimal buds during closure of the fetal fissure, implantation of surface ectoderm during lens formation, extension of lacrimal tissue before the closure of scleral defects during fetal life, and aberrant differentiation of pluripotent intraocular cells {218}.

Localization

Ectopic lacrimal gland in the iris is found in the stroma of the iris.

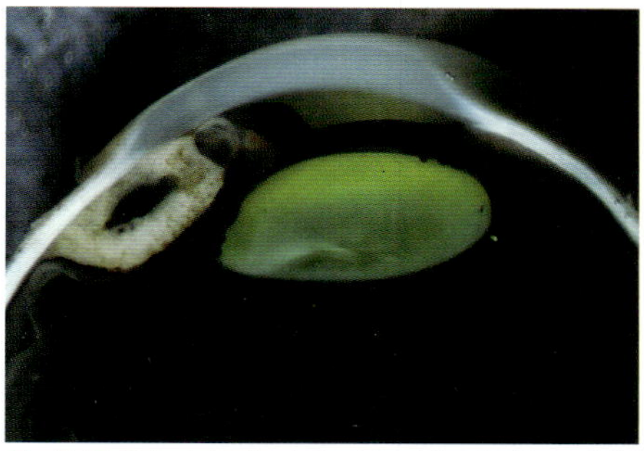

Fig. 2.17 Ectopic lacrimal gland involving the iris and ciliary body. In this case, the bulk of the lesion is localized within the pars plicata of the ciliary body, with involvement of the iris root; cysts can be discerned within the iris component.

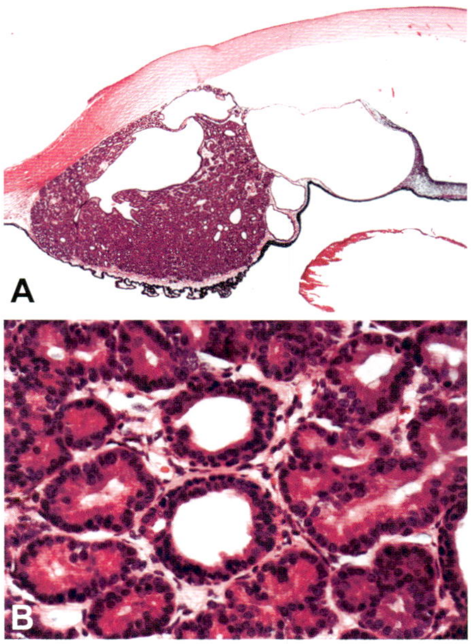

Fig. 2.18 Ectopic lacrimal gland involving the iris and ciliary body. **A** Low-power microscopy confirms the presence of a well-circumscribed mass composed of lacrimal tissue, involving the pars plicata and iris root; prominent, cystically dilated lacrimal ducts are present; the lesion obliterates the iridocorneal angle, which can lead to closed-angle glaucoma. **B** High-power microscopy reveals histologically normal lacrimal acini and ducts.

Clinical features

This ectopia is typically diagnosed in infants or children aged < 6 years. It presents as a fleshy pink mass with an irregular nodular surface and may appear vascularized {636,1140}. The lesion can become cystic and expand, obstructing the iridocorneal angle and leading to secondary closed-angle glaucoma {631}. In most reported cases, resection or enucleation of the eye was necessary for definitive histological diagnosis. In some cases, it may be possible to diagnose this lesion by fine-needle aspiration biopsy {636}.

Histopathology

Ectopic lacrimal tissue has the histological appearance of benign acini and ducts of the normal lacrimal gland. The ducts can become cystically dilated (dacryops), and their lining epithelium may become attenuated.

Differential diagnosis

A number of clinical differential diagnoses exist, but ectopic lacrimal gland in the iris is histologically distinctive and readily diagnosed.

Histogenesis

Lacrimal gland ectopias consist of benign lacrimal tissue in an ectopic site. They may arise during fetal life or as a result of aberrant differentiation of pluripotent intraocular cells.

Prognosis and predictive factors

Clinical follow-up is recommended, to prevent vision loss due to lesional growth and secondary glaucoma {1134}. Phthisis of the eye can result in cases not being treated. Malignant transformation has not been reported.

Histiocytic tumours of the iris

Iacob C.E.
Kivelä T.T.
Margo C.
Meyer P.
Singh A.

Definition

Histiocytic tumours of the iris include involvement by several histiocytic disorders, all of which are rare except for juvenile xanthogranuloma.

Juvenile xanthogranuloma is a benign, self-healing, cutaneous proliferation of macrophages and Touton-type multinucleated giant cells with a variable degree of lipidization, in the absence of a metabolic disorder.

Rosai–Dorfman disease is a non-neoplastic histiocytic proliferation that usually has an indolent clinical course.

Langerhans cell histiocytosis is a neoplastic clonal expansion of myeloid-derived Langerhans cell histiocytes categorized as antigen-presenting dendritic cells.

Erdheim–Chester disease is a clonal systemic proliferation of macrophages, commonly having a foamy xanthomatous component and containing Touton-type multinucleated giant cells.

A revised classification of histiocytoses and macrophage-dendritic cell neoplasms has been published {322A}. In the 2017 revision of the *WHO classification of tumours of haematopoietic and lymphoid tissues* {1231}, Langerhans cell histiocytosis and Erdheim–Chester disease are grouped with histiocytic and dendritic cell neoplasms because of the finding of activating mutations in the MAPK pathway, most commonly BRAF p.V600E mutations {322B}.

ICD-O codes

Langerhans cell histiocytosis	9751/1
Erdheim–Chester disease	9749/3

Synonyms

Juvenile xanthogranuloma: xanthogranuloma; solitary xanthogranuloma; naevoxanthoendothelioma

Langerhans cell histiocytosis: Langerhans cell granulomatosis; histiocytosis X; eosinophilic granuloma; Hand–Schüller–Christian disease; Letterer–Siwe disease

Erdheim–Chester disease: lipogranulomatosis; lipoid granulomatosis; polyostotic sclerosing histiocytosis

Epidemiology

Juvenile xanthogranuloma of the uvea occurs in > 70% of cases in the iris {262,1028} and accounts for about 3% of all paediatric iris tumours. It occurs in 0.3–0.4% of children with cutaneous juvenile xanthogranuloma {178,1092}. It usually appears in infants and only rarely in adults. The children at highest risk are aged ≤ 2 years, have multiple cutaneous lesions, and have newly diagnosed juvenile xanthogranuloma {178}. Intraocular involvement is rare in Rosai–Dorfman disease {77,509,1324}, Langerhans cell histiocytosis {45,127,604,737}, and Erdheim–Chester disease {2,1243}. Juvenile xanthogranulomas are diagnosed most commonly in infancy and childhood, with a slight male preponderance. The other diseases are rare, have a male-to-female ratio of about 3:1, and are usually diagnosed in adults.

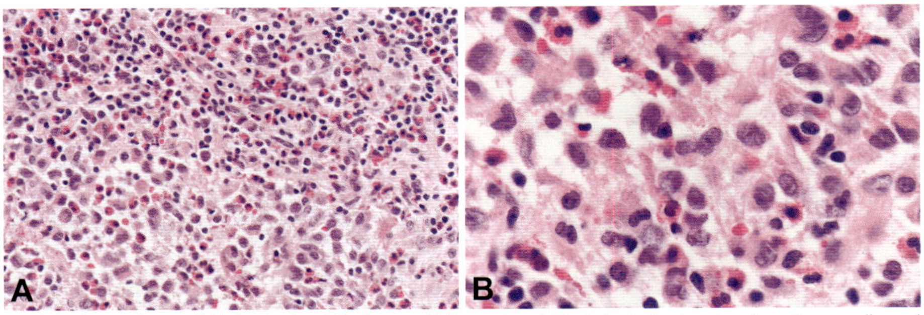

Fig. 2.19 Langerhans cell histiocytosis. **A** Background inflammatory infiltrate including lymphocytes, plasma cells, and numerous eosinophils. **B** Histiocytes with abundant pink (often vacuolated) cytoplasm and large vesicular nuclei with folds and grooves (oil immersion).

Localization

Histiocytic tumours can occur in any uveal location, although juvenile xanthogranulomas most often involve the iris {127}. Bilateral involvement can occur.

Clinical features

Juvenile xanthogranuloma of the iris is a localized nodular or diffuse tumour. The nodular type is a well-circumscribed orange mass. The diffuse type presents as a thin, transparent or heterochromic coat, usually on the iris surface. Spontaneous hyphaema is the presenting sign in 38% of iris lesions, and cells can shed into the aqueous humour {1092}. Ancillary diagnostic tests include anterior segment optical coherence tomography, ultrasound biomicroscopy, and fine-needle aspiration biopsy; these tests are especially useful when cutaneous lesions are absent, the presentation is atypical, or the response to steroids is poor {580,747,1027,1232}. Rosai–Dorfman disease has presented with a choroidal mass lesion {77,1324}. Intraocular Langerhans cell histiocytosis can present as a mass or can involve the uvea diffusely; spillover into the aqueous or vitreous mimics uveitis {1281}. Erdheim–Chester disease can cause a yellowish choroidal infiltrate or mass {2,1243}.

Histopathology

Juvenile xanthogranuloma is characterized by diffuse infiltration by foamy histiocytes, occasionally along with other inflammatory cells, including lymphocytes,

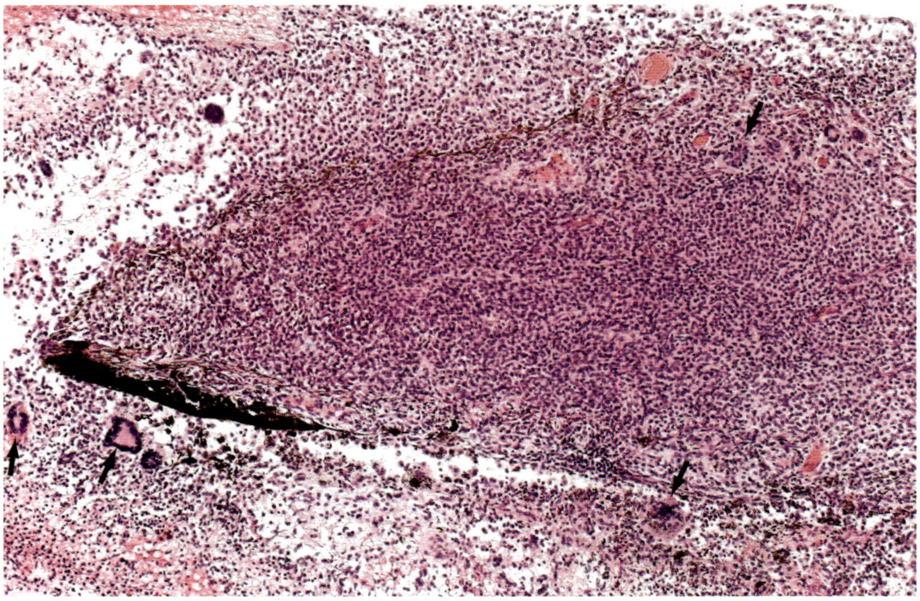

Fig. 2.20 Juvenile xanthogranuloma of iris in a 1-year-old child. There is diffuse infiltration of the iris by histiocytes and some Touton giant cells (arrows), with shedding into the anterior and posterior chamber; there are some thin-walled, engorged capillaries along the anterior surface of the iris.

eosinophils, and Touton giant cells. It often has thin-walled blood vessels. Immunohistochemistry is consistently positive for CD68, CD163, and fascin. There is usually positivity for CD4, CD11c, and factor XIIIa, and sometimes for CD31, whereas CD1a, CD21, CD34, langerin, and S100 protein are negative, except in interspersed cells {652,1030}.

In Rosai–Dorfman disease, there is a proliferation of histiocytes, including large cells with round vesicular nuclei and abundant pale eosinophilic cytoplasm. They are positive for S100 protein, CD68, and CD163 and negative for langerin and CD1a.

Langerhans cell histiocytosis is characterized by Langerhans cells with convoluted nuclei and a substantial amount of pink cytoplasm. Ultrastructurally, the cells contain Birbeck granules (pentalaminar tubules with dilated ends containing langerin). Immunohistochemistry is positive for histiocytic markers including CD68, CD163, and antichymotrypsin, and characteristically for HLA-DR, CD1a, S100 protein, and langerin (CD207). Ocular lesions usually have a mixed inflammatory background including lymphocytes, plasma cells, eosinophils, and neutrophils, with a variable number of Langerhans cells. Cytopathological diagnosis by fine-needle aspiration of the anterior chamber has been reported {1086}.

In Erdheim–Chester disease, the uvea is infiltrated by histiocytes with single small nuclei and foamy cytoplasm. Histiocytes with compact eosinophilic cytoplasm may be present. A few Touton giant cells and reactive inflammatory cells are frequently present. The neoplastic histiocytes express CD14, CD68, CD163, factor XIIIa, and fascin, and they are negative for S100 protein, CD1a, and langerin. Patients can simultaneously show other lesions consistent with Langerhans cell histiocytosis.

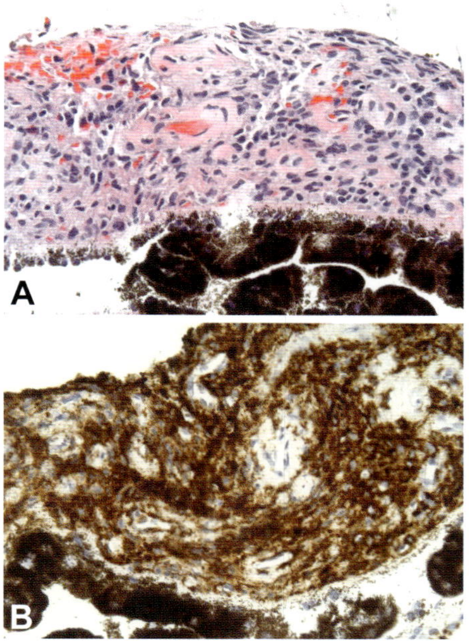

Fig. 2.21 Juvenile xanthogranuloma of iris in a child. **A** There is diffuse infiltration of the iris stroma by histiocytes and few eosinophils. **B** There is strong 3+ CD163 reactivity.

Differential diagnosis

The differential diagnosis includes diffuse so-called tapioca melanoma of the iris, choroidal melanoma and lymphoma, and uveal granulomas.

Histogenesis

These tumours develop from the macrophage/histiocyte lineage.

Genetic profile

The majority of Langerhans cell histiocytosis lesions show a BRAF p.V600E mutation responsible for activation of the MAPK/RAS/RAF/MEK/ERK cell signalling pathway {71,139,479,993}. The aberrant diffusion of Langerhans cells in the lymphoid system is driven by the upregulation of CCR7 (a chemokine receptor on the surface of Langerhans cells that binds to its specific ligands, CCL19 and CCL21, present in lymphoid tissue), with simultaneous downregulation of the normal epidermal Langerhans cell receptor CCR6 (a chemokine receptor on the surface of Langerhans cells that binds to its specific ligand, CCL20, present in skin and bone) {46,356}.

In Erdheim–Chester disease, activating mutations in MAPK pathway genes have been reported, most notably BRAF p.V600E (in > 50% of cases), as well as rarer mutations in *MAP2K1*, *ARAF*, *MAP2K2*, *NRAS*, and *KRAS*.

Genetic susceptibility

There is no known genetic susceptibility. Of note, juvenile xanthogranulomas occur in 20–30% of patients with neurofibromatosis type 1 {723}.

Prognosis and predictive factors

Juvenile xanthogranuloma of the iris can lead to blinding complications such as hyphaema, secondary glaucoma, and amblyopia. Treatment is usually nonsurgical, because topical or periocular corticosteroids eradicate juvenile xanthogranuloma {1028}. Refractory cases often respond to systemic corticosteroids; alternatively, intraocular anti-VEGF injection can be considered {57}.

The prognosis of other intraocular histiocytic tumours depends on the number and location of the lesions and the initial response to therapy.

Tumours of the ciliary body

Uveal melanocytoma

Eagle R.C. Jr
Kivelä T.T.
Laver N.
Loeffler K.U.
Pe'er J.
Salomao D.R.
Wilson M.

Definition
Uveal melanocytoma is an intensely pigmented subtype of ciliary body, iris, and choroidal naevi, composed of large, plump, polyhedral cells.

ICD-O code
Melanocytoma (of the ciliary body, iris, and choroid) 8726/0

Synonym
Magnocellular naevus

Epidemiology
The incidence of uveal melanocytomas is unknown. They account for 3% of iris naevi {268}. A total of < 100 ciliary body cases with pathological confirmation have been reported. Choroidal melanocytomas are equally rare. The reported patient age at presentation ranges from infancy to 90 years {697,1155}. In children and adolescents, melanocytomas account for 7% of melanocytic iris lesions {1092}. The median age at diagnosis is 40–45 years. About 9% of iris melanocytomas occur in Black patients, whereas only 2% of ordinary iris naevi occur in this population {268,1090}. A female-to-male ratio of 2:1 was noted in the largest reported series {268}. Aside from these findings, the distribution of melanocytomas by sex and in different races is reported to be nearly equal {330}. In dark-skinned individuals, uveal melanocytomas are more common than uveal melanomas {730,1155,1187}.

Etiology
The etiology is unknown, but melanocytoma is assumed to be congenital.

Localization
At this anatomical site, melanocytoma arises in the stroma of the iris, with or without extension to the chamber angle {268,689}, ciliary body {730}, or choroid {330}. See also *Melanocytoma of the optic disc and optic nerve* (p. 142).

Clinical features
Most iris melanocytomas are asymptomatic, and 70% are incidental findings {268}. About 15% of patients are first alerted by a dark spot on the iris; the rest by symptoms such as blurred vision. At the time of diagnosis, about 50% of iris melanocytomas have seeded the adjacent iris surface, chamber angle, or both, and some have formed satellites {268}. At baseline and by 15 years after diagnosis, respectively, approximately 5% and 50% of cases have caused secondary glaucoma. Most iris melanocytomas are nodular with an irregular surface and lack visible blood vessels, but one fifth are diffuse {268,588}. The majority of ciliary body melanocytomas probably go unrecognized; the diagnosed cases are typically those that erode through the iris root, seed the anterior chamber and trabecular meshwork, focally shallow the anterior chamber, induce a sectoral cataract, extend extraocularly, or have sentinel episcleral vessels. The clinical appearance of choroidal melanocytomas may be similar to that of a choroidal naevus or a small melanoma {980,1155}. In most cases, they form a discoid or dome-shaped dark-grey or black mass that elevates the retina. In a few cases, the presence of overlying orange pigment and subretinal fluid makes the distinction from choroidal melanoma even more difficult {330}. Ultrasound biomicroscopy and anterior segment optical coherence tomography are useful ancillary examinations for iris and ciliary body melanocytomas {106,292,1155}. Fine-needle aspiration or cutter biopsy may aid in the diagnosis {65,268,804}.

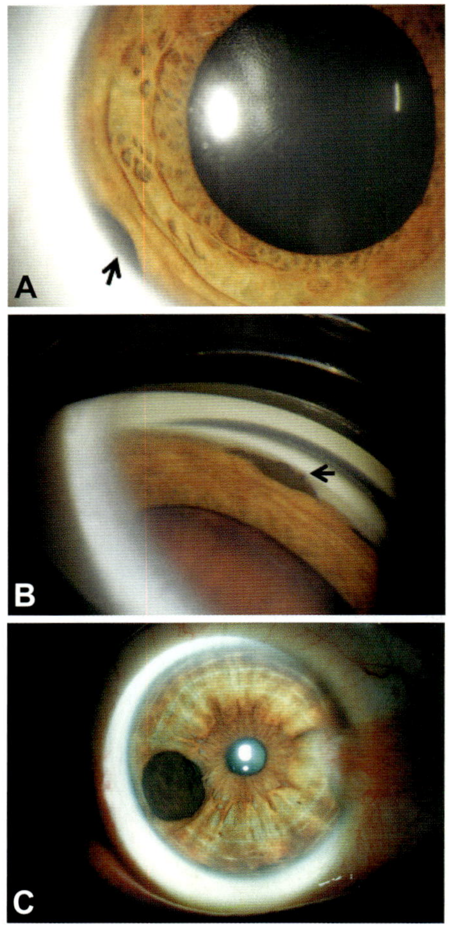

Fig. 2.22 Uveal melanocytoma. **A,B** Ciliary body melanocytoma; there is dark pigment at the 7 o'clock position (**A**); gonioscopy shows the mass to be eroding through the angle to involve the iris root (**B**). **C** Iris melanocytoma; a dark-brown dome-shaped tumour in the 8 o'clock meridian of the iris in a 58-year-old patient.

Histopathology
On gross examination, the tumour appears dark brown to jet black, with full thickness. Most iris melanocytomas measure 1–5 mm in diameter. Choroidal and ciliary body melanocytomas usually replace the normal uvea and measure 1–5 mm in thickness. Ciliary body lesions may be larger than other melanocytomas because they must attain a larger size before they can be detected. Their abundant intracytoplasmic melanin pigment obscures cellular details. Foci of spontaneous necrosis may be seen in larger melanocytomas. Paraffin-embedded sections must be bleached to reveal the cytological detail and identify plump

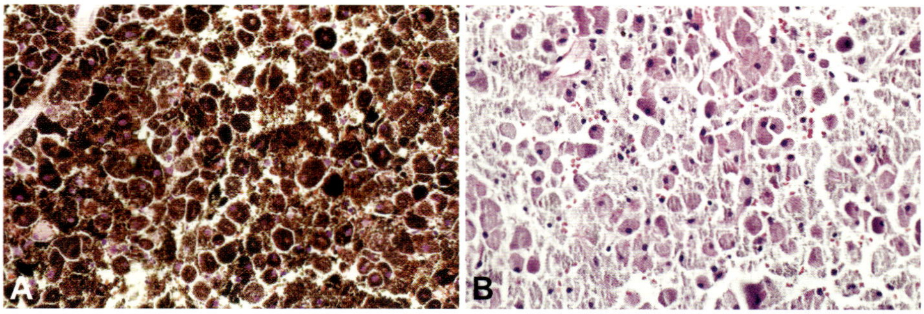

Fig. 2.23 Choroidal melanocytoma. **A** The neoplasm is composed of large polyhedral cells with abundant intracytoplasmic melanin pigment obscuring nuclear details. **B** Bleaching reveals tumour cells with abundant cytoplasm and small nuclei with inconspicuous nucleoli without nuclear atypia; no mitoses are seen.

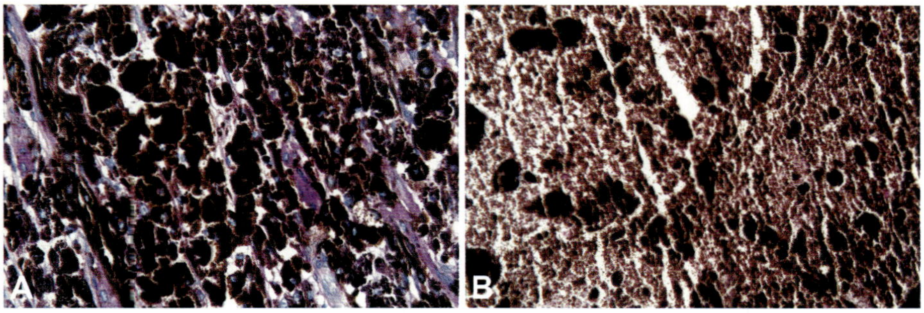

Fig. 2.24 Iris melanocytoma. **A** Periodic acid–Schiff (PAS) staining highlights large polyhedral melanocytes in which the cellular detail and even the nuclei are mostly obscured by very heavy pigmentation. **B** An adjacent area with spontaneous necrosis.

polyhedral cells with bland nuclei, small nucleoli, and a low N:C ratio. Pigment dispersion and melanophages are frequent. Mitotic figures are absent or rare.

Differential diagnosis
The differential diagnosis includes iris, ciliary body, and choroidal melanomas; ordinary naevi in these locations; adenoma and adenocarcinoma of the pigmented iris and ciliary epithelium or retinal pigment epithelium; and cysts of the pigmented iris epithelium.

Histogenesis
Melanocytomas arise from melanocytes of neural crest origin.

Genetic profile
A genetic study of two ciliochoroidal melanocytomas revealed *GNAQ* mutations {828}, which were also present in 2 of 6 cases in another series: an iridociliary melanocytoma and an optic nerve melanocytoma {372}. Melanocytomas with *GNAQ* mutations can rarely progress to melanoma; those that do so have been found to have *BAP1* mutations {372}.

Prognosis and predictive factors
Iris and ciliary body melanocytomas may be monitored with clinical examination, photography, ultrasound biomicroscopy, and optical coherence tomography. Those that involve, extend to, or seed the chamber angle must be followed up for secondary melanocytomalytic glaucoma {268,672,1117,1155}. Growth (sometimes rapid) and spontaneous necrosis can occur {672,1073}. Resection may be warranted if the tumour grows or induces secondary glaucoma. The prognosis for survival is excellent, except in rare instances of malignant transformation to melanoma {81,506,670,698,828,1019}.

Adenocarcinoma of the ciliary body

Moulin A.
Eagle R.C. Jr

Definition
Adenocarcinoma of the ciliary body is a malignant epithelial tumour arising from the pigmented or non-pigmented ciliary epithelium.

ICD-O code
Ciliary body adenocarcinoma 8140/3

Synonyms
Malignant non-pigmented or pigmented ciliary body adenocarcinoma; pleomorphic ciliary body adenocarcinoma

Epidemiology
The incidence of non-pigmented and (rarer) pigmented ciliary body adenocarcinomas is highest among adults in the fifth decade of life, with no clear sex predilection. Pleomorphic ciliary body adenocarcinoma usually affects patients in their eighth decade of life. Few cases have been reported in Black {433,754} or Asian {694,1226} patients.

Etiology
The etiology is unknown. Several cases have been reported in phthisical eyes several years after a trauma or chronic inflammation {299,460,687}.

Localization
At this anatomical site, adenocarcinomas arise within the ciliary body and can infiltrate the iris and angle and eventually exteriorize to the ocular surface anteriorly with formation of an epibulbar mass {23,433,460,687,985} or posteriorly via the scleral channels.

Clinical features
The symptoms range from decreased visual acuity to incidental discovery of

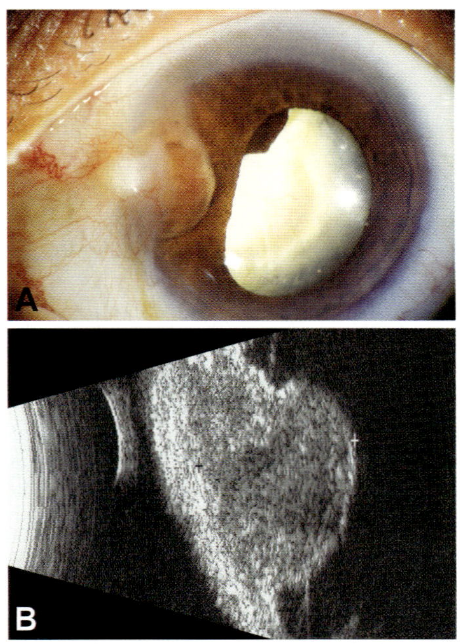

Fig. 2.25 Ciliary body adenocarcinoma. **A** A partially pigmented ciliary body mass extending to the iris surface. **B** B-scan ultrasonography shows a mass with abrupt borders.

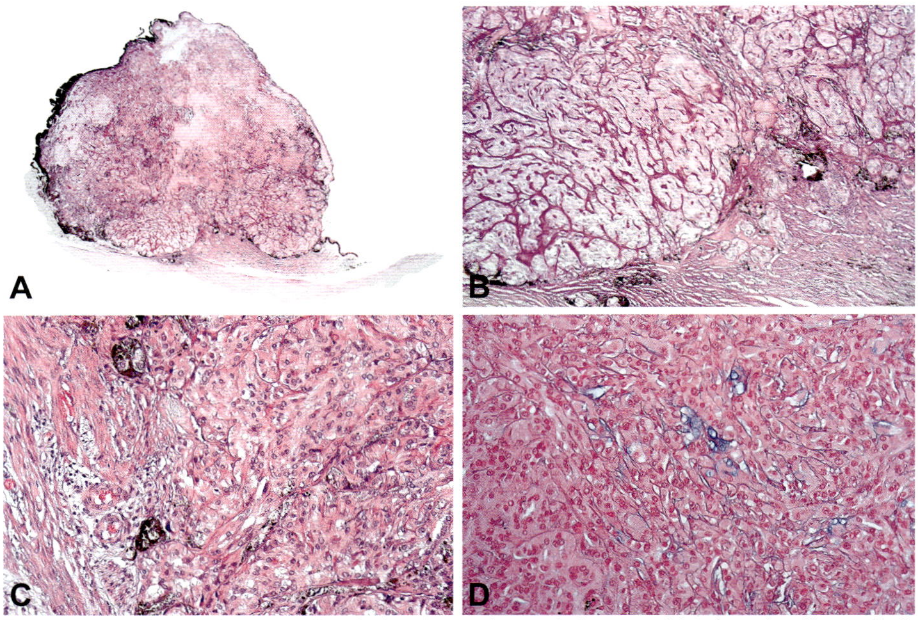

Fig. 2.26 Low-grade non-pigmented ciliary body adenocarcinoma. **A** A mass arising from the ciliary epithelium. **B** Strands and cords of cuboidal and epithelioid cells with moderate pleomorphism surrounded by a basal membrane network that gives a positive periodic acid–Schiff (PAS) reaction. **C** The cells infiltrate the ciliary body stroma and muscle. **D** Occasional intracellular and extracellular mucopolysaccharides can be highlighted with Alcian blue staining.

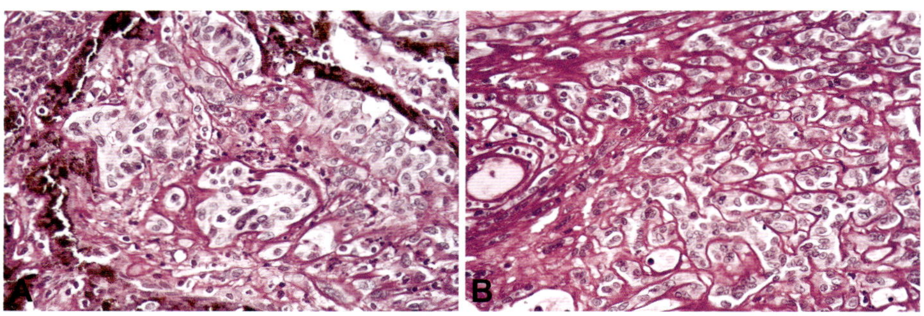

Fig. 2.27 Pleomorphic ciliary body adenocarcinoma. **A,B** Strands of epithelioid cells with irregular nuclei containing prominent nucleoli; there is a dense network of basal membrane that gives a positive periodic acid–Schiff (PAS) reaction.

an iris mass. Ciliary body adenocarcinomas can appear as a greyish, yellowish, or pinkish mass, or as a dark mass with an irregular surface, sometimes associated with lens subluxation, cataract, or mild inflammation. Ultrasonographically, these tumours are hyper-reflective and show a solid homogeneous aspect with abrupt borders.

Histopathology

Non-pigmented ciliary body adenocarcinomas are composed of strands, cords, and duct-like structures of cuboidal to epithelioid cells with enlarged and irregular nuclei with prominent nucleoli. The cells are frequently surrounded by a meshwork of basal membrane material that gives a positive periodic acid–Schiff (PAS) reaction. Papillary, solid, and pleomorphic variants have been described {1422}. Mucopolysaccharides (mostly extracellular) can be seen {541}. Pigmented ciliary body adenocarcinomas are populated by heavily pigmented cells commonly associated with vacuoles (which are thought to be extracellular) {1221}. Local tissue invasion and necrosis are elements suggestive of malignancy.

The cells are immunoreactive for epithelial markers such as pancytokeratin (AE1/AE3), CK8/18, and CK5/6. In pigmented cases, expression {1226} and absence of expression {1040} of melanocytic markers (e.g. melan-A, MITF, and HMB45 antigen) have both been documented.

Differential diagnosis

The differential diagnosis includes ciliary body melanoma. In small biopsy specimens, the differential diagnosis with a ciliary body adenoma can be difficult if the atypia is not striking.

Histogenesis

The histogenesis is unknown. Adenocarcinoma of the ciliary body is presumed to arise de novo or from longstanding reactive hyperplasia or adenoma {1129}.

Genetic profile

Comparative genomic hybridization has been performed on only one case, in a patient with a non-pigmented ciliary body adenocarcinoma showing 6p gains and 6q losses {858}. *BRAF* mutations are found in some cases {823}.

Prognosis and predictive factors

The prognosis is usually good. A few fatal cases of exteriorized tumour, usually associated with intracranial invasion {299,687}, and more rarely with metastasis {687}, have been described.

Ciliary body adenoma

Rao N.
Croxatto J.O.
Loeffler K.U.
Li B.

Definition

Ciliary body adenoma is a benign neoplasm of the pigmented ciliary epithelium (pigmented epithelial adenoma) and/or the non-pigmented ciliary epithelium (non-pigmented epithelial adenoma).

ICD-O code

Ciliary body adenoma	8140/0

Epidemiology

These rare tumours generally occur in middle-aged individuals, with no sex predilection {183}.

Localization

Ciliary body adenoma occurs in the ciliary epithelium.

Clinical features

These tumours are often asymptomatic, but they may be associated with visual disturbances due to local inflammation, secondary glaucoma, cataract, or lens subluxation. They can protrude into the posterior chamber and may extend

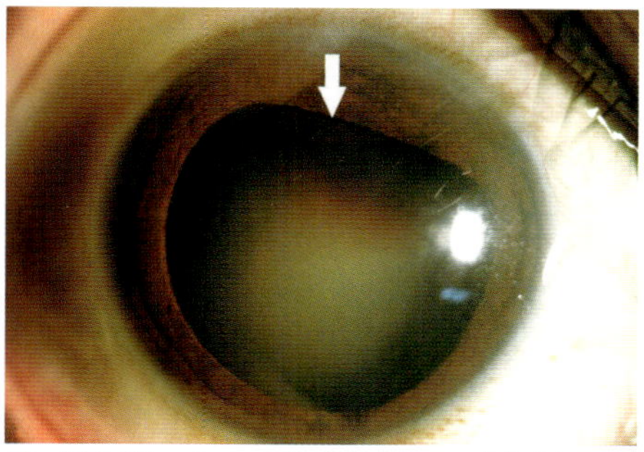

Fig. 2.28 Ciliary body epithelial adenoma. A dark-brown, well-defined, solid mass (arrow) located behind the iris.

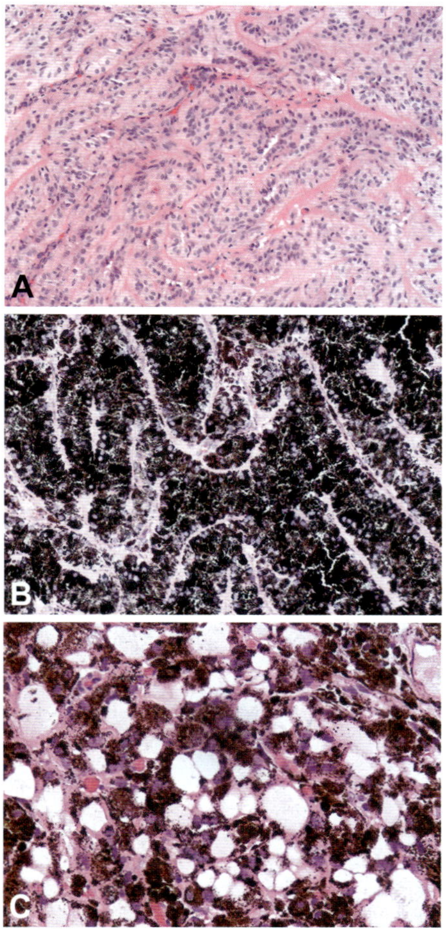

Fig. 2.29 Ciliary body epithelial adenoma. **A** Non-pigmented adenoma; the neoplastic cells exhibit a glandular pattern, with hyalinized stroma. **B** Pigmented adenoma; the tumour consists mostly of cords and nests of pigmented epithelial cells separated by prominent septa of vascularized fibrous connective tissue. **C** Pigmented adenoma; the vacuolated tumour cells contain numerous intracellular melanin granules.

anteriorly to involve the iris and anterior chamber {1133,1138}.
Pigmented epithelial adenomas are dark grey to black, and they block light on globe transillumination. Non-pigmented adenomas are greyish-white, vascularized, multilobular masses that transmit light on transillumination.
Ultrasound of both pigmented and non-pigmented epithelial adenomas reveals a well-circumscribed mass with medium to high internal reflectivity. The median diameter of these tumours is about 5 mm. On MRI, non-pigmented epithelial adenoma is T1 isointense and T2 isointense to hyperintense relative to lacrimal gland tissue, whereas pigmented epithelial adenomas are T1 hyperintense and T2 hypointense relative to brain tissue {183,1385}.

Histopathology
Both pigmented and non-pigmented adenomas are composed of nests, cords, and tubules of polygonal epithelial cells containing round to oval, rarely pleomorphic nuclei with small nucleoli {1390}. The tumours can exhibit solid, papillary, and pleomorphic features, with delicate fibrous septa and basement membrane. Pigmented epithelial adenomas contain large spherical melanin granules, and the neoplastic cells can be vacuolated. Both non-pigmented and pigmented adenomas show immunopositivity for S100 protein and neuron-specific enolase. Expression of cytokeratins is variable {708,843,1131}.

Differential diagnosis
For non-pigmented epithelial adenomas, the differential diagnosis includes adenomatous hyperplasia of the ciliary body, ciliary body amelanotic melanoma, leiomyoma, primary and metastatic adenocarcinomas, and medulloepithelioma. Pigmented epithelial adenomas must be distinguished from pigmented ciliary body melanoma and rare malignant ciliary epithelial tumours.

Histogenesis
Ciliary body adenoma is derived from ciliary epithelium.

Genetic profile
The findings of one cytogenetics study suggest an imbalance of chromosome 6 in non-pigmented epithelial adenoma. Non-pigmented epithelial adenomas may also be associated with loss of opticin expression {61,858}. *BRAF* mutations are found in some cases {823}.

Prognosis and predictive factors
Local resection is usually curative. Enucleation may be necessary when a tumour is large and there is loss of vision due to tumour-related complications {1133}.

Adenomatous hyperplasia of the ciliary body

Roberts F.
Li B.
Loeffler K.U.

Definition
Adenomatous hyperplasia of the ciliary body is a benign proliferation of the pars plicata epithelium of the ciliary body.

ICD-O code
None

Synonyms
Fuchs adenoma; coronal adenoma

Epidemiology
Adenomatous hyperplasia is associated with age; it is found in about 60% of autopsied eyes from individuals aged > 80 years, but in only about 5% of autopsied eyes from individuals aged < 50 years {1129}.

Etiology
This benign proliferation of the non-pigmented ciliary epithelium is associated with ageing.

Localization
These proliferations are located in the pars plicata of the ciliary body and are usually confined to a single ciliary process.

Clinical features
Adenomatous hyperplasia of the ciliary body is often an incidental finding

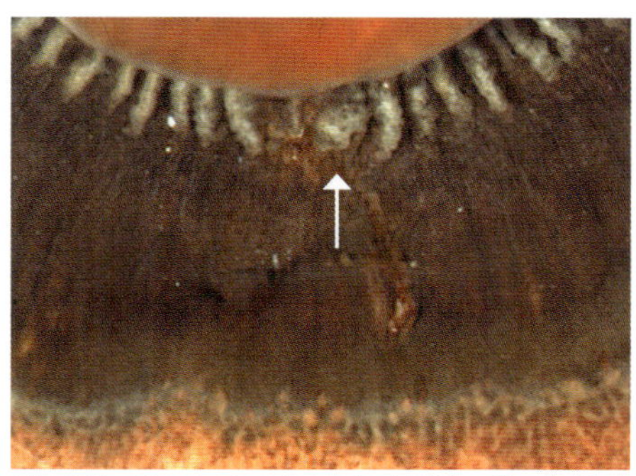

Fig. 2.30 Adenomatous hyperplasia of the ciliary body. A macroscopic image of an example presenting as a small nodular expansion of a single ciliary process (arrow).

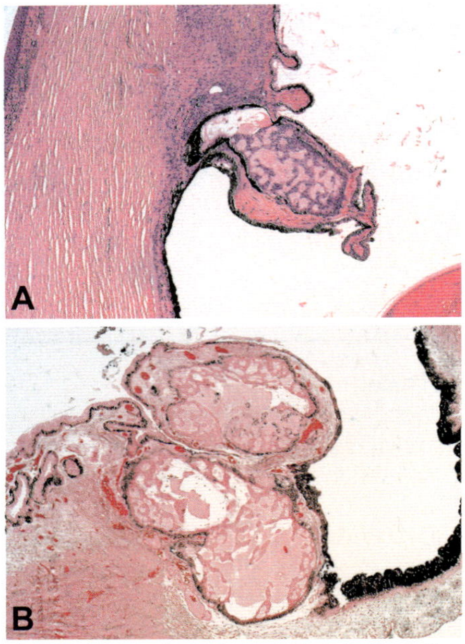

Fig. 2.31 Adenomatous hyperplasia of the ciliary body. **A** A single ciliary process is expanded by non-pigmented cells (derived from the ciliary epithelium) in interlacing cords separated by hyaline extracellular material. **B** Rarely, larger nodules composed of non-pigmented ciliary epithelium with variable amounts of extracellular matrix can extend behind the iris.

in enucleated eyes, because it is generally small and asymptomatic. The proliferations, which can be solitary or multiple (and unilateral or bilateral), occur as yellowish-white nodules or slightly pigmented nodules in the pars plicata.

Histopathology

These small nodules are composed of interlacing cords of uniform, non-pigmented ciliary epithelial cells surrounded by amorphous extracellular hyaline material that gives a positive periodic acid–Schiff (PAS) reaction. The nodules may be pedunculated, countersunk, or embedded in the ciliary body stroma. In some cases, the extracellular material may be the predominant feature, with only occasional strands of epithelial cells. The extracellular material has been shown by immunohistochemistry to be collagen IV and laminin {1129}.

Differential diagnosis

For larger lesions, the clinical differential diagnosis includes ciliary body melanoma, acquired neoplasm of the non-pigmented ciliary epithelium, tumours of the pigmented epithelium, and leiomyoma.

Histogenesis

This form of hyperplasia of the non-pigmented ciliary epithelium results in a nodular growth pattern.

Genetic profile

Adenomatous hyperplasia of the ciliary body appears to be associated with ageing, but no genetic profile has been published.

Prognosis and predictive factors

These reactive proliferations are usually an incidental finding in enucleated eyes. Occasionally, they can cause sectoral cataract or grow to sufficient size to involve the iris root and simulate a malignant neoplasm of the ciliary body, necessitating removal.

Reactive epithelial hyperplasia of the ciliary body

Roberts F.
Kivelä T.T.
Loeffler K.U.

Definition

Reactive epithelial hyperplasia of the ciliary body is an increase in cell number and volume of the ciliary epithelium, usually in response to injury.

ICD-O code

None

Synonym

Pseudoadenomatous hyperplasia

Epidemiology

The incidence is unknown. Reactive epithelial hyperplasia is seen mostly in eyes that have been subject to various forms of insult.

Etiology

Reactive epithelial hyperplasia can occur in reaction to physical trauma, surgery (including cyclocryotherapy), inflammation, or longstanding retinal detachment. It can also occur in an end-stage blind, phthisical eye.

Localization

At this anatomical site, reactive epithelial hyperplasia occurs in the pars plana or pars plicata of the ciliary body, often with extension into the adjacent posterior chamber or vitreous cavity.

Clinical features

Reactive epithelial hyperplasia is typically an incidental finding in enucleated eyes with other substantial pathology. It is usually clinically obscured by opaque media of the diseased eye.

Histopathology

The ciliary epithelium proliferates either as cords and strands or as pseudoacinar structures. The proliferation consists predominantly of cells of the inner non-pigmented epithelial layer but may also contain cells from the outer pigmented epithelial layer. These cells are entrapped within a variable amount of fibrous stroma induced by the underlying insult, and the epithelial cells may appear stretched within this fibrous tissue. Together, the epithelial cells and the fibrous stroma may form a tumorous mass or (more commonly) a diffuse proliferation covering the pars plana and extending behind the lens (called a cyclitic membrane) {1008}.

Differential diagnosis

The differential diagnosis includes adenoma and adenocarcinoma of the ciliary body. Cytological and histological evaluation helps with this distinction; adenocarcinoma is associated with tissue invasion and other features of malignant behaviour.

Histogenesis

Reactive hyperplasia may be induced by growth factors released during the inciting insult.

Prognosis and predictive factors

The prognosis depends on the inciting pathology and its effect on the eye.

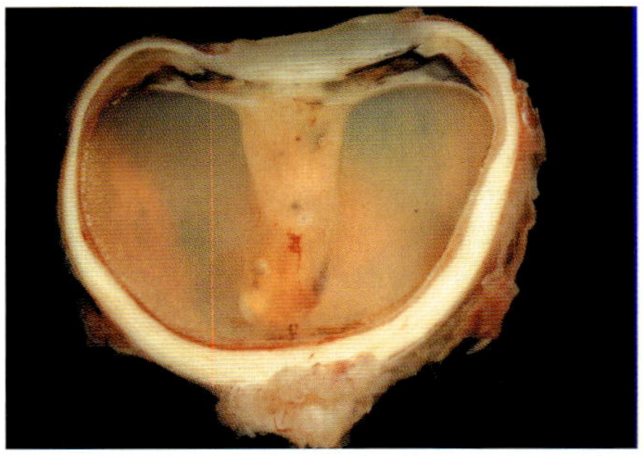

Fig. 2.32 Cyclitic membrane showing reactive epithelial hyperplasia. A macroscopic photo of an aphakic eye with longstanding retinal detachment and a cyclitic membrane forming a fibrous sheet extending from the ciliary body.

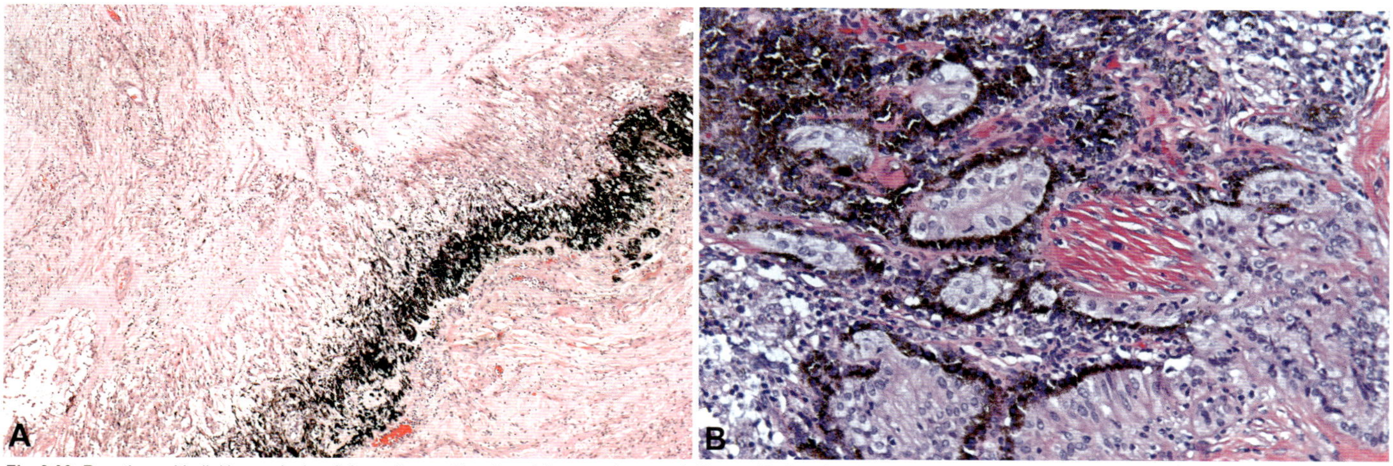

Fig. 2.33 Reactive epithelial hyperplasia. **A** A reactive proliferation of the non-pigmented ciliary epithelium forming cords and glandular structures within the fibrous tissue of a cyclitic membrane in an enucleation specimen after failed treatment of retinal detachment. **B** A multilayered proliferation of cells of the non-pigmented inner layer of the ciliary epithelium flanked by its non-proliferating pigmented outer layer, in an enucleated eye from a 3-year-old child with persistent fetal vasculature (previously called persistent hyperplastic primary vitreous).

These proliferations become increasingly fibrous with time and after the inciting pathology has been dealt with.

Medulloepithelioma of the ciliary body

Eagle R.C. Jr
Biswas J.
Edward D.P.
Verdijk R.M.
Chan A.S.Y.

Definition

Medulloepithelioma of the ciliary body is a primary intraocular embryonal tumour characterized by cords of multilayered neuroepithelial cells resembling the medullary epithelium of the optic cup.

ICD-O codes

Medulloepithelioma, benign	9501/0
Medulloepithelioma, malignant	9501/3
Teratoid medulloepithelioma, benign	9502/0
Teratoid medulloepithelioma, malignant	9502/3

Synonyms

Diktyoma; teratoneuroma

Epidemiology

Most cases occur in children aged 2–5 years, but rare cases in adults have been reported (patient age range: < 1 year to 66 years) {21}; 63% of cases occur in females {567}. There is no race predilection.

Etiology

Medulloepitheliomas are considered to be congenital tumours, thought to arise from anlagen of the medullary epithelium of the optic cup {136,1129,1136}. There are no known risk factors for intraocular medulloepithelioma. Most intraocular medulloepitheliomas occur sporadically and are not associated with congenital malformations or cytogenetic abnormalities. Rare cases have occurred in patients with pleuropulmonary blastoma family tumour and dysplasia syndrome caused by germline mutations in *DICER1* {651,676,931}.

Localization

Most tumours are located on the inner surface of the ciliary body. Rare cases have been reported in the optic nerve and retina {108,190,417,938}.

Clinical features

The most common presenting symptoms are poor vision or blindness (present in 27% of cases), leukocoria (in 20%), strabismus (in 12%), and a red painful eye (in 20%) {567}. Intratumoural cysts, which may be helpful diagnostic clues, are present in 61% of patients. Lens notching or lens coloboma caused by segmental loss of zonular fibres is present in 20% of cases {567,909}. A neoplastic cyclitic membrane is present in half of all patients {909,1071}, 44% have secondary glaucoma, and 51% have iris neovascularization. Ophthalmoscopy reveals a fleshy pink, tan, whitish-grey, or yellow ciliary body mass.

Treatment and diagnosis are often delayed. In one series, the average age at presentation was about 4 years, but the age at diagnosis and treatment was 5 years {136}. Before diagnosis, some patients have been treated for cataract or glaucoma. Extraocular extension of tumour cells has been observed after misguided tube shunt surgery for neovascular glaucoma {566}. In some cases, the tumour is found incidentally in a blind, painful eye after enucleation or

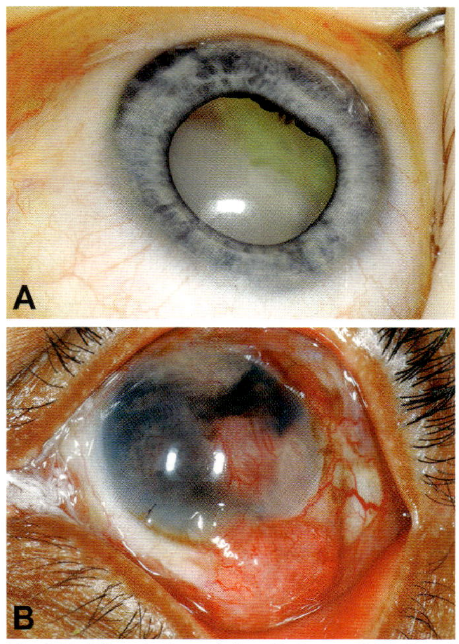

Fig. 2.34 Ciliary body medulloepithelioma. **A** Dilation of the pupil discloses a yellow ciliary body mass and cyclitic membrane. **B** Malignant medulloepithelioma in an adult has extended extraocularly, producing an epibulbar mass; the patient developed metastases.

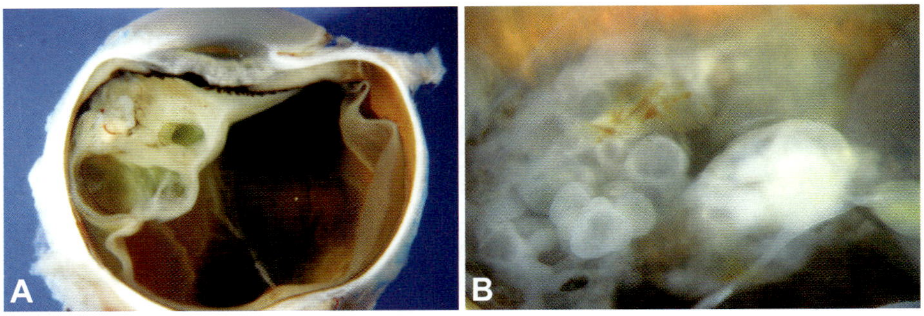

Fig. 2.35 Ciliary body medulloepithelioma. **A** A tumour on the inner surface of the ciliary body; intralesional cysts, a cyclitic membrane, and a persistent hyaloid vessel are present. **A** Whitish tumour on the inner surface of the ciliary body contains numerous cysts.

evisceration. An epibulbar mass may be present in cases with extraocular extension. Most cases are enucleated. Local resection is an option in some cases, but the tumour often recurs as a result of incomplete resection. The role of plaque brachytherapy has not been clearly established.

Histopathology

Medulloepithelioma is centred on the ciliary body and typically rests on the ciliary body's inner surface. Iris and anterior chamber involvement occurs in some cases. The mean tumour size is 11 mm (range: 2–30 mm). The tumour is composed of anastomosing cords, bands, and ribbons of polarized neuroepithelial cells that resemble embryonic medullary epithelium. A net-like pattern composed of thinner interweaving strands of neuroepithelium characterizes the rare diktyomatous pattern. The polarized neuroepithelial elements are surrounded by relatively acellular myxoid stroma that is rich in hyaluronidase-sensitive mucopolysaccharide (called neoplastic vitreous). The myxoid stroma abuts a thin basement membrane on the inner surface of the neuroepithelium, and the lumina of the neuroepithelial clefts and rosettes contain zonulae adherentes analogous to the retina's external limiting membrane {305}. Intralesional cystoid spaces are present in about half of the tumours, and one third contain areas of intrinsic pigmentation {567,1137}. Sheets of poorly differentiated neuroblastic cells resembling retinoblastoma are a histopathological criterion for malignancy; these areas may contain Homer Wright or Flexner–Wintersteiner rosettes. Additional criteria for malignancy include invasion of ocular tissues (including the uvea, cornea, sclera, and optic nerve), extraocular extension, sarcomatous change in areas of heterologous tissue, pleomorphism, atypia, and mitotic activity. About 66–80% of medulloepitheliomas are classified as malignant {136,567}.

Because the current criteria for malignancy do not correlate with clinical behaviour, and because molecular studies have identified no differences between histologically benign and malignant medulloepitheliomas, a simple grading scheme has been proposed to replace the current dichotomous classification {1318}. The proposed grading scheme comprises grade I tumours (corresponding to the current WHO designation "benign"), grade II tumours (with progression evidenced by pleomorphism, increased mitotic activity, and local invasion), and grade III tumours (with malignant transformation and metastatic potential, evidenced by extrascleral extension or metastasis). Metastatic disease occurs only in cases with extraocular extension {1318}.

Heteroplastic elements (including hyaline cartilage, muscle, myoblasts, and brain-like tissue) are found in 37% of cases {567}. Medulloepitheliomas with heteroplastic elements are designated as teratoid. Approximately one fifth of benign medulloepitheliomas and half of malignant medulloepitheliomas contain heteroplastic elements {136,567}. Hyaline cartilage is the most common heteroplastic element. The presence of heteroplastic elements has no effect on prognosis. Sheets of medulloepithelioma can grow posteriorly on the inner surface of the retina, reaching the posterior pole of the eye.

The non-teratoid component of medulloepithelioma is typically immunoreactive for vimentin and neuron-specific enolase. Limited and conflicting results have been reported for chromogranin, synaptophysin, GFAP, S100 protein, and HMB45 antigen. Immunoreactivity for pancytokeratin and CK18, with no reactivity for CK7, CK20, or epithelial membrane antigen, has been described {531,1037}. Almost all medulloepitheliomas stain positively for LIN28A protein, and the intensity of staining correlates with aggressive behaviour {528}. LIN28A staining is specific for medulloepithelioma; it is uniformly negative in retinoblastoma.

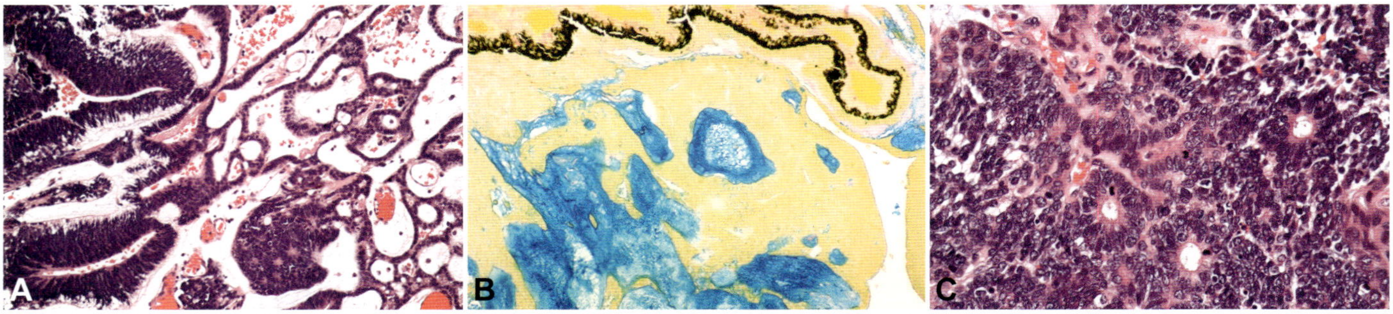

Fig. 2.36 Ciliary body medulloepithelioma. **A** Thick bands of polarized epithelium resembling medullary epithelium and a diktyomatous pattern made up of thinner cellular strands are present; pools of hyaluronic acid surround epithelial elements. **B** Colloidal iron staining for acid mucopolysaccharides discloses pools of hyaluronidase-sensitive mucopolysaccharide within the tumour. **C** A poorly differentiated focus in malignant ciliary body medulloepithelioma resembles retinoblastoma; several Flexner–Wintersteiner rosettes are present.

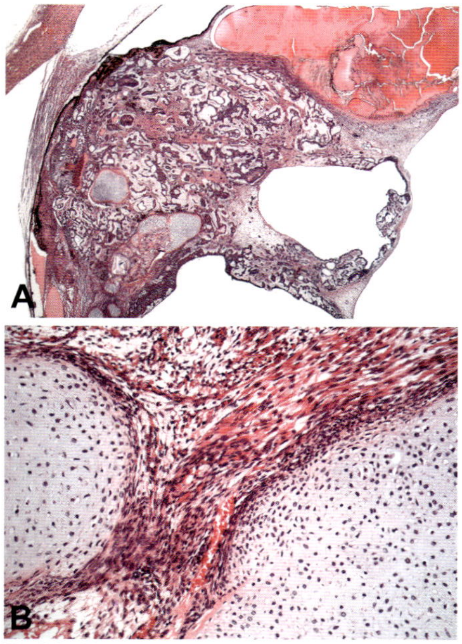

Fig. 2.37 Teratoid ciliary body medulloepithelioma. **A** Teratoid tumour on the inner surface of the ciliary body contains foci of hyaline cartilage and multiple cystoid spaces; it abuts the posterior surface of the lens. **B** Teratoid tumour contains islands of hyaline cartilage and muscle.

Differential diagnosis

The differential diagnosis includes retinoblastoma, persistent fetal vasculature, and cataract.

Histogenesis

The tumour and its multilaminar medullary epithelium appear to arise from a simple pre-medullary epithelial monolayer of S100-positive cells {539}. Positive staining for CRX and the neuronal marker NeuN suggests that the most anterior layers of the optic cup retain the potential for retinal and neuroglial differentiation. Intraocular medulloepithelioma shares histomorphological features with CNS medulloepithelioma, a rare entity currently grouped with several other primitive neuroectodermal tumours as embryonal tumours with multilayered rosettes. Both ocular and CNS medulloepitheliomas express LIN28A, but intraocular tumours show numerous copy-number aberrations that involve either whole chromosomes or chromosome arms. They show no amplification of the C19MC cluster of microRNA and have DNA methylation patterns that are strikingly different from those of CNS tumours, suggesting that the ocular and CNS neoplasms do not share common origins or biological behaviours {528,648,1213}.

Genetic profile

Cytogenetic analysis of intraocular medulloepithelioma shows recurrent aberrations in chromosomes 1p, 4, 8, and 16p {648}. Intraocular medulloepithelioma has occurred in patients with pleuropulmonary blastoma family tumour and dysplasia syndrome caused by germline mutations in *DICER1*. Recurrent somatic *DICER1* mutations have been reported in some cases of sporadic intraocular medulloepithelioma {302,309,676,1020}. MicroRNA profiling in intraocular medulloepitheliomas shows markedly upregulated and downregulated microRNAs. The microRNA dysregulation has profiles similar to those seen in glioblastomas and retinoblastomas {309}. Recurrent mutations in the histone methyltransferase gene *KMT2D* have also been reported {1020}. Unsupervised hierarchical clustering of DNA methylation has shown that intraocular medulloepitheliomas have signatures distinct from those of intracranial medulloepithelioma {648}. The targetable epigenetic tumour protein EZH2 is enriched in intraocular medulloepithelioma {64}.

Genetic susceptibility

Rare cases of intraocular medulloepithelioma have occurred in patients with pleuropulmonary blastoma family tumour and dysplasia syndrome caused by germline mutations in *DICER1* {651,676,931}, but most cases are sporadic.

Prognosis and predictive factors

The prognosis for life is excellent if the tumour remains confined to the interior of the eye. Metastases (which may be fatal) can develop if there is extraocular extension of the tumour. The prognosis for vision is poor, because enucleation of the affected eye is often necessary.

Leiomyoma of the ciliary body

Rao N.
Croxatto J.O.
Mudhar H.S.

Definition

Leiomyoma of the ciliary body is a benign smooth muscle tumour. The mesectodermal variant shows hybrid histological features of neuroglial and smooth muscle cell differentiation {527}.

ICD-O code

Leiomyoma 8890/0

Epidemiology

Most patients are in the second to fourth decade of life at the time of diagnosis. The female-to-male ratio is 3:1.

Localization

Most leiomyomas arise in the ciliary body, but they can also occur in the iris and choroid.

Clinical features

Leiomyoma of the ciliary body presents with progressive blurred vision. It is a fleshy mass rarely exceeding 10 mm, and it readily transmits light on transillumination. Fluorescein angiography reveals a vascularized tumour pattern, and ultrasonography shows a well-circumscribed mass with low to medium internal reflectivity. CT depicts a mass with soft tissue density, and MRI reveals hyperintensity on T1-weighted imaging, with enhancement after gadolinium administration.

Histopathology

Leiomyomas are well-circumscribed, greyish-white or yellow, non-pigmented masses. The ciliary epithelium overlying the tumour is mostly intact. The tumours range from 4 mm to 22 mm in greatest diameter, with most cases not exceeding 10 mm {640}. The tumour is composed of spindle-shaped cells with abundant eosinophilic cytoplasm containing round to

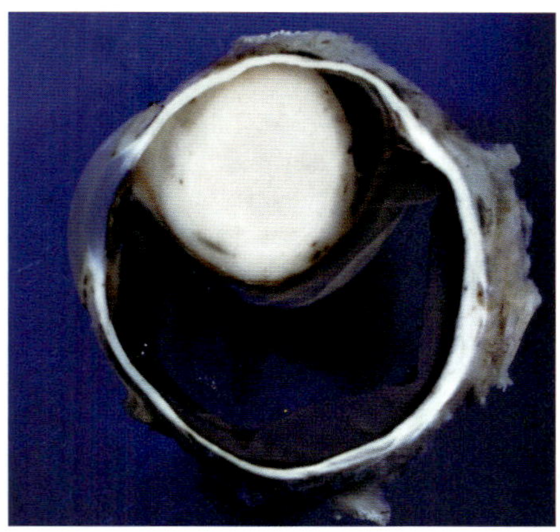

Fig. 2.38 Mesectodermal leiomyoma of the ciliary body. This macroscopic image shows a well-circumscribed white solid mass under the choroid, directly apposed to the sclera.

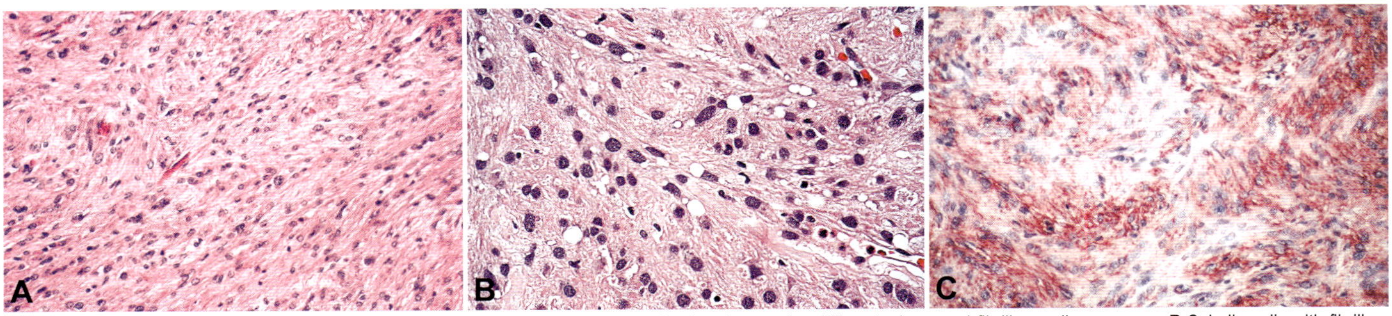

Fig. 2.39 Mesectodermal leiomyoma. **A** The tumour exhibits round to oval nuclei with abundant eosinophilic cytoplasm and fibrillary cell processes. **B** Spindle cells with fibrillary eosinophilic cytoplasm contain oval, granular nuclei, some of which are indented by cytoplasmic perinuclear vacuoles. **C** Several neoplastic cells show immunopositivity for MSA.

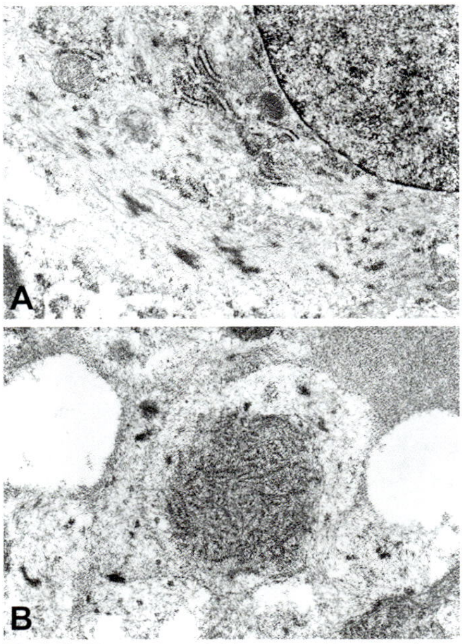

Fig. 2.40 Mesectodermal leiomyoma. Electron microscopy reveals smooth muscle densities (**A**) and skeinoid fibres in the cytoplasm (**B**).

oval, finely granular, slightly pleomorphic nuclei. Perinuclear cytoplasmic vacuoles can often be seen. Mitosis is rarely present. Scattered melanocytes can be present. Leiomyoma shows immunoreactivity for SMA, MSA, caldesmon, calponin, and desmin. The mesectodermal variant of leiomyoma can show a fibrillar background with positivity for CD56 and neuron-specific enolase. Leiomyomas are negative for GFAP, S100 protein, HMB45 antigen, and melan-A. Some cases express nuclear sex hormone receptors {943}. Transmission electron microscopy demonstrates typical cytoplasmic smooth muscle densities. The mesectodermal variant can additionally show skeinoid fibres, which are seen in some neural tumours {154}; this finding supports the notion that this variant has hybrid smooth muscle and neural features.

Differential diagnosis

The main differential diagnoses are amelanotic melanoma, peripheral nerve sheath tumour, and astrocytoma. For the mesectodermal variant, addition differential diagnoses are epithelioid and vascular leiomyomas.

Histogenesis

Leiomyoma of the ciliary body has two possible derivations. Mesectodermal leiomyomas are thought to derive from the ciliary body muscle that originates from the neural crest {527}. The other possible derivation is from the smooth muscle of ciliary body blood vessels, which are of mesodermal origin {371,1157}.

Prognosis and predictive factors

There are no reported cases of tumour metastasis. Local resection of the entire tumour (if possible) or observation is the treatment of choice, and the prognosis is good.

Schwannoma of the ciliary body

Mudhar H.S.
Croxatto J.O.

Definition

Schwannoma of the ciliary body is a benign nerve sheath tumour composed of Schwann cells.

ICD-O code

Schwannoma 9560/0

Synonyms

Neurilemmoma; benign peripheral nerve sheath tumour

Epidemiology

Most cases occur in females in the second to sixth decade of life {1403}.

Etiology

Pure ciliary body schwannomas are sporadic and not associated with neurofibromatosis, schwannomatosis, or Carney complex.

Localization

Ciliary body schwannomas most commonly occur in the inferior or inferonasal ciliary body {662,914,998,1201}.

Clinical features

Patients present with decreased vision. The tumours are typically solitary, unilateral, dome-shaped, and amelanotic. Schwannomas in this anatomical site are often mistaken for ciliary body melanoma, but they can usually be distinguished from melanoma by an absence of sentinel vessels and by increased light transmission {662,914,998,1201}.

Histopathology

Conventional schwannoma comprises benign neoplastic Schwann cells

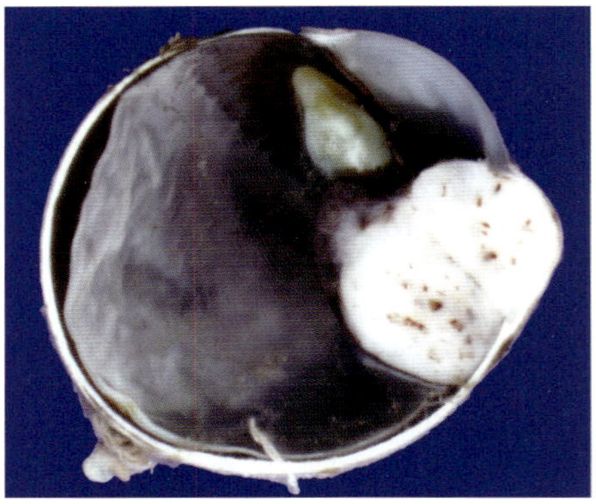

Fig. 2.41 Ciliary body schwannoma. The tumour effaces the iris, expanding into the anterior chamber, with associated scleral thinning and lens subluxation; its cut surface is solid and white, punctuated by blood vessels.

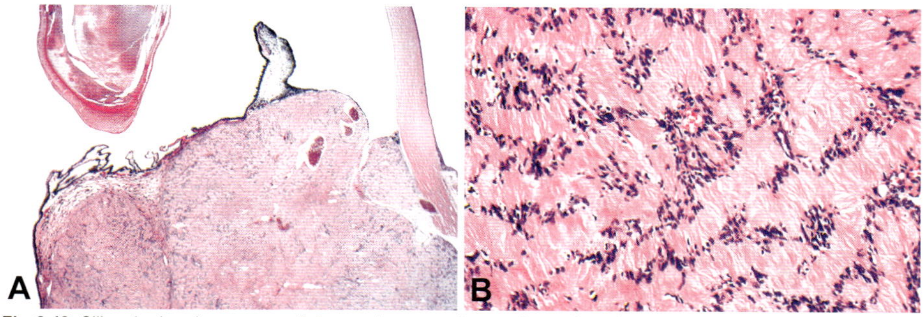

Fig. 2.42 Ciliary body schwannoma. **A** A scanning-power image shows the schwannoma expanding out of the ciliary body and effacing the iris; the lens is above and the cornea to the right. **B** An Antoni A area showing Verocay bodies (nuclear palisades).

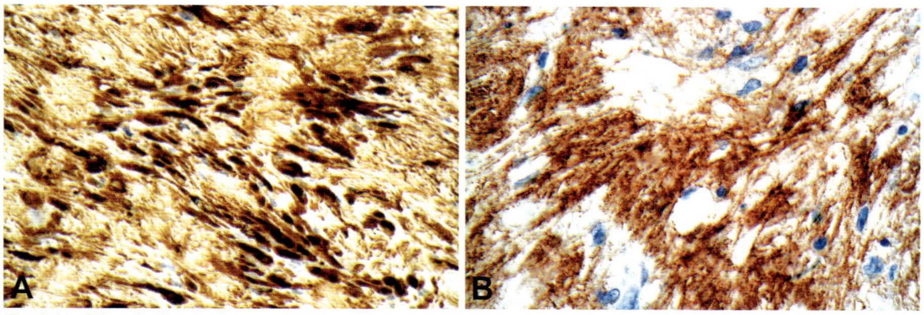

Fig. 2.43 Ciliary body schwannoma. **A** The tumour cells show strong and diffuse nuclear and cytoplasmic staining for S100 protein. **B** The Verocay bodies stain for fibrillar collagen IV.

arranged in an alternating pattern of hypercellular Antoni A areas and hypocellular Antoni B areas. In the Antoni A areas, the Schwann cells are oval and spindle-shaped, with twisted, tapering nuclei and often with intranuclear vacuoles. The spindle cells are arranged as short fascicles. Nuclear palisading may be present, and Verocay bodies may be seen. In Antoni B areas, the Schwann cells are spindle or oval (with round to oval-shaped nuclei); they are loosely arranged within the stroma, which can show hyalinized blood vessel walls {1403}. Plexiform schwannoma involving the ciliary body has also been reported {1011}.
The tumour cells are diffusely and strongly positive for S100 protein, with both nuclear and cytoplasmic staining {1357}. They can also express SOX10, CD57 (LEU7), calretinin {352,905}, GFAP {786}, collagen IV, and laminin {873}.
Transmission electron microscopy shows prominent, continuous basal lamina surrounding long cytoplasmic processes. Stromal Luse bodies (long-spaced collagen) are a common feature {1403}.

Differential diagnosis
The differential diagnosis includes leiomyoma, neurofibroma, malignant peripheral nerve sheath tumour, melanoma, and fibrous histiocytoma {662,914,998,1201}.

Histogenesis
Ciliary nerve–derived Schwann cells are the likely origin of the tumour.

Genetic profile
There are no genetic data for intraocular schwannoma. Sporadic cases of conventional schwannoma occurring at other anatomical sites have been found to be caused by loss of merlin (the *NF2* gene product) {518}.

Genetic susceptibility
Ciliary body schwannomas have not been reported in association with any syndrome, but some choroidal schwannomas have been reported in association with neurofibromatosis type 2 {376,778,1310}.

Prognosis and predictive factors
This is a benign lesion with no risk of metastasis. Local resection can be curative {501,662}, although one case of post-resection recurrence has been reported {501}. Enucleation should be performed in cases difficult to distinguish from melanoma.

Glioneuroma of the ciliary body

Kivelä T.T.
Croxatto J.O.
Rao N.

Definition
Glioneuroma of the ciliary body is a congenital choristoma that consists of a mass of mature glial and neuronal cells without neoplastic potential in an otherwise healthy child; there is usually an adjacent coloboma of the anterior uvea and retina {622,1208}.

ICD-O code
Glioneuroma	9490/0

Epidemiology
There have been 5 reported cases in children aged 1–6 months and 1 reported case in a 20-year-old woman {7,622,750,1208}.

Etiology
Glioneuroma of the ciliary body is a random congenital developmental malformation of unknown origin {622,1208}.

Localization
Glioneuroma of the ciliary body typically occurs in a temporal quadrant of the eye, with extension to the adjacent iris and retina {7,622,750,1208}.

Clinical features
Patients present with a tan-coloured, growing mass in one eye, which may be smaller or larger than the fellow eye. Minor pigmented elements and an extraocular extension along blood vessels may be present. The intraocular pressure can be high, and the adjacent cornea and lens can be cloudy. A persistent pupillary membrane and chorioretinal coloboma may be present {622,1208}. On CT, the mass enhances with contrast medium {622}.

Histopathology
The tumour contains fibrillary astrocytes with finely dispersed chromatin, an eosinophilic matrix of glial and neuronal processes, clusters of neuronal cells with small round nuclei, dysplastic rosettes and tubules composed of several rows of cells (resembling Homer Wright and Flexner–Wintersteiner rosettes), and

scattered large ganglion cells and calcospherites. Mitotic figures are rare or absent. The glial component is immunopositive for GFAP and the neuronal component for synaptophysin and NFP. The ciliary epithelium over the mass shows reactive proliferation in a loose extracellular matrix, which stains with Alcian blue. The adjacent retina is dysplastic, and it often extends over to the chorioretinal coloboma when one is present {622,1208}. The adjacent iris epithelium may have a fetal appearance {622}.

Differential diagnosis

Glioneuroma of the ciliary body must be distinguished from teratoid medulloepithelioma of the ciliary body containing mature brain tissue {136,622,750}.

Histogenesis

There are two possible modes of histogenesis: a dysgenetic glioneuromatous mass may interfere with the normal development of adjacent retina, choroid, ciliary body, and iris, resulting in a secondary coloboma, or a mass may arise secondary to faulty differentiation of the pigmented layer of the optic cup, resulting in a coloboma and abnormal neuroepithelial development of the iris and ciliary body {622}.

Prognosis and predictive factors

These glioneuromas are managed by surgical excision and do not recur {7,622,750,1208}.

Tumours of the choroid

Choroidal and ciliary body melanomas

Grossniklaus H.E.
Eagle R.C. Jr
Albert D.
Harbour J.W.
Mendoza P.
Schoenfield L.
Verdijk R.M.
White V.A.

Definition

Choroidal and ciliary body melanomas are primary malignant melanocytic tumours.

ICD-O codes

Mixed epithelioid and spindle cell uveal melanoma	8770/3
Epithelioid cell uveal melanoma	8771/3
Spindle cell uveal melanoma NOS	8772/3
Spindle cell uveal melanoma, type A	8773/3
Spindle cell uveal melanoma, type B	8774/3

Synonyms

Uveal melanoma (less specific, because the choroid and ciliary body are different parts of the uveal tract, which also includes the iris); intraocular melanoma (less specific, because the iris is also intraocular tissue); ocular melanoma (inaccurate and discouraged, because the term also includes extraocular conjunctival melanoma)

Epidemiology

The worldwide incidence of uveal melanoma is uncertain, but it is estimated to be about 7000 cases per year {618}, accounting for 5% of all primary melanomas {310}. Choroidal and ciliary body melanomas are most common in White populations (in which 65% of all cases are reported, although only 12% of the world's population is White); they are rare in Asian and African populations {310,497,574,1186}. Among Asians, the risk of developing uveal melanoma is 1.2 times the risk among African-Americans; among Hispanic and non-Hispanic White people, the risk is 5 times and 19 times (respectively) the risk among African-Americans {496}. Worldwide, the incidence rate is about 2–8 cases per 1 million person-years – lower at lower latitudes (1.3–2.9 cases per 1 million person-years) and increasing with latitude (to 6.1–8.6 cases per 1 million person-years) {1329,1402}. This incidence has been relatively stable over a 25-year period {1179,1329}. The mean patient age at diagnosis, which has increased because of rising life expectancy, is currently 60–64 years in White populations and 45 years among Asians {109,277,666,1254}. These melanomas are rare in people aged < 20 years, accounting for only 0.4–0.8% of all cases {15,1184}. There is no sex predilection {246}. Choroidal and ciliary body melanomas are more common among lightly pigmented than darkly pigmented individuals {310,498,760,1185}.

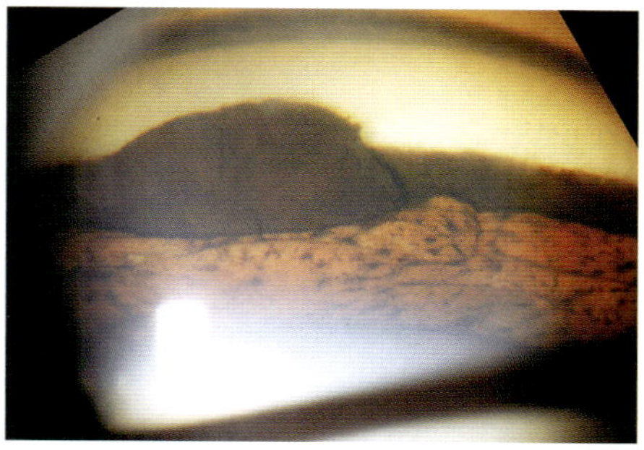

Fig. 2.44 Ciliary body melanoma invading the anterior chamber. Gonioscopic examination shows pigmented melanoma invading the periphery of the anterior chamber; a band of tumour blankets the trabecular meshwork.

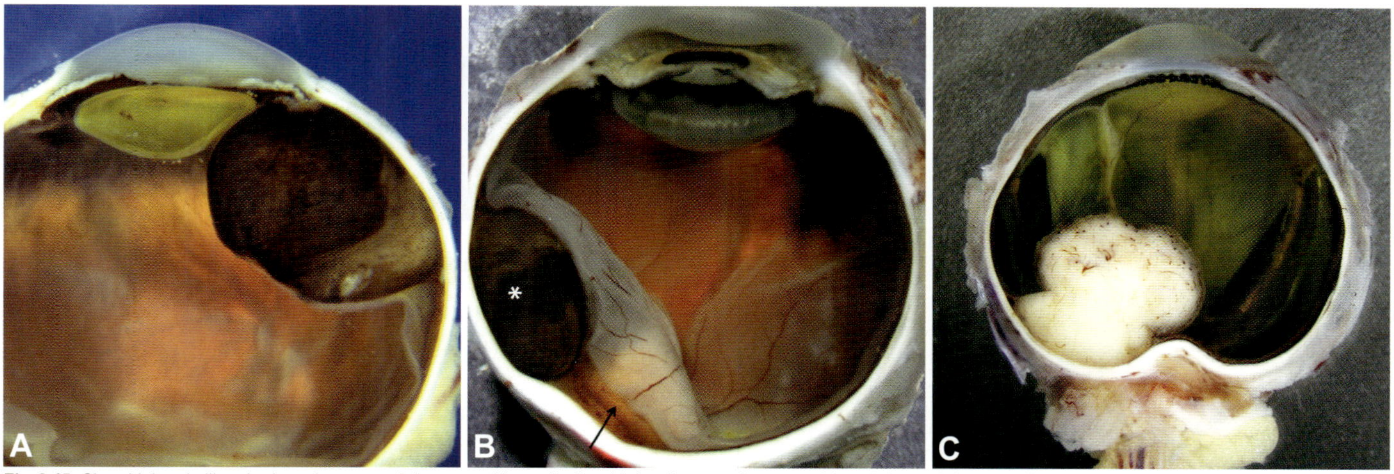

Fig. 2.45 Choroidal and ciliary body melanomas. **A** Lens moulding; ciliochoroidal melanoma distorts and has dislocated the crystalline lens. **B** This variably pigmented choroidal melanoma is heavily pigmented in one area (asterisk) and amelanotic in another (arrow). **C** This amelanotic choroidal melanoma has broken through the Bruch membrane and assumed a mushroom-like or collar-button shape; there are congested vascular channels in the portion of the tumour internal to the Bruch membrane, and a serous retinal detachment is present.

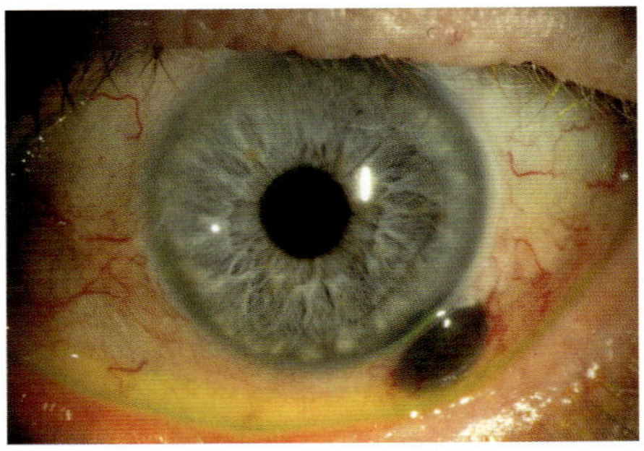

Fig. 2.46 Ciliary body melanoma. Clinical appearance of a bulbar conjunctival extension of an underlying melanoma through the collecting ducts.

Etiology

Some choroidal and ciliary body melanomas develop de novo. Others develop from melanocytes in uveal naevi (with a lifetime risk of 1 in 400) {327,621,1181} or from melanocytes in congenital ocular or oculodermal melanocytosis (naevus of Ota; with a lifetime risk of 1 in 400) {1180}. Risk factors include light skin pigmentation, blond or red hair, light-coloured irides {388,1058}, dysplastic naevus syndrome {1179}, and *BAP1* tumour predisposition syndrome {161,1180,1367}. There is no definite role of ultraviolet (UV) radiation exposure in the development of uveal melanoma {290,1186}.

Localization

Melanoma can arise anywhere in the choroid and ciliary body, and it can extend from one to the other. Choroidal and ciliary body melanomas can also extend to the iris, chamber angle, retina, vitreous nerve, and optic nerve, as well as extraocularly {1329,1402}.

Clinical features

Approximately 25% of patients with ciliary body or choroidal melanoma have no symptoms and are diagnosed during routine eye examination {1093}. Symptoms include photopsia (perceived flashes of light), floaters, and loss of vision {653}. Occasionally, large choroidal and ciliary body melanomas result in pain, redness of the eye, and glaucoma {1093}. Multifocal uveal melanomas have been reported {285}. Bilateral primary uveal melanoma occurs rarely {448,1223}.

Ciliary body melanomas are usually circumscribed and nodular. Diagnosis is often delayed because the tumour is hidden behind the iris and is not apparent on routine examination. These melanomas often encroach on and distort the crystalline lens, producing lens dislocation, astigmatism, and unilateral cataract. The tumour can also produce focal shallowing of the anterior chamber. Some ciliary body melanomas grow through the iris root and invade the anterior chamber, simulating a primary iris melanoma. Anterior chamber seeding and iris heterochromia can develop in such cases, and secondary glaucoma is another complication. Glaucoma mechanisms include anterior displacement of the lens-iris diaphragm, tumour seeding, and iris neovascularization. Annular or ring melanomas usually involve more than 180° of the ciliary body and show disproportionately less anteroposterior growth. The aqueous outflow pathways can be obstructed by a ring melanoma {695,1212,1415}. Rare cases of melanomalytic glaucoma develop when melanophages containing necrotic tumour debris physically obstruct the trabecular meshwork {150}. In contrast, some eyes become hypotonous when the tumour disrupts the ciliary epithelium, causing decreased production of aqueous humour. Hyphaema and vitreous haemorrhage occur rarely when the tumour disrupts blood vessels or undergoes necrosis. Ultrasonography, anterior segment optical coherence tomography, and transillumination are helpful diagnostic techniques. External ocular signs that can suggest the diagnosis include dilated episcleral blood vessels (so-called sentinel vessels) overlying the tumour and episcleral nodules from extrascleral extension through emissary canals in the anterior sclera.

Choroidal melanomas appear as a mass that is dome-shaped (in 75% of cases), mushroom-shaped (in 20%), or diffuse (in 5%). They are pigmented in 55% of cases, non-pigmented in 15%, and of mixed colour in 30% {1089}. Their mean size is 11.3 mm in basal diameter by 5.5 mm in thickness {1084}. The mass is deep to the retina, without feeder vessels, and there may be an overlying exudative retinal detachment, which is an important presenting sign. Necrotic tumours cause painful uveitis, glaucoma, or both. Extraocular extension may also occur, via vortex veins or emissary canals in the sclera and around the optic disc. The tumour can also invade the optic nerve sheath, orbit, or both. Optic nerve invasion occurs in 5–6% of cases {714,715}.

The most common way to localize a choroidal melanoma is by direct visualization with direct and indirect ophthalmoscopy. The tumour should be documented using fundus photography and measured using A-scan and B-scan ultrasonography. Optical coherence tomography is

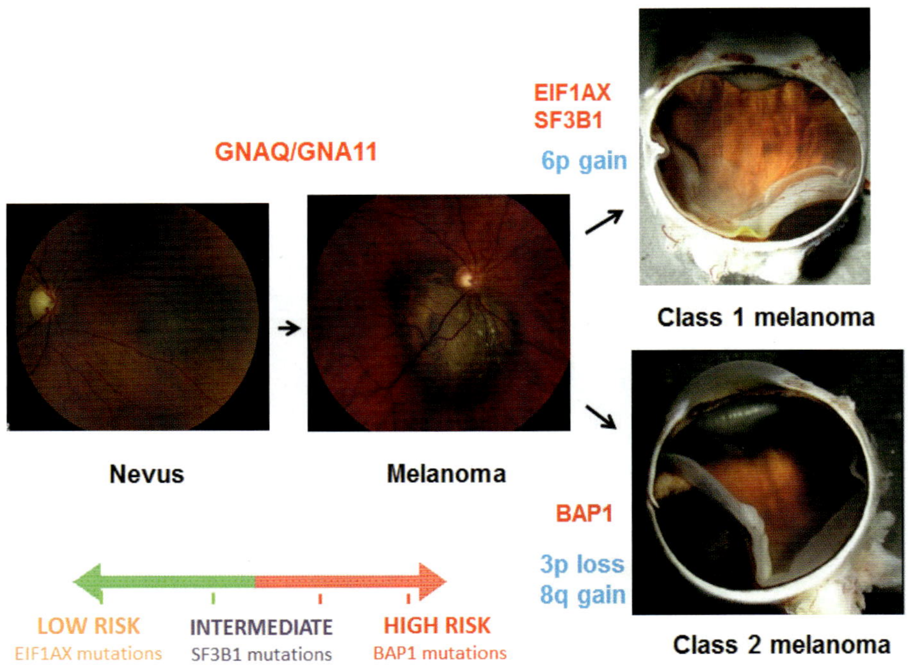

Fig. 2.47 Progression of choroidal naevus to melanoma. A *GNAQ/GNA11* mutation appears to occur early in the progression. After the tumour is a melanoma, it may acquire further mutations; mutations in *EIF1AX* or *SF3B1* (also 6p gain) result in class 1 melanomas with a low or intermediate risk (respectively) of metastasis, whereas mutations in *BAP1* (3p loss, 8q gain) result in class 2 melanomas with a high risk of metastasis.

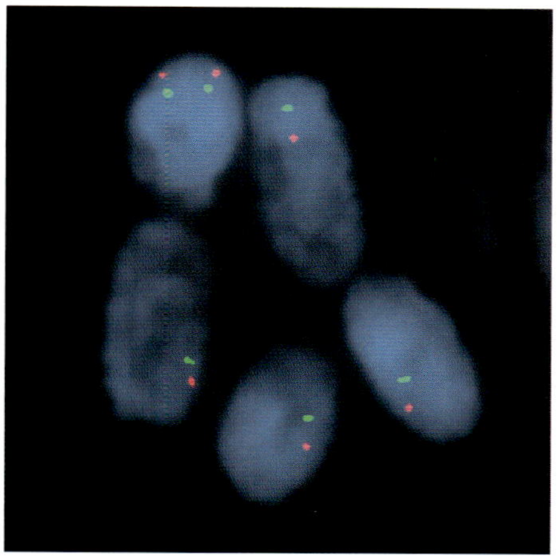

Fig. 2.48 Choroidal melanoma. FISH shows nuclei with monosomy 3, with only single copies of red and green probes (the normal finding is two copies of each); the FISH probe included D3Z1 (centromere CEN3; red) and *BCL6* (3q27; green).

generally used to determine the effect of the tumour on the overlying and surrounding retina, including to evaluate subretinal fluid. Fundus autofluorescence imaging can reveal orange lipofuscin pigment overlying the tumour. According to the TNM classification system {132}, choroidal and ciliary body melanomas are grouped by size as small (T1), medium (T2), large (T3), or very large (T4), and they are staged (stage I–IV) according to size, ciliary body involvement, extraocular extension, and presence of metastasis (see the TNM classification table on p. 63).

Histopathology

Macroscopically, ciliary body melanomas are either dome-shaped or circumferential ring-shaped tumours. Choroidal melanomas may exhibit a flat to domed shape when confined by the Bruch membrane, or they may exhibit a characteristic so-called collar-button or mushroom-like shape when they break through the Bruch membrane; the portion of the tumour that has broken through is choked off by the membrane, resulting in vascular congestion.

Microscopic examination should be used to assess for invasion of ocular structures (e.g. the chamber angle, iris, sclera, retina, and optic nerve), as well as for extrascleral extension.

Variable amounts of melanin pigment are produced by these melanomas, which range from amelanotic to mildly, moderately, or heavily pigmented. The cytological description of choroidal melanoma was traditionally based on the Callender system, which in its modified form included four types of tumours: spindle A (naevus-like) cell, spindle B cell, epithelioid cell, and mixed (spindle B and epithelioid) cell {779}. Spindle A cells are fusiform and cohesive, and they have poorly defined cell borders. Their spindle-shaped nucleus contains a central nuclear envelope fold (or groove). Spindle B cells are fusiform and cohesive, and they contain spindle-shaped or cigar-like nuclei and prominent nucleoli; this is the most frequent cell type in most choroidal melanomas. Epithelioid cells are noncohesive and contain large, round nuclei and abundant, prominent eosinophilic cytoplasm; this cell type is associated with a high risk of metastasis. Intermediate cells (small epithelioid cells) are intermediate between spindle B and epithelioid melanoma cells. Uveal melanomas may undergo spontaneous necrosis. Tumours that exhibit 90–100% necrosis are composed of so-called ghost melanoma cells; this phenomenon is probably due to a sequence of events that starts with vascular insufficiency within the tumour, followed by cytokine release, tumour necrosis, and secondary glaucoma {1252}. So-called balloon cells are sometimes seen in uveal melanoma {597}. These cells have foamy, vacuolated cytoplasm because of faulty production of melanin or degradation of melanosomes, and their cytoplasm contains lipid. Balloon cells are often seen in choroidal melanoma after plaque brachytherapy or proton beam irradiation {1032}. Both dendritic and scavenger tumour-infiltrating macrophages are ubiquitous in uveal melanomas, and they can constitute a substantial portion of the tumour mass {742}.

Although the cut-off points are arbitrary, spindle cell melanoma is defined as being composed of spindle B cells in ≥ 90% of the tumour, and epithelioid cell melanoma is defined as being composed of epithelioid cells in ≥ 90% of the tumour; all other tumours are mixed cell melanomas (the most common type in many series) {619}. Epithelioid cell melanomas are associated with the worst prognosis, and pure spindle cell melanomas are associated with the best prognosis {781}. Because of the association between epithelioid cells and poor prognosis, some pathologists favour simplifying the reporting to two categories: presence or absence of epithelioid cells in the tumour {619}.

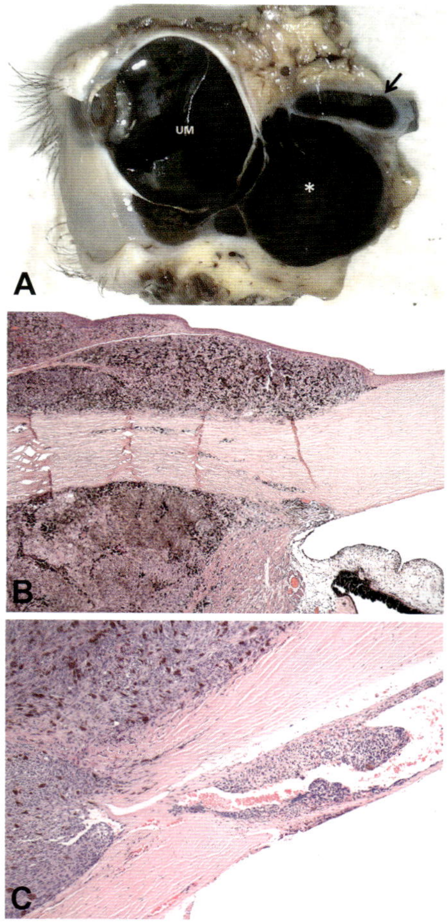

Fig. 2.49 Choroidal and ciliary body melanomas. **A** This exenteration specimen contains a heavily pigmented choroidal melanoma that fills the eye (UM), invades the optic nerve (arrow), and extends beyond the sclera, where it forms a nodule (asterisk). **B** In this ciliary body melanoma specimen, tumour is seen within the trabecular meshwork and intrascleral collector channels, deep to the focus of anterior extraocular extension. **C** This choroidal melanoma extends through a vortex vein in the sclera.

A number of special variants of choroidal and ciliary body melanomas may need to be considered. Diffuse uveal melanoma is defined as being < 5 mm in thickness and occupying at least one quarter of the uveal tract {188}. This growth pattern may be associated with a higher risk of metastasis and extraocular growth, although the tumour is relatively thin. Retinoinvasive uveal melanoma tends to evolve from a melanoma of the ciliary body, then invades the vitreous, the retina, and through these tissues into the optic nerve {413,623}. Other mechanisms of optic nerve invasion by choroidal melanoma include via the retina after retinal invasion, directly from the peripapillary

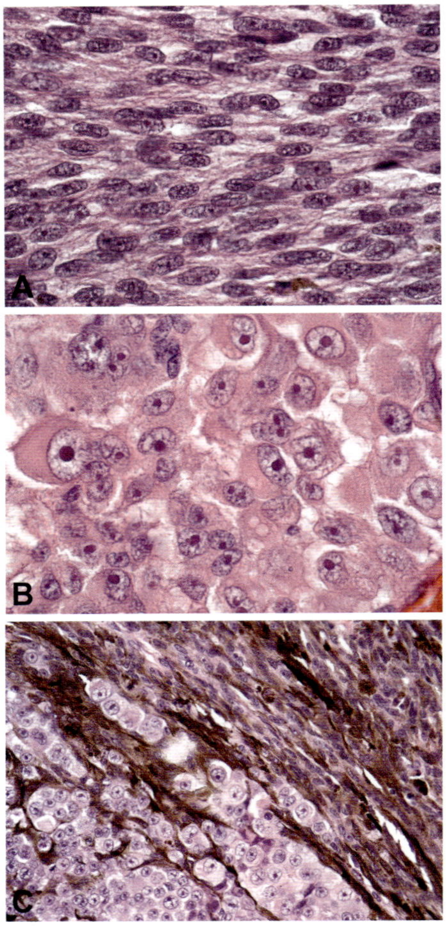

Fig. 2.50 Uveal melanoma. **A** Spindle cell type; spindle B cells have nucleoli and form a syncytium. **B** Epithelioid cell type; epithelioid cells have distinct cytoplasmic margins and large round or oval nuclei with prominent reddish-purple nucleoli and peripheral margination of chromatin. **C** Mixed cell type; mixed cell melanoma comprises clones of pigmented spindle cells (top right) and amelanotic epithelioid cells (bottom left).

choroid, and a combination of these mechanisms. A rare variant of ring melanoma is anterior chamber angle melanoma, which leads to secondary glaucoma with minimal involvement of the uveal tract {273,1212}. Another rare variant of uveal melanoma is clear cell melanoma {427}; the tumour cells have oval, centrally located nuclei and clear cytoplasm (due to the dissolution of glycogen granules during fixation). Clear cell melanomas must be distinguished from renal cell carcinoma metastatic to the choroid. Cavitary melanomas of the ciliary body contain extensive cavitary spaces {727}.
Choroidal melanomas are positive for HMB45 antigen, S100 protein, melan-A, MITF, tyrosinase, and SOX10 {345,826,868,992}. When using immunohistochemical stains to identify choroidal melanoma, it is advisable to use at least two, such as HMB45 and S100 protein, in case one is negative. Additionally, MIB1 staining for Ki-67, a nuclear proliferation marker, may be used to assess proliferative activity and has some prognostic relevance {583,821}. Mitotic activity should be reported as the number of mitoses/mm^2 {235}.
A number of other prognostic features of choroidal and ciliary body melanomas may also be considered for reporting to the clinician. A lack of nuclear immunostaining for the BAP1 protein in choroidal melanoma is strongly associated with an increased rate of metastasis {571,647,1302}. The following extravascular matrix patterns have been identified, listed from least to most complex: normal, silent, straight, parallel, parallel with cross-linking, arcs, arcs with branching, closed vascular loops, and vascular networks; the last three patterns are associated with an increased risk of metastasis {361,741}. It has been proposed that the extravascular matrix patterns constitute vasculogenic mimicry {358,369}. Large tumour cell nucleoli {16,780} and a high microvascular density also are associated with shorter survival {195,370,740}. Prominent tumour-infiltrating lymphocytes and tumour-associated macrophages have been associated with an increased likelihood of metastasis, and they are associated with high-risk chromosomal abnormalities (in particular monosomy 3) {134,135,399,742}.

Differential diagnosis

Choroidal and ciliary body melanomas must be differentiated from uveal naevus and melanocytoma (magnocellular naevus), paraneoplastic bilateral diffuse uveal melanocytic hyperplasia {815}, uveal metastasis, and primary spindle cell neoplasms. The differential diagnosis of ciliary body melanomas also includes mesectodermal leiomyoma, iris and ciliary body cysts, and adenoma and adenocarcinoma of the ciliary epithelium. Choroidal melanomas must be distinguished from peripheral exudative haemorrhagic chorioretinopathy {881}, circumscribed choroidal haemangioma, age-related macular degeneration with disciform scars and haemorrhage, retinal pigment epithelial adenoma and adenocarcinoma, and congenital hypertrophy of the retinal pigment epithelium {1144}.

Histogenesis

Melanoma at this anatomical site is thought to arise from uveal melanocytes. Most cases develop de novo, but uveal naevi can also transform into melanoma {327,621,1181}.

Genetic profile

Two recurrent, mutually exclusive G protein driver mutations (in *GNAQ* and *GNA11*) have been identified in uveal melanoma by mutation analysis {263,1306}. *GNAQ* and *GNA11* encode heterotrimeric G protein alpha subunits of the Gq class {499} that are 90% identical at the amino acid level and play redundant roles. Q209 and R183 mutations activate the MAPK pathway and the Hippo tumour suppressor pathway {196,344,1405}. Q209 mutations are more common than R183 mutations in uveal melanoma {1306}. These mutations appear to be an early event, and they are also present in blue naevi, choroidal naevi {1297}, and naevi of Ota. *BRAF* mutations, which are a characteristic finding in cutaneous melanoma, are very exceptional in uveal melanoma.
Loss of chromosome 3 (monosomy 3), in particular when associated with polysomy 8q, is associated with metastasis in choroidal melanoma {1305}. *BAP1*, a gene located on chromosome 3 (at 3p21.1), has been found to carry inactivating mutations in about 80% of metastasizing uveal melanomas {455}. BAP1 is a ubiquitin carboxy-terminal hydrolase. Some mutations affect the catalytic domain of the enzyme; others are frameshift or nonsense mutations resulting in a non-functional protein that is excluded from the nucleus. BAP1 appears to be involved with chromatin remodelling {1045} and cell-cycle control {318}. BAP1-deficient cells exhibit stem cell–like qualities {769}. BAP1 also appears to be involved in transendothelial migration and extravasation from the eye to the systemic circulation {874}. Once the neoplastic cells have entered the systemic circulation, a variety of factors, including receptor/ligand gradients (e.g. between c-Met and its ligand HGF/SF) {73,278,279,476} and the stoichiometric properties of the liver {426,432}, are involved in the propensity of uveal melanoma to metastasize to the liver.
Mutations of codon 625 of *SF3B1* on chromosome 2 are also found in some uveal melanomas {456}. SF3B1 is a splice factor involved in intron excision

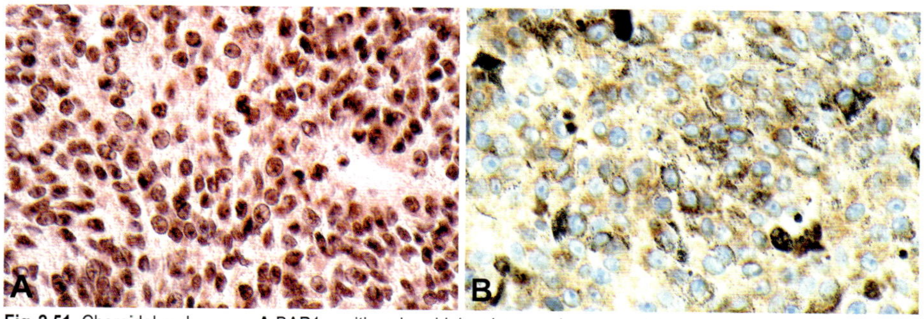

Fig. 2.51 Choroidal melanoma. **A** BAP1-positive choroidal melanoma; immunostaining for BAP1 is positive in the nuclei. **B** BAP1-negative choroidal melanoma; immunostaining for BAP1 is negative.

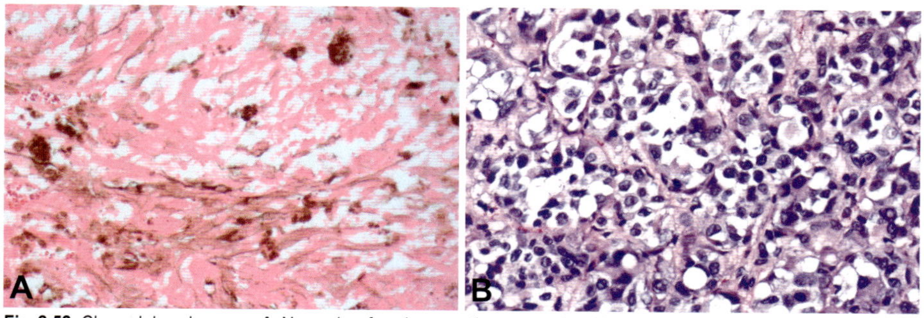

Fig. 2.52 Choroidal melanoma. **A** Necrosis of melanoma tissue can be difficult to diagnose (particularly in cases without substantial pigmentation) and may occur spontaneously. **B** This melanoma has undergone treatment-induced changes, with vacuolation of melanoma cells, after plaque radiotherapy.

from pre-mRNA, and it may also be associated with chromatin remodelling {456}. Another frequently mutated gene in uveal melanoma is *EIF1AX*, located at Xp22.1 {761}; this gene encodes a translation initiation factor. *BAP1*, *SF3B1*, and *EIF1AX* mutations appear to be mutually exclusive in uveal melanoma {263}.

Gene expression profiling has identified a set of differentially expressed genes in class 1A and 1B (low and intermediate metastatic risk, respectively) versus class 2 (high metastatic risk) uveal melanoma {875} Further work has shown that class 1 melanomas retain a differentiated melanocytic phenotype and transcriptome, whereas class 2 melanomas have a dedifferentiated, cancer stem cell–like phenotype and transcriptome {179}. As the tumour progresses, it may undergo *SF3B1* or *EIF1AX* mutation (which appears to be associated with a class 1 gene expression profile) or hemizygous *BAP1* mutation (which, when associated with monosomy 3, is associated with a class 2 gene expression profile) {351}. The preferentially expressed antigen in melanoma (PRAME) has also been shown to be a biomarker for metastases in class 1 melanomas {351}.

In the liver, the tumour forms relatively dormant micrometastases that have the potential to grow into clinical metastases {426,432}. These metastases may form nodules (the nodular pattern), infiltrate the hepatic parenchyma (the infiltrative pattern) {432}, or both. A variety of factors may contribute to the growth of micrometastases into large metastases, including likely abrogation of the host immune response (in particular NK cell function) {286,1013} and an increased local VEGF-to-PEDF ratio {685}.

A recent study by The Cancer Genome Atlas (TCGA) categorized 80 uveal melanomas into four subsets: two associated with poor-prognosis monosomy 3 and two with better-prognosis disomy 3 {979}. The poor-prognosis monosomy 3 uveal melanomas were characterized by a distinct global DNA methylation pattern and had distinct genomic, signalling, and immune profiles.

Genetic susceptibility

To date, the only known specific genetic susceptibility for choroidal and ciliary body melanomas is *BAP1* tumour predisposition syndrome, which is estimated to be present in approximately 2% of all patients with uveal melanoma and 20% of those with familial cases {442,862,913,949,1290}. In this syndrome, there is a germline mutation in *BAP1*. The syndrome includes an increased risk of developing uveal melanoma, atypical Spitz tumours of the skin, mesothelioma, cutaneous melanoma, clear cell renal cell carcinoma, and basal cell carcinoma {913,949}. Other cancers suspected to be associated with the syndrome include breast cancer, cholangiocarcinoma, non-small cell lung adenocarcinoma, meningioma, and neuroendocrine carcinoma {913}. *BAP1* tumour predisposition syndrome is inherited in an autosomal dominant pattern. Diagnosis of the syndrome is based on the identification of a heterozygous germline pathological variant in *BAP1* by molecular genetic testing {913}.

White patients with ocular or oculodermal melanocytosis (naevus of Ota) have a 1 in 400 lifetime risk of developing melanoma {1180}.

Prognosis and predictive factors

Tumour size, ciliary body involvement, and extraocular extension of the melanoma are of prognostic significance. The risk of metastasis increases with increasing tumour size, and from invasion of the ciliary body through extraocular invasion to invasion of both compartments {507,619,663}.

As many as 50% of patients in whom ciliary body or choroidal melanoma is diagnosed ultimately die from haematogenous metastasis of the tumour, most commonly (in 90% of cases) to the liver {60,664}. The prognosis for survival is worse for patients with melanomas of the ciliary body and anterior choroid {706} and with larger tumours {619}. Other common (often secondary) sites of metastasis are lung (affected in 24% of cases) and bone (in 16%) {60}. The median survival after detection of metastasis is 4–17 months, depending on how advanced the metastases are when detected {144,625}. In the past, when the liver was not imaged during surveillance, the reported median survival rates for patients with metastases were 15–20% at 6 months and 10% at 1 year {60}; in a recent study in which most patients underwent regular liver imaging, the reported rates were 75% at 6 months and 50% at 1 year {625}. Liver function tests and imaging, including MRI, PET-CT, and ultrasound, have been used to detect liver metastases {564}. Older age is a risk factor for decreased survival in patients with uveal melanoma {149}. Patients with metastasis confined to extrahepatic sites have longer survival

times (of 19–28 months) than patients with hepatic metastases {60}.
The reported 5-year survival rates are 88% for the spindle cell type and 60% for the epithelioid or mixed cell type overall {60}, but melanomas that have monosomy 3, are of gene expression profile class 2, or show loss of nuclear BAP1 expression are associated with 5-year survival rates of only about 30% {1303}. Disomy 3 melanomas have a worse prognosis if there is amplification of 8q {1191}. Other negative prognostic factors include larger tumour size {222,289,663,1347}, extravascular matrix loops and networks {569,1002}, high microvascular density {195,370,740}, high numbers of tumour-infiltrating macrophages {134,135,399,742}, and large tumour cell nucleoli {16,780}.

Choroidal and ciliary body naevi

Salomao D.R.
Eagle R.C. Jr
Grossniklaus H.E.
Kivelä T.T.
Wilson M.

Definition
Choroidal and ciliary body naevi are benign neoplasms arising from choroidal and ciliary body melanocytes.

ICD-O code
Uveal naevus 8720/0

Epidemiology
The prevalence of ciliary body naevi is unknown, because data are available only from autopsy and archival studies. In 152 consecutive autopsies, a ciliary body naevus was found in 3% of the 200 eyes studied {450}. In the Armed Forces Institute of Pathology (AFIP) registry, 6% of 102 uveal naevi in 100 enucleated eyes were located in the ciliary body {845}. A number of studies have reported the prevalence of choroidal naevi in adults {420,557,844,853}. The highest prevalence, estimated at 4–7%, is found in White populations {420,1228}.

Etiology
The etiology is unknown, but choroidal and ciliary body naevi are generally assumed to be congenital lesions that may grow slowly during childhood and early adulthood {766}.

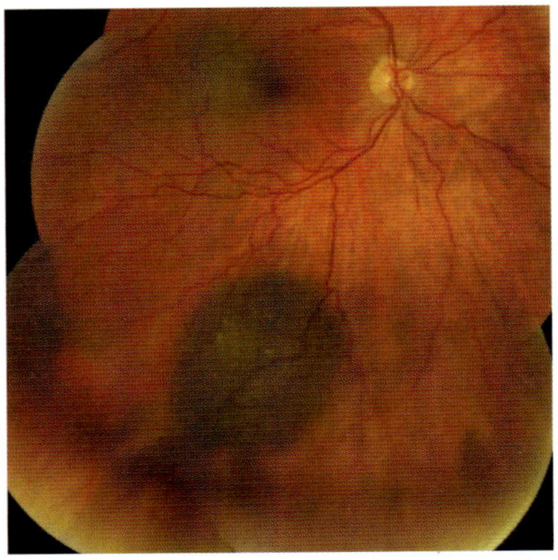

Fig. 2.53 Choroidal naevus. Fundus photography shows a flat lesion with overlying drusen, inferior to the macula.

Localization
These naevi occur in the pars plicata or pars plana of the ciliary body or choroid, most often in the post-equatorial choroid outside the foveolar region {200}.

Clinical features
Ciliary body naevi typically go undetected unless they are associated with anterior extension of the lesion through the iris root, focal shallowing of the anterior chamber, a sectoral cataract, episcleral sentinel vessels, or extraocular extension {284,637,1187}. Ultrasound biomicroscopy and anterior segment optical coherence tomography are useful ancillary examinations {465,1314,1356}. Choroidal naevi typically appear as a flat or slightly elevated patch of increased pigmentation or a yellowish amelanotic lesion measuring < 5 mm in diameter and < 2 mm in thickness {1083}; they often have irregular or feathered borders.

Histopathology
Choroidal and ciliary body naevi are composed of bland-looking cells that are generally plumper than normal melanocytes. Four histological types of naevus cells can be identified: (1) plump polyhedral cells, (2) slender spindle cells, (3) plump fusiform and dendritic cells, and (4) balloon cells {845}. Naevus cells have oval or cigar-shaped nuclei that usually lack nucleoli and nuclear membrane folding. The degree of cytoplasmic pigmentation is variable. Cytological atypia and mitotic figures are absent.

Differential diagnosis
The main differential diagnoses are choroidal and ciliary body melanocytomas and melanomas of spindle cell type, from which naevi can generally be differentiated on the basis of their smaller size and the absence of cellular atypia and mitotic figures. Amelanotic naevi must additionally be distinguished from other bland-looking spindle cell neoplasms, such as solitary fibrous tumour, schwannoma, and neurofibroma. For ciliary body naevi, the differential diagnosis additionally includes mesectodermal leiomyoma and adenoma or adenocarcinoma of the pigmented or non-pigmented ciliary epithelium. Immunopositivity for markers such as melan-A and SOX10 has proved helpful in confirming the melanocytic nature of uveal naevi.

Histogenesis
The naevus cells are derived from melanocytes of neural crest origin.

Genetic profile
In one study, mutually exclusive *GNAQ* and *GNA11* mutations were detected in 15 of 16 choroidal naevi, at a low frequency {1297}.

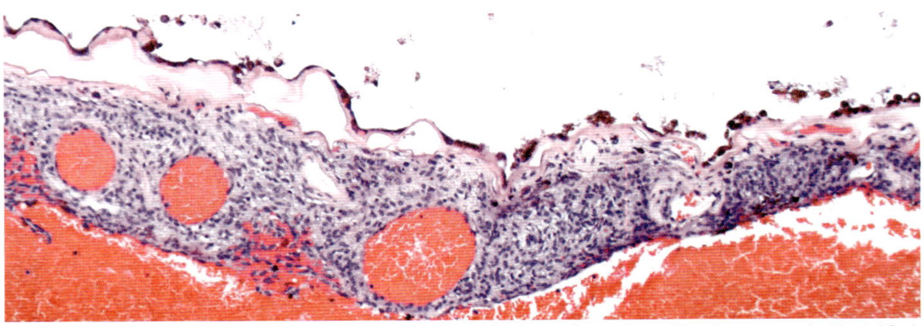

Fig. 2.54 Choroidal naevus. This example, characterized by a benign melanocytic proliferation, was an incidental finding in an enucleation specimen removed after ocular trauma with marked intraocular haemorrhage and retinal detachment; the entire lesion measured 2 mm.

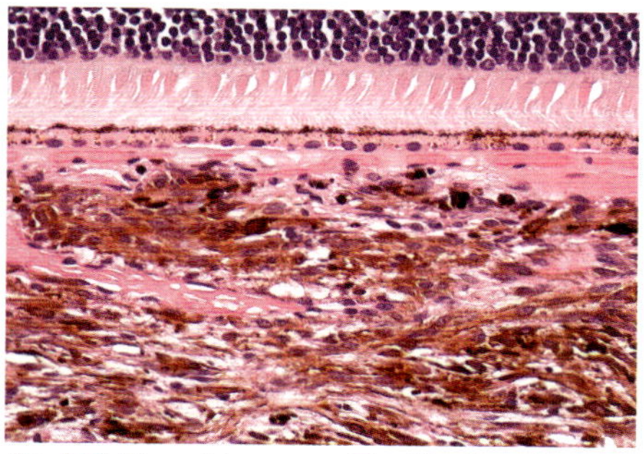

Fig. 2.55 Choroidal naevus. Bland-looking elongated pigmented cells nuclear atypia, nucleoli, and mitoses are absent.

Prognosis and predictive factors

Choroidal and ciliary body melanocytic naevi are benign lesions. They are monitored with clinical observation and repeat diagnostic imaging with ultrasound and optical coherence tomography to measure their thickness {465,1314,1356}. Approximately one third of choroidal naevi show minor, slow growth during long-term follow-up {766}, but only a few undergo malignant transformation {1181}. It is estimated that the lifetime risk for malignant transformation of a choroidal naevus is about 0.2% {621}.

Bilateral diffuse uveal melanocytic hyperplasia

Salomao D.R.
Eagle R.C. Jr
Mudhar H.S.

Definition

Bilateral diffuse uveal melanocytic hyperplasia is a paraneoplastic syndrome characterized by diffuse proliferation of benign melanocytes in the uvea, in patients with an underlying extraocular malignancy {393,867}.

ICD-O code

None

Synonyms

Bilateral diffuse uveal melanocytic proliferation (BDUMP); paraneoplastic uveal melanocytic hyperplasia

Epidemiology

The exact incidence of bilateral diffuse uveal melanocytic hyperplasia is unknown. The syndrome seems to have an equal sex distribution and an average patient age at presentation of 63 years (range: 34–89 years) {170}.

Etiology

In patients with bilateral diffuse uveal melanocytic hyperplasia, the IgG fraction contains a serum factor called cultured melanocyte elongation and proliferation (CMEP) factor, which selectively stimulates melanocyte proliferation {800}, although the exact mechanism is unknown.

Localization

Bilateral diffuse uveal melanocytic hyperplasia arises in the iris, ciliary body, and choroid.

Clinical features

Patients present with otherwise inexplicable rapid onset of bilateral vision loss refractory to treatment. Unilateral ocular involvement is rare {1207}. Important signs of bilateral diffuse uveal melanocytic hyperplasia include multiple subtle red patches at the level of the retinal pigment epithelium corresponding to areas of hyperfluorescence {635}, serous retinal detachment, and rapidly progressive cataract {393,867}. These ocular findings are associated with (and often precede) the finding of underlying malignancy, most commonly carcinoma from the ovary or endometrium in women and from the lung in men {170}. Less common primary sites of the underlying primary neoplasm are the pancreas, lung, colon, and kidney {635,829,867}. Other paraneoplastic symptoms may coexist.

Histopathology

The uvea shows diffuse thickening secondary to proliferations of melanocytic cells in the choroid, ciliary body, and iris. These proliferations consist of spindle-shaped cells with elongated oval nuclei, inconspicuous nucleoli, and scant intracytoplasmic melanin pigment. Occasional cellular atypia has been described, but mitoses are rare. The melanocytes stain positively for melan-A and HMB45 antigen, but do not overexpress p53 {759}, and they show a low proliferation rate {815,867}. A serous detachment of the retina may overlie choroidal lesions.

Differential diagnosis

The differential diagnosis includes diffuse uveal melanoma.

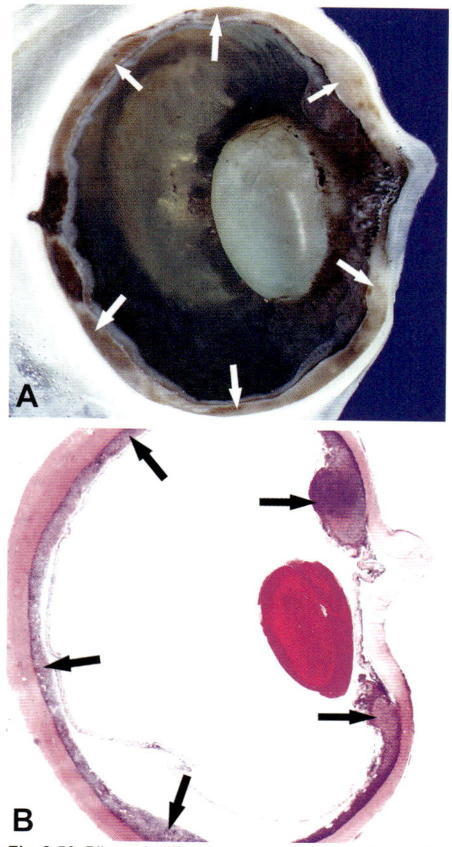

Fig. 2.56 Bilateral diffuse uveal melanocytic hyperplasia. **A** An enucleation specimen shows diffuse melanocytic hyperplasia (arrows) of the entire uvea. **B** This is also demonstrated in a low-power view of the same specimen.

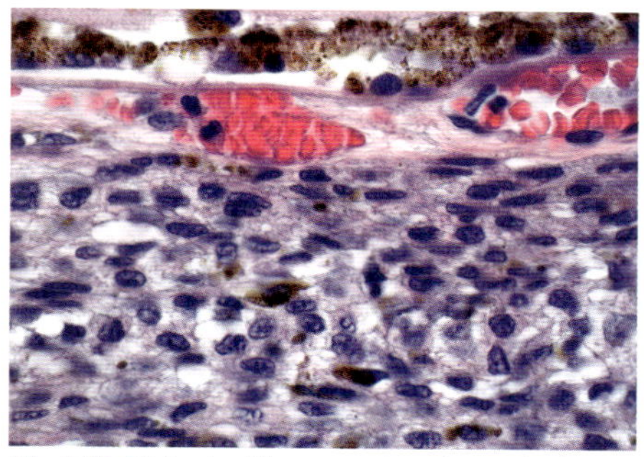

Fig. 2.57 Bilateral diffuse uveal melanocytic hyperplasia. The uveal melanocytes show elongated nuclei, inconspicuous nucleoli, and scant intracytoplasmic melanin pigment.

Histogenesis

Bilateral diffuse uveal melanocytic hyperplasia arises due to hyperplasia of uveal melanocytes; in patients with this syndrome, melanocytes of the dermis, mucous membranes, and conjunctiva are also affected {746,933}.

Genetic profile

Recent molecular studies have shown gains in chromosomes 6 {829} and 5

{948}, as well as polysomy 8q {815}. Bilateral diffuse uveal melanocytic hyperplasia cells do not show the chromosome 3 abnormalities or *GNAQ* mutations seen in uveal melanoma {815,829}.

Prognosis and predictive factors

The prognosis depends on the response of the primary tumour to therapy. Most patients die within a year of the diagnosis, although there have been rare reports of longer survival {867}. Until recently, the vision loss resulting from bilateral diffuse uveal melanocytic hyperplasia was considered to be progressive and irreversible, but recent studies have shown stabilization of ocular symptoms in patients treated with plasmapheresis {548}.

Neurofibroma and ganglioneuroma of the choroid

Rodriguez F.
Eagle R.C. Jr
Moulin A.
Croxatto J.O.
Kase S.
Mudhar H.S.

Definition

Neurofibroma of the choroid is a benign peripheral nerve sheath tumour composed of a mixture of Schwann cells, perineurial-like cells, and intraneural fibroblasts. Ganglioneuroma of the choroid differs from neurofibroma in that it additionally contains a variable number of mature ganglion cells.

ICD-O codes

Neurofibroma	9540/0
Ganglioneuroma	9490/0

Epidemiology

Choroidal lesions in the setting of neurofibromatosis type 1 (NF1) may develop in paediatric patients, and they appear to increase in frequency with age.

Etiology

NF1 gene mutation is a likely initiation event.

Localization

Diffuse/multifocal choroidal involvement is typical, and there is a predilection for the posterior pole {1298}. Associated involvement of small ciliary nerves is variable.

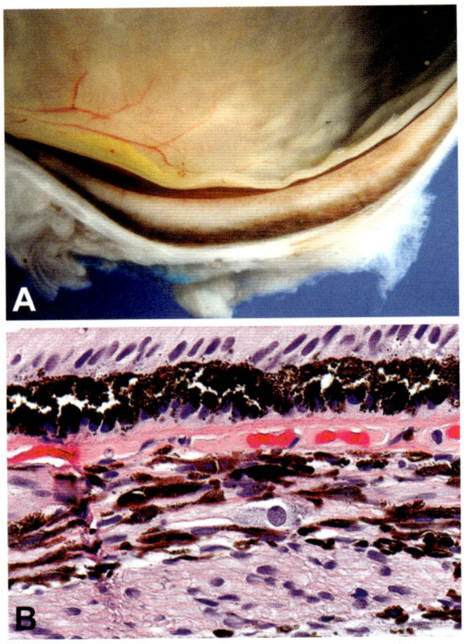

Fig. 2.58 A Choroidal neurofibroma in neurofibromatosis type 1 (NF1); uveal neurofibromas typically cause diffuse expansion of the choroid. **B** Choroid in NF1; rare ganglion cells are a normal component of the choroid, but numerous ganglion cells are often encountered in choroidal lesions of NF1 in association with a Schwann cell proliferation; when the aggregate of ganglion cells is florid, these lesions are termed ganglioneuroma.

Clinical features

Recent studies using modern imaging techniques (i.e. indocyanine green angiography, infrared fundus autofluorescence, and enhanced depth imaging optical coherence tomography) suggest that choroidal involvement is very common in NF1 and might be a potential diagnostic criterion for the disease {1298,1328,1395}. MRI is helpful for identifying choroidal tumours in patients with NF1, revealing circumscribed or diffuse thickening of the choroid {512}.

Histopathology

Histopathology often reveals diffuse thickening of the uveal stroma by a Schwann cell proliferation, fibroblasts, and choroidal melanocytes. This thickening is massive in some cases; parts of the choroid may be several times as thick as the sclera. The lesion may contain ovoid bodies that resemble tactile corpuscles, ultrastructurally composed of Schwann cells arranged in lamellae {671}. Ganglion cells, which are a normal constituent of the choroid, are fairly numerous in some cases, to which the term "ganglioneuroma" has been applied.

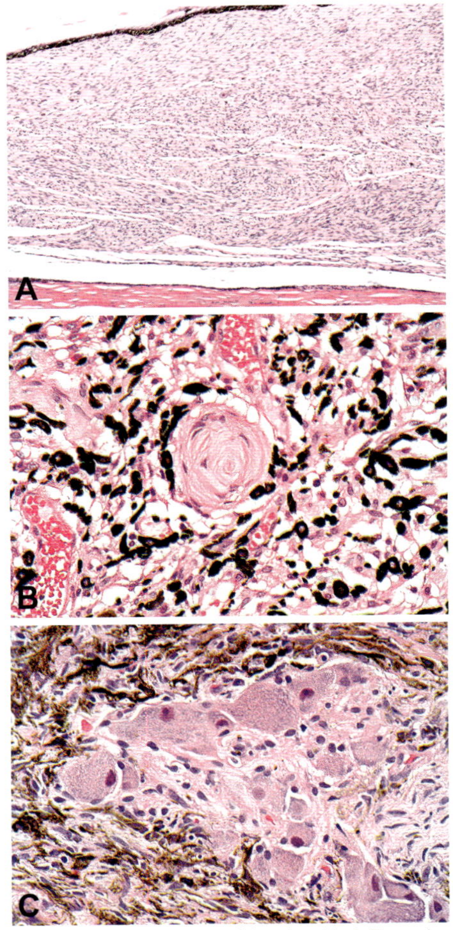

Fig. 2.59 Ganglioneuroma of the choroid. **A** Expansion of the choroid by a proliferation of Schwann and ganglion cells; the patient had a germline *PTEN* mutation. **B** Ovoid bodies resembling Meissner (tactile) corpuscles are composed of concentric Schwann cell processes. **C** A florid aggregate of abnormal ganglion cells in the choroid, consistent with the diagnosis of ganglioneuroma.

Differential diagnosis

The differential diagnosis is limited, because the clinical and histological features are distinctive.

Histogenesis

Neurofibroma and ganglioneuroma probably originate from neural crest–derived precursors.

Genetic profile

Genetic characterization of these lesions is lacking.

Genetic susceptibility

Patients with NF1 are predisposed to the development of these lesions, and the number of choroidal nodules is increased in the presence of truncating *NF1* mutations {166}. One reported

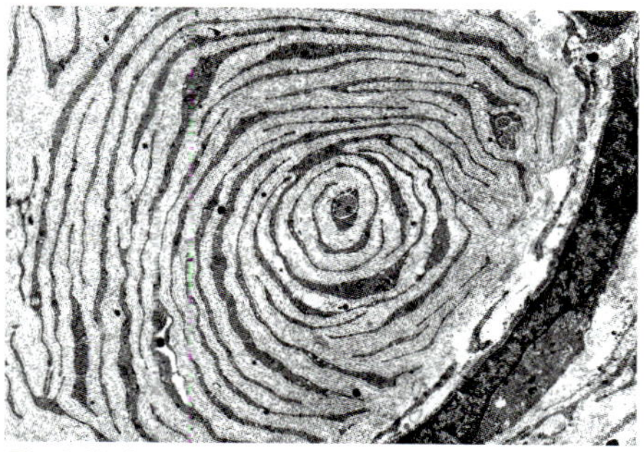

Fig. 2.60 Choroidal neurofibroma in neurofibromatosis type 1. Ovoid bodies are composed of elongated cells with Schwann cell properties, including a fragmented basal lamina.

example developed in a patient with germline *PTEN* mutation (Cowden syndrome) {275}.

Prognosis and predictive factors

Diffuse uveal tract abnormalities are typically found incidentally during histopathological examination of blind, painful, buphthalmic eyes enucleated from patients with NF1.

Schwannoma of the choroid

Rodriguez F.
Eagle R.C. Jr
Moulin A.

Definition

Schwannoma of the choroid is a benign circumscribed nerve sheath tumour composed exclusively of neoplastic Schwann cells.

ICD-O code

Schwannoma 9560/0

Synonyms

Neurilemmoma; benign peripheral nerve sheath tumour

Epidemiology

The average patient age at presentation is 37 years (range: 9–76 years), and these tumours are more common in women, with a female-to-male ratio of 3:1 {1403}.

Etiology

These tumours are sporadic; they are not associated with neurofibromatosis, schwannomatosis, or Carney complex.

Localization

Approximately 60% of uveal tract schwannomas develop in the choroid and 40% in the ciliary body {1403}. There may be overlap, because a ciliary body schwannoma can extend into the choroid and vice versa.

Clinical features

Patients may present with vision loss and/or an amelanotic intraocular mass {1403} that is ovoid or dome-shaped. Rarely, the tumours are lobulated, mushroom-shaped, and pigmented – an appearance clinically similar to that of uveal melanoma. Schwannomas can usually be distinguished from melanoma by an absence of sentinel vessels and by increased light transmission, but this is not always the case {662,914,998}.

Histopathology

Schwannomas are composed exclusively of neoplastic Schwann cells. Unlike schwannomas at other sites, uveal schwannomas often lack a capsule. The neoplastic cells are arranged in an alternating pattern of compact areas with or without Verocay bodies (Antoni A areas) and areas with variable amounts of loosely arranged cells with a myxoid stroma and lipidization (Antoni B areas). Degenerative nuclear atypia (so-called ancient change) may be present, but this finding has no clinical significance {824}. Almost all uveal schwannomas are of the conventional type, although a rare example of melanotic schwannoma has been reported {1139}. No cellular cases have been reported.

Schwannomas uniformly express S100 protein (nuclear and cytoplasmic), SOX10, CD57 (LEU7), and calretinin {552,905,1357}. They may also express GFAP {786}, collagen IV, and laminin {873}. Except in melanotic schwannoma, melanocytic markers (e.g. melan-A, MITF, and HMB45 antigen) are negative. Transmission electron microscopy shows prominent, continuous basal lamina surrounding long cytoplasmic processes. Stromal Luse bodes (long-spaced collagen) are a common feature {1403}.

Differential diagnosis

The main differential diagnosis is uveal melanoma {1146,1201}, but leiomyoma, neurofibroma, and fibrous histiocytoma should also be ruled out {662,914,998,1201}.

Histogenesis

In the uvea, schwannoma presumably originates from the nerve sheath of ciliary nerves {1403}.

Genetic profile

Because of their rarity, uveal schwannomas have not been well characterized at the genetic level. However, it is likely that they have genetic traits similar to those of their extraocular counterparts, including *NF2* mutation/chromosome 22 loss.

Genetic susceptibility

Most uveal schwannomas are sporadic; occurrence in the setting of presumed neurofibromatosis type 2 is rare {376}. However, some choroidal schwannomas have been reported in association with

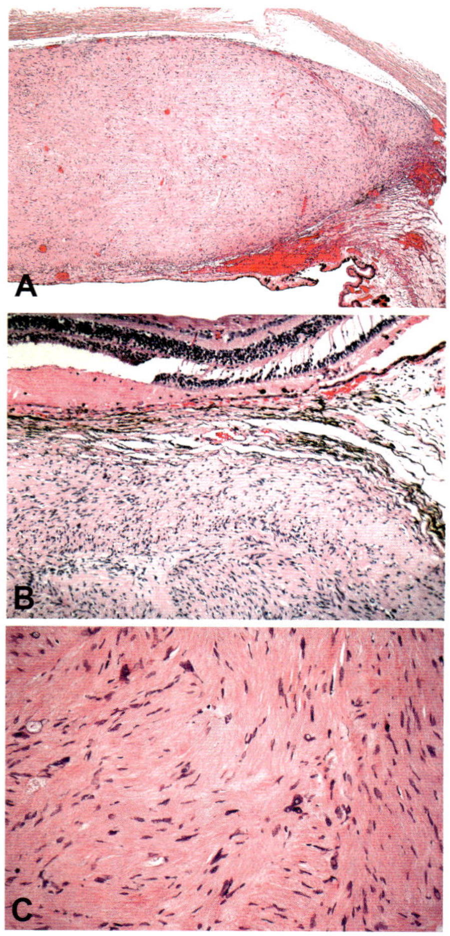

Fig. 2.61 Choroidal schwannoma. **A** Schwannomas form well-circumscribed but unencapsulated intraocular masses. **B** An intimate association with the choroid is typical of intraocular schwannomas. **C** Compact Antoni A areas predominate in schwannomas of the uveal tract; degenerative atypia (so-called ancient change) may be present.

neurofibromatosis type 2 {376,778,1310}. A single choroidal schwannoma has been reported to have developed in the context of *PTEN* hamartoma tumour syndrome {1317}.

Prognosis and predictive factors

Schwannomas arising in the uveal tract have an excellent prognosis, although the tumours may rarely recur after local resection {501}.

Haemangioma of the choroid

Eagle R.C. Jr
Rao N.
Materin M.A.

Definition

Haemangioma of the choroid is a vascular hamartoma.

ICD-O code

Haemangioma	9120/0

Epidemiology

Most circumscribed cases (92%) are diagnosed in White adults (mean patient age: 47 years); there is a slight male predominance, with 58% of cases reported in males {1087}. Diffuse haemangioma in Sturge–Weber syndrome (SWS) is diagnosed in children with ipsilateral naevus flammeus or retinal detachment.

Etiology

Diffuse choroidal haemangioma occurs in patients with SWS.

Localization

Circumscribed choroidal haemangiomas involve the posterior choroid, with 67% located in the macula. Diffuse haemangioma may involve the half of the choroid posterior to the equator, and it is often thickest in the macula {1087}.

Clinical features

Circumscribed haemangioma appears as a discrete reddish-orange mass in the posterior choroid. The tumour may present with vision loss secondary to a subfoveal location, secondary retinal detachment, or induced hyperopia. The overlying retina often shows cystoid oedema or retinoschisis {764,1087}. The tumour vessels are hyperfluorescent in the pre-arterial phase of intravenous fluorescein angiography, with late staining. Indocyanine green angiography shows early filling and characteristic washout of hyperfluorescence in later frames {1087}. The tumour vessels show high internal reflectivity and acoustic solidity, respectively, on A-scan and B-scan ultrasonography. On MRI, choroidal haemangioma is hyperintense to vitreous on T1-weighted imaging and isointense on T2-weighted imaging. Choroidal haemangioma shows little intrinsic autofluorescence {950}. Enhanced depth imaging optical coherence tomography shows a smooth, acutely dome-shaped mass with subretinal fluid and/or cystoid retinal oedema {1101}. Diffuse haemangioma in SWS causes a so-called tomato ketchup fundus, with diffuse reddish-orange thickening of the choroid obscuring normal anatomical features ipsilateral to the port wine mark. About 75% of SWS patients with diffuse haemangioma have glaucoma, the mechanisms of which include iris neovascularization, pupillary block, maldevelopment of angle structures, and elevation of episcleral venous pressure secondary to abnormal episcleral vasculature {912}.

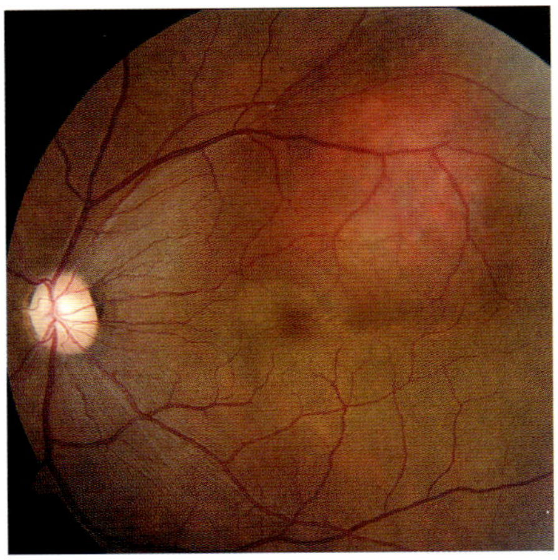

Fig. 2.62 Choroidal haemangioma. On ophthalmoscopy, the lesion appears as a reddish tumefaction superotemporal to the fovea.

Histopathology

The tumour is composed of thin-walled vascular channels lined by endothelial cells with scant intervening stroma {1168,1373}. Haemangiomas can be classified as cavernous, capillary, or mixed depending on the size of their vascular channels. Sporadic tumours have sharply demarcated pushing margins that compress adjacent normal choroid. In diffuse lesions, the vascular tumour is intermixed with engorged pre-existing vascular channels. In chronic cases, there is often cystoid oedema of the overlying retina, and the tumour may be capped by fibrous metaplasia of the retinal pigment epithelium or even a plaque of bone.

Differential diagnosis

The differential diagnosis includes other primary choroidal neoplasms, in particular amelanotic choroidal melanoma and orange-coloured metastases from thyroid tumours, renal cell carcinoma, or neuroendocrine tumours {1087,1094}.

Genetic profile

The somatic *GNAQ* mutation c.548G>A (p.R183Q) is consistently found in the port wine stains of SWS {842}.

Genetic susceptibility

There is no evidence of hereditary transmission.

Prognosis and predictive factors

Although choroidal haemangioma is a benign neoplasm, the visual prognosis is guarded. Visual acuity of 20/200 or less occurs in approximately half of patients, usually as a result of chronic subretinal fluid and macular oedema {1087}. Vision-threatening haemangioma is usually

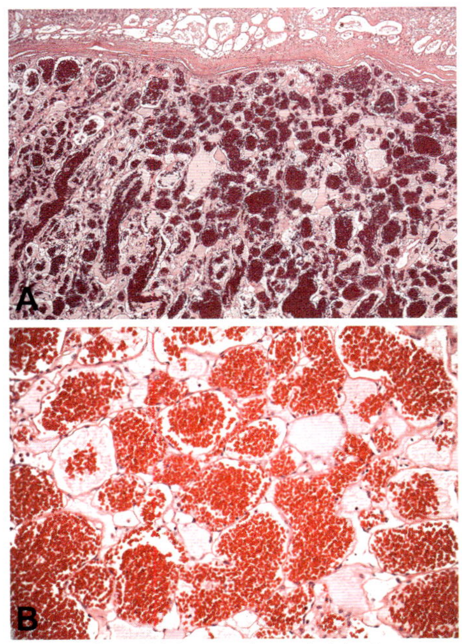

Fig. 2.63 Choroidal haemangioma. **A** A benign vascular neoplasm in choroidal stroma is capped by fibrous metaplasia of the epithelium; the overlying retina shows cystoid oedema and atrophy of its outer layers. **B** Haemangioma is composed of thin-walled vascular channels; the tumour contains very little stroma.

treated with a variety of therapeutic modalities, including transpupillary thermotherapy, photodynamic therapy, and radiotherapy using radioactive plaques or external beam or proton beam radiotherapy {52,880,1123}.

Osteoma of the choroid

Meyer P.
Eagle R.C. Jr
Materin M.A.

Definition
Osteoma of the choroid is a benign, often slow-growing tumour of mature bone.

ICD-O code
Osteoma 9180/0

Synonym
Choroidal osseous choristoma (obsolete)

Epidemiology
Osteoma is rare, but its precise prevalence is unknown. It occurs in all races, and two thirds of patients are women. Patient age ranges from a few months to late in the sixth decade of life, but most patients are in their late teens or early twenties at the time of diagnosis. About 20% of cases are bilateral {18}.

Localization
Osteoma of the choroid is mostly localized in the juxtapapillary and macular areas of the choroid.

Clinical features
The most common signs and symptoms are blurred vision, metamorphopsia, photophobia, and visual field defects, which are generally related to partial deossification. About 8–30% of cases are asymptomatic; in many such cases, deossification has not occurred {66,1120}.
Choroidal osteoma is a deep, orangish-yellow (orangish-red in early stages) placoid lesion with distinct geographical or well-defined scalloped borders and branching vessels on the tumour surface. Deossification leads to degeneration of the overlying retinal pigment epithelium. Important ancillary diagnostic tests include ultrasonography and optical coherence tomography. Ultrasound imaging reveals a calcified component with high acoustic reflectivity and shadowing {1110}, and optical coherence tomography can reveal a wide range of appearances, including a lamellar pattern, speckled hyper-reflective lines, and tubule formation; photoreceptor loss over deossified areas has also been reported {1077}. CT reveals a hyperdense choroidal plaque with the same density as bone, but this imaging modality is not recommended, because the other imaging methods mentioned are sufficient for diagnosis.

Histopathology
The only histopathological information about this lesion comes from a single case reported by two groups of authors {394,1369}. Choroidal osteoma contains dense interconnected trabeculae of mature bone with numerous osteocytes and focal osteoblastic rimming, with intervening spaces filled with loose connective tissue containing large, cavernous, endothelial-lined vascular channels and small capillary-type blood vessels connected to a rich capillary network beneath the Bruch membrane; there is a focally depigmented and degenerated pigment epithelium. The bone is present within the choroid, not on the inner surface of the Bruch membrane as is seen in osseous metaplasia of the retinal pigment epithelium (a relatively common type of intraocular ossification often found in blind, phthisical eyes).

Differential diagnosis
The differential diagnosis includes amelanotic choroidal melanoma {1110} and naevus, choroidal haemangioma (focal ossification may overlie a solitary lesion), metastatic carcinoma and lymphoma, posterior scleritis, and choroidal granuloma.
In practice, a frequent differential diagnosis is sclerochoroidal calcification {1085}, an idiopathic nodular deposition of calcium in the sclera extending into the choroid. Sclerochoroidal calcification is asymptomatic and is typically found in elderly patients on routine eye examination. Like choroidal osteoma, sclerochoroidal calcification is a yellowish lesion with high acoustic reflectivity and shadowing, and it is often bilateral; but sclerochoroidal calcification is typically located between the retinal vascular arcades and the equator (near the insertions of the oblique muscles) rather than in the posterior pole. Rarely, sclerochoroidal calcification can

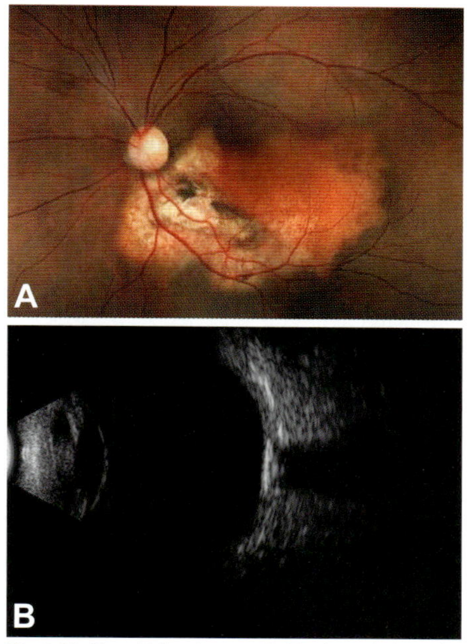

Fig. 2.64 Choroidal osteoma. **A** Fundus photography of the left eye revealed a large choroidal osteoma in the inferior macula, with a peripapillary atrophic scar and partial atrophy of the retinal pigment epithelium. **B** B-scan ultrasonography of the same case reveals focal subretinal calcification, with shadowing.

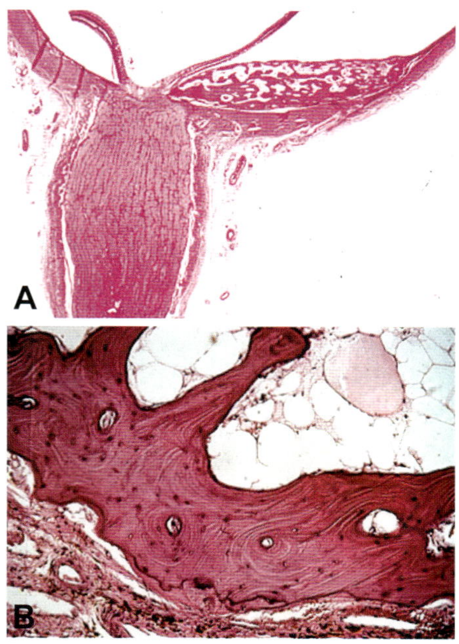

Fig. 2.65 Choroidal osteoma. **A** A juxtapapillary osseous choroidal tumour containing numerous bony trabeculae. **B** Interconnecting bony trabeculae and occasional fibrofatty marrow.

be associated with systemic disease (e.g. renal disease), hyperparathyroidism, hypercalcaemia, hypomagnesaemia, diuretic or calcium intake, Bartter syndrome, and Gitelman syndrome.

Genetic susceptibility

The genetic susceptibility is unknown, but familial cases have been reported {1284}.

Prognosis and predictive factors

On long-term follow-up, tumour growth has been found to occur in 51% of cases, and partial or complete deossification in 46%, followed by choroidal neovascularization, which occurs in 31–47% of eyes, with visual acuity loss to 20/200 vision or worse in 56–58% of eyes {66,1120}. If asymptomatic, osteomas are not treated. In the event of choroidal neovascularization, regression of neovascularization and subretinal fluid can be achieved with intravitreal anti-VEGF treatment, with or without additional modalities such as photodynamic therapy or transpupillary thermotherapy.

Primary choroidal lymphoma

Grossniklaus H.E.
Coupland S.E.

Definition

Primary choroidal (uveal) lymphoma is a low-grade (indolent) lymphocytic neoplasm in the uveal tract {226}.

ICD-O code

Primary choroidal lymphoma 9699/3

Synonyms

Reactive lymphoid hyperplasia; uveal lymphoid infiltrate {429}

Epidemiology

This lesion occurs primarily in adults, with both sexes equally affected.

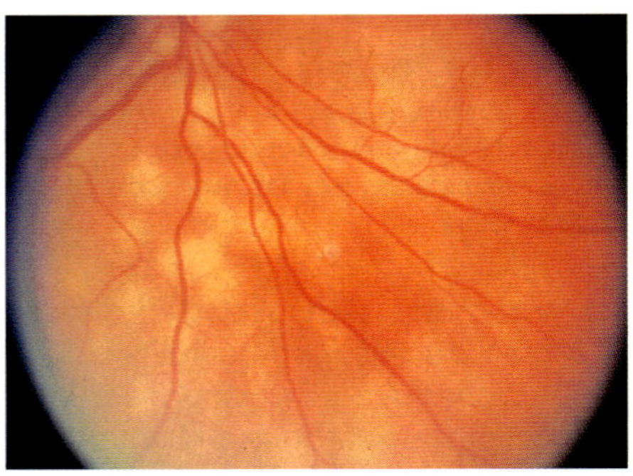

Fig. 2.66 Primary choroidal lymphoma. This image of the fundus shows that the choroid contains patchy beige infiltrates.

Etiology

The lesion occurs spontaneously, with no known etiology.

Localization

Primary uveal lymphoma is mainly located in the choroid, although it may extend anteriorly to the ciliary body and possibly the iris.

Clinical features

The lesion appears as creamy beige infiltrates in the uveal tract {429}; it may also give rise to confluent thickening of the uvea, which can be demonstrated by ultrasonography. There may be focal serous detachments of the retina overlying the lesion. The lesion may also extend via emissary canals into the subconjunctival space, giving a fleshy nodular appearance to the conjunctiva {429}. It may extend along peripapillary emissary canals, resulting in an ultrasonographic appearance of peripapillary nodules on the external scleral surface {181}. The ultrasonographic appearance of the lesion along with the optic nerve is known as the whale tail sign.

Histopathology

Primary choroidal lymphoma, which was once considered to be reactive in nature {1010}, consists of a diffuse infiltrate of small, round lymphocytes, and the infiltrate may contain follicles with germinal centres. A study of the initially examined cases revealed that the majority contained clonal B lymphocyte populations {211}. This lesion is now considered to be a low-grade B-cell lymphoma, similar to extranodal marginal zone lymphoma of mucosa-associated lymphoid tissue (MALT lymphoma) {226}.

Differential diagnosis

The main differential diagnosis for this condition is reactive lymphocytic infiltration in the uveal tract, including Vogt–Koyanagi–Harada disease, sympathetic ophthalmia, and sarcoidosis. These conditions must be ruled out by clinical tests and examination of biopsy specimens. If the primary choroidal lymphoma extends into the subconjunctival space, a conjunctival biopsy may be performed for tissue diagnosis {181}. A choroidal biopsy may also be performed, although this is usually not necessary, because the diagnosis can typically be made on clinical grounds.

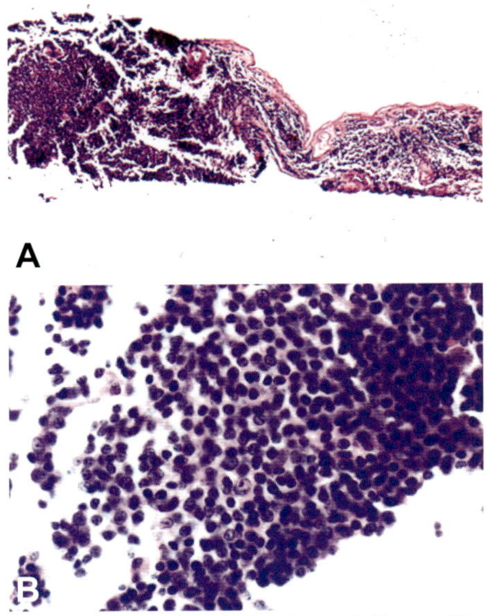

Fig. 2.67 Primary choroidal lymphoma. **A** Biopsy of the choroid shows a diffuse lymphocytic infiltrate. **B** Higher magnification shows that the lesion is composed mainly of sheets of small, round lymphocytes.

Histogenesis

This entity is idiopathic in nature. It is possible that an inflammatory/reactive lymphocytic infiltrate in the uveal tract may transform into a low-grade lymphoma after a clonal population of B lymphocytes emerges.

Prognosis and predictive factors

Patients with this lesion have an excellent prognosis; they usually respond favourably to systemic corticosteroid administration or low-dose external beam radiation therapy. There have been only rare instances of systemic low-grade lymphocytic infiltration associated with this lesion.

Secondary lymphomatous infiltration of the choroid

Coupland S.E.
Meyer P.
Rašić D.M.

Definition

Secondary lymphomatous infiltration of the choroid is secondary involvement of the choroid by systemic lymphoma, typically a non-Hodgkin lymphoma.

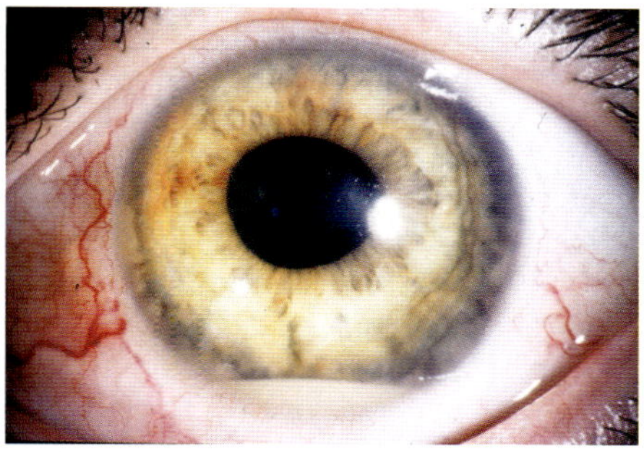

Fig. 2.68 Secondary uveal lymphoma. This 44-year-old woman with secondary involvement of her uveal tract developed a pseudohypopyon in her left eye.

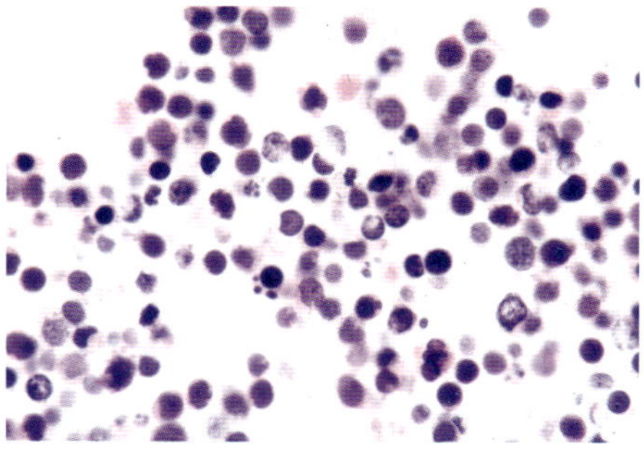

Fig. 2.69 Secondary uveal lymphoma. Anterior chamber aspirate from the patient shown in Fig. 2.68 is composed of large, round lymphocytes and occasional tingible body macrophages.

ICD-O codes

Code according to the lymphoma subtype.

Synonyms

Secondary choroidal lymphoma; metastatic choroidal lymphoma

Epidemiology

The exact incidence is unknown. Secondary lymphomatous infiltration can occur at any age, but tends to occur in middle-aged to elderly patients. Advanced aggressive systemic lymphoma is associated with an increased risk, particularly in immunosuppressed patients. There is no sex or race predilection {228,629,765}.

Localization

Secondary lymphomatous infiltration can occur in any part of the choroid.

Clinical features

In most cases (~80%), there is a known underlying systemic lymphoma at presentation, but in as many as 1 in 5 cases, the secondary choroidal lymphoma may be the first clinical manifestation of the disease. As many as one third of patients with secondary uveal lymphoma have bilateral disease {228,295,375,629,765}.

Secondary choroidal lymphomas may present with a variety of signs and symptoms, depending on the location of the infiltration and its extent. Some patients may have minimal symptoms despite extensive intraocular disease. Most patients present with blurred or decreasing vision due to involvement of the choroid adjacent to the fovea, or with vitreous haze {226,765,1420}.

The neoplastic cells, which are contained within the choroid by the Bruch membrane, can penetrate the sclera via exit routes such as nerves and veins, and they form extraocular nodules or masses either anteriorly or posteriorly. These masses result in episcleral masses, episcleral vascular congestion, proptosis, and diplopia {226,295,765}.

Secondary lymphomatous infiltration that extends from the choroid into the ciliary body can also involve the ciliary processes, causing their distortion and destruction; in very advanced cases, the tumour cells then spill over into the vitreous, causing extensive haze {226,440}.

Choroidal lymphomatous infiltration may also extend into the iris and cause either discrete nodules or masses, leading to floating cells within the anterior chamber or keratic precipitates {226,440}. Diffuse iridal involvement can lead to angle closure and subsequent glaucoma. Secondary lymphomatous infiltration of the iris can present as hyphaema or pseudohypopyon {226,440}.

Other (unusual) manifestations of secondary choroidal lymphoma include optic disc swelling and serous macular detachment {226,440}.

Histopathology

In enucleation specimens, extensive infiltration of the anterior and posterior choroid by neoplastic cells is typically seen. As noted above, invasion of adjacent intraocular and extraocular structures can be seen. Although the tumour cells are usually contained by the Bruch membrane, the overlying retinal pigment epithelium can show secondary effects, such as detachment, clumping, and proliferation. Similarly, the neural retina may be detached and demonstrate atrophy and cell loss.

The morphology, immunophenotype, and genotype of secondary choroidal lymphomas depend on the underlying lymphoma subtype. In order of decreasing frequency, the secondary choroidal lymphoma subtypes are diffuse large B-cell lymphoma, chronic lymphocytic leukaemia/small lymphocytic lymphoma, myeloma, lymphoplasmacytic lymphoma (including Waldenström macroglobulinaemia), extranodal marginal zone lymphoma of mucosa-associated lymphoid tissue (MALT lymphoma; usually arising

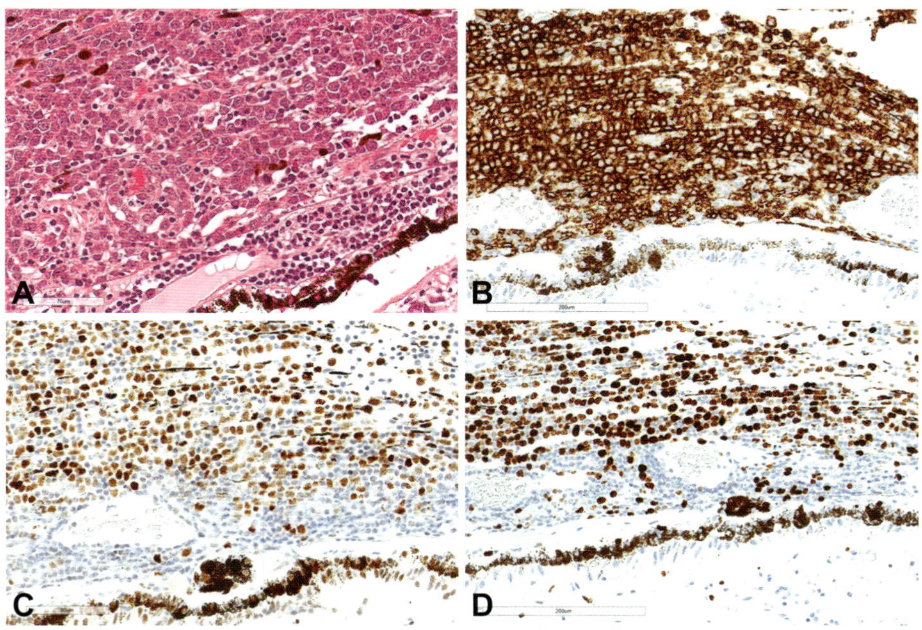

Fig. 2.70 Secondary choroidal lymphoma. **A** Diffuse and dense infiltration of the anterior choroid by large atypical lymphoid cells, causing disruption of the overlying retinal pigment epithelium and detachment of the peripheral retina. **B** CD20 immunoreactivity of the neoplastic B cells. **C** Clear nuclear positivity of the diffuse large B-cell lymphoma cells for the immunoglobulin transcription factor BCL6. **D** High Ki-67 proliferation index of viable tumour cells, reflecting the high-grade nature of lymphoma secondarily infiltrating the choroid.

in the lung), and plasmablastic lymphoma {226,228,295,765}. Rarely, intravascular lymphoma with secondary involvement of the eye (particularly the choriocapillaris), sometimes leading to secondary choroidal haemorrhage, can occur {692,830}. Secondary involvement of the choroid by a T-cell or NK-cell lymphoma is exceptionally rare {186,227,711,1237}.
The morphological, immunophenotypic, and genotypic characteristics of these secondary choroidal lymphoma entities are covered in more detail in the volume *WHO classification of tumours of haematopoietic and lymphoid tissues* {1231}.
Increasingly, choroidal and chorioretinal biopsies are being undertaken to aid confirmation of the clinical diagnosis of secondary choroidal lymphoma and to exclude infectious causes {375,440,615,709,1006,1033}.

Differential diagnosis
The main differential diagnosis is primary MALT lymphoma arising in the choroid {226}. Reactive or infectious causes include uveitis due to Vogt–Koyanagi–Harada disease, sarcoidosis, tuberculosis, syphilis, Behçet disease, Sweet syndrome, and disseminated bacterial or fungal infection {709,770,1006}.

Histogenesis
The histogenesis depends on the lymphoma subtype and the putative neoplastic cell of origin {226}. The histogenesis of both B-cell and T-cell non-Hodgkin lymphomas is often related to recurrent genetic abnormalities, which are covered in the volume *WHO classification of tumours of haematopoietic and lymphoid tissues* {1231}.

Genetic profile
The genetic profile depends on the lymphoma subtype.

Prognosis and predictive factors
The prognosis of secondary choroidal lymphomatous involvement depends on the lymphoma subtype and clinical stage. Unlike primary choroidal lymphomas, secondary choroidal lymphomas usually demonstrate a rapidly progressive course. Although no standard treatment for secondary choroidal lymphoma has yet been established, most patients are treated with low-dose external beam radiation therapy to slow disease progression and delay the onset of pain while chemotherapy is being initiated {226,295,765}.

Leukaemic infiltration of the choroid

Coupland S.E.
Meyer P.
Rašić D.M.

Definition
Leukaemic infiltration of the choroid is secondary involvement of the choroid by a systemic leukaemia of either acute or chronic form.

ICD-O codes
Code according to the leukaemia subtype.

Synonym
Secondary choroidal leukaemia

Epidemiology
Ocular involvement is common in all types of leukaemia; it has been estimated to occur in 30–70% of leukaemia cases overall, depending on the geographical area surveyed {701,966,1072,1242}. The prevalence in acute leukaemias appears to be about 5 times that seen in chronic forms. Ocular involvement in leukaemia can affect patients of any age, has a slight predilection for males, and is often bilateral {257,966}. No race predilection has been observed.

Etiology
Leukaemic infiltration of the choroid tends to occur in advanced disease, possibly as a relapse. It has been posited that the choroid may act as a sanctuary for the leukaemic cells, allowing them to escape the effects of radiation and systemic cytotoxic therapy {859}.

Localization
The posterior choroid is typically affected.

Clinical features
Choroidal involvement presents as a serous retinal detachment, which is generally shallow and located at the posterior pole. These detachments have been reported in patients with lymphoblastic leukaemia {825,885,1424}, acute myeloid leukaemia {400}, chronic lymphocytic leukaemia {228,850}, and chronic myeloid leukaemia {484}, and they are detected using a variety of imaging techniques, including fluorescein angiography, indocyanine green angiography, and optical coherence tomography {198,966,1072,1242}. Serous retinal detachment may in turn lead to changes in the retinal pigment epithelium, such as depigmentation and proliferation {610}.
Because choroidal lesions can also be detected in many asymptomatic leukaemia cases, some authors suggest that eye examinations should be part of the routine evaluation at initial diagnosis for all patients with leukaemia {1072}.

Histopathology
In enucleated eyes, the choroid can be variably thickened {610}. The morphology, immunophenotype, and genotype of the infiltrating leukaemic cells usually correspond to the bone marrow–derived leukaemia; however, blastic (high-grade) transformation has been described in some patients with relapsed chronic leukaemia {437}.
The choroidal involvement by leukaemic cells tends to be perivascular, and it may be patchy or diffuse {610,701}. Rarer complications of dense leukaemic infiltration within the choriocapillaris include thrombosis and haemorrhage, which can be extensive on histology, extending into the retina and causing tissue destruction. The leukaemic cells themselves tend to respect the Bruch membrane, but histopathological examination may reveal secondary alterations of the overlying retinal pigment epithelium, such as displacement, clumping, atrophy, hypertrophy, and hyperplasia {610,701}. The neural retina often displays alterations (e.g. photoreceptor atrophy and cell loss) as a result of serous effusion and cystoid oedema {610}.
Increasingly, chorioretinal biopsies are being performed to diagnose malignancies disseminated to the choroid, including secondary leukaemias.

Differential diagnosis
Patients with leukaemia are susceptible to a wide variety of infections by viral, fungal, protozoal, and bacterial organisms, and any of these may result in choroidal thickening, a posterior uveitis picture, or serous detachment. Leukaemic infiltration of the choroid can also mimic scleritis {898}. Patients who receive an allogeneic bone marrow transplant as part

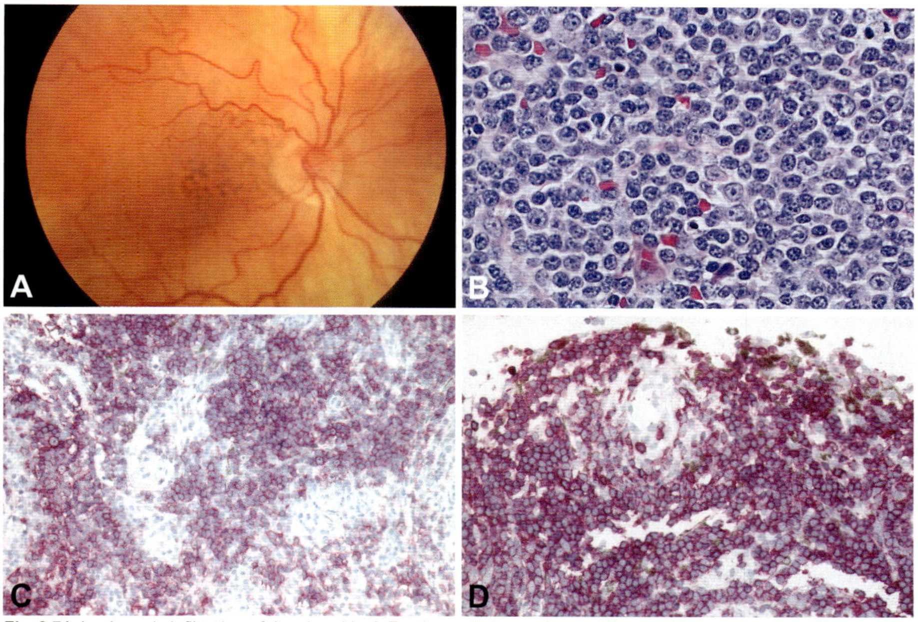

Fig. 2.71 Leukaemic infiltration of the choroid. **A** Funduscopic image from a 77-year-old man, showing diffuse yellowish-white choroidal infiltration. **B** Chorioretinal biopsy revealed an infiltrate of small atypical lymphocytes with clumped chromatin and discrete nucleoli. **C** The tumour cells are immunoreactive for CD20. **D** The neoplastic B cells are positive for CD5 and CD23 (not shown), in the absence of cyclin D1.

of their leukaemia treatment may have a complicating graft-versus-host reaction, which has been observed to present as central serous chorioretinopathy {516,561,807,1072}. Less common differential diagnoses include uveal effusion syndrome and primary uveal lymphoma.

Histogenesis

Leukaemias are malignant neoplasms of the haematopoietic stem cells, characterized by diffuse replacement of the bone marrow by neoplastic cells. The histogenesis of both acute and chronic leukaemias is often related to recurrent genetic abnormalities, which are covered in the volume *WHO classification of tumours of haematopoietic and lymphoid tissues* {1231}.

Genetic profile

The genetic profile depends on the leukaemic subtype.

Prognosis and predictive factors

Leukaemic infiltration of the choroid is usually not treated directly; rather, systemic chemotherapy is administered in an attempt to control the underlying disease, with the treatment tailored to the histological type and clinical stage of the leukaemia. However, low-dose local radiation therapy may be necessary to improve response {1072}. If left untreated, leukaemic infiltration of the choroid can cause substantial vision loss and pain (e.g. due to secondary glaucoma), but it is usually responsive to systemic treatment with chemotherapy and/or local radiation therapy to the eye {898}.

Secondary tumours of the iris, ciliary body, and choroid

Roberts F.
Bechrakis N.E.
Meyer P.
Wilson M.

Definition

Secondary tumours of the iris, ciliary body, and choroid are tumours that have metastasized to these locations from a distant site.

ICD-O codes

Code according to the originating tumour type.

Epidemiology

Uveal metastases are the most common intraocular malignancy, occurring in 8–10% of patients with metastatic disease {641}. Because of the high-flow choroidal vasculature, metastases are most common in the choroid (accounting for 88% of cases), with less-frequent involvement of the iris (9% of cases) and ciliary body (2% of cases) {1113}. The age and sex distribution varies depending on the primary origin of the tumour.

Clinical features

Most patients have known systemic cancer at the time of ocular diagnosis, but in as many as 34% of patients, uveal metastases may precede the primary cancer diagnosis. In patients without a known cancer, the primary site is identified as lung in 35% of cases and breast in 7% of cases, and it remains unknown in about 50% of cases {1113}.

The most common presenting symptoms are blurred vision and vision loss due to associated exudative retinal detachment {641}. Anterior uveal metastases may abut and tilt the lens, causing visual disturbance. Pain is a presenting feature in as many as 5–12% of cases {269,1065}, with floaters and photopsia occurring in 5–14% {641}; 9–13% of patients are asymptomatic {1113}.

Choroidal metastases are predominantly postequatorial, with as many as 40% located in the macular region {641}. The mean number of metastases per eye is 1.4–1.6, with multiple and bilateral tumours more commonly reported in breast cancer {642,1113}. Unilateral and unifocal metastases are more commonly found with lung cancer {1065}.

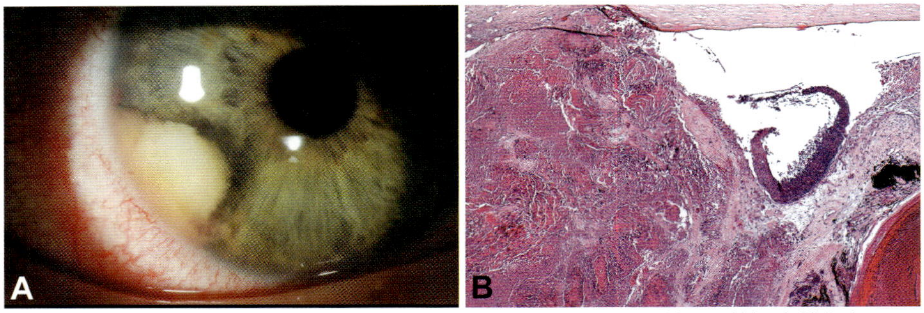

Fig. 2.72 Oropharyngeal squamous cell carcinoma metastatic to the ciliary body and base of iris. **A** Clinical appearance. **B** Histology of the same case, showing metastatic squamous cell carcinoma in the ciliary body and chamber angle.

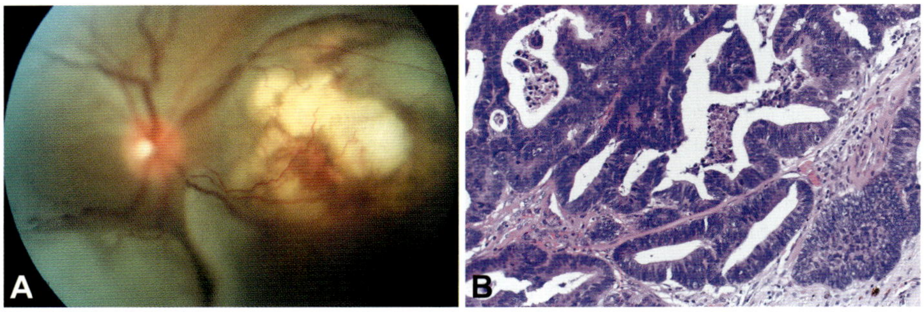

Fig. 2.73 Metastatic colorectal carcinoma. **A** Funduscopic view showing an irregular white mass with overlying haemorrhage and concomitant exudative retinal detachment in the inferior part of the fundus. **B** Histology of the same case, showing malignant garland-like glands with central dirty necrosis.

Secondary tumours in the choroid usually appear as cream-coloured or pale-yellow dome-shaped or rounded masses. They may be associated with haemorrhage, necrosis, and/or subretinal fluid. When the tumour appears orange in colour, an origin from renal carcinoma, thyroid carcinoma, or neuroendocrine tumour should be considered {641}. Metastatic cutaneous melanoma may be brownish-grey or amelanotic {641}.

Ciliary body metastases are usually amelanotic, and may be flat or dome-shaped. Secondary iris tumours are usually white, but secondary renal or thyroid carcinoma may be pink or orange, and melanoma may appear brown {641}.

Secondary iris tumours may present as stromal nodules or poorly defined thickening of the iris, or they may be associated with feeder vessels, secondary glaucoma, corectopia, pseudohypopyon, and hyphaema {785}.

Secondary choroidal tumours may show autofluorescence due to lipofuscin accumulation {31}; although this can be a useful identifying feature in some cases, it may also be seen in choroidal melanoma. Compared with choroidal melanoma, secondary tumours have a higher reflectivity on A-scan ultrasonography and are acoustically solid on B-scan. The height-to-base ratio is typically much lower than in melanoma {50}.

Optical coherence tomography shows that these metastases are usually undulating, associated with thickening of the retinal pigment epithelium and subretinal fluid {13}.

Fluorescein angiography typically shows hypofluorescence in the early stages and hyperfluorescence in the late stages (usually later than choroidal melanoma) {31}. Indocyanine green angiography is also useful; it facilitates visualization of tumours through the retina and can

provide information about the surrounding vasculature.
CT is not usually useful, because of poor definition. On MRI, the choroidal mass usually appears isointense on T1-weighted imaging and hypointense on T2-weighted imaging {50,641}.
Biopsy may be useful, in particular if no primary site can be identified by systemic investigations {50,641}.

Histopathology

Enucleation is relatively uncommon for secondary tumours of the uveal tract. Secondary tumours can usually be distinguished from melanoma because they appear flatter and more undulating and are often associated with serous retinal detachment and exudation. Occasionally, tumours may spread through the Bruch membrane and develop a mushroom or collar-button shape, similar to that of uveal melanoma. However, secondary tumours are usually yellow or cream-coloured, in contrast to the majority of melanomas, which are usually at least in part pigmented.
The pathology of secondary tumours depends on the primary site of origin. Metastatic breast carcinoma is most commonly of the invasive ductal type, but lobular and other subtypes have also been described {269}. For metastatic lung carcinoma, both small cell carcinoma and non-small cell carcinoma have been described, but metastases from non-small cell carcinoma predominate, accounting for 80% of cases (with metastases from small cell carcinoma accounting for the other 20%); this corresponds with the primary cancer incidence {1065}. The most common type of non-small cell lung carcinoma is adenocarcinoma, followed by squamous cell carcinoma. Metastatic colorectal adenocarcinoma has a characteristic histology, often showing necrotic debris (so-called dirty necrosis) in glands, whereas tumours of the upper gastrointestinal and pancreaticobiliary tracts may be morphologically indistinguishable from lung or breast carcinoma. Renal carcinoma may have classic clear cell morphology or may be more poorly differentiated, even sarcomatoid. Thyroid carcinoma may show colloid production. Neuroendocrine tumours typically have a packeted architecture, with a rich vascular supply. Cutaneous melanoma may be indistinguishable from uveal melanoma on morphology.

Table 2.01 Immunohistochemical markers used to distinguish different tumour types and the primary origin of tumours

Origin	Markers		
	CK7	CK20	Other
Carcinomas			
Breast	+	− or (+)	ER, PR, GATA3
Lung (NSCLC)	+	− or (+)	TTF1, napsin A
Stomach	+	− or (+)	CDX2
Colon	− or (+)	+	CDX2
Prostate	− or (+)	− or (+)	PSA, PSAP, NKX3-1
Kidney	− or +	−	PAX8, RCCm, vimentin
Thyroid	+	−	Thyroglobulin, PAX8, TTF1
Bladder	+	+	GATA3
Ovary	+	− or +	ER, PR, PAX8
Non-carcinomas			
Testis (EC or S)	+ or −	−	CD30 (EC), OCT3/4, KIT (CD117) (S), PLAP
Melanoma	−	−	S100 protein, melan-A, MITF, HMB45 antigen, SOX10
Sarcoma	−	−	Vimentin[a]
Lymphoma	−	−	LCA (CD45)[a]
Neuroectodermal neoplasm	− or +	−	Chromogranin, synaptophysin, CD56

+, positive; (+), weakly positive; −, negative; EC, embryonal carcinoma; ER, estrogen receptor; LCA, leukocyte common antigen; NSCLC, non-small cell lung carcinoma; PR, progesterone receptor; PSA, prostate-specific antigen; PSAP, prostate-specific acid phosphatase; RCCm, renal cell carcinoma marker; S, seminoma.
[a]The full immunohistochemical staining panel is outside the scope of this volume.

Morphological features may give clues as to the primary origin, but immunohistochemical staining is the most useful ancillary technique for ascertaining the primary site of origin. The most commonly used immunohistochemical markers are shown in Table 2.01.

Histogenesis

Breast cancer is the most common secondary uveal tumour, accounting for 40–53% of choroidal metastases {269}, with concurrent systemic metastases present in 92% of patients. Lung cancer is the second most common secondary uveal tumour, accounting for 20–29% of cases {1065}.
Less common primary sites for secondary carcinoma of the uveal tract are the gastrointestinal tract (accounting for 4% of cases), prostate (2%), and kidney (2–4%). Rarer origins of metastasis include the thyroid, testis, ovary, and bladder. Non-carcinoma primaries of secondary tumours include cutaneous melanoma, neuroendocrine tumours, sarcomas, and lymphomas.

Genetic profile

The genetic profile can be useful in certain circumstances. It may be helpful in distinguishing secondary cutaneous melanoma from primary uveal melanoma. Cutaneous melanoma commonly shows *BRAF* mutations, which are not usually present in choroidal or ciliary body melanoma (although they may occur in iris melanoma). Uveal melanomas may show chromosome 3 loss, which does not occur in cutaneous melanoma. FISH for 1p36 and 8q is less helpful, because amplification of these DNA regions can occur in cutaneous melanoma.
The genetic profile may also be useful for choosing therapeutic interventions in certain settings, for example, *ERBB2*

(*HER2*) status in breast carcinoma, *ALK* and *EGFR* status in non-small cell lung carcinoma, and *KRAS* status in colorectal adenocarcinoma; therefore, it is recommended where possible to reserve some of the diagnostic sample (e.g. an intraocular biopsy) for molecular testing, to aid in the further care of the patient.

Prognosis and predictive factors

Uveal metastases tend to become apparent late in the course of malignancy, and they are associated with disseminated disease and poor prognosis. With choroidal metastasis, the median survival time is 6 months (range: 0.5–47 months) {642}. Patients with metastatic lung cancer have a shorter survival time than do patients with breast cancer, and survival time is shorter when there are also extraocular sites of metastasis.

The most common treatment modality is external beam radiation therapy, which results in tumour regression in about 94% of cases, with conservation of vision in about 75% {50,641}; bilateral treatment should be considered, because metastasis may later occur in the other eye. Other local treatments include brachytherapy, photodynamic therapy, VEGF inhibitors, and surgical resection {50,641}. Systemic treatments may be administered in the case of relapsed disseminated disease.

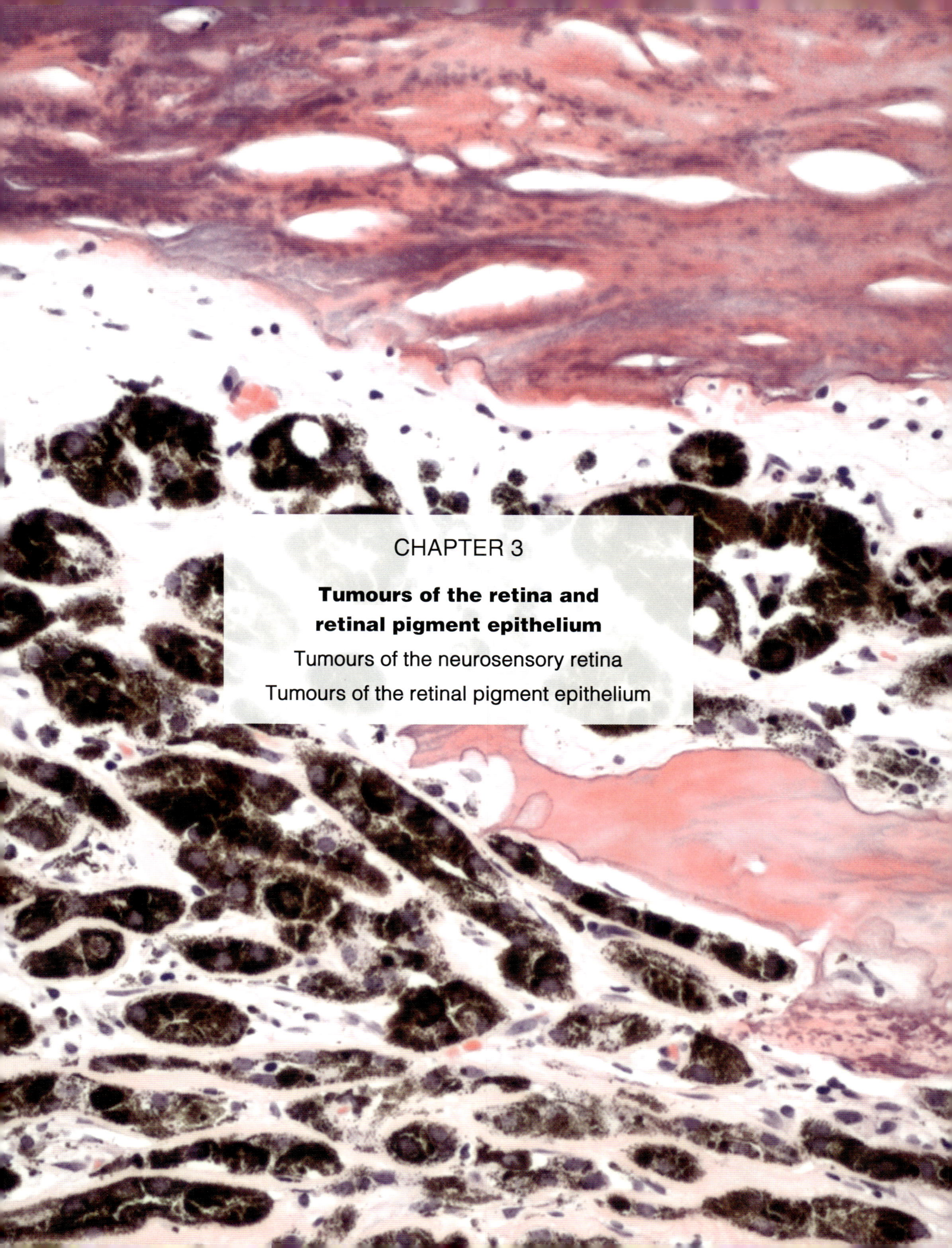

CHAPTER 3

Tumours of the retina and retinal pigment epithelium

WHO classification of tumours of the retina and retinal pigment epithelium

Tumours of the neurosensory retina	
Retinoblastoma	9510/3
Retinocytoma	9510/0
Astrocytoma NOS	9400/3
Nodular and massive retinal gliosis	None
Haemangioblastoma	9161/1
Cavernous haemangioma	9121/0
Vitreoretinal lymphoma	9680/3
Leukaemia NOS	9800/3
Secondary tumours	See note[a]
Tumours of the retinal pigment epithelium	
Retinal pigment epithelial adenocarcinoma	8140/3
Retinal pigment epithelial adenoma	8140/0
Reactive hyperplasia	None
Simple and combined hamartomas	None
Congenital hypertrophy	None

[a]Code secondary tumours according to the originating tumour type.

The morphology codes are from the International Classification of Diseases for Oncology (ICD-O) {381}. Behaviour is coded /0 for benign tumours; /1 for unspecified, borderline, or uncertain behaviour; /2 for carcinoma in situ and grade III intraepithelial neoplasia; and /3 for malignant tumours.

The classification is modified from the previous WHO classification, taking into account changes in our understanding of these lesions.

TNM classification of retinoblastoma

Retinoblastoma

(ICD-O-3 C69.2)

TNM Clinical Classification

T – Primary Tumour

- TX Primary tumour cannot be assessed
- T0 No evidence of primary tumour
- T1 Tumour confined to the retina with subretinal fluid no more than 5 mm from the base of any tumour, without retinal detachment
  - T1a No tumour in either eye is greater than 3 mm in largest dimension or located closer than 1.5 mm to the optic nerve or fovea
  - T1b At least one tumour is greater than 3 mm in largest dimension or located closer than 1.5 mm to the optic nerve or fovea. No retinal detachment or subretinal fluid beyond 5 mm from the base of the tumour
- T2 Tumour with vitreous or subretinal seeding or retinal detachment
  - T2a Tumour with subretinal fluid more than 5 mm from the base of any tumour
  - T2b Tumour with vitreous and/or subretinal seeding
- T3 Severe intraocular disease
  - T3a Phthisis or prephthisis bulbi
  - T3b Invasion of: choroid, pars plana, ciliary body, lens, zonules, iris or anterior chamber
  - T3c Raised intraocular pressure with neovascularization and/or buphthalmos
  - T3d Hyphema and/or massive vitreous haemorrhage
  - T3e Aseptic orbital cellulitis
- T4 Extraocular tumour
  - T4a Invasion of optic nerve or orbital tissues
  - T4b Extraocular invasion with proptosis and/or orbital mass

N – Regional Lymph Nodes

- NX Regional lymph nodes cannot be assessed
- N0 No regional lymph node metastasis
- N1 Regional lymph node metastasis

M – Distant Metastasis

- M0 No distant metastasis
- M1 Distant metastasis
  - M1a Single or multiple metastasis to sites other than CNS or brain
  - M1b Metastasis to the CNS including brain

pTNM Pathological Classification

T – Primary Tumour

- pTX Primary tumour cannot be assessed
- pT0 No evidence of primary tumour
- pT1 Tumour confined to eye with no optic nerve or choroidal invasion
- pT2 Tumour with intraocular invasion
  - pT2a Focal choroidal invasion and pre- or intralaminar invasion of the optic nerve head
  - pT2b Tumour invasion of stroma of iris and/or trabecular meshwork and/or Schlemm's canal
- pT3 Tumour with significant local invasion
  - pT3a Choroidal invasion larger than 3 mm in diameter or multiple foci of invasion totalling more than 3 mm or any full-thickness involvement
  - pT3b Retrolaminar invasion of optic nerve without invasion of transected end of optic nerve
  - pT3c Partial-thickness involvement of sclera within the inner two-thirds
  - pT3d Full-thickness invasion into outer third of the sclera and/or invasion into or around emissary channels
- pT4 Extraocular extension: Tumour invades optic nerve at transected end, in meningeal space around the optic nerve, full-thickness invasion of the sclera with invasion of the episclera, adipose tissue, extraocular muscle, bone, conjunctiva, or eyelid.

N – Regional Lymph Nodes

- pNX Regional lymph nodes cannot be assessed
- pN0 No regional lymph node involvement
- pN1 Regional lymph node involvement

pM – Metastasis

- pM0 No distant metastasis
- pM1 Distant metastasis
  - pM1a Single or multiple metastasis to sites other than CNS
  - pM1b Metastasis to CNS parenchyma or cerebrospinal fluid

Stage

(Continued on next page)

Retinoblastoma

(Continued)

Stage

Clinical Stage

Stage I	T1, T2, T3	N0	M0
Stage II	T4a	N0	M0
Stage III	T4b	N0	M0
	Any T	N1	M0
Stage IV	Any T	Any N	M1

Pathological Stage

Stage I	T1, T2, T3	N0	M0
Stage II	T4	N0	M0
Stage III	Any T	N1	M0
Stage IV	Any T	Any N	M1

The information presented here has been excerpted from the 8th edition of the *TNM classification of malignant tumours* (2017) {132}.
A help desk for specific questions about the TNM classification is available at http://www.uicc.org/resources/tnm/helpdesk.

Tumours of the retina and retinal pigment epithelium: Introduction

Kivelä T.T.
Grossniklaus H.E.
Eberhart C.G.

The complex neuroretina and the simple monolayer of hexagonal retinal pigment epithelial (RPE) cells derive from the embryonic inner and outer walls of the optic cup, respectively. The neuroretina has nine layers: (1) the inner limiting membrane, composed of periodic acid–Schiff (PAS)-positive basement membrane secreted by footplates of Müller radial glial cells; (2) the nerve fibre layer, composed of axons of retinal ganglion cells; (3) the ganglion cell layer; (4) the inner plexiform layer, containing synapses between ganglion, bipolar, and amacrine cells; (5) the inner nuclear layer, consisting of the cell bodies of bipolar, amacrine, horizontal, and Müller cells; (6) the outer plexiform layer, containing synapses between bipolar, horizontal, and photoreceptor cells; (7) the outer nuclear layer, containing the cell bodies of rod and cone photoreceptors; (8) the outer limiting membrane, corresponding to junctional complexes between photoreceptor and Müller cells; and (9) the photoreceptor layer, which consists of inner segments and of outer segments that intermingle with the microvilli of the RPE, immersed in the interphotoreceptor matrix. The inner retinal layers (from the inner limiting membrane to the inner nuclear layer) contain astrocytes surrounding branches of the central retinal vessels, which are non-fenestrated and form the inner blood–retina barrier. The outer blood–retina barrier is formed by the occluding junctions of the RPE. The myelin sheaths of the ganglion cell axons begin just behind the lamina cribrosa. The neuroretina extends posteriorly to the optic nerve and anteriorly to the non-pigmented inner ciliary epithelium. The RPE extends posteriorly around the optic disc and anteriorly to the pigmented outer ciliary epithelium.

As neuronal, non-proliferating tissues, the neuroretina and RPE are not particularly prone to producing tumours, except retinoblastoma, which is an embryonic developmental cancer of childhood. Retinoblastoma results from loss of both copies of *RB1*, followed by increasing genomic instability {283}, and it has a worldwide incidence of 1 case per 16 000–18 000 live births. Retinoblastoma is the most common primary intraocular cancer in infants and young children; although this tumour shows no race predilection, the very large paediatric populations in Africa and Asia and the high birth rates in Africa have resulted in retinoblastoma being the most common intraocular cancer worldwide overall, slightly exceeding uveal melanoma in predicted incidence {620}. Rarely, the same *RB1* mutations can result in a stable benign retinocytoma, although most retinocytomas eventually degenerate into retinoblastoma {283,304}. Exceptional cases of retinoblastoma develop in the absence of *RB1* mutations, instead resulting from high-level *MYCN* oncogene amplification {1005}. The retinal glia can produce acquired astrocytomas, astrocytic hamartomas in tuberous sclerosis, and reactive proliferations that can reach tumour-like dimensions (including retinal nodular and/or massive retinal gliosis). Capillary, cavernous, and racemose haemangiomas and haemangioblastomas are additional retinal vascular tumours. Secondary retinal tumours include lymphoma, leukaemia, and metastases.

The most common RPE lesion is congenital hypertrophy, which (like reactive hyperplasia of the RPE) may produce

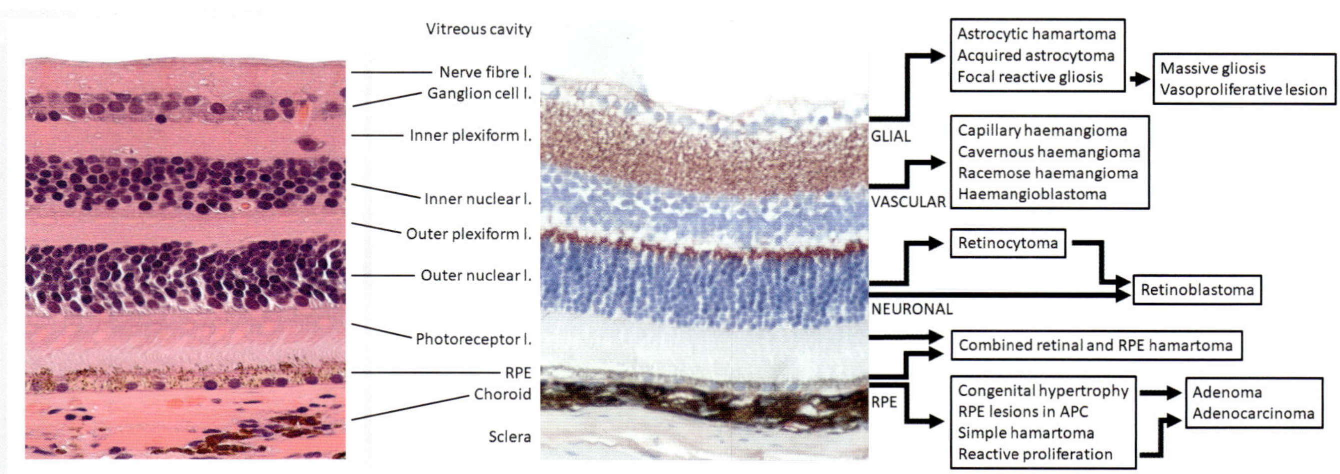

Fig. 3.01 Anatomy of the retina and spectrum of retinal tumours. The retina consists of nine layers (l.; the inner and outer limiting membranes are not labelled in this figure) and the retinal pigment epithelium (RPE); it is bordered by the vitreous cavity internally and the choroid externally (synaptophysin staining with nuclear haematoxylin counterstaining to highlight the plexiform layers). The primary tumours of the retina can be categorized as being of glial, vascular, neuronal, or RPE origin. APC, (familial) adenomatous polyposis coli.

RPE adenomas and adenocarcinomas. Other congenital lesions include simple and combined hamartomas (the latter of which also involve retinal glia and adjacent vitreous) and RPE hypertrophy associated with familial adenomatous polyposis {866,1153}. Various growth factors can induce the RPE to migrate and proliferate, including over choroidal tumours, under retinal detachments, and (most commonly) in disorganized blind eyes undergoing phthisis {1315}. The proliferating cells typically become metaplastic. This metaplasia is first evidenced by immunopositivity for SMA {383}; in phthisical eyes, it is also eventually evidenced by the proliferating cells' transdifferentiation into fibroblast-like cells, which may form bone {1022,1315}.

Retinal and RPE tumours are generally not biopsied (except to confirm vitreoretinal lymphoma by vitreous or chorioretinal biopsy) {768}; however, some vascular tumours may be resected piecemeal using vitrectomy instrumentation {579,1396}.

Tumours of the neurosensory retina

Retinoblastoma

Eagle R.C. Jr
Chévez-Barrios P.
Li B.
Al Hussaini M.
Wilson M.

Definition

Retinoblastoma is a malignant neoplasm of the neurosensory retina, almost exclusively affecting young children. Hereditary cases are typically bilateral with multiple tumour foci in one or two eyes and, more rarely, intracranially at midline.

ICD-O code

Retinoblastoma 9510/3

Synonym

Glioma retinae (obsolete)

Epidemiology

Retinoblastoma is the most common primary intraocular malignant tumour in infants and young children, and it is thought to be the most common primary malignant intraocular neoplasm overall {620}. It accounts for approximately 3% of all cancers occurring in young children {48} There is no race or sex predilection. The reported incidence of retinoblastoma is 1 case per 16 000–18 000 live births {1327}, with approximately 7000–8000 new cases worldwide each year {133,620}. The diagnosis is made in 80% and 95% of cases before the ages of 3 years and 5 years, respectively {48}. The mean patient age at diagnosis is 18 months overall and 1–2 months in familial cases. Rare cases that occur in older children and adults are often misdiagnosed. The incidence of retinoblastoma appears to be higher in Africa, in India, and among children of Native American descent {1220}, possibly because of socioeconomic factors {259,336}. In developed countries, the survival rate of retinoblastoma approaches 95%, and > 90% of children with the disease have at least one eye with visual function; worldwide, the average survival rate may be as low as 50% {157,620}.

Etiology

Retinoblastoma is caused by germline and somatic mutations in the *RB1* gene or (rarely) somatic amplification of *MYCN*.

Localization

Retinoblastoma is a neoplasm of the neurosensory retina. Tumour progression leads to involvement of the vitreous, anterior chamber, uvea, and optic nerve, as well as extension through the sclera into periocular tissues.

Clinical features

The hallmark of retinoblastoma is leukocoria (white pupillary reflex), which parents often bring to the attention of their health care providers. The second most common presenting sign is strabismus; disruption of the child's developing visual pathway can manifest as either esotropia or exotropia. Clinical features associated with later presentation of retinoblastoma include iris heterochromia, glaucoma with buphthalmos, pseudohypopyon, hyphaema, and aseptic orbital cellulitis. In advanced cases, extraocular disease extension may present with proptosis, a fungating orbital mass, or enlarged regional lymph nodes.
Although the diagnosis can be suspected clinically during a routine dilated eye examination, optimal evaluation usually requires detailed examination under anaesthesia. Ocular ultrasonography can help to confirm the diagnosis by highlighting dystrophic calcifications within the tumour. The diameter and clarity of the cornea and the intraocular pressures should be recorded, and the anterior segment is evaluated for the presence of tumour cells, iris neovascularization, and lens opacification. The number and location of the tumours in each eye, the presence of associated serous retinal detachment, and vitreous and subretinal

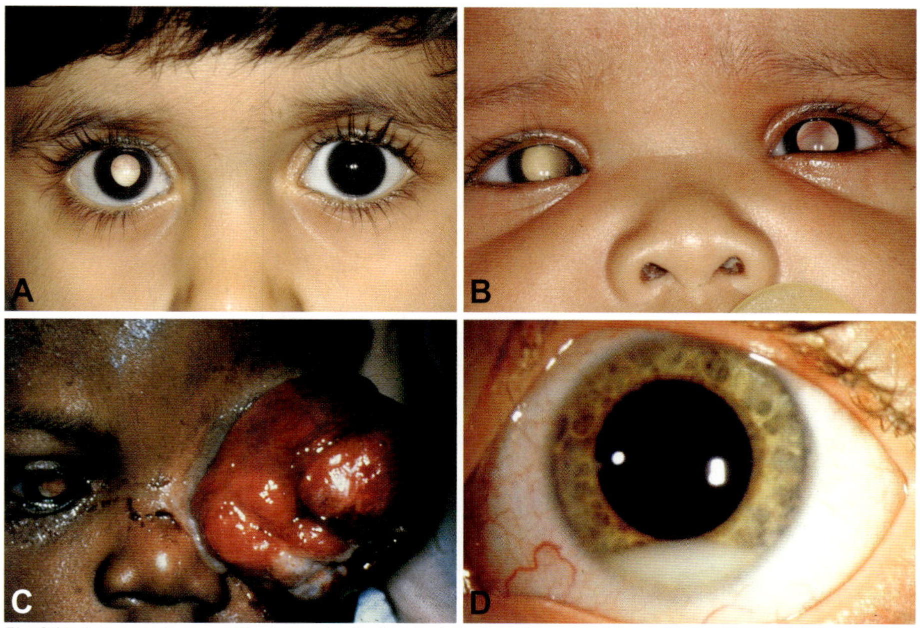

Fig. 3.02 Retinoblastoma. **A** The hallmark of retinoblastoma is leukocoria (white pupillary reflex), evident here in the right eye. **B** Bilateral leukocoria indicates bilateral retinoblastoma in this infant with germline *RB1* mutation. **C** In another patient with germline *RB1* mutation, neglected retinoblastoma has extended extraocularly in the left eye, forming a massive fungating orbital mass; leukocoria in the right eye indicates that the disease is bilateral. **D** Diffuse infiltrative retinoblastoma; pseudohypopyon of tumour cells in the inferior anterior chamber was the presenting manifestation; the eye shows no inflammatory signs.

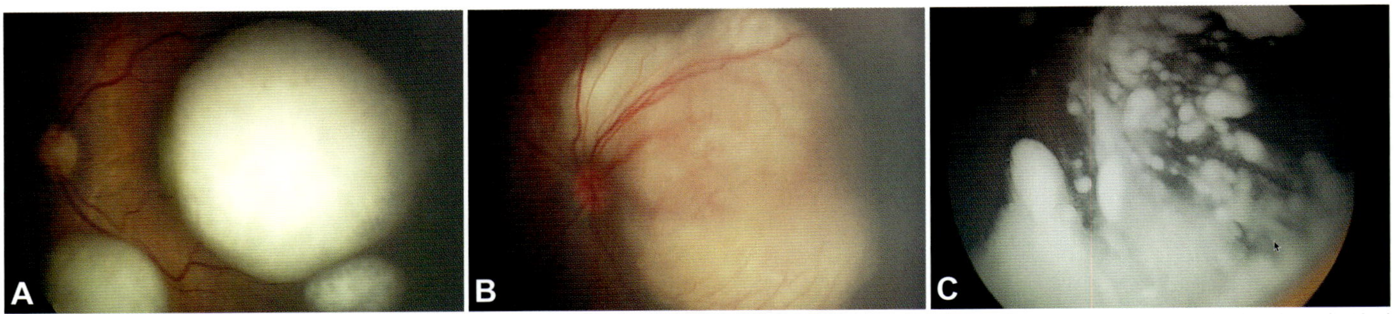

Fig. 3.03 Retinoblastoma. **A** Endophytic growth pattern; a fundus photograph shows multiple encephaloid tumours projecting into the vitreous from attached retina; the patient had bilateral tumours and germline *RB1* mutation. **B** Exophytic growth pattern; a fundus photograph shows vascularized retina covering tumour that has arisen from the retina's posterior layers. **C** A fundus photograph show numerous tumour seeds in the vitreous humour, dispersed from endophytic retinoblastoma.

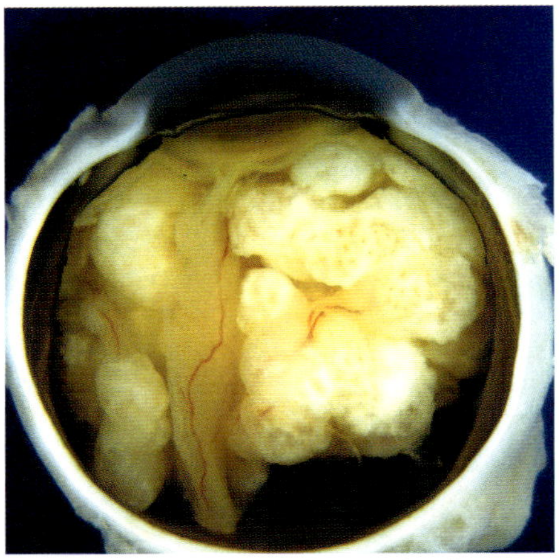

Fig. 3.04 Retinoblastoma. In this example with an exophytic growth pattern, encephaloid lobules of tumour fill most of the subretinal space beneath the totally detached retina.

seeding are documented by a fundus drawing or photography.

Retinoblastoma appears as a non-pigmented, often whitish mass. Exophytic tumours grow from the outer layers of the retina towards the subretinal space, and they are often associated with serous retinal detachment. Exophytic tumours often seed the subretinal space, resulting in satellite tumour foci. Endophytic tumours grow into the vitreous cavity, producing vitreous seeds that can have the appearance of dust, spheres, or clouds. Vitreous seeding has the worst prognosis for eye preservation. Diffuse infiltrating retinoblastoma is a rare variant that has a predilection for children aged > 5 years.

MRI of the orbits and brain should be performed on each patient and the images evaluated for evidence of extraocular extension into the orbital soft tissues and tumour invasion into the optic nerve. Brain images should be reviewed closely for evidence of pineoblastoma or suprasellar neuroblastic tumour, which can develop in patients with germline *RB1* mutations. Although MRI continues to improve as a diagnostic modality, histopathology remains the gold standard for assessing the high-risk features that predispose patients to the development of metastatic disease. The detection of calcification by imaging studies is very helpful in confirming the diagnosis clinically.

The tumour is separately classified in each eye, to stratify prognosis for ocular salvage and guide treatment. The now-outdated Reese–Ellsworth Classification (published in the 1960s) grouped eyes based on tumour size, tumour location, and the presence of vitreous seeding. Outcomes were assessed on the basis of response to external beam radiation therapy. The International Classification of Retinoblastoma (ICRB) groups eyes on the basis of tumour size, tumour location, the extent of serous fluid, and the presence of vitreous and subretinal seeding. In addition to the ICRB grouping, the TNM classification {132} incorporates several additional findings: extraocular extension (clinical or radiographical), proptosis, regional lymph node involvement, and metastatic disease. The International Retinoblastoma Staging System stages the patient rather than the individual eye, on the basis of eye salvage with no disease dissemination versus enucleation with complete resection or microscopic residual tumour, versus orbital, systemic, and CNS disease.

Exophytic retinoblastoma may be confused clinically with Coats disease and vice versa.

Histopathology

Grossly, the tumour has a white or encephaloid appearance. Endophytic retinoblastomas arise from the inner layers of the retina (which typically remains attached) and grow into the vitreous cavity. Anterior chamber seeding may occur and can be misdiagnosed as inflammatory disease. Exophytic retinoblastomas arise from the outer retinal layers, proliferate in the subretinal space, and often cause a high bullous retinal detachment that may abut the posterior surface of the lens, causing anterior displacement of the lens–iris diaphragm and secondary closed-angle glaucoma. The growth pattern may be indeterminate when large tumours fill the vitreous cavity. In many cases, macroscopic examination discloses white flecks of dystrophic calcification that develops within necrotic parts of the tumour. Calcification can be quite intense in regression scars that are found in eyes enucleated after chemotherapy or radiotherapy. In such cases, decalcification may be necessary before microtomy. Calcification is usually absent in diffuse infiltrative retinoblastoma (the rarest growth pattern), which accounts for about 1.5% of cases and is typically found in older children (mean age: 6–7 years) {103}. Such tumours diffusely thicken the retina and do not form a distinct tumefaction. In many cases of diffuse infiltrative retinoblastoma, tumour cells circumferentially blanket the pars plana and zonules. Patients present with vitreous clumps or a pseudohypopyon of tumour cells in the anterior chamber; clinical misdiagnosis as inflammation may result in patients undergoing vitreous biopsy. Despite the pseudohypopyon, affected eyes lack other signs of inflammation, such as ocular injection, perilimbal flush, posterior synechiae, and vitreous membranes. Tumours in eyes enucleated from patients with advanced disease who present with aseptic orbital cellulitis {1167} often have a reddish or orange tinge, reflecting necrosis and bloodstaining. Such eyes typically have severe neovascular glaucoma that has caused extensive necrosis of intraocular structures. Involvement of anterior-segment structures or massive invasion of the posterior uvea may be evident grossly as a white infiltrate. In developing countries with limited access to medical care, patients often present in the late stages of the disease with an orbital mass, reflecting scleral erosion and extraocular extension. Lemon-coloured foci of haematoidin pigment may be present in these neglected tumours.

Histopathologically, retinoblastoma is a small blue cell tumour composed of primitive neuroblastic cells with basophilic nuclei and scant cytoplasm. Numerous mitotic figures and apoptotic cells are present. Retinoblastoma cells have a propensity to outgrow their blood supply and undergo necrosis. This typically occurs when the cells have grown 90–110 µm away from a nutrient vessel {148}. A characteristic pattern of basophilic sleeves and cuffs of viable basophilic tumour cells separated by sheets of necrotic tumour results. The necrotic tumour appears eosinophilic because cells have lost their nuclear DNA. Foci of dystrophic calcification typically develop within the necrotic foci. In eyes with extensive tumour necrosis, the released DNA may form basophilic deposits around retinal vessels, the lens capsule, and the wall of the Schlemm canal {147,726}. Occasionally, amorphous globules of DNA are found in subretinal fluid.

Various degrees of retinal differentiation are evident in retinoblastoma as Homer Wright and Flexner–Wintersteiner rosettes and fleurettes, which represent photoreceptor differentiation. Homer Wright rosettes represent neuroblastic differentiation and appear as a tangle of neurofilaments ringed by nuclei. They also occur in other tumours, such as neuroblastoma. Flexner–Wintersteiner rosettes are characteristic of retinoblastoma, but they also occur in other neoplasms, such as medulloepithelioma. Flexner–Wintersteiner rosettes represent early retinal differentiation and have a central lumen that corresponds to the subretinal space {1277}. Rosettes are more common in retinoblastomas that are enucleated from younger children {304}. Tumours typically become less well differentiated as the age of the patient increases.

Foci of photoreceptor differentiation, called fleurettes, are found histopathologically in at least 15–20% of retinoblastomas {283,304,1279}. Photoreceptor differentiation occurs in areas of viable

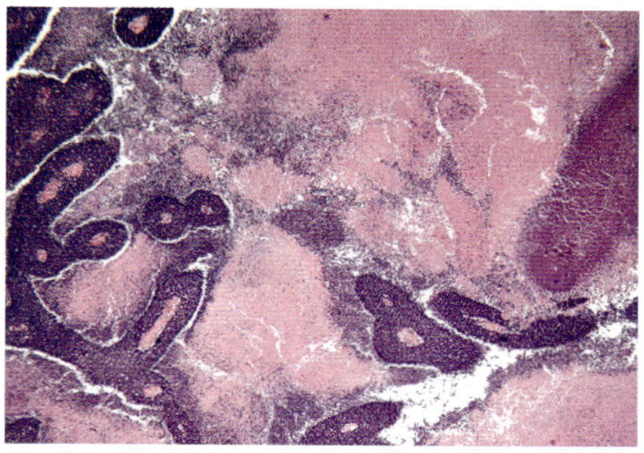

Fig. 3.05 Retinoblastoma. Necrotic tumour containing foci of dystrophic calcification surrounds perivascular cuffs and sleeves of viable retinoblastoma cells.

tumour that appear more eosinophilic than typical retinoblastoma. A retinal neoplasm composed entirely of photoreceptor differentiation is called a retinoma (clinically) or retinocytoma (histopathologically), and it is considered to be a benign, often transient, precursor of retinoblastoma {283}. Foci of photoreceptor differentiation are found in the basal portions of endophytic retinoblastomas, supporting the contention that they may be precursor lesions. Bland nuclei with finely dispersed chromatin are found in areas of photoreceptor differentiation, and mitoses and apoptosis are absent. Unlike in retinoblastomas, calcification occurs within viable parts of retinocytomas. Photoreceptor differentiation is evident as bouquet-like aggregates of eosinophilic structures called fleurettes (French for "small flowers"), which correspond to the inner segments of photoreceptors and are often aligned along segments of neoplastic external limiting membrane. Electron microscopic studies have disclosed early outer segment differentiation in some cases.

Various degrees of anaplasia are found in retinoblastoma, and it has been suggested that severe anaplasia is a risk factor for metastasis {789}. Severely anaplastic tumours are poorly differentiated and have cells with large, very pleomorphic nuclei that are angular, rhomboid, or fusiform in shape. Cell wrapping and numerous mitotic figures are also present.

Retinoblastoma arises from the retina and initially invades the vitreous cavity and subretinal space. Eventually, the tumour may breach the Bruch membrane and invade the choroidal stroma, gaining access to vessels that serve as a route for distant haematogenous metastasis. Retinoblastoma also has a marked propensity to invade the optic nerve. The tumour may travel along the nerve to the brain or be dispersed in the cerebrospinal fluid. The posterior uvea and optic nerve must be carefully assessed during the pathological examination of enucleated eyes with retinoblastoma, because massive posterior uveal invasion and retrolaminar optic nerve invasion are high-risk features that are indications for adjuvant chemotherapy in many centres. Invasion of anterior-segment structures is also thought to increase the risk of metastasis. Deposits of retinoblastoma cells often collect on the inner surface of the Bruch membrane, causing focal detachments of the retinal pigment epithelium. These detachments do not constitute choroidal invasion and do not increase the risk of metastasis. During assessment of eyes containing retinoblastoma, pathologists must take care to distinguish true choroidal invasion from artefactual contamination, which is quite common and comprises an admixture of necrotic and viable tumour cells that form irregular aggregates instead of infiltrative sheets of cells. Iris neovascularization and neovascular glaucoma with synechial blockage of the iridocorneal angle are other common findings. Retinoblastoma does not stain for RB1 protein. Positive immunoreactivity for synaptophysin {624} can help to confirm the presence of optic nerve invasion when routine histopathology is equivocal, and this finding also serves to differentiate choroidal invasion from extramedullary haematopoiesis.

Differential diagnosis

Histopathologically, the differential diagnosis includes retinocytoma, medulloepithelioma, leukaemia, primitive neuroectodermal tumour, retinal dysplasia, and small round blue cell tumour metastases. Clinically, retinoblastoma should be differentiated from inflammatory, congenital, and neoplastic disorders. Ocular toxocariasis is the most common inflammatory condition that simulates retinoblastoma {1426}. It is usually unilateral and occurs in children towards the end of the first decade of life {1122}. Granulomatous inflammation containing many eosinophils surrounding necrotic larval fragments is seen {983}. Serial sectioning may be needed to demonstrate the parasite. A negative enzyme-linked immunosorbent assay (ELISA) test for *Toxocara* antigen essentially excludes the diagnosis; however, a positive ELISA test does not exclude retinoblastoma {321,1122}. Other inflammatory diseases include endogenous endophthalmitis, congenital toxoplasmosis, cytomegalovirus retinitis, herpes simplex virus retinitis, and peripheral uveoretinitis {1157}. Persistent fetal vasculature (previously called persistent hyperplastic primary vitreous) is usually a unilateral congenital disorder. A plaque of fibrovascular tissue that resembles primary vitreous adheres to the posterior lens capsule, the hyaloid artery is often patent {1209}, and the tips of the ciliary processes typically adhere to the margins of the retrolenticular plaque and are drawn centrally {784}. Intraocular adipose tissue and even bone have been reported {367}. Coats disease is often confused with exophytic retinoblastoma {519,1147}; it is usually unilateral and occurs more commonly in boys aged about 5–10 years {311}. Eyes with Coats disease have high bullous retinal detachments that typically abut the posterior surface of the lens and ciliary body. Large, abnormal telangiectatic vessels are seen in parts of the inner retina {311}, exudates massively thicken the outer retinal layers, and intravenous fluorescein angiography reveals capillary nonperfusion. The subretinal space contains densely proteinaceous, lipid-rich fluid with cholesterol crystals and aggregates of foamy histiocytes {1148}. In the setting of bilateral disease, cerebroretinal microangiopathy with calcifications and cysts (so-called Coats plus) and facioscapulohumeral muscular dystrophy should be considered {37,923,1121}. Retinopathy of prematurity, originally called retrolental fibroplasia, shares two features with retinoblastoma: bilaterality and rare presentation at birth. It usually develops in premature infants who have received supplemental oxygen therapy {58}. Vascular proliferation and secondary vitreous fibrosis lead to an organized vitreous and to retinal detachment, with the formation of a fibroneural mass {339}. End-stage disease is marked by total retinal detachment, leukocoria, blindness, and phthisis bulbi. In children presenting with retinal detachment and vitreous haemorrhage, the possibility of retinoblastoma should always be considered {1107}. Appropriate preoperative investigations, including ultrasonography and MRI, should be performed. If vitrectomy is performed, the specimen should always be submitted for cytological examination. Incontinentia pigmenti (Bloch–Sulzberger disease) is an X-linked dominant disease that manifests in females {468} and in males with Klinefelter syndrome (XXY) or XXY mosaicism. The ocular manifestations, which include a retrolental mass of organized chronically detached retina, can be confused with retinoblastoma {468}. Histopathological features are nonspecific {339}. Norrie disease is an X-linked recessive disorder characterized by bilateral leukocoria caused by masses of detached malformed retina {1050}. Retinal dysplasia, along with persistent fetal vasculature, is a characteristic

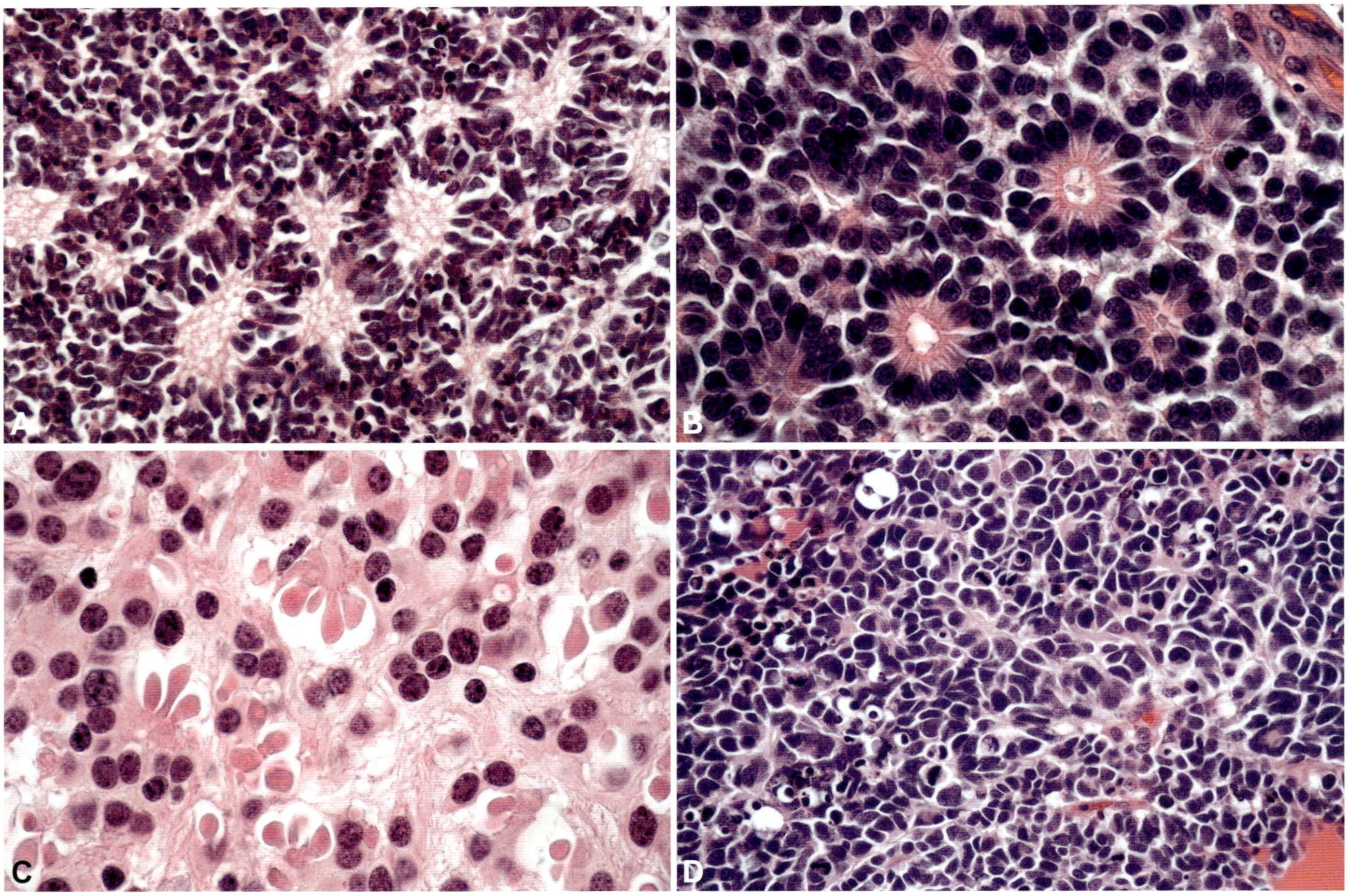

Fig. 3.06 Retinoblastoma. **A** Primitive Homer Wright rosettes lack a central lumen. **B** Consistent with early retinal differentiation, Flexner–Wintersteiner rosettes have a central lumen that corresponds to the subretinal space. **C** Fleurettes comprise eosinophilic bouquet-like aggregates of neoplastic photoreceptor inner segments; the nuclei are bland, and mitotic activity and apoptosis are absent. **D** A severely anaplastic focus contains large, extremely pleomorphic nuclei, cellular wrapping, and mitotic figures.

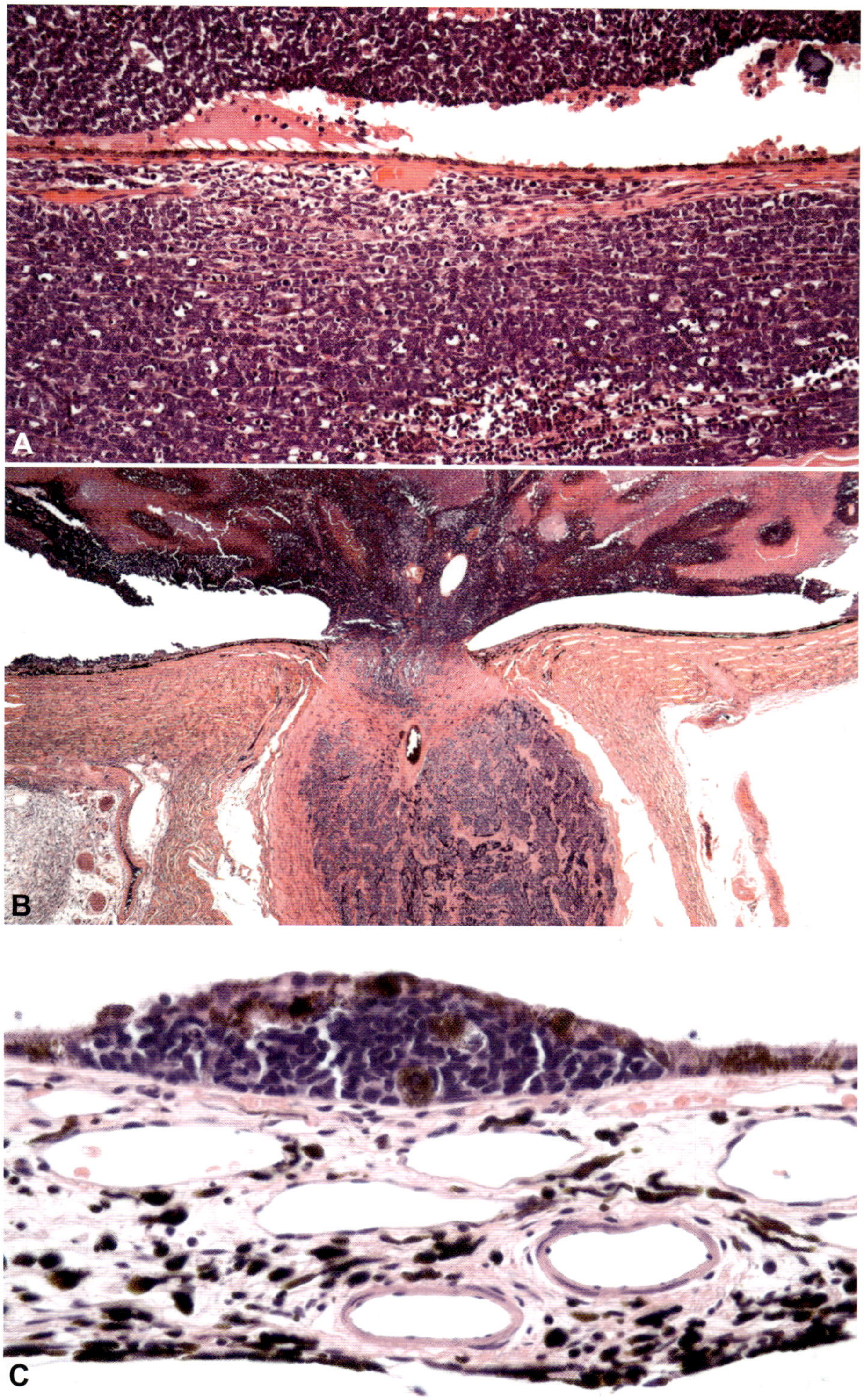

Fig. 3.07 Retinoblastoma. **A** A sheet of tumour cells infiltrates the full thickness of the posterior choroid; massive posterior choroidal invasion is defined as > 3 mm. **B** Tumour invading optic nerve extends posterior to the lamina cribrosa; postlaminar invasion is a high-risk feature. **C** A segment of retinal pigment epithelium has been detached by retinoblastoma; the tumour is located on the inner surface of the Bruch membrane and does not represent choroidal invasion.

feature of trisomy 13 {487}. Dysplastic rosettes are generally larger than the neoplastic Flexner–Wintersteiner rosettes of retinoblastoma, and they comprise multiple retinal layers {675}. Medulloepithelioma and various astrocytic lesions (including astrocytoma, astrocytic hamartoma, glioneuroma, and massive gliosis) are also important considerations in the differential diagnosis with retinoblastoma, as are cataract, choroidal coloboma, and myelinated nerve fibres as other possible causes of leukocoria.

Histogenesis

Retinoblastoma arises from retinal precursor cells {1387}.

Genetic profile

RB1 mutations are responsible for initiating almost all cases of retinoblastoma. *RB1* is a tumour suppressor gene located in chromosome 13 (13q14.2), and its mutation conforms to the Knudson two-hit hypothesis for the development of tumours {19,130,298}. In 2% of patients with unilateral cases, the *MYCN* oncogene is amplified ($RB1^{+/+}MYCN^{A}$) in the tumours {1005}. Additional genetic alterations thought to be associated with tumour progression have been described {645}.

Genetic susceptibility

Approximately 40% of retinoblastoma cases are caused by heterozygous de novo or inherited germline mutations in *RB1*. The offspring of affected individuals have a 50% chance of inheriting the pathogenic variant. The inheritance pattern is autosomal dominant. Retinoblastoma caused by germline mutations is typically bilateral, but 40% of patients with familial germline mutations have unilateral tumours. Tumours in patients who harbour germline mutation tend to arise at an earlier age (12 months in sporadic cases) than retinoblastomas that arise from somatic mutations in retinal cells (24 months). Germline status is associated with patient outcomes, including cancer-related morbidity and mortality. Occasionally, the first person in a family with inherited retinoblastoma to present with the disease presents with a unilateral tumour {1203}; in most such instances, the family members have *RB1*-null alleles that are altered by frameshift or nonsense variants. The majority of these *RB1*-null alleles display > 95% penetrance; < 10% of families have a low-penetrance phenotype with reduced expressivity, and therefore with an increased prevalence (of ~25%) of unilateral retinoblastoma, with incomplete penetrance. This phenotype is usually associated with mutated *RB1* alleles with missense or in-frame mutations, distinct splice-site variants, certain indel variants in exon 1, or pathogenic variants in the promoter region. Pathogenic variants in the promoter region show differential penetrance within families, depending on the parental origin of the pathogenic allele (the parent-of-origin effect) {1203}. In a small percentage of cases, cytogenetically visible deletions of 13q14 include deletions of additional genes in the same chromosome region as *RB1*. In these patients, the deletions may cause developmental delay and facial dysmorphism or may uncover latent pathogenic alleles in nearby genes {771}. These large deletions of 13q14 have reduced expressivity; most patients develop unilateral retinoblastoma or no tumours at all {816}.

In 60% of cases, retinoblastoma is sporadic and unilateral, and the pathogenic variant of *RB1* occurs only within retinal cells. For retinocytoma or retinoblastoma to develop, both alleles must have the pathogenic variant. Because retinocytomas already have pathogenic variants of the *RB1* gene in both alleles, additional mutations are necessary to develop retinoblastoma {283}.

In 2% of patients with unilateral retinoblastoma who have no detectable mutation in *RB1*, there is amplification of the *MYCN* gene (28–121 DNA copies). These children develop unilateral retinoblastoma and have tumours with distinctive histopathological features and advanced features at the time of diagnosis (at a median patient age of 4.5 months) {1005}. *MYCN* amplification can also occur in tumours with *RB1* mutations {334}.

Prognosis and predictive factors

The feature most prognostic of successful treatment, especially for sporadic retinoblastomas, is early diagnosis, when the tumour is still small and entirely contained within the eye and has not invaded the ocular coats. The cure rate for such cases is > 95% {1203}.

Clinical factors: Patients whose tumours have extended extraocularly have a worse prognosis, because there may be extension into lymph nodes and an increased chance of systemic metastasis. Extraocular extension may occur if diagnosis is delayed, presentation is atypical, or the patient has undergone inappropriate surgical intervention due to misdiagnosis. Large tumours that have associated neovascular glaucoma and buphthalmos often harbour high-risk histopathological features for metastasis. The eighth edition of the TNM classification {132} incorporates the tumour characteristics of size and location (ICRB groups A–E), imaging findings, and the status of systemic metastasis. Children with an associated midline intracranial tumour (trilateral retinoblastoma) have a worse prognosis {255}.

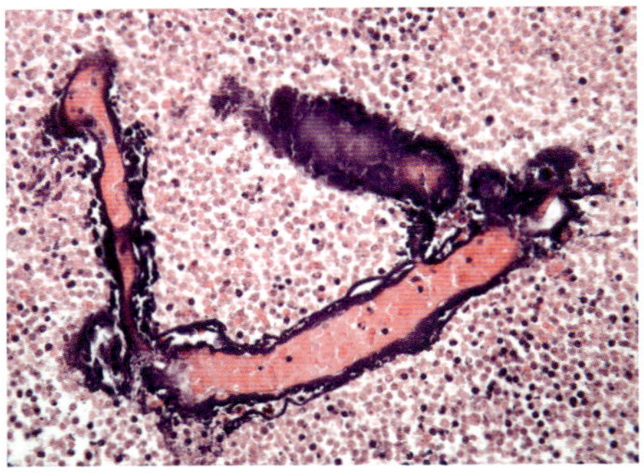

Fig. 3.08 Retinoblastoma. Basophilic deposits of DNA surround vessels within necrotic tumour.

Histopathological factors: Enucleated eyes with retinoblastoma may harbour histopathological prognostic factors for metastasis. Lymph node or systemic metastasis often complicates extraocular invasion of tumour through the sclera into the orbit. The presence of tumour at the surgical margin of the optic nerve or its meninges results in local recurrence in the orbit and in the CNS. In such cases, the incidence of CNS involvement is > 90%, and survival is dismal {1035}. A prospective trial sponsored by the Children's Oncology Group (COG) studied > 300 enucleated eyes with unilateral retinoblastoma and identified two histopathological features as prognostic of metastasis: massive uveal invasion (≥ 3 mm in maximum dimension) and retrolaminar optic nerve invasion {304,1035}. The most important prognostic factor for recurrence and death was extensive retrolaminar optic nerve invasion concomitant with massive choroidal invasion. Anterior chamber invasion alone did not appear to have a prognostic value for metastasis. However, the number of such cases was small, because most eyes with anterior chamber invasion also have massive choroidal or optic nerve invasion, or both. Other histopathological factors associated with metastasis include neovascularization of the iris with secondary glaucoma, buphthalmos, and extensively necrotic retinoblastoma (defined as > 90% tumour necrosis with necrotic intraocular tissues) {206}. These features are often seen in patients who present with the clinical picture of aseptic orbital cellulitis due to delayed diagnosis and therapy {206}. Severe anaplasia in tumour cells has been identified as a potential risk factor for metastasis, especially in the absence of optic nerve or massive choroidal infiltration {789}.

Genetic and molecular factors: In the eighth edition of the American Joint Committee on Cancer (AJCC) TNM classification {33}, genetic status (H) has been added to the staging system for the first time. A retinoblastoma is classified as H0 if there is no history of hereditary retinoblastoma and the patient is not known to have a germline mutation. H1 denotes hereditary retinoblastoma or the presence of a germline mutation. Tumours classified as H1 should be carefully monitored for the development of new retinoblastoma tumours, including bilateralization, trilateral retinoblastoma, and secondary malignancies. Genetic counselling of family members and screening of children at risk for developing retinoblastoma is recommended in these cases.

The molecular identification of minimal disease in cerebrospinal fluid or blood may aid in predicting recurrence and possibly implementing aggressive treatment {1265}. The identification of the specific *RB1* mutation originally found in the eye tumour may confirm the presence of metastatic extraocular tumour, in particular in children with germline mutations who develop second malignancies that may mimic retinoblastoma {944}.

The treatment of retinoblastoma should be focused on preserving the life of the child. Treatment decisions are made based on patient age, laterality and severity of disease, and potential toxicity. For advanced unilateral retinoblastoma in eyes with limited visual potential, enucleation provides the hope of complete curative resection with no need for additional therapy. The extent of intraocular disease predicts the likelihood of treatment success for an eye with retinoblastoma. Historically, eye salvage treatment relied on external beam radiation therapy, but because of the cosmetic deformities and risk of radiation-induced second malignancies associated with that modality, chemotherapy is now the treatment of choice. The delivery of chemotherapy has rapidly evolved from systemic {568,1097} to intra-arterial {5,1042,1106} and intravitreal {832,833,1081}. Chemotherapy is paired with focal consolidating treatments to the eye, which include cryotherapy, transpupillary thermotherapy, and episcleral plaque brachytherapy {1112}. The preferred treatment regimens vary among retinoblastoma specialists, but the various regimens achieve comparable efficacies. Treatment of extraocular retinoblastoma requires systemic chemotherapy and radiation to the orbit and regional lymph nodes (if they are involved). Metastatic retinoblastoma is best treated with high-dose chemotherapy with bone marrow rescue {884,989}. However, the prognosis for CNS metastases remains poor.

Retinocytoma

Marco C.
Al Hussaini M.
Moulin A.
Tso M.O.M.

Definition

Retinocytoma is a benign tumour that arises from retinal precursor cells and may transform into retinoblastoma.

ICD-O code

Retinocytoma	9510/0

Synonyms

Retinoma (clinical); spontaneously regressed retinoblastoma (archaic)

Epidemiology

Approximately 2% of people with a mutant *RB1* allele are estimated to have retinocytoma {283}. Of 920 consecutive patients with retinoblastoma seen at an oncology referral centre, 17 (1.8%) were found to have retinocytoma {1183}. Because this lesion is usually asymptomatic, the patient age at presentation is older than for retinoblastoma. In one clinical series, the median age at presentation of retinocytoma was 15 years {1183}; in another series (of 36 cases), the average age was 29 years {4}. The reported age at diagnosis ranges from < 1 year to 45 years. There appears to be no race or sex predilection, but the total number of reported cases is low.

Etiology

Like retinoblastomas, retinocytomas result from the loss of both *RB1* tumour suppressor gene alleles, but they differ from retinoblastomas in that they demonstrate low levels of genomic instability and high expression of senescence-associated proteins {283}.

Localization

Retinocytomas are primary tumours of the neurosensory retina.

Clinical features

Most retinocytomas occur unilaterally, but they can develop bilaterally when associated with germline *RB1* mutation {752,1183}. Some retinocytomas are associated with otherwise typical retinoblastoma in the same or the contralateral eye, and some are discovered after conservative treatment with chemotherapy or radiation. Retinocytomas can cause blurred vision in older children and strabismus in younger children. Some cases are detected during a screening examination in individuals with a family history of retinoblastoma.

On retinal examination, the tumours often resemble treated retinoblastomas that have partially regressed {4,1183}. They appear semi-translucent, surrounded by mild to moderate pigmentary changes at the level of the retinal pigment epithelium. White globular opacities (dystrophic calcium) are commonly observed, along with surrounding chorioretinal atrophy. Most retinocytomas are relatively small (4–9 mm in greatest diameter), but tumours as large as 15 mm in greatest diameter have been reported. Some retinocytomas contain cysts {4}. Some cases present as diffuse retinal thickening in which neurosensory retina is replaced by a totally photoreceptor-differentiated tumour {1279}. Retinocytoma is typically stable, showing no enlargement or growth when examined serially over time. Tumour enlargement is suggestive of malignant transformation {306}.

Histopathology

Retinocytomas are composed of a uniform population of cells that often exhibit photoreceptor differentiation in the form of elongated, eosinophilic cytoplasmic processes. The cellular proliferation replaces the neurosensory retina and expands into the vitreous but does not invade choroid. Individual cells with prominent eosinophilic cytoplasmic processes are found singly, in small clusters, or in linear arrays called fleurettes (French for "small flowers"). These cytoplasmic processes are often surrounded by extracellular matrix that stains with Alcian blue and is resistant to digestion with hyaluronidase. The nuclei are round

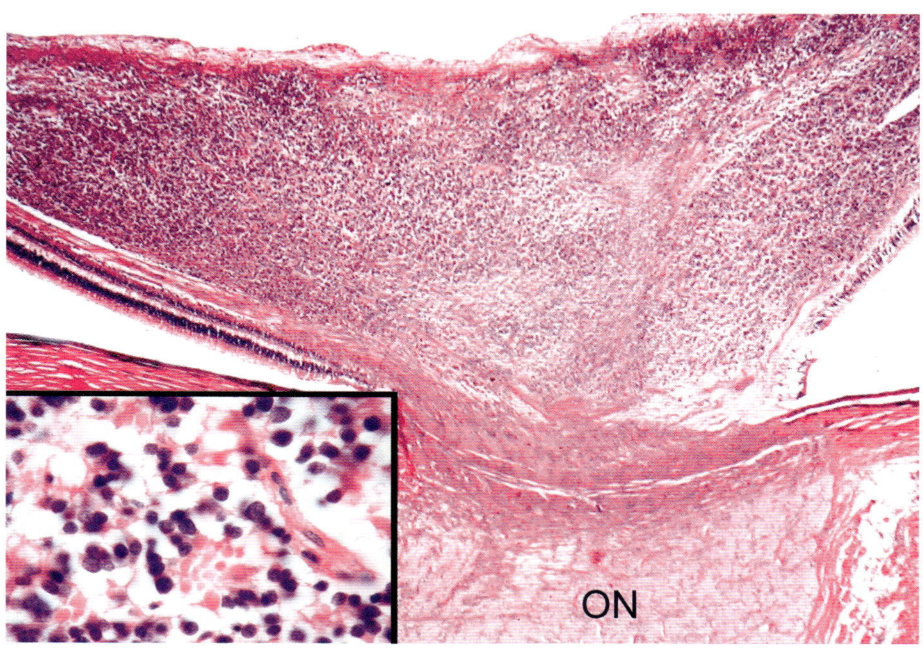

Fig. 3.09 Retinocytoma. Juxtapapillary tumour overlying an optic nerve (ON); at low magnification, the proliferation of cells has a pinker appearance than retinoblastoma. At higher magnification (**inset**), the cells have bland round nuclei and poorly defined clear cytoplasm; the eosinophilic bodies clustered near the centre are probably inner segments of photoreceptors.

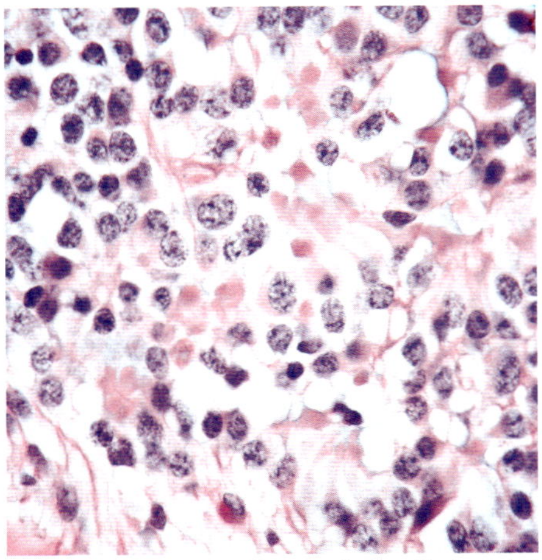

Fig. 3.10 Retinocytoma. Clusters of cells with elongated cytoplasmic projections; these extensions of cytoplasm correspond to inner segments of photoreceptors.

to oval, are relatively uniform in size, and contain evenly dispersed chromatin. Mitotic figures are not seen. In some cases, the cytoplasm is clear rather than eosinophilic. Focal dystrophic calcium deposits are common, but necrosis is unusual. Although Flexner–Wintersteiner rosettes are considered a manifestation of retinal differentiation, they are not generally observed in retinocytomas. Retinocytomas do not express Ki-67 or p53 {282}. Ultrastructurally, most of the cells are neuronal cells with photoreceptor differentiation {752,1282}.

In addition to occurring as an independent retinal tumour, retinocytoma has also been described as a minor component of otherwise typical retinoblastoma. In one retrospective study of archival material from 128 retinoblastomas, investigators detected retinocytomas buried within 20 (16%) of the tumours {283}. Retinocytomas can also be encountered after eye-conserving treatment for retinoblastoma, as a residual mass persisting after therapy {282,1279}; these solid remnants of the primary tumour are relatively unresponsive to the therapy that successfully destroyed the contiguous retinoblastoma {1279}. These findings add to the accumulating evidence that the relative rarity of retinocytoma is due to the fact that the vast majority of cases rapidly progress to retinoblastoma after tertiary mutations occur in critical cancer pathways {283,787}.

Differential diagnosis

The differential diagnosis is similar to that of retinoblastoma. Retinocytoma is differentiated from a small retinoblastoma by its bland, speckled nuclear chromatin; lack of mitotic activity and necrosis; and pink cytoplasmic processes, including fleurette formation. Retinal astrocytomas (which occur in patients with tuberous sclerosis and sporadically) often contain dystrophic calcium and lack mitotic activity; however, they are composed of glial cells and lack photoreceptor differentiation. Intraocular medulloepithelioma is composed of cells organized in ribbons, sheets, and cysts, resembling medullary epithelium during embryonic development. The benign variant is considered a choristoma. Its netlike appearance at low magnification is a key feature distinguishing it from retinocytoma. Medulloepitheliomas do not display fleurettes or other signs of photoreceptor differentiation, but they can display rosettes.

Histogenesis

Retinocytomas, like retinoblastomas, are thought to arise from neuroectodermal cells in the inner layer of the optic cup, so-called retinal precursor cells {578}. These precursor cells have the ability to differentiate into a variety of retinal cells, such as horizontal cells and photoreceptors. Gene expression studies suggest that a cone precursor cell may be a more immediate antecedent {1387}. The presence of glial tissue within retinocytomas has raised questions as to whether this entity is a manifestation of neoplastic differentiation or a reactive process {1278}.

Genetic profile

Our current understanding of retinocytoma involves the model of tumour induction through mutational alterations of both *RB1* alleles {1255}. Retinocytoma remains arrested at this quiescent phase of tumorigenesis until additional mutation events drive progression towards a highly proliferative retinoblastoma. The low level of genomic instability is attributed in part to high expression of the senescence-associated proteins p16 (p16INK4a) and p130 {282}.

Genetic susceptibility

There are two clinical forms of retinocytoma, with distinct patterns of genetic susceptibility: bilateral/multifocal and unifocal {787}. Retinocytoma occurring in conjunction with a tumour in the opposite eye (either another retinocytoma or a retinoblastoma), or arising multifocally in one eye, is caused by germline mutation of the retinoblastoma gene (*RB1*). Even in the absence of a family history, affected individuals are at risk of transmitting the trait in an autosomal dominant manner. Patients with a sporadic, unilateral, unifocal retinocytoma have a 15% chance of being a carrier of a germline *RB1* mutation.

Prognosis and predictive factors

With a small retinocytoma, the prognosis for vision is good if the tumour is located outside the macula, where a scotoma may go largely unnoticed. The risk of progression to retinoblastoma depends on whether additional mutation events occur that might trigger transformation. Because there is currently no way to predict these events, patients with retinocytoma must be monitored for changes in the tumour. Genetic counselling for patients with retinocytoma can be carried out using an algorithm similar to that used for patients with retinoblastoma.

Astrocytic hamartoma and astrocytoma of the retina

Eberhart C.G.
Van Ginderdeuren R.
Wilson D.

Definition

Astrocytic hamartoma and astrocytoma of the retina are low-grade astrocytic neoplasms arising in the retina or optic nerve head.

ICD-O code

Astrocytoma NOS	9400/3

Synonyms

Astrocytic hamartoma of the retina; intraocular glioma; acquired retinal astrocytoma; retinal phakoma

Epidemiology

Astrocytic hamartoma and astrocytoma of the retina are often associated with a phakomatosis, most commonly tuberous sclerosis or neurofibromatosis. Tuberous sclerosis has an estimated incidence of 1 case per 6000–10 000 live births, and retinal astrocytomas are detected in one third to one half of patients {54}. A few cases have been reported in patients with retinitis pigmentosa, but most such reports lack histopathological confirmation of the diagnosis {731}. Retinal

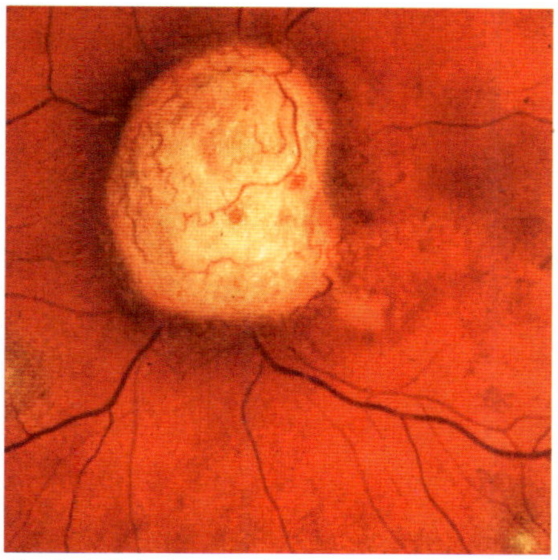

Fig. 3.11 Retinal astrocytic hamartoma. This heavily calcified retinal tumour contains larger cells, similar to those of subependymal giant cell astrocytoma in the brain.

astrocytomas generally arise in children or young adults, although some cases have been first noted at an older age.

Etiology
Aside from the syndromic associations listed above, little is known about the etiology of these neoplasms.

Localization
Astrocytic hamartomas in tuberous sclerosis are generally discrete, slightly elevated lesions arising in the inner retina; they are found most commonly along the arcades, and less commonly in locations adjacent to the optic nerve and in the periphery {54}. Most tumours grow by direct extension, but vitreous seeding has also been reported {213}.

Clinical features
In one cohort of 83 patients with tuberous sclerosis, 30 patients (36%) were found to have retinal astrocytic hamartomas; the tumours were bilateral in 13 patients (43%) and multiple in 12 patients (40%) {54}. A study of 15 retinal astrocytic hamartomas by optical coherence tomography identified a gradual transition between normal retina and the optically hyper-reflective mass, with associated retinal disorganization, so-called motheaten spaces, and posterior shadowing as characteristic features {1078}.

Histopathology
These are generally well-circumscribed lesions. Two main histopathological patterns have been described {936,1149}. In the first, the tumour is composed of fascicles of spindle-shaped, GFAP-positive astrocytes with cytologically bland nuclei. In the second, sometimes termed giant cell astrocytoma of the retina, the tumour comprises larger cells with abundant eosinophilic cytoplasm, round nuclei, and prominent nucleoli, morphologically similar to subependymal giant cell astrocytoma in the brain. As is the case with subependymal giant cell astrocytoma, both glial and neuronal immunohistochemical markers can be expressed. In this second type of tumour, calcification and necrosis are common. Although mitotic figures are rare or absent, these tumours can begin to grow and can eventually fill the posterior globe; such cases are termed aggressive retinal astrocytoma. Rosenthal fibres, eosinophilic granular bodies, and other features of pilocytic astrocytoma are generally absent. However, pilocytic astrocytoma of the optic nerve can very rarely extend into the retina {988}.

Differential diagnosis
Retinal astrocytomas must be distinguished from reactive retinal astrocytic proliferations, which lack abundant eosinophilic cytoplasm and other features similar to those of subependymal giant cell astrocytoma. Retinal astrocytomas can also clinically mimic retinoblastoma in children, amelanotic melanoma, haemangioblastoma, and metastatic carcinoma, particularly in patients lacking other syndromic manifestations.

Histogenesis
The histogenesis of these tumours is unclear, but many are centred in the inner retina, a finding consistent with an origin

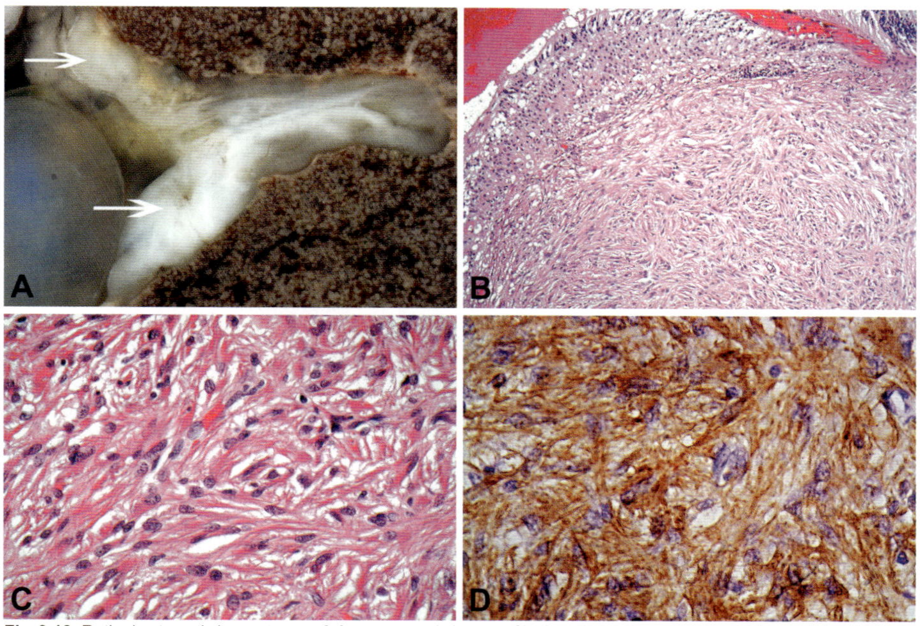

Fig. 3.12 Retinal astrocytic hamartoma. **A** A macroscopic image of lesions (arrows) in a patient with tuberous sclerosis; the eye was enucleated because of subretinal haemorrhage and ocular pain. **B** A low-power view showing the hamartoma emanating from the inner retina. **C** A high-power view of the whorled astrocytes making up the lesion. **D** Positive immunohistochemical staining for GFAP.

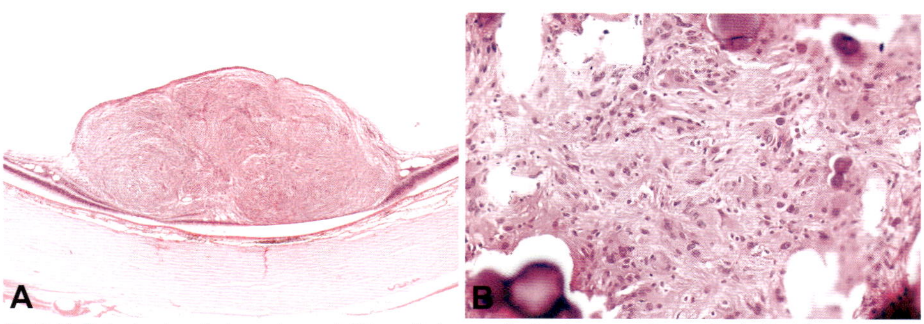

Fig. 3.13 Retinal astrocytic hamartoma. **A** This well-circumscribed lesion arose in a patient with tuberous sclerosis. **B** A lesion in a patient with tuberous sclerosis, composed mainly of spindled glial cells with calcifications.

from astrocytes of the nerve fibre layer. Ultrastructural analysis of one large giant cell astrocytoma suggested a possible origin from Müller radial glial cells {524}.

Genetic profile
Aside from syndromic associations suggesting roles for the *TSC1*, *TSC2*, and *NF1* genes, little is known about the genetic alterations in these tumours.

Genetic susceptibility
One review of 42 histologically documented astrocytic tumours of the retina found that 24 (57%) of the patients had tuberous sclerosis and 6 (14%) had neurofibromatosis; in the remaining 12 patients (29%), the astrocytic tumours were an isolated finding {1292}.

Prognosis and predictive factors
Astrocytic hamartomas are generally not clinically aggressive, but progressive growth and severe local complications have been reported in exceptional cases; these cases are often associated with large gemistocytic cells and necrosis {438,1135}. One such tumour, which also featured more-common mitoses, invaded into the optic nerve and choroid {438}. Resolution has been reported with verteporfin in combination with photodynamic therapy {328,494,1286}.

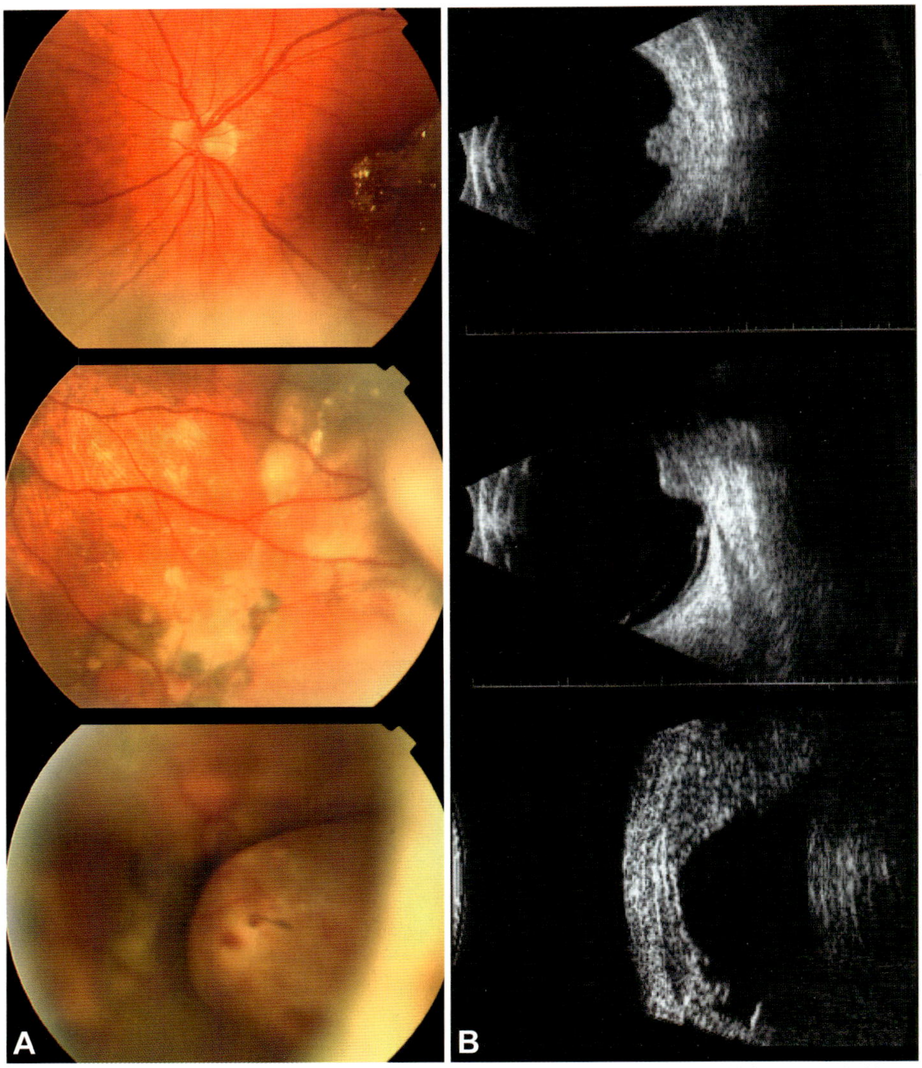

Fig. 3.14 Focal reactive (nodular) gliosis. **A** The initial fundus appearance shows an elevated inferotemporal white-to-yellow mass anterior to the equator, with an associated shallow, exudative retinal detachment. **B** Ultrasound images show a solid lesion with medium internal reflectivity.

Nodular and massive retinal gliosis

Grossniklaus H.E.
Eberhart C.G.
Edward D.P.
Mendoza P.
Chan A.S.Y.

Definition
Nodular and massive retinal gliosis encompasses a spectrum of discrete glial proliferations surrounding blood vessels, ranging in size from small nodules to massive lesions that fill the eye {538}.

ICD-O code
None

Synonyms
Vasoproliferative tumour/lesion {1111}; peripheral retinal angioma {500}; angioma-like mass {82}; retinal angiomatous mass {415}; neovascular fundus abnormalities {342}; peripheral nodular retinal telangiectasis {72}; angioma-like lesion {387}; presumed acquired retinal haemangioma {1124}

Epidemiology
These lesions generally occur in adults, and there is no sex or hereditary predilection {924}.

Etiology
Focal reactive (nodular) gliosis and larger lesions on this spectrum can be idiopathic or related to etiological factors such as neurofibromatosis {530}, retinitis pigmentosa, uveitis, retinopathy of prematurity, Coats disease, retinal detachment surgery, cryotherapy, physical trauma, infection (e.g. toxoplasmosis and toxocariasis), and idiopathic inflammatory retinal diseases {1111}.

Localization
These lesions are usually located in the inferotemporal pre-equatorial retina.

Clinical features
The lesion may be asymptomatic and incidentally discovered during dilated fundus examination, or it may cause decreased vision, primarily due to exudative retinal detachment or macular exudation. The lesion is a pink to yellow or orange nodule that often appears vascular in nature (hence the term "vasoproliferative lesion"); it is associated with subretinal exudation, shallow non-bullous retinal detachment, and retinal pigment epithelial hyperplasia at its base. These

lesions leak fluorescein on fluorescein angiography.

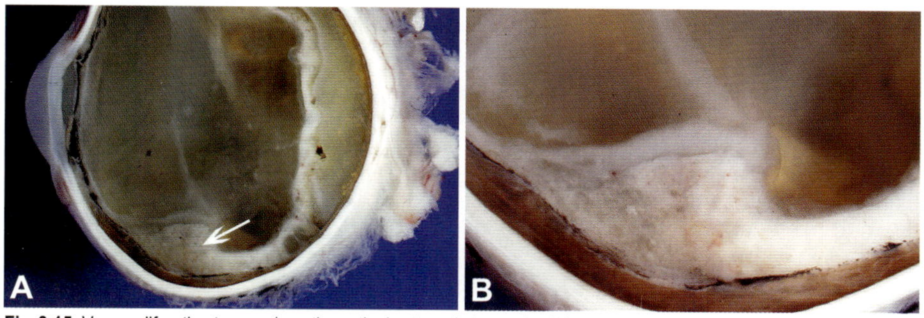

Fig. 3.15 Vasoproliferative tumour (reactive retinal astrocytic tumour). **A** A macroscopic view of a discrete glial proliferation (arrow) surrounding blood vessels in the eye. **B** At higher magnification.

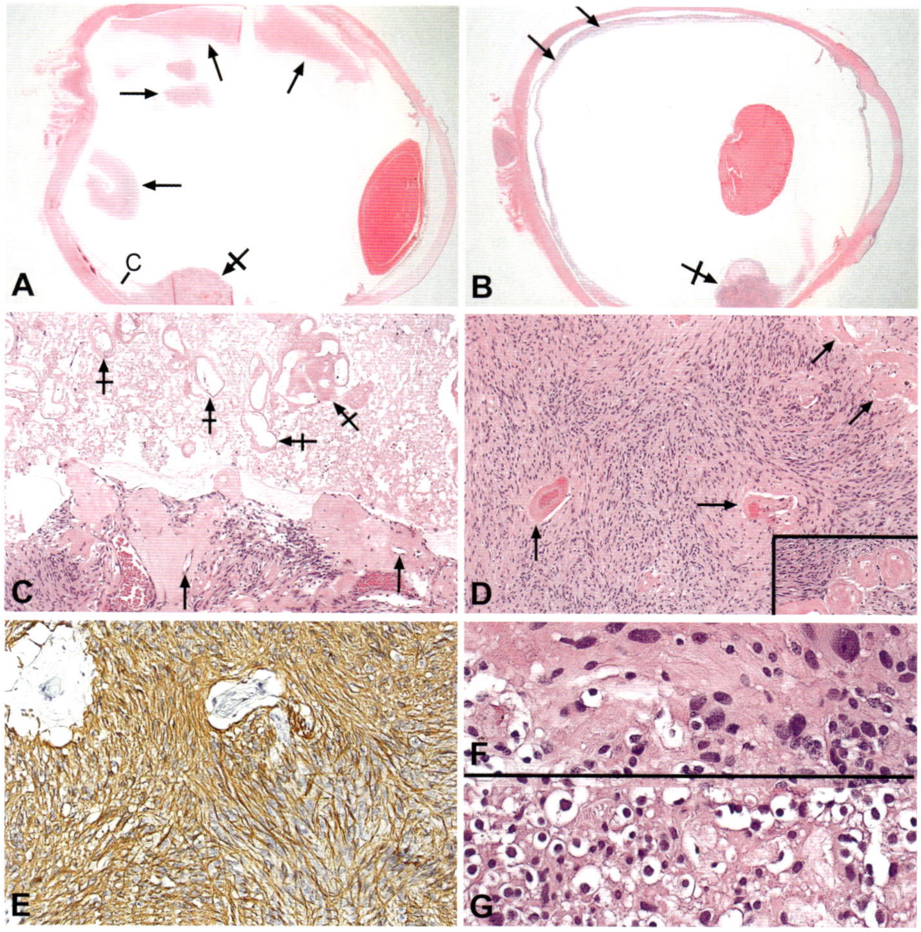

Fig. 3.16 Focal nodular gliosis in enucleated eyes. **A** There is a moderately elevated inferotemporal mass (crossed arrow), with an eosinophilic exudate in the vitreous (arrows) and an intraretinal cyst (c) posterior to the mass. **B** Another example shows the tumour (crossed arrow) with an area of apical necrosis; there is diffuse placoid fibrous material (arrows) in the subretinal space on the side opposite the tumour. **C** There is no inflammation within the necrotic area of the tumour (top right); ghost-like vascular outlines (crossed arrows) are present, and there are severely sclerotic vessels (arrows) at the interface with the tumour. **D** The tumour is composed of interweaving bundles of bipolar spindle cells with regularly spaced sclerotic vessels (arrows), shown as a cluster in the **inset**. **E** Immunohistochemical staining for GFAP is strongly positive within the tumour. **F** The tumour may contain cells with mildly atypical nuclei and occasional nucleoli. **G** The tumour may contain cells with clear cytoplasm, resembling oligodendroglia.

Histopathology

The lesion is composed of spindle-shaped fibrous astrocytes and may contain hair-like (piloid) processes or Rosenthal fibres. There are often scattered sclerotic vascular channels and capillaries within the lesion. Subretinal proteinaceous exudates associated with the lesion may extend beyond its borders, and these exudates may contain cholesterol clefts or even a granulomatous response. Fibrous (or even osseous) metaplasia of the retinal pigment epithelium at the base of the lesion can be prominent, along with an inflammatory lymphocytic infiltrate in the choroid. The astrocytic cells are immunopositive for GFAP and S100 protein; mitotic figures are absent or rare, and the Ki-67 proliferation index is < 5%. The hyalinized blood vessels, which give a positive periodic acid–Schiff (PAS) reaction, may be highlighted by immunohistochemical staining for CD31 and CD34. The perivascular orientation of glial cells led one group to suggest that these lesions constitute retinal ependymoma, but this hypothesis has not been generally accepted {1246}. Ultrastructural features include interweaving cells with intermediate cytoplasmic filaments correlating with GFAP, as well as small cellular processes that contain lysosomes.

Differential diagnosis

The histological differential diagnosis includes pilocytic astrocytoma, diffuse astrocytoma, giant cell (gemistocytic) astrocytoma, astrocytic hamartoma (phakoma), and retinal haemangioblastoma {924}.

Histogenesis

These lesions are reactive in nature, arising from retinal astrocytes or Müller radial glial cells, and they form a spectrum of reactive retinal astrocytic proliferations {924}. There is a well-documented case of the clinical progression of focal nodular (reactive) gliosis to massive gliosis {500}.

Genetic profile

One case of massive retinal gliosis was shown to be polyclonal, a finding supporting a reactive etiology {505}. In one series of 4 cases, neither the *KIAA1549-BRAF* fusion gene commonly seen in pilocytic astrocytomas nor the mutation *IDH1* c.395G>A (p.R132H) seen in many low-grade infiltrating astrocytomas was detected {924}. Genes associated with astrocytes (but not vascular genes) have been found to be upregulated {1074}.

Prognosis and predictive factors

The prognosis for focal reactive (nodular) gliosis is guarded. The disease often has a long, protracted course, and it may require treatments such as laser photocoagulation, cryotherapy, plaque brachytherapy, vitreoretinal surgery, and in some cases enucleation. Vision may be threatened by either vascular exudation or retinal detachment. Although massive retinal gliosis generally remains confined to the eye, one reported case extended outside the sclera, but it still retained microscopic features consistent with a reactive process {221}.

Haemangioblastoma of the retina

Wilson D.
Chévez-Barrios P.
Roberts F.

Definition

Haemangioblastoma of the retina is a tumour derived from developmentally arrested angioblasts {1339}; it is generally caused by mutation of the *VHL* gene.

ICD-O code

Haemangioblastoma	9161/1

Synonyms

von Hippel's tumour; retinal capillary haemangioma; angiomatosis retinae; angioblastoma

Epidemiology

Retinal haemangioblastomas can occur sporadically or as part of von Hippel–Lindau syndrome (VHL) along with CNS haemangioblastomas. Sporadic tumours are generally solitary and unilateral, whereas haemangioblastomas occurring in VHL are frequently multiple with bilateral involvement. The median patient age at diagnosis of sporadic cases has been reported to be 36 years, and in VHL, 17 years {1182}. No sex difference was found in prevalence {197,1182}. Approximately 50% of patients with *VHL* mutations develop retinal haemangioblastoma {197}.

Etiology

Retinal haemangioblastomas result from mutations in the *VHL* gene. In VHL, there is a germline defect in one copy of the gene; random loss of the normal allele (loss of heterozygosity) predisposes patients to developing haemangioblastomas. In sporadic cases, presumably there is somatic loss of both normal copies of the *VHL* gene, resulting in a similar but solitary tumour {197,1046}.

Localization

Haemangioblastomas can occur anywhere in the retina, but they are most common in the temporal quadrants {1182}. Haemangioblastomas can also occur in the optic nerve, both in the nerve head and in the retrobulbar nerve {197,795,1182}. In addition, haemangioblastomas can occur in the cerebellum, spinal cord, and retroperitoneal space.

Clinical features

Small haemangioblastomas appear as flat or slightly raised clumps of capillary-sized vessels. Prominently dilated vascular channels may be seen within these clumps, and some white gliotic tissue may be seen at the surface of the lesion. Juxtapapillary lesions have a similar appearance, but they often have an indistinct margin where they abut the optic nerve, and they are often associated with serous retinal detachment. Larger haemangioblastomas are elevated, and lipid exudate surrounds the lesion because of vascular leakage. The dense capillary plexus acts as a shunt, causing the feeding artery and draining vein to become dilated and resulting in a very characteristic clinical appearance. Larger haemangioblastomas often also have a fibrotic so-called glial component, and the overlying vitreous may become adherent to the lesion. Vascular leakage may progress to the point of exudative retinal detachment, with the vitreous adhesion providing a tractional component to the detachment as well. A small proportion of patients develop retinal neovascularization {197}. In the most extreme cases, progressive exudative retinal detachment can lead to phthisis bulbi.

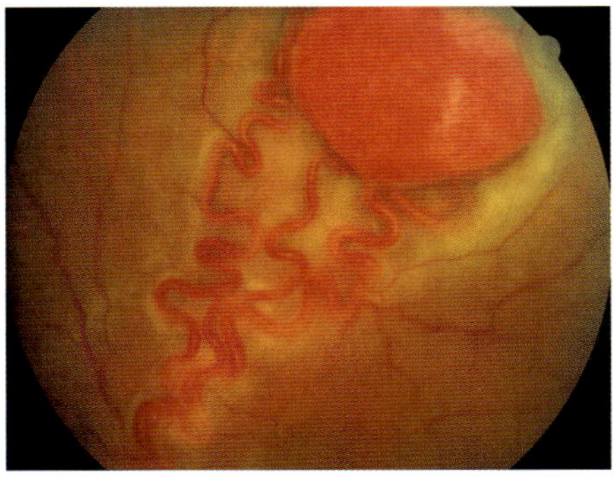

Fig. 3.17 Haemangioblastoma of the retina. This large haemangioblastoma is elevated and contains very prominent feeder vessels and surrounding lipid exudate.

Histopathology

Haemangioblastomas are composed of capillary-sized vascular channels surrounding stromal cells, which characteristically have prominently vacuolated cytoplasm; in ocular and cerebellar haemangioblastomas, small clusters of angiomesenchymal cells, called tumourlet cells, have also been described {175}. The stromal cells and tumourlet cells may express CD133, a marker present on haematopoietic, endothelial, and neural progenitor cells. Only the stromal cells harbour genetic alterations in the *VHL* gene; these alterations are not present in the vascular or glial components. This observation suggests that only the stromal cells are truly neoplastic cells {175}. The abnormal VHL protein that the stromal cells produce results in abnormal regulation of hypoxia-inducible factor, with subsequent effects on the growth factors VEGF, TGF, PDGF, FGF, EGF, and CXCR4. Clusterin may also play a role in tumour suppression by the VHL protein; it is markedly decreased in the haemangioblastoma cells compared with in the retinal and optic nerve cells {1417}.

Differential diagnosis

Early lesions must be distinguished from retinal microaneurysms due to any cause. For medium to large retinal haemangioblastomas, the main differential diagnosis is reactive retinal astrocytic proliferation (nodular and/or massive retinal gliosis). Retinal astrocytic tumours are generally not as well circumscribed as haemangioblastomas, and they have a less prominent feeding artery and draining vein. For haemangioblastomas in which an exudative retinal detachment has occurred, Coats disease is a differential diagnostic concern. The differential diagnosis for papillary and parapapillary haemangioblastomas includes papillitis and inflammatory tumours such as sarcoidosis.

Genetic profile

Retinal haemangioblastomas are associated with germline and sporadic mutations in *VHL*, a tumour suppressor gene located on chromosome 3p25.3.

Genetic susceptibility

Germline mutations in the *VHL* gene are inherited in an autosomal dominant pattern. Patients are susceptible to benign and malignant tumours of multiple

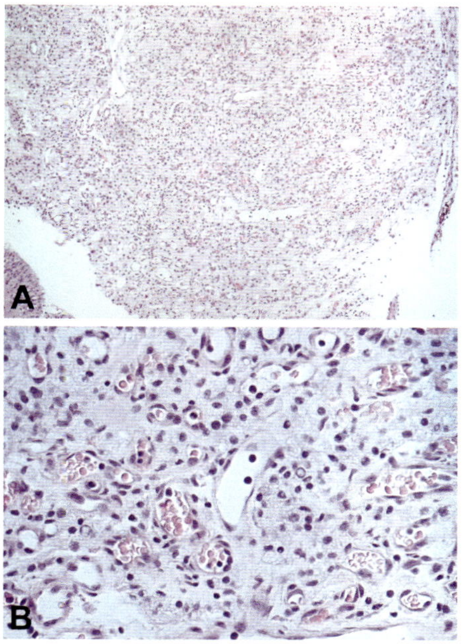

Fig. 3.18 Haemangioblastoma of the retina. **A** A low-magnification photomicrograph of a resected tumour; there are numerous capillary-sized vessels, with sparse interstitial cells. **B** The lesion consists of capillary-sized vessels surrounding sparse stromal cells with prominently vacuolated cytoplasm; small cells with a spindled to crescent-shaped nucleus (called tumourlet cells) are present adjacent to some vessels.

organs, most notably to renal cell carcinomas. Common tumour sites include the eye, CNS, kidney, inner ear, pancreas, broad ligament, and epididymis; more rarely affected sites include the liver, lung, and ovary.

Prognosis and predictive factors

The disease phenotype depends on the type of germline mutation present in the *VHL* gene. Deletions and truncating mutations are associated with type 1 VHL, which is characterized by renal cell carcinoma and haemangioblastoma (but not phaeochromocytoma). Missense mutations are associated with type 2 VHL, which is characterized by renal cell carcinoma and phaeochromocytoma. Retinal haemangioblastomas occur in 45% of patients with partial deletions, simple missense mutations, or nonsense mutations of the *VHL* gene; they are much less common in patients with complete deletion of the *VHL* gene, occurring in only 9% {197}.

The prognosis for vision in patients with VHL is good: 88% of patients retain 20/20 (or better) vision in at least one eye {197}. Laser therapy and cryotherapy are effective treatments for small to medium-sized intraocular haemangioblastomas that do not involve the optic nerve. Surgical resection of unresponsive and large retinal haemangioblastomas is becoming increasingly common, with good visual outcomes {1046}. Treatment of haemangioblastomas involving the optic nerve remains challenging.

In terms of systemic morbidity and overall survival in VHL, the prognosis depends on the treatment of the associated cerebellar haemangioblastoma and renal cell carcinoma.

Cavernous haemangioma of the retina

Wilson D.
Grossniklaus H.E.
Kivelä T.T.

Definition

Cavernous haemangioma of the retina is a vascular hamartoma that occurs both sporadically and in a familial fashion.

ICD-O code

Cavernous haemangioma	9121/0

Synonym

Vascular hamartoma of the retina

Epidemiology

Precise incidence estimates are not available, but cavernous haemangioma of the retina is a rare disorder. Most of the reported cases have occurred in White patients, in a roughly equal number of males and females. The lesions are congenital, but because of the lack of symptoms, the median age at diagnosis is 21 years {1350}.

Etiology

Most cases are sporadic and occur without identifiable predisposing factors. However, approximately 20% of patients have a family history of the disorder, and several patients have been found to have a mutation in the *KRIT1* (*CCM1*) gene {965}.

Localization

Cavernous haemangiomas of the retina affect the peripheral retina in 70% of cases, but they can also affect the posterior retina and the optic nerve head {1350}. The temporal quadrant of the retina is the most common quadrant of involvement. The dilated vessels arise from the retinal circulation, but they may extend to the full thickness of the retina. CNS involvement is present in 14% of patients, and it occurs with a greater frequency in patients with a family history of the disorder {392,1350}. Cutaneous involvement, characterized by capillary haemangiomas of the skin, is also seen in some patients {288,392}.

Clinical features

Cavernous haemangiomas of the retina are characterized by multiple thin-walled saccular aneurysms evident on the retinal surface. The aneurysms are filled with dark blood, and in many cases there is white fibrous tissue evident between the vascular channels. Retinal and/or vitreous haemorrhage may be present and may be related to vitreous traction on the thin-walled surface vessels. Fluorescein angiography may demonstrate a separation of the serum and cellular components of the blood, consistent with a low flow rate through the dilated vascular channels. There are no dilated feeder or draining vessels associated with the lesion, and the surrounding retina is normal in appearance. No lipid exudates are present.

Patients are generally asymptomatic, and the lesions are detected on routine eye examination. However, vision is decreased when a haemangioma affects the macula. Vitreous haemorrhage may also lead to diminished vision. Patients with CNS lesions may present with headaches, seizures, and/or visual field abnormalities.

Histopathology

The histopathology is similar to that of other cavernous haemangiomas. Dilated thin-walled interconnected vascular spaces are lined by a continuous non-fenestrated endothelial lining {392,791}. Occasional areas of partially organized thrombus may be present. The adjacent retina may exhibit gliosis.

Differential diagnosis

Other vascular anomalies, such as Coats disease, Leber miliary aneurysms, retinal haemangioblastomas, retinal racemose angioma (Wyburn–Mason syndrome), and reactive glial cell tumours, should be considered, but they are generally easily distinguished from cavernous haemangioma on the basis of clinical appearance.

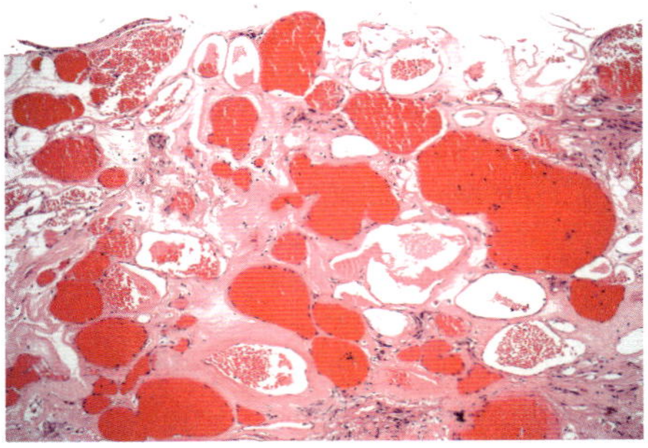

Fig. 3.19 Cavernous haemangioma of the retina. Large, irregularly shaped and sized vascular channels surrounded by thick walls; gliotic retina is interspersed between the channels.

Genetic profile

Most cases of cavernous haemangioma of the retina are sporadic. Familial cases are inherited in an autosomal dominant pattern {392,409,704}.

Genetic susceptibility

Familial cases are more likely to be bilateral and to be associated with CNS cavernous haemangiomas. Familial cases can also manifest as a neuro-oculo-cutaneous haemangioma syndrome.

Prognosis and predictive factors

The visual prognosis is largely dependent on the location of the haemangioma. These lesions are non-progressive and are not associated with exudative changes; therefore, when the lesion is not in the macula, the prognosis for vision is excellent. Vitreous haemorrhages generally affect vision only temporarily and clear spontaneously. Patients with retinal cavernous haemangiomas should be evaluated for CNS haemangiomas because of the risk for seizures.

Vitreoretinal lymphoma

Wilson D.
Chévez-Barrios P.
Coupland S.E.
Laver N.
Loeffler K.U.

Definition

Vitreoretinal lymphoma is a high-grade malignant lymphoproliferative disease in which atypical lymphocytes infiltrate the retina and vitreous in the absence of lymph node or visceral involvement. It is frequently accompanied by involvement of the CNS.

ICD-O code

Vitreoretinal lymphoma	9680/3

Synonyms

Intraocular lymphoma; primary intraocular lymphoma

Epidemiology

The true incidence of primary vitreoretinal lymphoma (PVRL) is difficult to estimate because of its rarity and the effect of improvements over time in the diagnostic techniques used. The observed incidence is reported to have steadily increased from 0.23 cases per 1 million population in 1990 to 0.48 cases per 1 million population in 2010 {702}. A slight predominance of females relative to males is reported {702,975}. The mean patient age at diagnosis is 58 years {975}.

Etiology

HIV and EBV infections are believed to be predisposing factors for the development of PVRL, given the overlap with primary CNS lymphoma. No other environmental risk factors are known.

Localization

By definition, PVRL is localized to the retina and vitreous. More specifically, it tends to present as cells circulating within the vitreous and aqueous humour, accumulating in the subretinal space, or both. These modes of presentation are associated with subclinical retinal involvement, as can be seen in retinal biopsy specimens (when available).

Clinical features

The symptoms most commonly associated with PVRL are decreased vision and floaters. In patients with concomitant CNS lymphoma, additional symptoms and signs include headaches, seizures, altered mental status, hemiplegia, and hemianopia. The most common sign is scattered cell infiltration in the vitreous, anterior chamber, or both. This relatively nonspecific clinical presentation is responsible for delayed diagnosis in many patients, who are treated with immunosuppression after an unrevealing evaluation for posterior uveitis. A partial or complete response to immunosuppression may occur, only to be followed by a relapse upon tapering or cessation of immunosuppressive therapy. A minority of patients develop subretinal pigment epithelial (sub-RPE) accumulation of lymphoma cells. This finding, which is characteristic of PVRL, may facilitate earlier diagnosis. The cells in the sub-RPE space may resolve spontaneously, with their disappearance leaving an RPE defect. Ultimately, this may result in extensive areas of focal RPE defects.

Less commonly, PVRL may cause ischaemic retinopathy. The angiocentric nature of the lymphomatous infiltrate in the retina is responsible for this appearance. The main differential diagnosis is acute retinal necrosis due to retinal infection with cytomegalovirus, herpes simplex virus, or varicella zoster virus. Retinal biopsy may be required to make the diagnosis of PVRL.

Rarely, PVRL presents with optic nerve involvement, showing an elevated and oedematous optic nerve head, often with vascular congestion. In most such cases, vitreous cells are present.

Occasionally, most commonly in patients with recurrent or advanced disease, anterior chamber cellular infiltrates develop; these can be associated with characteristic stellate keratic (corneal) precipitates.

Histopathology

The pathological diagnosis of PVRL often relies on a combination of diagnostic tests. Initial testing is generally performed on vitreous removed by vitrectomy, and

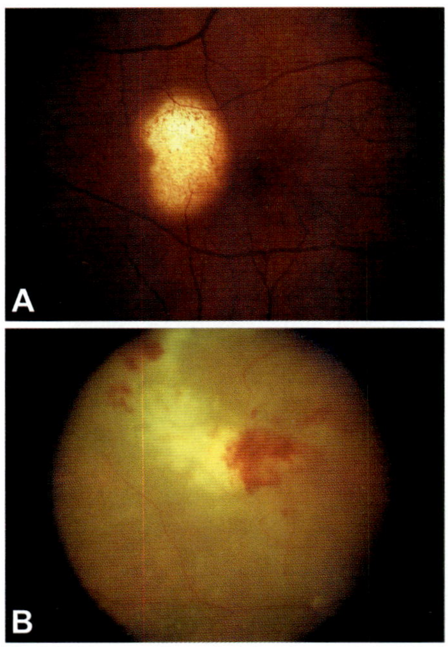

Fig. 3.20 Primary vitreoretinal lymphoma. **A** A clinical photograph of characteristic subretinal pigment epithelial infiltrates. **B** Ischaemic retinopathy, with intraretinal whitening and haemorrhage.

can include cytology, immunophenotyping, flow cytometry, cytokine analysis, and molecular diagnostic techniques {957}. These tests are complementary, and the combination of results is often necessary to establish a definitive diagnosis. Each pathology laboratory potentially has a different battery of testing that they have determined to result in the highest diagnostic yield {783}. Evaluation of vitrectomy samples is sometimes insufficient for diagnosis, and a subretinal aspirate or retinal or combined chorioretinal biopsy is necessary for additional analyses to be performed, including histopathology.

Most PVRLs are diffuse large B-cell lymphomas. Immunophenotyping indicates that most PVRLs are of the activated B-cell subtype of diffuse large B-cell lymphoma {49}. However, PVRL is recognized as a specific lymphoma entity in the *WHO classification of tumours of haematopoietic and lymphoid tissues* {1231}. Rarely, PVRL is of T-cell type {186,225}.

Cytology: Since the development of vitrectomy in the 1970s, vitreous cytology has facilitated the diagnosis of PVRL in many cases {49,796}. The atypical lymphoid cells are generally medium-sized to large cells with a condensed chromatin pattern and prominent nucleoli. The nucleus is often irregular in shape, with finger-like projections. The neoplastic lymphocytes are usually admixed with reactive inflammatory cells, such as T cells and macrophages {957}. In some cases, small, mature T lymphocytes predominate and can mask the presence of neoplastic B cells. PVRL cells are typically friable, with numerous apoptotic bodies; therefore, vitreous samples often contain abundant lytic cell remnants or ghosts, often within macrophages. Such cell ghosts are uncommon in other diseases associated with vitreous infiltrates, so their presence is highly suggestive of PVRL.

Immunophenotyping: Immunophenotyping can be carried out by flow cytometry, immunocytology on cytospins of fluid samples, or immunohistology of cell blocks. The neoplastic B cells of PVRL have a high cell proliferation rate and are positive for CD79a, CD20, PAX5, BCL2, BCL6, MUM1, and IgM {232}.

Flow cytometry: Although a limited number of cells are available in most vitrectomy specimens, the number is typically sufficient to determine the ratio of B cells to T cells, and to enable testing for light chain restriction {250,1370}. Most lymphoid infiltrates in inflammatory conditions are T-cell dominant; therefore, infiltrates containing atypical B cells are suggestive of lymphoma. Lambda or kappa light chain restriction is very useful in identifying B-cell monoclonal expansions. Because many vitrectomy samples are paucicellular, oligoclonal or monoclonal expansions (e.g. of T cells) can also be seen as a result of a benign immunological response to an infectious agent; therefore, the presence of clonality should be considered supportive, but not stand-alone diagnostic evidence of PVRL.

Cytokine analysis: The ratios of IL-10 to IL-6 and interferon-γ within vitreous or aqueous fluids have been used to support the diagnosis of lymphoma in suspected cases. An IL-10/IL-6 ratio of > 1 is suggestive of PVRL {176}. Including the IL-10/interferon-γ ratio in this analysis may increase the sensitivity of the analysis in distinguishing lymphoma from reactive inflammation {354}. Cytokine analysis of aqueous humour specimens has been proposed as a screening tool for patients at risk of PVRL and for treatment monitoring of patients with PVRL {160,167}.

Molecular diagnosis: Monoclonal expansion of B lymphocytes can be assessed using IGH PCR. IGH PCR can be performed on fluid and tissue samples (fresh frozen or fixed) and is very useful in PVRL diagnosis as an adjunct to cytomorphology and immunophenotyping {49}. It is also of value in monitoring B-cell clone progression and somatic mutation analysis of the variable region of the immunoglobulin molecule {230}. Recently, evaluation for *MYD88* mutation has confirmed its presence in 70% of cases of PVRL {122}. In addition to conventional sequencing approaches, targeted next-generation sequencing panels may be used to detect this and other mutations on small biopsy specimens, improving the turnaround time in the diagnosis of PVRL.

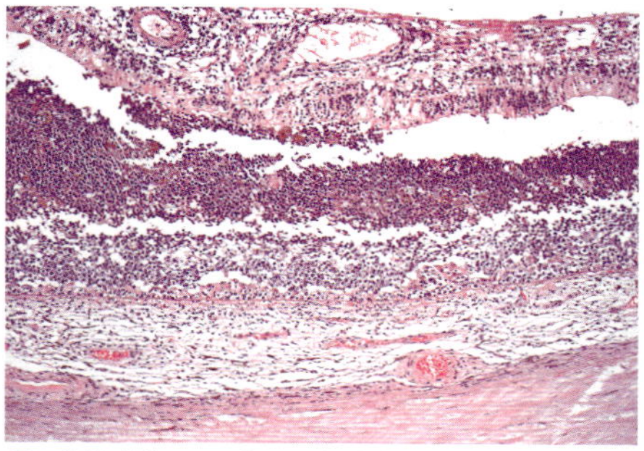

Fig. 3.21 Primary vitreoretinal lymphoma. There is marked accumulation of atypical lymphocytes in the subretinal pigment epithelial and subretinal spaces; scattered atypical lymphocytes are evident in the retina and the vitreous; the choroid is spared from involvement.

Histopathology: Microscopic examination of chorioretinal biopsy specimens and enucleated eyes reveals atypical lymphocytes in the vitreous, in the neural retina, and/or beneath the RPE. The highly characteristic sub-RPE infiltrates (of variable thickness) consist of neoplastic B cells accumulating anterior to the Bruch membrane, which acts as a barrier to their infiltration into the choroid. There is perivascular accumulation of atypical lymphocytes in PVRL cases with the appearance of ischaemic retinopathy, often with occlusion of retinal vessels. In autopsied cases of PVRL, subclinical residual disease may be evident.

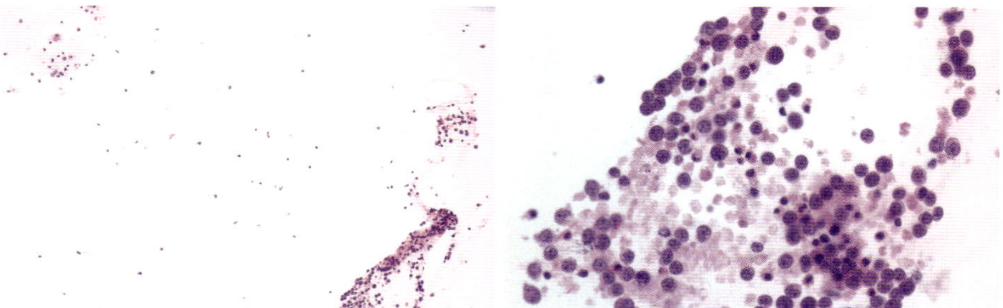

Fig. 3.22 Vitreoretinal lymphoma. **A** Low power shows the hypocellularity of a typical vitreous cytology specimen, with scattered clusters of cells. **B** High power shows large malignant lymphocytes with pleomorphic, hyperchromatic nuclei and prominent nucleoli in a background of pyknotic, necrotic, and inflammatory cells.

Differential diagnosis

PVRL presents with a constellation of clinical signs and can masquerade as other conditions. The main differential diagnoses are summarized here.

Anterior and posterior uveitis: The many and varied causes of infectious and non-infectious uveitis are in the differential diagnosis for PVRL.

Sub-RPE infiltrates: Adult vitelliform dystrophy, drusenoid pigment epithelium detachment, and confluent drusen should be considered in the differential for patients with posteriorly located sub-RPE deposits.

Ischaemic retinopathy: Cytomegalovirus retinitis and acute retinal necrosis have a very similar clinical appearance to PVRL that is causing an ischaemic retinopathy.

Optic nerve infiltration: Optic nerve involvement by PVRL resembles neuropathies seen in sarcoidosis and optic nerve leukaemic infiltration.

Histogenesis

Immunophenotypic and molecular studies suggest that PVRLs are derived from cells at a late stage in germinal centre B-cell differentiation {230,232}.

Genetic profile

MYD88 mutations are found in about 70% of cases of PVRL; there is a high somatic mutation load in the variable region of immunoglobulin.

Prognosis and predictive factors

The prognosis of PVRL patients is generally poor; it is dependent on the presence and/or subsequent development of CNS lymphoma. CNS involvement is present in 15% of patients at the initial diagnosis of PVRL, and secondary CNS lymphoma has been reported to develop in a high proportion of patients with PVRL during follow-up. To date, there are no prognostic factors for the development of CNS involvement. Steady improvement in the survival of patients with primary CNS lymphoma has been observed with the development of various chemotherapeutic regimens {607}. Currently, the median overall survival is close to 5 years {423}.

Leukaemic infiltration of the retina

Coupland S.E.
Laver N.
Wilson D.

Definition

Leukaemic infiltration of the retina is secondary involvement of the retina by a systemic leukaemia, of either acute or chronic type.

ICD-O code

Leukaemia NOS 9800/3

Synonyms

Secondary retinal leukaemia; leukaemic retinopathy

Epidemiology

Retinal involvement is common in leukaemia; its exact frequency is unknown, but it has been estimated to occur in 9–70% of leukaemia cases in various studies {29,447,581,610,966,997,1072}. These divergent findings may reflect the transient nature of leukaemic findings in the eye, which can wax and wane with time and treatment {966}. In an autopsy study, about 30% of eyes from patients who had fatal leukaemia were involved by the leukaemia {701}.

Etiology

Leukaemic infiltration of the retina tends to occur in advanced disease, but it can also present as a relapse. It is often related to a coexisting anaemia {997}.

Localization

Retinal leukaemic infiltration can occur anywhere in the retina, but it is particularly common at the posterior pole of the eye. Rarely, the infiltrates are localized to the optic nerve head.

Clinical features

Retinal leukaemic involvement leads to prominent haemorrhages of various sizes and shapes (e.g. dot, blot, blotch, and flame shapes); these haemorrhages can be preretinal, intraretinal, or subretinal, and they can occur in the macular area and the peripheral retina. Some retinal haemorrhages, called Roth spots, have a pale white centre due to the accumulation of leukaemic cells. These retinal haemorrhages commonly break through the inner limiting membrane into the vitreous. Other frequent retinal changes include dilated tortuous veins, cotton-wool spots (microinfarctions), perivascular infiltration with sheathing, and exudative retinal detachment {29,447,581,610,966}. Less common retinal lesions (e.g. peripheral retinal microaneurysms {543} and peripheral neovascularization) have been described in chronic leukaemia {373}. They are attributed to hyperviscosity changes {966}. Isolated optic nerve infiltration {563,1075} and papilloedema from CNS involvement have also been well documented {610,966}.

Histopathology

The extent of the secondary leukaemic infiltration varies considerably, with infiltrates ranging from scattered neoplastic cells to large aggregates of blasts within the retina. Haemorrhages are found at all levels of the retina, but most commonly within its inner layers, together with local tissue destruction (which can be extensive). Perivascular and intravascular leukaemic infiltrates are often observed, with associated necrosis. Occasional cytoid bodies have also been described {610,701}.

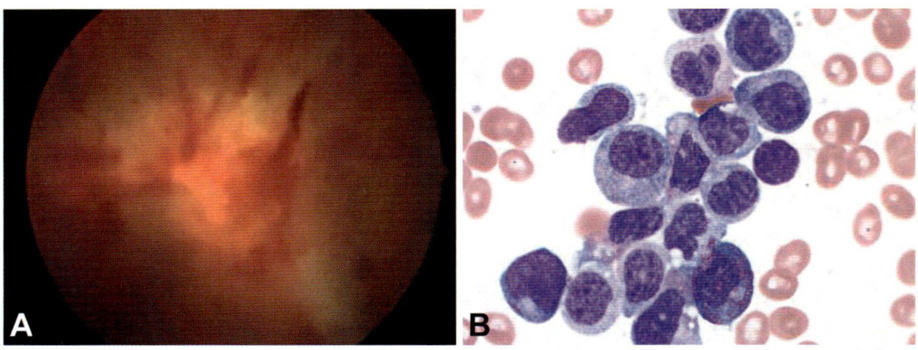

Fig. 3.23 Retinal infiltration by acute myeloid leukaemia. **A** Funduscopic image from a 42-year-old woman with flame haemorrhages due to leukaemic infiltration. **B** Vitreous biopsy reveals characteristic atypical myeloid blasts, some with Auer rods (May–Grünwald–Giemsa staining).

Differential diagnosis

Infectious retinitis is an important differential diagnosis, because opportunistic infections (e.g. cytomegalovirus, herpesvirus, and fungal infections, as well as toxoplasmosis) are common in immunosuppressed patients {1072}. Bone marrow transplantation as part of leukaemia treatment can lead to ischaemic retinopathy, mimicking a relapse of disease {1353}.

Histogenesis

Leukaemias are malignant neoplasms of the haematopoietic stem cells, characterized by diffuse replacement of the bone marrow by neoplastic cells. The histogenesis of both acute and chronic leukaemias is often related to recurrent genetic abnormalities, which are covered in the volume *WHO classification of tumours of haematopoietic and lymphoid tissues* {1231}.

Genetic profile

The genetic profile depends on the underlying leukaemia.

Prognosis and predictive factors

Retinal leukaemia is usually not treated directly; rather, systemic chemotherapy is administered in an attempt to control the underlying systemic disease. However, low-dose local radiation therapy is often recommended when leukaemic infiltration fails to respond promptly to systemic chemotherapy {491,563}.

The prognosis of retinal leukaemia depends on the leukaemia subtype and clinical stage. Studies have identified a relationship between survival and certain retinal changes; for example, one study of acute leukaemia cases showed that the mean survival was significantly shorter for patients with cotton-wool spots than for those without them {142}. Another study's findings suggested that intraretinal haemorrhages were associated with a worse outcome in acute leukaemia {967}, an association also found in childhood leukaemia {872}. The 5-year survival rate among patients with leukaemic retinopathy at the time of their initial presentation with leukaemia is lower than that among patients without ocular involvement at presentation. Therefore, patients with clinical evidence of leukaemic retinopathy at the initial diagnosis of leukaemia may benefit from more-aggressive therapy.

Secondary tumours of the retina

Bechrakis N.E.
Eagle R.C. Jr
Thaung C.

Definition

Secondary tumours of the retina are tumours metastatic to the retina and the vitreous.

ICD-O codes

Code according to the originating tumour type.

Epidemiology

Vitreoretinal metastasis has been described from a variety of primary carcinomas and from cutaneous melanoma. Because most reported cases have been published only as single cases and small case series, detailed epidemiological evaluation of this rare pathology is not possible {630,928,1100,1178,1363, 1388}.

Clinical features

Loss of visual acuity, floaters, and metamorphopsia have been reported in association with retinal and vitreous metastases. In rare instances, retinal and choroidal metastases can coexist {630}. Optical coherence tomography, echography, and wide-angle retinal imaging reveal whitish retinal thickening in areas of retinal infiltration by pigmented or amelanotic lesions. Amelanotic retinal metastases can masquerade as inflammatory lesions, such as parasitic or fungal infections, lymphoma, or herpetic retinitis (e.g. acute retinal necrosis).

Histopathology

Retinal metastases are usually non-pigmented and can cause retinal vasculopathy, such as branch retinal artery occlusion or branch retinal vein thrombosis with typical signs of intraretinal haemorrhage. Melanoma lesions metastatic to the retina can be pigmented and invade endophytically towards the vitreous cavity or exophytically towards the subretinal space.

Metastatic lesions infiltrate within the retina and invade towards the vitreous cavity by breaking through the inner limiting membrane. They may exhibit a pagetoid spread on the surface of the retina. In some instances, they can invade into the vitreous cavity and form an infiltrative network between vitreous elements. They can also invade towards the lamina cribrosa on the optic nerve head, invade through it, and infiltrate into the optic nerve. Retinal metastases can also invade towards the subretinal space, producing an exudative retinal detachment and mimicking choroidal tumours.

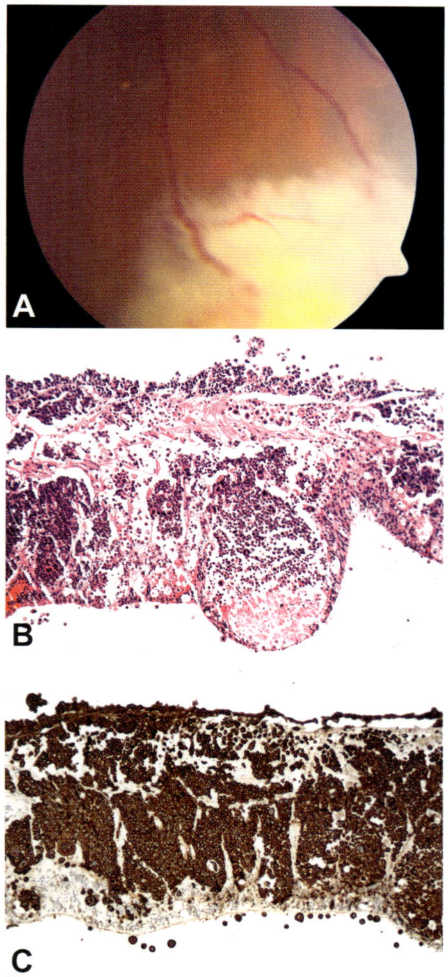

Fig. 3.24 Bladder carcinoma metastatic to the retina. **A** Funduscopic view. **B** H&E staining. **C** CK7 immunostaining.

Histogenesis

Metastases to the retina and vitreous have been reported from cutaneous melanoma, small cell carcinoma of the lung, oesophageal carcinoma, and liver carcinoma (cholangiocarcinoma).

Prognosis and predictive factors

Ocular morbidity and mortality are associated with the stage of the primary tumour and depend on the extent of retinal infiltration.

Tumours of the retinal pigment epithelium

Adenocarcinoma of the retinal pigment epithelium

Eagle R.C. Jr
Loeffler K.U.
Kivelä T.T.

Definition
Adenocarcinoma of the retinal pigment epithelium (RPE) is a malignant neoplasm derived from the RPE.

ICD-O code
Retinal pigment epithelial adenocarcinoma 8140/3

Synonyms
Retinal pigment epithelial carcinoma; malignant epithelioma of the retinal pigment epithelium

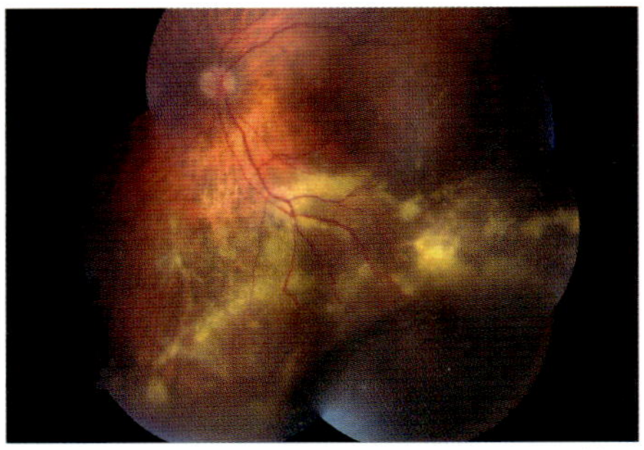

Fig. 3.25 Adenocarcinoma of the retinal pigment epithelium. Characteristic lipid exudation surrounds the deeply pigmented tumour, which has perforated the retina and developed a prominent retinal blood supply.

Epidemiology
There is no race predilection or notable male or female predisposition. These tumours occur in adults; the mean patient age at diagnosis is 53 years (range: 28–79 years) {1161}.

Etiology
Some histopathologically confirmed adenocarcinomas of the RPE have arisen from congenital hypertrophy of the RPE {1132,1159,1273}. Others may arise from reactive RPE proliferations in blind, disorganized eyes.

Localization
There is no predilection for retinal location or laterality.

Clinical features
It is usually impossible to differentiate benign RPE adenomas from RPE adenocarcinomas clinically. Although RPE tumours are typically dark grey to jet-black in colour, amelanotic variants do occur {627,1161}. RPE neoplasms are located on the inner surface of the choroid, are dome-shaped with abruptly elevated margins, and frequently perforate the overlying retina {1161}; many develop

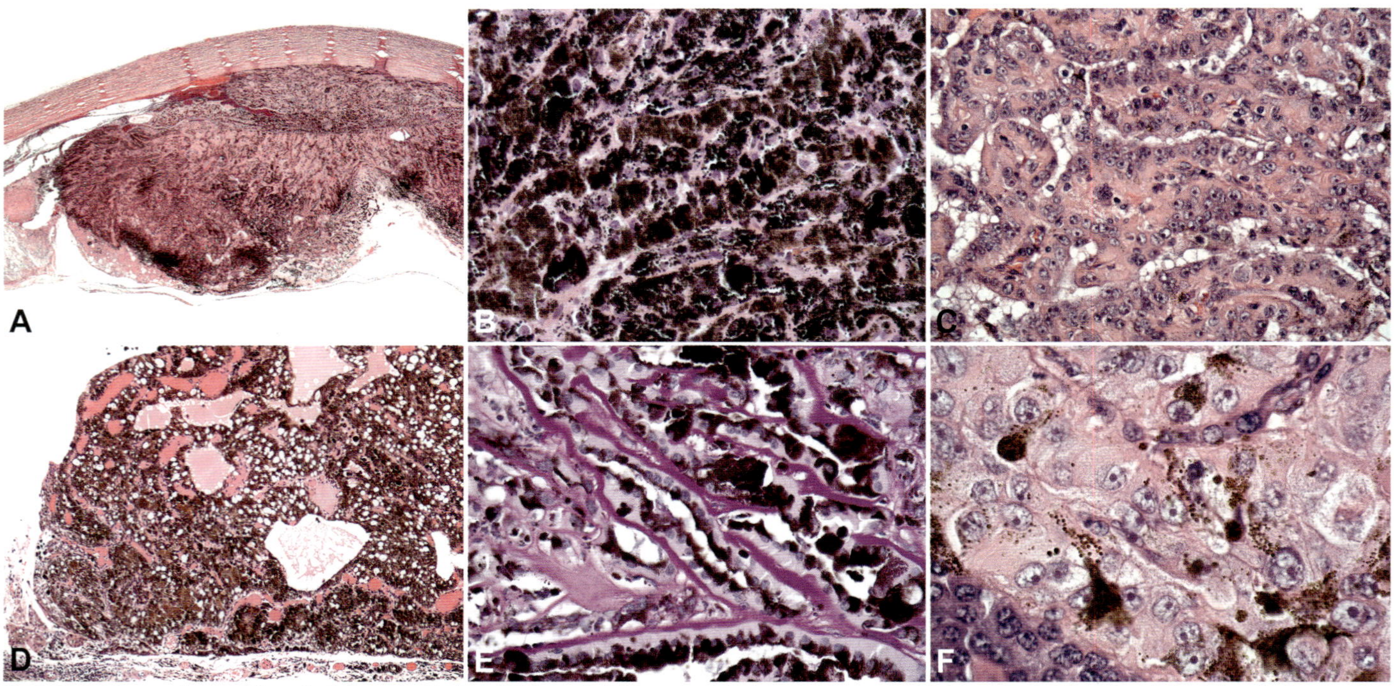

Fig. 3.26 **A** Adenocarcinoma of the retinal pigment epithelium (RPE); most of this moderately pigmented tumour, which has perforated the retina, is located on the inner surface of Bruch membrane; invasion of the choroidal stroma is a histological criterion for malignancy. **B** Adenocarcinoma of the RPE; the cells of this heavily pigmented tumour form characteristic linear arrays; the pigmentation includes macromelanosomes. **C** Adenocarcinoma of the RPE; cells forming linear arrays in this amelanotic example have prominent nucleoli. **D** Cystic RPE neoplasm; this peripheral tumour rests on the inner surface of the Bruch membrane; many of the cells are vacuolated. **E** Adenocarcinoma of the RPE; linear strands of neoplastic RPE cells rest on prominent septa that give a positive periodic acid–Schiff (PAS) reaction. **F** Anaplasia in adenocarcinoma of the RPE; the anaplastic RPE cells in this amelanotic adenocarcinoma resemble epithelioid melanoma cells.

a retinal blood supply and are supplied by dilated and tortuous retinal feeder vessels. Unlike uveal melanomas, RPE tumours often produce exudative retinal detachments with prominent intraretinal and subretinal lipid exudates {1161}. The tumours show high internal reflectivity and acoustic solidity on A-scan and B-scan ultrasonography. RPE tumours tend to be relatively hypofluorescent on intravenous fluorescein angiography, and they lack the extensive internal vascularity of double circulation found in many melanomas.

Histopathology

Tumours arising from the peripheral RPE often have vacuolated cells similar to those in pigmented ciliary epithelial tumours {1161}. The cells of posterior RPE tumours are often arranged in linear arrays or strands that rest on prominent septa of connective tissue that gives a positive periodic acid–Schiff (PAS) reaction {337,1128,1161,1204}. Important features that differentiate RPE tumours from melanoma on routine histopathological examination include the septa, the linear arrangement of cells, and the tumour's location on the inner surface of the choroid. The tumour cells may also form tubules, lobules, or pseudoglandular structures. Choroidal invasion occurs in some cases, and it is one of the histological criteria for malignancy; other criteria are nuclear atypia, cellular pleomorphism, and mitotic activity (which may be scarce). The cells of RPE carcinomas can look quite atypical, with nuclear pleomorphism and prominent nucleoli, and they can easily be confused with epithelioid melanoma cells in fine-needle aspiration biopsy specimens {1128}.

The neoplastic RPE cells are typically immunoreactive for the commonly used melanocytic markers melan-A (MART1), MITF, and SOX10. They also stain for epithelial markers, including CK7, pancytokeratin (AE1/AE3 and CAM5.2), and epithelial membrane antigen {1128}, as well as for vimentin.

Differential diagnosis

The differential diagnosis includes reactive RPE hyperplasia, RPE adenoma, and uveal melanoma (in particular of the epithelioid cell type).

Histogenesis

These tumours arise from the RPE.

Prognosis and predictive factors

The prognosis for life is generally excellent if the tumour has not extended extraocularly. There are very few documented cases of metastatic RPE adenocarcinoma {474}. Visual complications can arise if more-aggressive lesions are not treated {1161}.

Adenoma of the retinal pigment epithelium

Dubovy S.
Eagle R.C. Jr
Heegaard S.

Definition

Adenoma of the retinal pigment epithelium (RPE) is a benign neoplasm that arises from the RPE.

ICD-O code

Retinal pigment epithelial adenoma 8140/0

Synonym

Benign epithelioma

Epidemiology

Adenoma of the RPE is typically diagnosed during adulthood {1153} and shows no race predilection. In some cases, these neoplasms arise in patients with a history of eye inflammation or injury, and they may develop from prior reactive RPE hyperplasia {1153}.

Etiology

Adenoma of the RPE is an acquired neoplasm arising from the neuroepithelium {1153}.

Localization

These neoplasms typically affect the peripheral retina, but some occur adjacent to the optic disc.

Clinical features

Adenoma of the RPE presents as a solitary, unilateral, oval, abruptly elevated, usually pigmented mass arising from adjacent normal RPE. The tumour grows slowly, invades the overlying retina, and develops a retinal feeding artery and draining vein. Intraretinal and (eventually) subretinal yellow lipid exudate can accumulate around the lesion {1153}.

Histopathology

The tumour consists of cords and tubules of variably pigmented proliferating RPE cells, separated by fibrous stroma and prominent basement membrane septa that give a positive periodic acid–Schiff (PAS) reaction. Bleached sections show large, polyhedral tumour cells with eccentric round to oval bland nuclei and abundant granular cytoplasm. Immunohistochemistry may reveal expression of both melanocytic and epithelial markers {1128}. The lesions can extend into emissary canals, but invasion and mitotic activity are absent.

Differential diagnosis

Adenoma of the RPE must be distinguished from adenocarcinoma of the

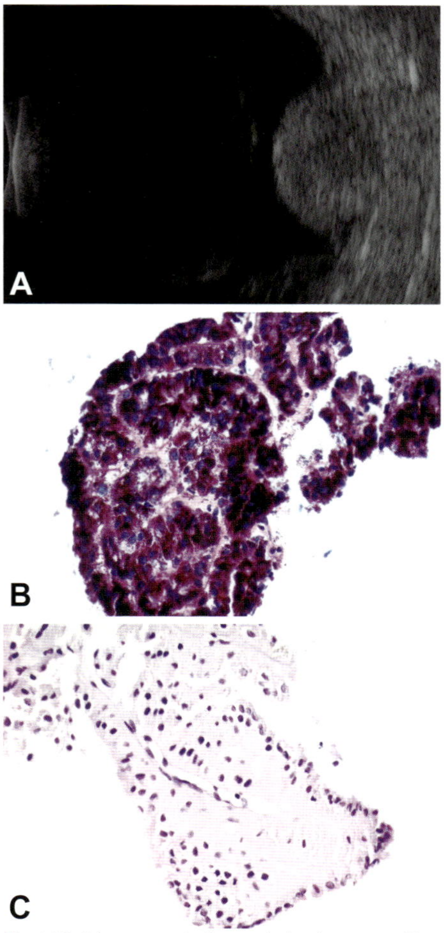

Fig. 3.27 Adenoma of the retinal pigment epithelium. **A** B-scan ultrasonography shows a mound-shaped posterior intraocular mass. **B** Biopsy of the mass reveals cords of heavily pigmented cells arranged in gland-like configurations. **C** A bleached section of the tumour shows bland nuclear features.

RPE, choroidal melanoma, congenital hypertrophy of the RPE, combined hamartoma of the RPE, and hyperplasia of the RPE.

Histogenesis
Most RPE adenomas arise in otherwise healthy eyes. Some arise at the site of previous ocular inflammation or injury {1161}.

Prognosis and predictive factors
Treatment is individualized. Small asymptomatic tumours can typically be safely observed. Plaque radiotherapy or local resection may be required for larger lesions anterior to the equator that exhibit progression. Lesions posterior to the equator can cause exudative retinal detachment {1153}. Malignant transformation is rare.

Reactive hyperplasia of the retinal pigment epithelium

Eagle R.C. Jr
Wilson D.

Definition
Reactive hyperplasia of the retinal pigment epithelium (RPE) is a non-neoplastic proliferation of RPE cells.

ICD-O code
None

Synonyms
Pseudoepitheliomatous hyperplasia; pseudoadenomatous hyperplasia; reactive hyperplastic lesion of the retinal pigment epithelium (nodular); Ringschwiele {1283}

Epidemiology
The incidence is unknown. Reactive hyperplasia of the RPE can occur in patients of any age and either sex. Multifocal hyperplasia may be seen in older people.

Etiology
The etiology of primary hyperplasia is unknown. Secondary hyperplasia can occur secondary to congenital abnormalities, inflammation, degenerative diseases, intoxications, radiation-induced choroiditis, chronic retinal detachment, subretinal haemorrhage, sequelae of traumatic retinopathy, or retinitis pigmentosa {374,472}. There may be a chronic vitreous base and zonular traction (Ringschwiele).

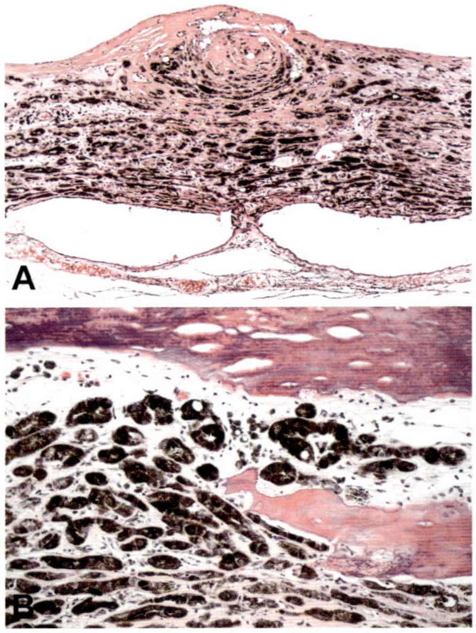

Fig. 3.28 Reactive hyperplasia of the retinal pigment epithelium. **A** Layers of proliferating pigmented retinal pigment epithelial cells over the choroid (lower field) alternate with extracellular basement membrane material. **B** Cords and tubules of proliferating retinal pigment epithelial cells are seen adjacent to metaplastic bony tissue in a phthisical eye.

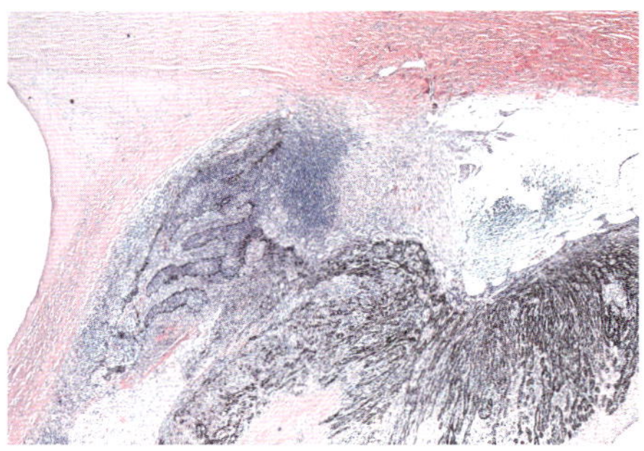

Fig. 3.29 Reactive hyperplasia of the peripheral retinal pigment epithelium. The Ringschwiele shows lymphocytic infiltration close by, a possible source of growth factors.

Localization
Reactive hyperplasia of the RPE can occur anywhere in the retina; examples occurring in the ora serrata and pars plana are called "Ringschwiele" {472}.

Clinical features
RPE hyperplasia is classified as localized, multifocal, or diffuse. It presents as darkly pigmented deposits. The pigment may be associated with retinal blood vessels, resulting in a spiculated appearance.
Nodular reactive RPE hyperplasia can be confused with adenomatous RPE tumours or choroidal melanoma. On fluorescein angiography, reactive RPE hyperplasia shows early hypofluorescence, with areas of hyperfluorescence in the late phase. It shows high reflectivity on ultrasound {472}.

Histopathology
Reactive RPE hyperplasia can range from simple duplication of cells to massive proliferations with intervening basement membrane material; in advanced, late-stage cases, the hyperplasia may be accompanied by collections of connective and osteoid tissue {374}.
In nodular reactive proliferation of the RPE, the cells are arranged in a tubular pseudoadenomatous pattern, with a large amount of basement membrane–like material. Areas of extracellular material alternate with areas of cellular proliferation. Neoplastic features, mitotic figures, and necrosis are absent {1283}.

Differential diagnosis
Reactive hyperplasia of the RPE must be distinguished from choroidal melanoma, RPE adenoma, RPE adenocarcinoma, congenital hypertrophy of the RPE, combined hamartoma of the retina and RPE, and simple hamartoma of the RPE.

Histogenesis
The proliferation of RPE cells is induced by growth factors.

Prognosis and predictive factors
These lesions are benign; the survival prognosis is excellent. The visual prognosis depends on the underlying process. Longstanding RPE hyperplasia in disorganized, blind eyes may rarely give rise to RPE adenocarcinoma {308,474,725,1016}.

Simple and combined hamartomas of the retinal pigment epithelium

Wilson D.
Dubovy S.
Kivelä T.T.

Definition
Simple and combined hamartomas of the retinal pigment epithelium (RPE) are hamartomas composed of normal retinal elements but lacking the distribution and organization of the normal retina and RPE. Simple hamartomas of

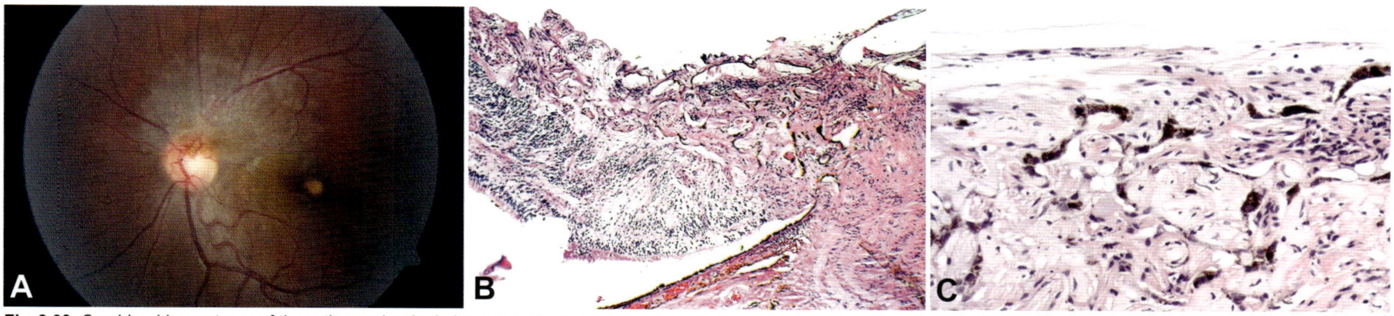

Fig. 3.30 Combined hamartoma of the retina and retinal pigment epithelium. **A** A colour photograph of a peripapillary lesion. **B** There is abnormal organization of the retinal layers of the juxtapapillary retina; pigmented cells are evident within the retinal layers. **C** There is a thin epiretinal membrane on the surface of the retina; the organization of the underlying retinal layers is abnormal, and pigmented cells are evident within the superficial retinal layers.

the RPE involve only the RPE, whereas combined hamartomas of the retina and RPE (CHR-RPEs) involve cellular elements of both the retina and the RPE.

ICD-O code

None

Synonyms

Retinal hamartomas; hyperplasias of the retinal pigment epithelium; juxtapapillary hamartomas of the retina

Epidemiology

Hamartomas of the RPE are rare lesions. Of the two largest series of cases, one series had a higher number of male patients than female patients {365}; the other showed no sex difference {1039}. The median patient age at initial diagnosis has been reported to be 13–15 years {365,1039}. The lesions are almost always unilateral and sporadic; however, CHR-RPE is associated with neurofibromatosis type 1 and type 2. CHR-RPE has also been reported in association with naevoid basal cell carcinoma syndrome (Gorlin syndrome) and branchio-oculo-facial syndrome {1153}.

Etiology

Simple and combined hamartomas of the RPE are probably congenital lesions; the median age at diagnosis is quite young, and the lesions have been observed in infants. Other than the association with neurofibromatosis, no other etiological factors are known.

Localization

These lesions occur most commonly in a peripapillary location, but they can also occur in the macula or the retinal periphery.

Clinical features

When symptomatic, combined hamartoma generally presents as decreased vision. Progressive loss of vision is common. The clinical appearance of the lesion is characterized by a variable amount of pigment, telangiectatic vessels, and white glial tissue. The white glial tissue may have the appearance of an epiretinal membrane, and it may distort the adjacent retinal vessels and lead to progressive decline in vision. The lesions may be slightly elevated, and their thickness can gradually increase over time. In rare instances, the lesions can be associated with haemorrhage and choroidal neovascularization. On fluorescein angiography, the vessels may leak fluorescein and be associated with intraretinal or subretinal fluid.
Simple hamartomas consist of a well circumscribed, mostly flat, pigmented lesion in the posterior pole {1115}. The pigmented cells are prominent on the surface of the retina and can extend throughout the full retinal thickness. Simple hamartomas are distinguished from combined hamartomas by a much less prominent vascular or glial component. These lesions tend to be less progressive.

Histopathology

Simple hamartomas of the RPE consist of normal retinal elements with abnormal distribution and organization.
CHR-RPEs are composed of disorganized glial tissue intermixed with numerous blood vessels and with cords and tubules of proliferated RPE. There is a glial epiretinal membrane on the surface of the retina. Pigmented cells may be present in the membrane.

Differential diagnosis

The differential diagnosis may be influenced by the patient's age at presentation. In younger patients presenting with leukocoria, retinoblastoma is an important differential diagnostic consideration. In older patients, the differential diagnosis of pigmented CHR-RPE includes uveal melanoma and melanocytoma. Most cases of CHR-RPE can be readily distinguished from retinoblastoma and uveal melanoma. Less common conditions that should also be considered are adenoma of the RPE, persistent fetal vasculature, and morning glory disc malformations.

Genetic susceptibility

There is an association with neurofibromatosis type 1 and type 2.

Prognosis and predictive factors

In one series of 41 patients, 10 patients lost ≥ 2 lines of visual acuity {1039}. Some patients have vision loss due to amblyopia and show improvement with treatment. In other patients, vision loss is due to progressive retinal traction, which can rarely improve with vitreoretinal surgery.

Congenital hypertrophy of the retinal pigment epithelium

Eagle R.C. Jr
Tso M.O.M.
Materin M.A.

Definition

Congenital hypertrophy of the retinal pigment epithelium (CHRPE) is a congenital patch of hypertrophic, benign retinal pigment epithelial (RPE) cells containing macromelanosomes.

ICD-O code

None

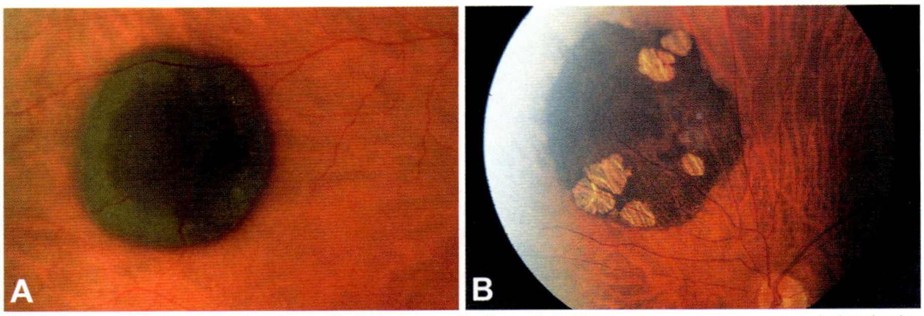

Fig. 3.31 Congenital hypertrophy of the retinal pigment epithelium. **A** Ophthalmoscopy discloses a round, deeply pigmented lesion with no lacunae. **B** A larger lesion has smooth, scalloped margins and multiple depigmented lacunae.

Synonym
Solitary congenital hypertrophy of the retinal pigment epithelium

Epidemiology
These lesions are believed to be congenital, but the mean patient age at diagnosis is 43 years (range: < 1 year to 83 years). There is no race predilection. A mild female predominance has been reported, with 64% of cases occurring in female patients {174,1098,1170}.

Etiology
CHRPE is generally believed to be a developmental lesion {724}.

Localization
These lesions usually affect the peripheral or midperipheral fundus, but 2% of cases occur in the macular or peripapillary region {62,658}.

Clinical features
CHRPE presents as a unilateral, sharply demarcated, flat or minimally elevated plaque of abnormally tall RPE cells {935,1098}. The lesions are typically asymptomatic and are found incidentally during ophthalmoscopy. Most lesions are round or oval, 13% are geographical with smooth margins marked by focal convexities, and 85% are jet black or dark brown. Rare non-pigmented cases in adults probably result from the confluence of characteristic depigmented intralesional lacunae, which develop in 43% of CHRPE lesions and have been documented to enlarge gradually in 32% of cases. The reported mean and median largest diameters are 4.7 mm and 4.5 mm, respectively (range: 1–13 mm). Most lesions are surrounded by a narrow, pigmented or depigmented ring or halo. Of lesions followed up for > 3 years, 83% have shown subtle enlargement {51,114,1098,1372}. Nodules develop in about 1% of cases and have been confirmed to be RPE adenocarcinomas in several instances {1132,1159,1165,1273}. Optical coherence tomography reveals thinning and photoreceptor loss in the overlying retina {261,385,626,877,1099}. Careful perimetry may disclose a focal scotoma corresponding to the lesion {935}. CHRPE appears dark on fundus autofluorescence imaging {1103,1238}.

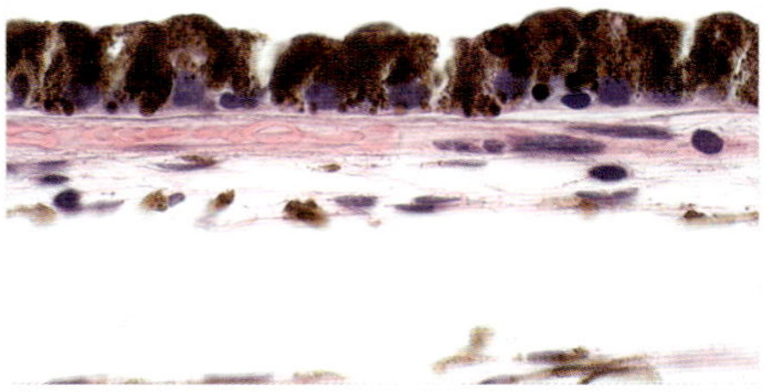

Fig. 3.32 Congenital hypertrophy of the retinal pigment epithelium. The cytoplasm of tall retinal pigment epithelial cells is packed with large round melanosomes (including macromelanosomes).

Histopathology
Light microscopy reveals a monolayer of thickened RPE cells. The cytoplasm is packed with large round melanosomes, which often obscure the nucleus {145,174,724,895}. Lacunae show segmental loss of the RPE and focal chorioretinal adhesions. Fluorescence microscopy confirms the absence of lipofuscin in dysfunctional RPE cells. The sharply circumscribed patches of abnormal RPE cells are readily apparent on scanning electron microscopy {174,724}.

An increased amount of melanin pigment is also found focally in RPE cells in congenital grouped pigmentation (so-called bear tracks), but the granules retain their normal ellipsoidal configuration and do not fill the entire cytoplasm {968,1169}.

Differential diagnosis
CHRPE must be distinguished from choroidal naevus, small choroidal melanoma, congenital grouped pigmentation (so-called bear tracks), adenoma and adenocarcinoma of the RPE, solitary hamartoma of the RPE, torpedo maculopathy, and pigmented ocular fundus lesion (POFL) or hamartoma of the RPE in familial adenomatous polyposis (FAP). Unfortunately, the term "congenital hypertrophy of the retinal pigment epithelium" is often used erroneously in the non-ophthalmic literature to designate POFLs or hamartomas of the RPE that occur in some kindreds with FAP. Unlike CHRPE, hamartoma of the RPE tends to be multiple and bilateral, and it has less well defined margins {1268,1269}. In a clinicopathological study, three types of POFLs were identified: one type similar to CHRPE and two types consistent with hamartomatous RPE malformations in a patient with FAP {1270}. In one patient with a POFL and FAP, optical coherence tomography disclosed retinal invasion {1291}.

Histogenesis
The lesion originates from the RPE.

Genetic profile
There is no genetic profile. No germline mutations have been found in the *APC* gene.

Prognosis and predictive factors
Most cases are benign and asymptomatic and require no treatment. Rarely, RPE adenoma or low-grade RPE adenocarcinoma may develop from CHRPE {1132,1159,1165,1273}. Typical CHRPE does not appear to be associated with FAP or colorectal adenocarcinoma {477,794,1164}.

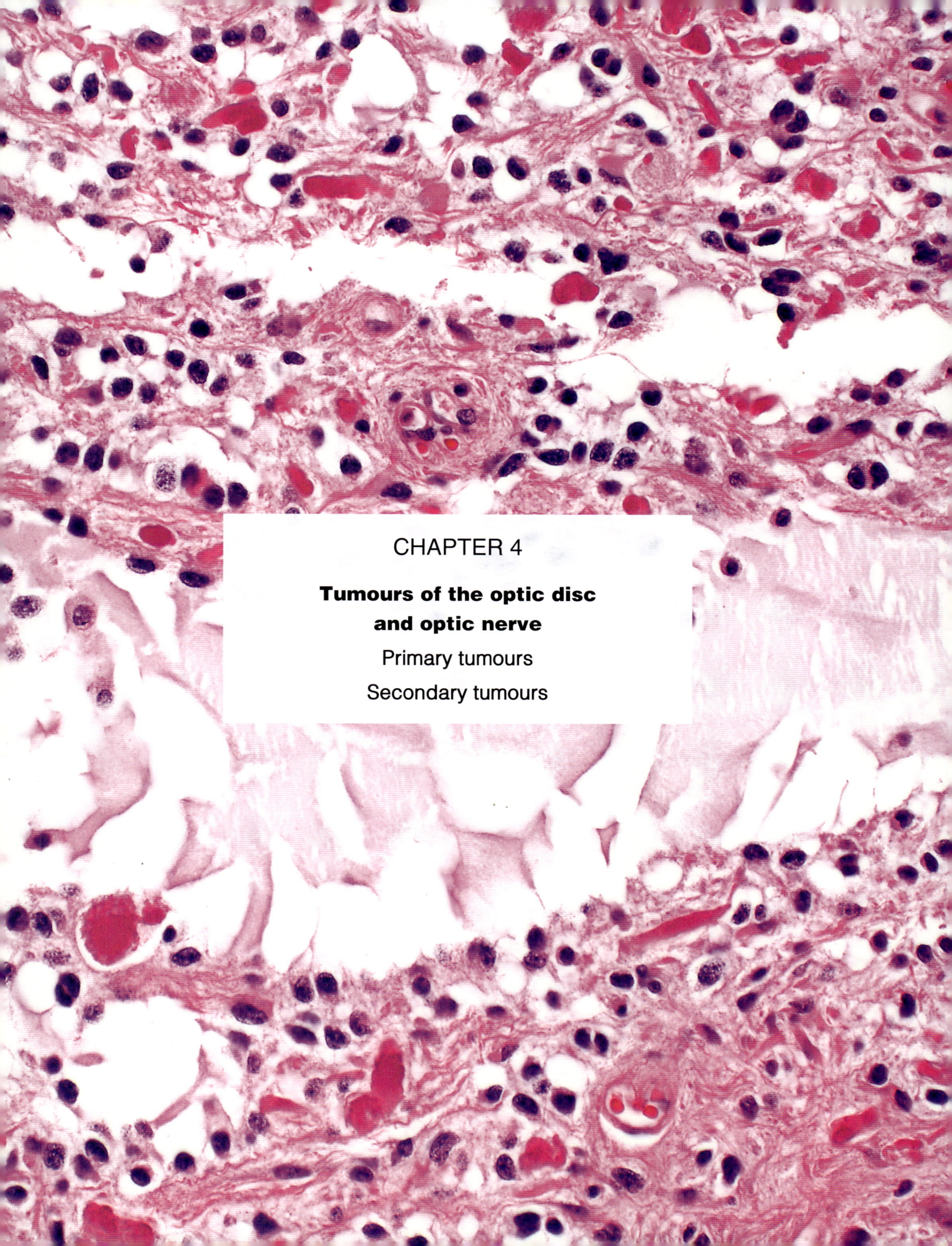

CHAPTER 4

Tumours of the optic disc and optic nerve

Primary tumours

Secondary tumours

WHO classification of tumours of the optic disc and optic nerve

Primary tumours	
Astrocytoma NOS	9400/3
Pilocytic astrocytoma	9421/1
Glioblastoma	9440/3
Meningioma NOS	9530/0
Medulloepithelioma, benign	9501/0
Medulloepithelioma, malignant	9501/3
Teratoid medulloepithelioma, benign	9502/0
Teratoid medulloepithelioma, malignant	9502/3
Solitary fibrous tumour NOS	8815/1
Melanocytoma	8726/0
Secondary tumours	See note[a]

[a]Code secondary tumours according to the originating tumour type.

The morphology codes are from the International Classification of Diseases for Oncology (ICD-O) {381}. Behaviour is coded /0 for benign tumours; /1 for unspecified, borderline, or uncertain behaviour; /2 for carcinoma in situ and grade III intraepithelial neoplasia; and /3 for malignant tumours.

The classification is modified from the previous WHO classification, taking into account changes in our understanding of these lesions.

Tumours of the optic disc and optic nerve: Introduction

Eberhart C.G.
Grossniklaus H.E.
Kivelä T.T.

The optic nerve arises from the embryonal optic stalk and contains axons extending from the retinal ganglion cells to the brain. These axons exit the globe through the lamina cribrosa, a connective tissue meshwork continuous with the sclera. Within the globe, the axons are unmyelinated; posterior to the lamina cribrosa, the axons are myelinated by oligodendroglial cells, with additional support provided by astrocytes and microglia. The optic nerve is surrounded by the same layers as the rest of the CNS (the dura mater, arachnoid mater, and pia mater), with invaginations of the pia dividing bundles of axons into individual fascicles.

Consistent with the derivation of the optic nerve from diencephalic extensions, tumours in the optic nerve comprise a subset of those seen in the CNS and its coverings. Astrocytomas most commonly arise in children, are of low grade, and have the microscopic features of pilocytic astrocytoma {379,969}. They are often associated with neurofibromatosis type 1, and they can be bilateral in such cases {987}. High-grade astrocytomas and gangliogliomas can also be encountered in the optic nerve, but only rarely {721,994}. High-grade B-cell lymphoma and medulloepithelioma can also involve the optic nerve. Interestingly, IDH-mutant gliomas, including infiltrating astrocytoma and oligodendrogliomas of various grades, are almost never found in the optic nerve. Meningioma, solitary fibrous tumour/haemangiopericytoma, melanocytoma, melanoma, and other neoplasms of the CNS coverings can also arise in the optic nerve.

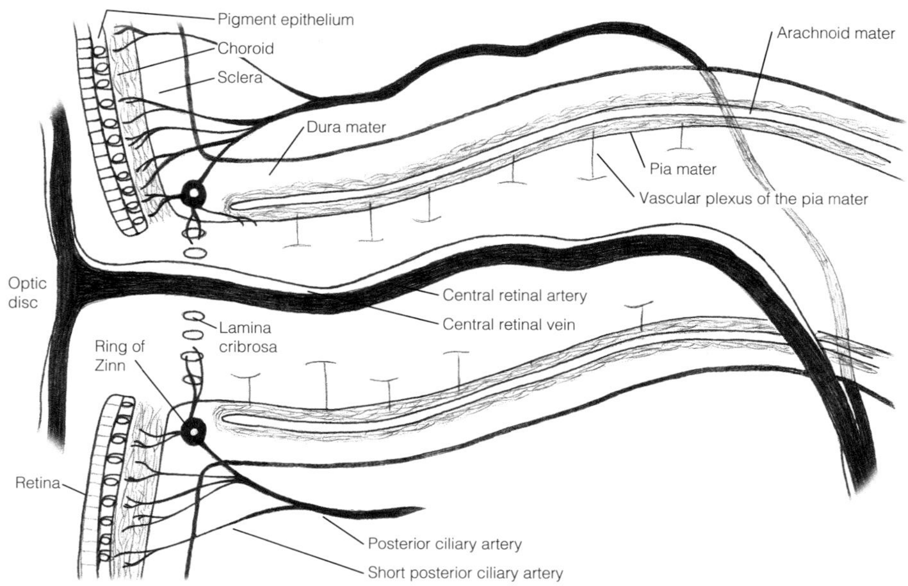

Fig. 4.01 The normal anatomy of the optic disc and optic nerve.

Primary tumours of the optic disc and optic nerve

Astrocytoma and glioblastoma of the optic disc and optic nerve

Cummings T.
Eberhart C.G.
Rushing E.J.
Specht C.S.
Stemmer-Rachamimov A.O.
Verdijk R.M.

Definition

Astrocytoma and glioblastoma of the optic disc and optic nerve are tumours derived from glial (astrocytic) cells within the optic nerve and chiasm. Optic nerve gliomas are most frequently pilocytic astrocytomas. However, both low-grade gliomas (pilocytic astrocytoma and diffuse astrocytoma) and high-grade gliomas (anaplastic astrocytoma and glioblastoma) may involve the nerve.

ICD-O codes

Astrocytoma NOS	9400/3
Pilocytic astrocytoma	9421/1
Glioblastoma	9440/3

Synonyms

Astrocytoma: optic nerve glioma; pilocytic astrocytoma

Glioblastoma: malignant optic nerve glioma; primary and secondary glioblastoma

Epidemiology

Optic nerve gliomas account for approximately 5% of all intracranial gliomas and 66% of primary optic nerve tumours {303,719,736,1171}. Approximately 90% are diagnosed within the first two decades of life. The median patient age at diagnosis is 7 years (range: from birth to the eighth decade of life). The female-to-male ratio is approximately 3:2. Both sexes appear to be equally affected when the neoplasm involves the optic chiasm.
Only 74 cases of malignant optic nerve glioma, including 33 confirmed cases of glioblastoma, have been reported in adults. There is a male predominance, with a mean patient age at diagnosis of 62 years (range: 26–83 years) {78,712,767}. Rare cases have been reported in children {1427}. Glioblastoma of the optic chiasm has been described in a 7-year-old child with a previous diagnosis of pilocytic astrocytoma {1427}.

Etiology

Optic nerve gliomas derive from glial cells within the optic nerve. Although the term "glioma" encompasses astrocytic, oligodendroglial, and ependymal neoplasms, ependymal tumours have not been reported in the optic nerve, and only rare putative cases of oligodendroglioma are reported in the literature. Radiation therapy has been implicated in the formation of some high-grade gliomas {1018}.

Localization

The most common location is the optic nerve or chiasm. Bilateral involvement can be seen in patients with neurofibromatosis type 1 (NF1) and low-grade lesions, as well as in high-grade astrocytoma. Intraocular tumour extension and vitreous spread are rare {1267}. Local recurrence of high-grade gliomas is inevitable, with frequent extension into the adjacent brain tissue. The tumour may spread via the optic radiations to the occipital pole. There have been 5 documented cases of malignant optic nerve glioma occurring in the context of multifocal glioblastomas {169,1267}. Transtentorial spread to the cerebellum has been documented {767}.

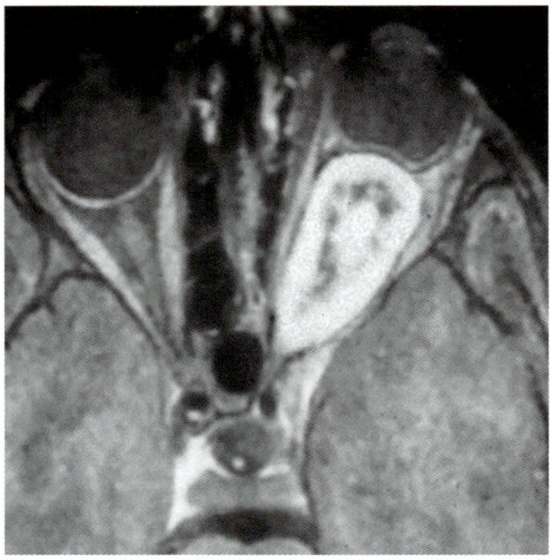

Fig. 4.02 Pilocytic astrocytoma. T1-weighted axial MRI shows a left optic nerve tumour with strong enhancement in an individual with neurofibromatosis type 1.

Clinical features

Individuals with optic nerve gliomas present clinically with a wide spectrum of ophthalmic abnormalities, including visual impairment, optic atrophy, and proptosis {312,596,839,863}. Patients with high-grade glioma present with rapidly progressive unilateral vision loss, often eventually developing bilateral blindness. Pain may be an accompanying symptom {1267}, along with headaches, motor deficits, and behavioural changes {767}.

Histopathology

Pilocytic astrocytomas expand the septa of the optic nerve and frequently exhibit a biphasic growth pattern. The tumour cells are characterized by delicate bipolar hair-like processes. Rosenthal fibres (eosinophilic cork-screw or beaded structures) are frequently found in pilocytic astrocytomas in addition to eosinophilic granular bodies and protein droplets {1001}. Verhoeff described three histological patterns of optic nerve pilocytic astrocytoma: coarsely reticulated, coarsely fibrillated, and finely reticulated {907}. The coarsely reticulated pattern is characterized by the classic biphasic pattern of bipolar astrocytic cells either tightly compacted around blood vessels or loosely woven around microcystic spaces containing abundant mucin. Tumours with this histological pattern are associated with Rosenthal fibres, eosinophilic granular bodies, and protein droplets. Blood vessels vary in number; in some cases, they may be thickened and hyalinized or may show glomeruloid vascular proliferation. The coarsely fibrillated pattern (also known as the spindle-cell type) consists of coarse neuroglial fibrils and spindle neuroglia cells, generally arranged in relatively definite bundles. The finely reticulated pattern resembles an expansion of the indigenous neuroglia of the optic nerve, in which small round or ovoid nuclei are embedded within a delicate reticulated syncytium of neuroglial fibres. This pattern can be confused histologically with diffuse astrocytoma. In some cases, the round nuclei can resemble oligodendroglioma. Immunohistochemical staining for GFAP highlights the tumour cells and their processes.

Anaplastic astrocytomas (WHO grade III) are cellular infiltrating lesions featuring brisk mitotic activity. Glioblastomas are WHO grade IV, and the microscopic picture of glioblastomas of the optic disc and optic nerve is identical to that of glioblastomas involving the brain and spinal cord; in addition to frequent mitoses, they contain microvascular proliferation and/or necrosis (with or without palisading). Abundant gemistocytes and so-called oligodendroglial-like features have been described {837}. Virtually all tumours are positive for GFAP {767}. Mitotic activity and the Ki-67 proliferation index are variable. Isolated cases have been found to be IDH-wildtype with intact *ATRX*, consistent with primary glioblastoma {767}; others are IDH-mutant with *ATRX* loss {721}.

Differential diagnosis

Piloid gliosis can mimic and be difficult to distinguish from pilocytic astrocytoma. Optic nerve gliosis may include arachnoid gliomatosis {1219} and diffuse hyperplastic gliosis, and may be seen in patients with or without NF1 {1004}. Diffuse leptomeningeal glioma can involve the optic nerve sheath {97}. Arachnoid enhancement of the optic nerve sheath on MRI may mimic optic nerve meningioma in some cases. Optic nerve gliomas can be associated with meningothelial hyperplasia, and a superficial biopsy of the meninges may result in an erroneous diagnosis of meningioma {220}. On a tiny biopsy specimen, it might not be possible to histologically distinguish pilocytic astrocytoma from a diffuse or fibrillary (WHO grade II) astrocytoma {987}.

Anaplastic pilocytic astrocytomas may exhibit an increased number of mitoses, vascular proliferation, and necrosis (with or without palisading) {674}; beware of misdiagnosing glioblastoma in such cases. Glioblastomas infiltrate more diffusely between axons, and they lack piloid cytomorphology, Rosenthal fibres, and eosinophilic granular bodies. Malignant optic nerve gliomas must also be distinguished from metastases, lymphoma, and meningioma. Attention to the clinical setting, radiographical appearance, and histological features is important in these cases.

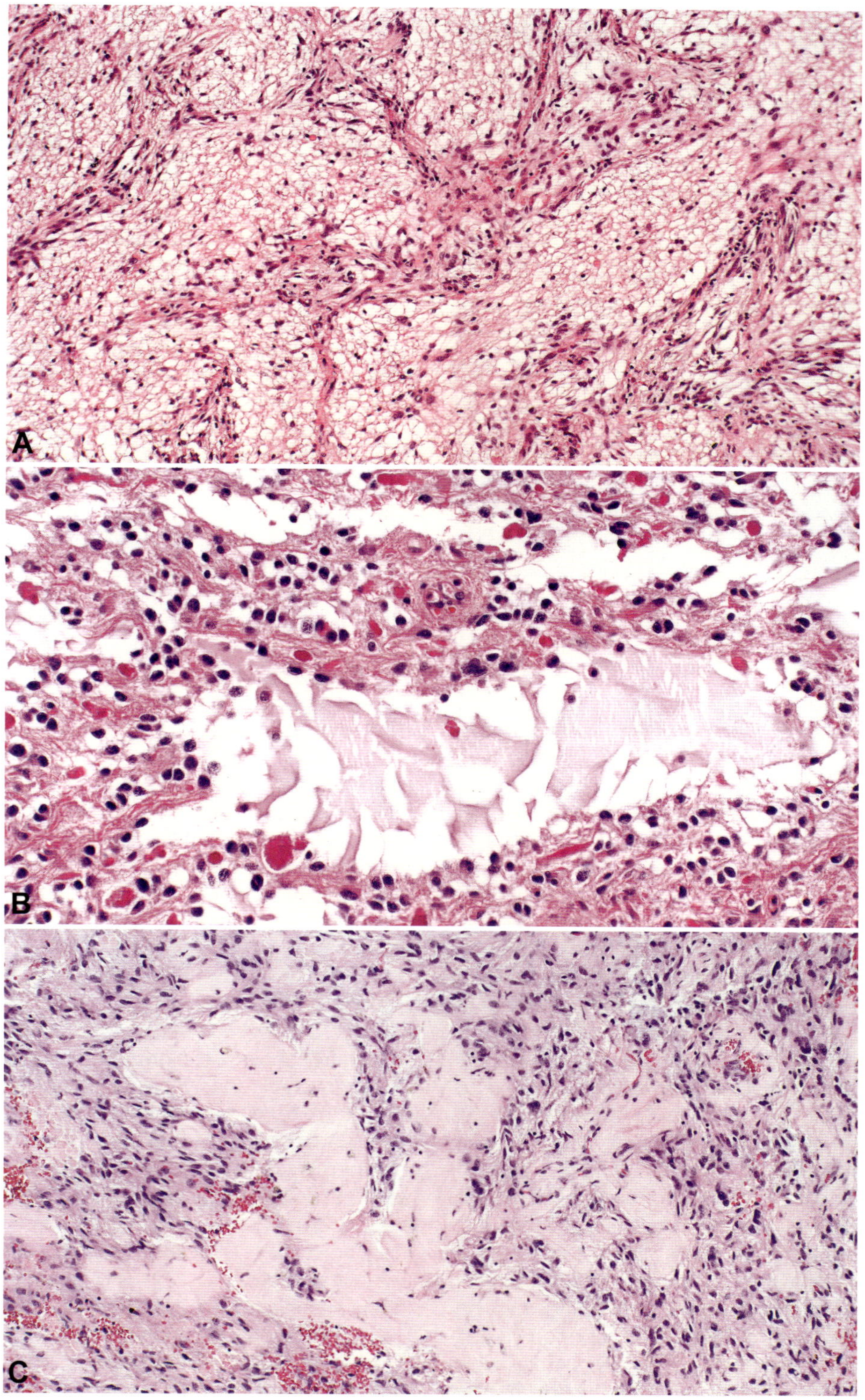

Fig. 4.03 Pilocytic astrocytoma. **A** An optic nerve tumour with a biphasic pattern and expansion of the optic nerve septa. **B** An example with mucin, Rosenthal fibres, and cells with round nuclei. **C** Hyalinized blood vessels are seen in some cases.

Pilomyxoid astrocytoma is closely related to pilocytic astrocytoma, but the pilomyxoid tumours are more aggressive and usually involve the hypothalamic/chiasmal region in young children. Rosenthal

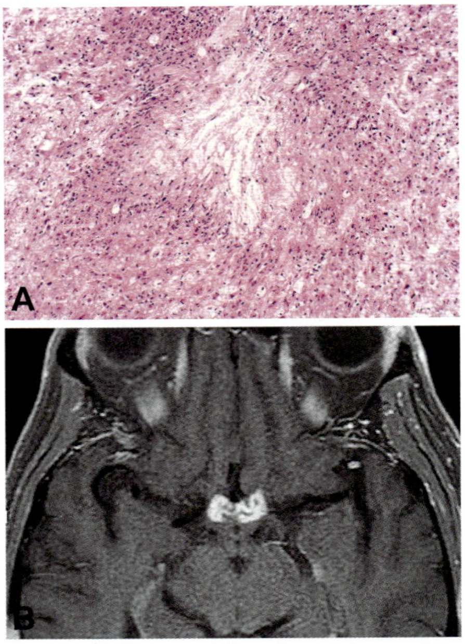

Fig. 4.04 Glioblastoma. **A** An optic nerve tumour showing palisading necrosis. **B** T1-weighted axial MRI shows a contrast-enhancing lesion in the optic chiasm; it was biopsied and diagnosed as glioblastoma.

fibres and eosinophilic granular bodies are absent, and the tumour cells have perivascular orientations that resemble ependymal perivascular pseudorosettes. Although oligodendrocytes are part of the normal cellular composition of the optic nerve, oligodendroglial neoplasms have rarely been reported to involve the optic nerve and chiasm {587,1001}. Gliomatosis cerebri is characterized by an extensive infiltration of neoplastic cells that do not form a defined mass lesion but can involve the supratentorial, infratentorial, and intraspinal compartments. The tumour cells diffusely invade the brain parenchyma and frequently migrate along myelinated white matter fibre tracts, including the optic pathway. Gliomatosis cerebri uncommonly involves the optic nerves and chiasm {1271}. A rare case of a chiasmal–optic nerve rosette-forming glioneuronal tumour occurring in a patient with NF1 has been reported {1043}.

Rare examples of ganglioglioma involving the optic nerve and chiasm have been reported, and they are histologically identical to similar tumours elsewhere in the CNS {994,1015}. They contain the same combination of neoplastic mature ganglion cells admixed with neoplastic glial cells that typically constitutes a pilocytic astrocytoma. Because the optic nerve is normally a pure white matter fibre tract that lacks ganglion cells, explanations for the presence of ganglion cells in optic nerve gangliogliomas include ectopic neurons {201} and undifferentiated neuroepithelium of the optic stalk lumen, which could conceivably differentiate concurrently into both glial and ganglionic derivatives with neoplastic potential {733}. When a ganglioglioma involves the region of the optic chiasm and hypothalamus, the pathologist must determine whether the neuronal component constitutes entrapped non-neoplastic hypothalamic neurons.

For glioblastoma, the most important aspect of the differential diagnosis is distinguishing malignant optic nerve gliomas from metastases, lymphoma, meningioma, ganglioglioma, and lower-grade gliomas (including pilocytic astrocytoma, diffuse astrocytoma, and anaplastic astrocytoma). Not surprisingly, biopsy specimens consisting largely of necrosis may pose a particular challenge {74}, as can the vascular proliferation commonly seen in pilocytic lesions.

Histogenesis

Optic nerve gliomas arise from glial cells of the optic nerve and chiasm. Glioblastomas are thought to derive from the supporting astroglial cells of the optic nerve, although the exact cell of origin remains unclear.

Genetic profile

Pilocytic astrocytomas of the optic pathway may show deletions and allelic losses involving the *NF1* gene on chromosome 17q and upregulation of *NF1* gene transcripts. It appears that various mechanisms involving the *NF1* tumour suppressor gene may play an important primary genetic role in the promotion or initiation of NF1-associated pilocytic astrocytomas {446,1371}. Pilocytic astrocytomas associated with NF1 typically lack the genetic changes associated with aggressive fibrillary astrocytomas {705}. Mutations of the *TP53* gene are rare {680}. Optic nerve pilocytic astrocytomas harbour *KIAA1549-BRAF* fusions typical of pilocytic astrocytomas in other locations. Unlike in diffuse or infiltrating astrocytomas, IDH mutations are absent in pilocytic astrocytomas {216,986}. Phosphorylated MAPK1 and p16 (CDKN2A) expression suggests that the MAPK pathway is active in optic nerve pilocytic astrocytomas {969}. One study showed that genes encoding cell motility proteins were expressed at lower levels in pilocytic astrocytomas than in glioblastomas, whereas genes involved in suppressing migration were expressed at higher levels {974}.

Very few optic pathway glioblastoma cases have been subjected to molecular genetic profiling. In a single case report, FISH/microsatellite analyses showed 1p36/19q13 loss in a high proportion of cells, deletion of *PTEN* on chromosome 10q23 in 28% of cells, monosomy 7 in 40% of cells, and polysomy 7 in 15%. No *EGFR* or *EGFRvIII* amplification or *MGMT* methylation was observed {1175}. *MGMT* promoter methylation was found in a case with transtentorial spread to the cerebellum {767}.

Genetic susceptibility

NF1 has a recognized association with gliomas of the optic pathways {265,718}. About 70% of optic pathway gliomas are associated with the syndrome {717}, and these tumours generally have a more favourable outcome than non-associated gliomas. Approximately 20% of optic nerve tumours in patients with NF1 affect both nerves {326}. Tumour enlargement and progressive visual impairment occasionally occur in children with NF1 {716,718}, and malignant change has exceptionally been reported in optic nerve gliomas in patients with NF1 or a family history of NF1 {124}.

Prognosis and predictive factors

Pilocytic astrocytomas are typically slow-growing and have a favourable prognosis. Some remain stable for extended periods of time, and some may regress. Others, despite years of relative quiescence, retain the ability to grow and invade the optic chiasm and hypothalamus, resulting in considerable morbidity and mortality and a worse prognosis {1382}. Malignant transformation is rare.

Like glioblastomas in the brain and spinal cord, glioblastomas in the optic pathways have a dismal prognosis, with most patients dying of the disease in < 2 years despite radiation and/or chemotherapy {767,1267}.

Meningioma of the optic nerve

Rodriguez F.
Cummings T.
Specht C.S.
Rushing E.J.

Definition

Meningioma of the optic nerve is a neoplasm arising from meningothelial cells of the optic nerve leptomeninges.

ICD-O code

Meningioma NOS 9530/0

Synonym

Optic nerve sheath meningioma

Epidemiology

Meningiomas of the optic nerve sheath and orbit are generally similar to those that arise elsewhere in the brain and spine. They are more frequent in females than in males, and the majority present in the fifth decade of life {521}. The higher incidence in females may be related to the expression of progesterone receptor and estrogen receptor in meningiomas {1349}. Some investigators have reported that as many as one quarter of primary orbital meningiomas become symptomatic before the age of 10 years, although other studies have not confirmed this early age of onset; in contrast, intracranial meningiomas are rarely apparent before the age of 20 years {585,790,1384}.

Etiology

The cause of meningiomas of the optic nerve sheath is unknown. A subset arise in the setting of the tumour predisposition syndrome neurofibromatosis type 2 (NF2) or after irradiation.

Localization

Meningiomas of the optic nerve can be subclassified as optic nerve sheath (i.e. primary) meningiomas or secondary meningiomas originating from an intracranial sphenoid wing tumour {803}. More rarely, meningiomas can develop ectopically in the orbit, unassociated with the optic nerve sheath {338}.

Clinical features

Primary optic nerve (i.e. optic nerve sheath) meningiomas account for about 2% of all orbital tumours. Approximately 92% of these tumours arise from the intraorbital optic nerve, and 8% are intracanalicular. The average patient age at presentation is 40 years, but cases have been reported in patients from childhood to the eighth decade of life. Nearly all optic nerve meningiomas are unilateral. Bilateral cases typically affect children, and they may be associated with NF2 {457,1068}. A female-to-male ratio of 2:1 has been reported, and tumour growth may accelerate during pregnancy {193,1068}.

Primary optic nerve meningioma causes symptoms primarily through compression of the nerve, and this may be associated with vascular compromise. The Hoyt–Spencer triad of progressive vision loss, optic disc atrophy, and optociliary shunt vessels is a classic but uncommonly seen clinical presentation. Vision loss (decreased colour vision or visual field defects) is common at presentation; these symptoms often develop over a 1–5 year period. Proptosis and strabismus may also occur {1068}.

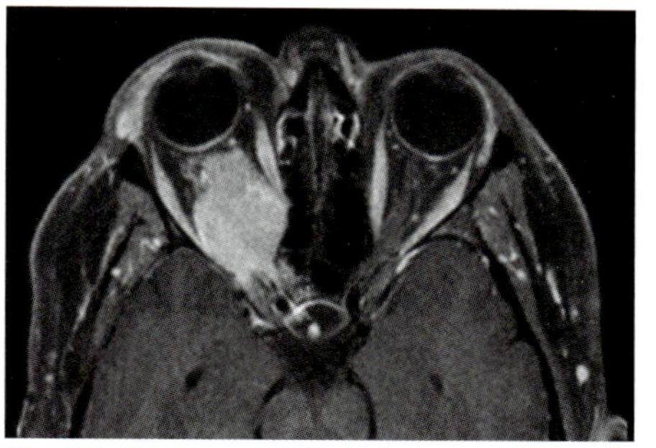

Fig. 4.05 Meningioma of the optic nerve sheath. T1-weighted postcontrast axial MRI demonstrates a tumour expanding the optic nerve sheath.

Histopathology

The morphological spectrum of meningiomas is wide; however, virtually all optic nerve examples belong to either the meningothelial or transitional subtype, WHO grade I {457,521}. Like intracranial and intraspinal meningiomas, optic nerve meningiomas may exhibit a variety of histological variants and WHO grades, which may correlate with biological behaviour; the most common type is WHO grade I meningothelial meningioma {521}. Meningothelial meningiomas are composed of lobulated or whorled aggregates of epithelioid cells with indistinct cell borders separated by collagenous septa. Nuclear pseudoinclusions are common. Transitional meningiomas contain a mixture of meningothelial and fibrous subtypes, often accompanied by psammoma bodies. In a series that included 21 optic nerve meningiomas, only 1 case with angiomatous features fulfilled the atypical (WHO grade II) criteria on the basis of increased mitotic activity. Focal microcystic and angiomatous changes were noted in otherwise typical transitional meningiomas. Several of these tumours showed dural invasion, with additional bone and nerve

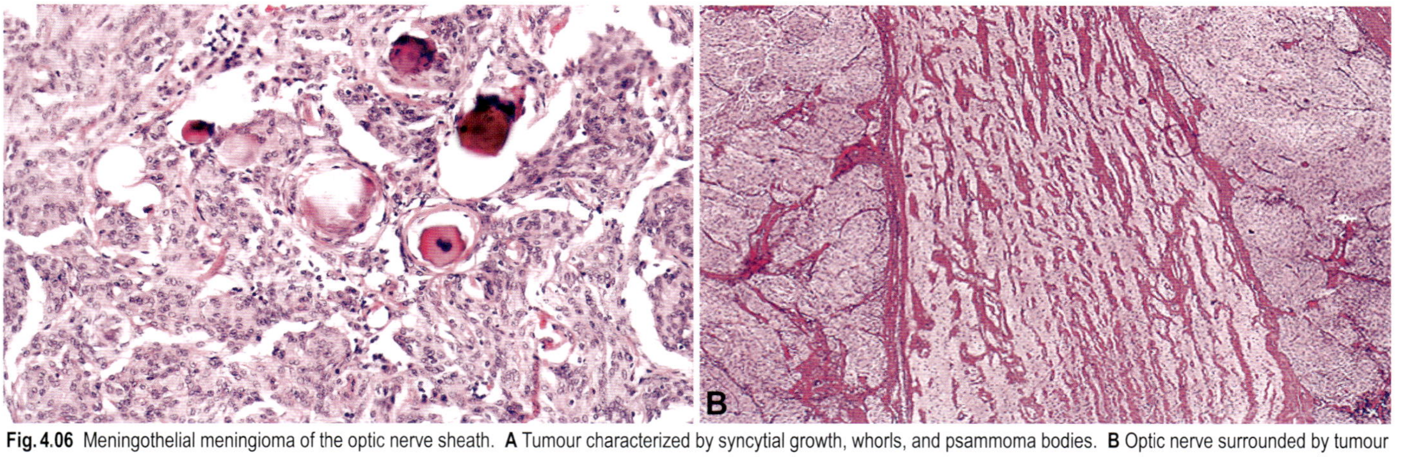

Fig. 4.06 Meningothelial meningioma of the optic nerve sheath. **A** Tumour characterized by syncytial growth, whorls, and psammoma bodies. **B** Optic nerve surrounded by tumour within the optic nerve sheath.

sheath invasion in 1 case and choroidal spread in another {521}. Other atypical examples have been reported {424}, including 2 cases in children {617,836}. With the exception of these rare cited cases, most tumours appear to surround the optic nerve without evidence of invasion of adjacent tissue {457,521,1068}.

Differential diagnosis

The differential diagnosis includes other primary meningeal tumours (solitary fibrous tumour/haemangiopericytoma, mesenchymal chondrosarcoma, and melanocytoma) {748,947,1391}, metastatic tumours (e.g. carcinoma and lymphoma) {775}, and inflammatory disorders (sarcoidosis, IgG4-related disease, and idiopathic hypertrophic pachymeningitis) {382,667,865}. Optic nerve seeding from intracranial atypical meningioma and optic nerve involvement by primary diffuse leptomeningeal gliomatosis have been reported {97,617}. Because primary optic nerve meningioma shares a common vascular supply with the optic nerve, complete surgical excision is often not an option, and biopsy specimens are small {1068}. However, the differential diagnosis can usually be evaluated histologically in conjunction with correlative clinical history and imaging findings.

Histogenesis

Meningiomas are thought to arise from arachnoid cap cells lining the intraorbital or intracanalicular portion of the optic nerve {457,521}.

Genetic profile

Primary optic nerve sheath meningiomas and secondary meningiomas extending from intracranial locations appear to be genetically distinct. Molecular cytogenetic studies in a small number of cases have demonstrated that sphenoid wing meningiomas frequently have monosomy 22 or 22q loss, as well as deletions involving chromosome arms 1p, 6q, and 19p. In contrast, chromosome 22 alterations were rare in meningiomas of the optic nerve sheath proper, which instead harboured uncommon alterations including abnormalities in chromosomes 17 and 19 {485}.

Genetic susceptibility

Most meningiomas of the optic nerve sheath develop sporadically, but a subset develop in patients with NF2. The incidence of optic nerve meningiomas in the setting of NF2 is 2–8% {125}.

Prognosis and predictive factors

Primary optic nerve meningioma is graded using the same WHO criteria used for other meningiomas; most cases are WHO grade I, but atypical meningioma is also (rarely) encountered {521}. Patients with primary optic nerve meningioma have an excellent prognosis for survival, but the visual prognosis is poor; most patients experience permanent vision loss in the affected eye {123, 1068}.

Medulloepithelioma of the optic disc and optic nerve

Eberhart C.G.
Biswas J.
Edward D.P.
Chan A.S.Y.

Definition

Medulloepithelioma of the optic disc and optic nerve is a primary intraocular embryonal tumour characterized by cords of multilayered neuroepithelial cells resembling the medullary epithelium of the optic cup.

ICD-O codes

Medulloepithelioma, benign	9501/0
Medulloepithelioma, malignant	9501/3
Teratoid medulloepithelioma, benign	9502/0
Teratoid medulloepithelioma, malignant	9502/3

Synonyms

Diktyoma; teratoneuroma

Epidemiology

Medulloepitheliomas of the optic disc and optic nerve are much less common than those of the ciliary body {539}. Most of the rare reported cases have presented in boys during the first 2–3 years of life, but optic disc medulloepitheliomas have been documented in children as old as 12 years {713,897}.

Etiology

Most intraocular medulloepitheliomas are sporadic and not associated with known risk factors. Medulloepitheliomas of the ciliary body (but not the optic nerve) have been reported in patients with pleuropulmonary blastoma family tumour and dysplasia syndrome caused by germline mutations in *DICER1* {567}.

Localization

Medulloepitheliomas occur in the ciliary body (most commonly), optic disc, and optic nerve {539}.

Clinical features

The presenting symptoms and clinical features include rapid vision loss, proptosis, strabismus, ptosis, and pain {713}. Ophthalmic examination may disclose raised intraocular pressure, disc swelling, an optic disc mass, and exudative retinal detachment {938}.

Histopathology

Medulloepitheliomas contain ribbons or cords of polarized neuroepithelial cells resembling the embryonic medullary epithelium lining the forebrain and optic vesicle. A thin basement membrane lines the inner surface of the elongated neuroepithelium and typically abuts myxoid stroma. Additional features may include so-called diktyomatous net-like growth of thin interweaving neuroepithelial strands, multilayered rosettes, and cystoid spaces.

Medulloepitheliomas are classified into teratoid and non-teratoid groups; tumours in both groups can be either benign or malignant. The heteroplastic elements that define teratoid lesions include cartilage (most common), muscle, and brain-like tissue {1037}. Poorly differentiated neuroblastic cell sheets are a histopathological criterion for malignant medulloepithelioma, and they may contain Homer Wright or Flexner–Wintersteiner rosettes. However, rosettes in medulloepithelioma are generally larger and multilayered. Additional criteria for malignancy include invasion of ocular tissues, extraocular extension, sarcomatous change, and prominent atypia and mitotic activity in the neuroepithelial component.

Differential diagnosis

The histological differential diagnosis of medulloepithelioma of the optic disc and optic nerve ranges from retinoblastoma, ganglioglioma, and sarcoma to retinal pigment epithelial adenoma and carcinoma. Extensive heteroplastic tissues should be distinguished from intraocular choristoma or teratoma.

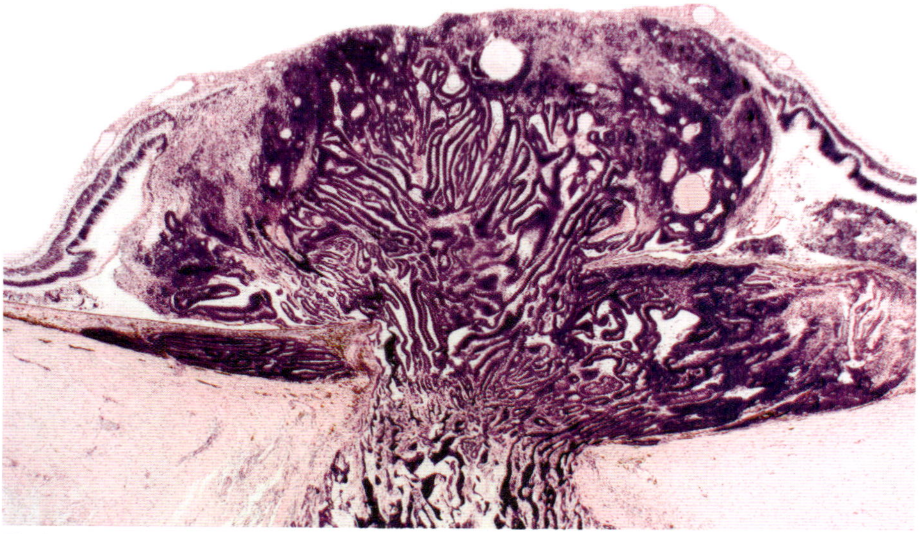

Fig. 4.07 Medulloepithelioma. Tumour extensively involves the optic nerve and optic nerve head.

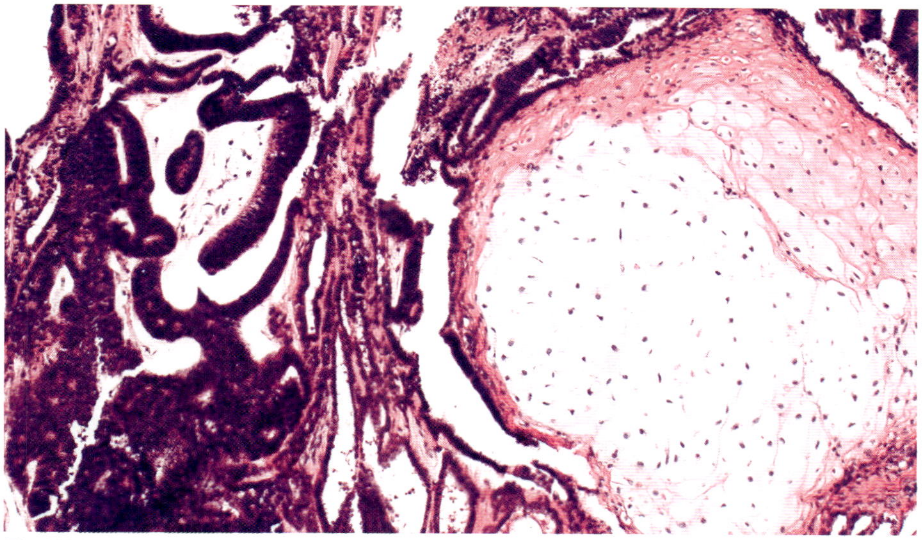

Fig. 4.08 Malignant teratoid medulloepithelioma. The tumour contains neuroepithelial and cartilaginous regions of differentiation.

Histogenesis
Medulloepitheliomas are thought to arise from the neuroepithelium lining the embryonic optic vesicle and optic nerve. Extensive immunohistochemical analysis of one posterior tumour associated with a coloboma suggested an origin from embryonic pigment epithelium {539}.

Genetic profile
The C19MC alterations common in intracranial medulloepithelioma are not present in intraocular tumours, and the lesions appear to be genetically distinct {648}. Mutually exclusive somatic mutations of *DICER1* and *KMT2D* are frequent in intraocular medulloepitheliomas of the ciliary body, but posterior lesions have not been analysed {1020}.

Genetic susceptibility
Rare ciliary body cases have occurred in patients with pleuropulmonary blastoma family tumour and dysplasia syndrome caused by germline mutations in *DICER1* {1020}.

Prognosis and predictive factors
In one series of 8 optic nerve or disc medulloepitheliomas, 2 patients died within 18 months of tumour resection; the remaining 6 survived the follow-up period (of 2–36 months) {713}. The relationship between malignant histopathological features and clinical outcome is not entirely clear {1318}.

Solitary fibrous tumour/ haemangiopericytoma

Mudhar H.S.
Rushing E.J.
Rodriguez F.
Vemuganti G.

Definition
Solitary fibrous tumour/haemangiopericytoma is a fibroblastic mesenchymal tumour, sometimes with a prominent haemangiopericytoma-like branching vascular pattern.

ICD-O code
Solitary fibrous tumour NOS 8815/1

Epidemiology
The true prevalence and incidence is unknown because of the rarity at this site. There is a predilection for women in the third and sixth decades of life {616,748,1055}.

Etiology
The tumour arises de novo, with no apparent causative factor.

Localization
Solitary fibrous tumour/haemangiopericytoma arises from the dura of the optic nerve.

Clinical features
Patients present with unilateral visual impairment, which may eventually lead to blindness and exophthalmos {616,748,1055}. Tumour growth is sometimes painful, and it may be accompanied by hypoglobus, optic atrophy, and optociliary shunt vessels {748}. Imaging studies typically demonstrate a well-circumscribed, intraconal, fusiform mass posterior to the eye {120,748}.

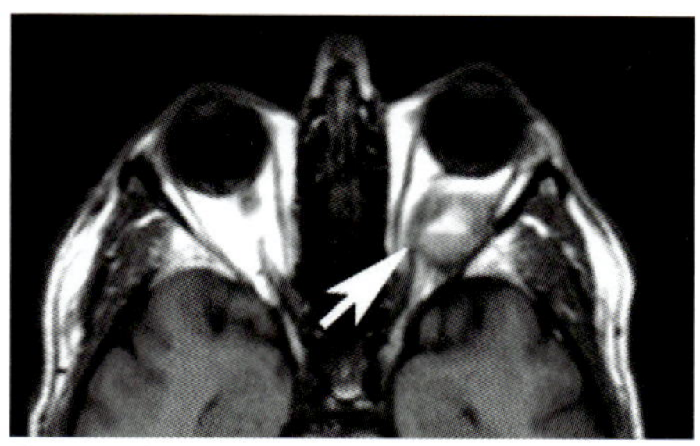

Fig. 4.09 Optic nerve solitary fibrous tumour/haemangiopericytoma. T1-weighted axial MRI shows optic nerve involvement (arrow) by tumour.

Histopathology
The microscopic appearance varies according to the ratio of tumour cells to stroma. Classic haemangiopericytoma is characterized by a patternless, often biphasic architecture with alternating paucicellular and hypercellular areas. Closely apposed fusiform tumour cells with indistinct borders are haphazardly arranged in a richly vascular stroma interrupted by branching, staghorn-shaped sinusoidal vessels. Individual and small groups of tumour cells are surrounded by reticulin fibres. Mitotic activity is variable, and focal necrosis is common. In the solitary fibrous tumour pattern, there is more-abundant intercellular collagen, lower cellularity, and mitotic activity {120,237}. The signature *NAB2-STAT6* fusion (detectable by STAT6 immunohistochemistry) shows nuclear positivity. Other variably positive markers include vimentin (positive in 85–100% of cases), BCL2, CD99, and CD34. Unlike meningioma, solitary fibrous tumour/haemangiopericytoma is usually negative for S100 protein, cytokeratins, and epithelial membrane antigen {616}.

Differential diagnosis
Solitary fibrous tumour/haemangiopericytoma may be confused with other mesenchymal tumours, such as meningioma, haemangioblastoma, synovial sarcoma, mesenchymal chondrosarcoma, and mesothelioma {1055}.

Histogenesis
The histogenesis remains uncertain.

Genetic profile
Solitary fibrous tumours/haemangiopericytomas are characterized by a novel *NAB2-STAT6* fusion resulting from a genomic inversion involving the 12q13 gene locus {202,981}. This alteration occurs independently of anatomical site, and it supports a morphological continuum independent of grade. The *NAB2-STAT6* fusion leads to nuclear localization of STAT6 protein, a highly specific biomarker for this tumour {266,296,1054}. On the basis of nuclear STAT6 immunoreactivity, giant cell angiofibroma, a neoplasm with a predilection for the orbit {264}, is now considered to be a morphological variant of solitary fibrous tumour/haemangiopericytoma (i.e. giant cell–rich solitary fibrous tumour) {1330}.

Prognosis and predictive factors
The prognosis depends on the extent of surgical resection and the presence of high-risk pathological features. The definition of high-risk features is controversial, but includes large size (> 5 cm), increased mitotic activity, hypercellularity, cellular atypia, haemorrhage, and/or necrosis {237}. Orbital and intracranial tumours with haemangiopericytoma features and increased proliferative activity require long-term follow-up, because local recurrence and late metastases may occur regardless of the extent of resection {1055}. The prognosis of haemangiopericytoma in the optic nerve sheath proper is difficult to assess given the rarity at this site; however, adjuvant therapy is recommended for high-risk tumours {748}.

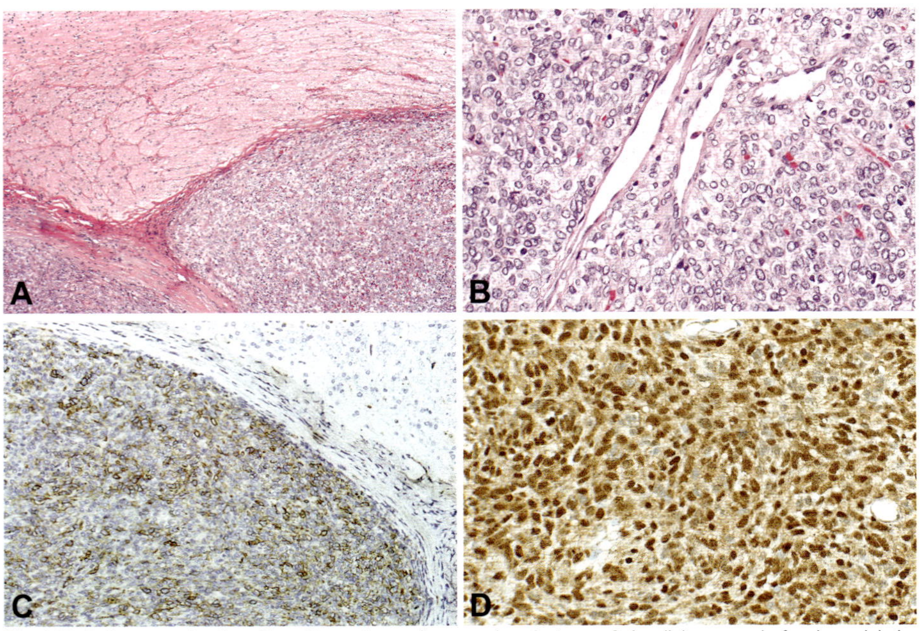

Fig. 4.10 Optic nerve sheath solitary fibrous tumour/haemangiopericytoma. **A** A cellular example forming a lobular mass (lower field) juxtaposed with the optic nerve parenchyma (upper field). **B** An example composed of oval cells, with a so-called jumbled architecture and staghorn vasculature. **C** CD34 expression. **D** Nuclear immunoreactivity for STAT6 is an immunophenotypic property highly specific for this entity.

Melanocytoma of the optic disc and optic nerve

Rushing E.J.
Cummings T.
Dubovy S.
Rodriguez F.

Definition
Melanocytoma is a benign melanocytic tumour that is classically located in the optic disc and anterior portion of the optic nerve, but it can also be found in the uveal tract.

ICD-O code
Melanocytoma 8726/0

Synonyms
Magnocellular naevus; hyperpigmented magnocellular naevus

Epidemiology
Optic nerve melanocytoma is proportionally more common than uveal melanoma in dark-skinned individuals. There is a slight female predilection, with a female-to-male ratio of approximately 1.5:1. The mean age at diagnosis is 50 years {1127,1155}.

Etiology
Melanocytoma is considered to be of congenital origin.

Localization
Melanocytoma is usually unilateral and found on or adjacent to the optic disc. The lesions average 1–2 disc diameters in size {316,1126,1127}. Rare giant examples may extend as far as the ora serrata {362}. Bilateral involvement is more common in children; 1 reported case occurred in a 10-month-old infant {271,1126}.

Clinical features

Melanocytoma is classically asymptomatic, with visual symptoms occurring in 24% of patients and pupillary defects in < 10%. The visual field is abnormal in 90% of patients, with enlargement of the blind spot ranging from minimal to marked. Vision loss is not necessarily related to malignant transformation {386,1126,1127}. Fluorescein angiography shows blocked fluorescence rather than alternating hyper- and hypofluorescence as seen in melanoma {1126}. Optical coherence tomography is characterized by a gradual transition from normal retina into nodular tumour. Optically empty internal details and a bright anterior border facilitate the distinction from melanoma {1102}.

Histopathology

Typical pathological features include a dark-brown to black gross appearance. Histologically, the tumours appear densely pigmented; bleaching is required in order to identify the round to oval or polyhedral cells with small nuclei, abundant cytoplasm, and generally inconspicuous nucleoli {730,1126,1155,1421}; see Fig. 2.23B (p. 77) for an example of a bleached melanocytoma. Mitoses are exceptional; however, necrosis is frequent, often accompanied by pigment-laden macrophages and lymphocytic inflammation {362,1126,1127,1421}. Although the diagnosis is based on routine histology, numerous giant round melanosomes are characteristic at the ultrastructural level {558}.

Differential diagnosis

The most important differential diagnosis is melanoma. Other differential diagnoses include juxtapapillary choroidal naevus and hypertrophy or adenoma of the retinal pigment epithelium {659,1026,1126}.

Histogenesis

Melanocytomas of the optic nerve may be related to other melanocytic lesions of the uveal tract and CNS. They are hypothesized to originate from extraepithelial melanocytes derived from the cranial neural crest {85}.

Genetic profile

Little is known about genetic predisposition to optic nerve melanocytomas. *BAP1* mutations were found in 2 cases with transformation to melanoma; in at least 1 of these cases, the mutation was probably somatic {372}. Some cases may develop in the setting of *BAP1* tumour predisposition syndrome, although this is not yet confirmed.

Genetic susceptibility

Few intraocular melanocytomas have been subjected to genetic analysis. In a targeted sequencing study that included 5 melanocytomas of the optic nerve, a mutation in the *GNAQ* gene was present in 1 case {372} – *GNAQ* and *GNA11* encode alpha subunits of the Gq class, and are frequently mutated in uveal melanoma and melanocytomas of the CNS. Interestingly, 2 cases that had a *BAP1* mutation plus monosomy 3 (one of which was the case with the *GNAQ* mutation) progressed to melanoma. In another study, gene expression profiling of 3 optic nerve melanocytomas revealed that all 3 cases showed a class 1A genetic signature, which is associated with a low risk of metastatic disease in uveal melanoma {252}.

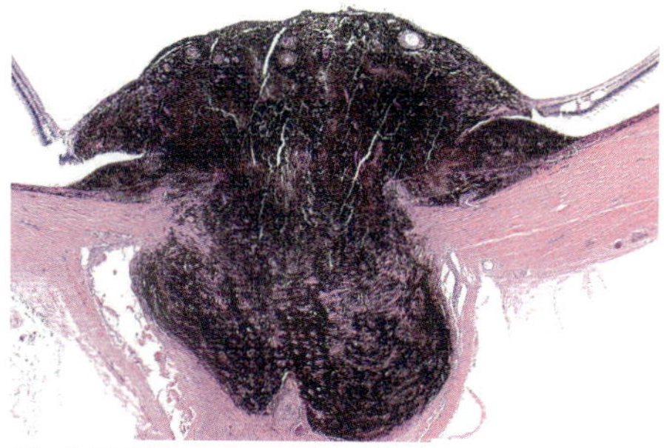

Fig. 4.11 Melanocytoma. Heavily pigmented tumour infiltrates the optic nerve and peripapillary retina.

Prognosis and predictive factors

Progressive growth with local invasion is common, with minor enlargement seen in as many as one third of all patients by 10 years after diagnosis. Malignant transformation is reported in 1–2% of cases, usually within 5 years of the initial diagnosis {1126,1127}; however, malignant transformation has been documented as late as 33 years after diagnosis {47,1173}.

Secondary tumours of the optic disc and optic nerve

Cummings T.
Eberhart C.G.
Materin M.A.
Rushing E.J.
Stemmer-Rachamimov A.O.

Definition

Secondary tumours of the optic disc and optic nerve are tumours that originate elsewhere and involve the optic disc and/or nerve by extension from neighbouring structures or by metastasis from another site.

ICD-O codes

Code according to the originating tumour type.

Epidemiology

Secondary involvement of the optic nerve occurs most frequently via extension of intraocular malignancies {137,208}. Metastases to the optic disc and nerve are exceedingly uncommon. Isolated examples are exceptional, with most showing contiguous choroidal deposits. Bilateral optic nerve metastasis occurs in about 18% of the patients. The mean reported age is 55 years, with women more commonly affected than men {348,384,606,1166}.

Isolated optic nerve lymphoma is rare, with < 10 reported cases; most lymphomas at this site are of the diffuse large B-cell type and associated with brain or eye lesions {90,251,774,801,1222}. Only 3 cases of biopsy-confirmed isolated optic nerve involvement from systemic lymphoma have been documented {520,590,606}; the patients were in the fifth and sixth decades of life {606}.

Clinical features

Metastases are typically painless and heralded by unilateral visual impairment. Rarely, bilateral involvement occurs {348,976,1206}. Only 10% are associated with pain due to elevated intraocular pressure {137,1166}. Afferent pupillary defects are common. Tumours can appear diffuse or nodular on funduscopic examination, often accompanied by swelling and flame-shaped haemorrhages {208,1166}. Fluorescein angiography results are variable, with reports of early-phase hypofluorescence and late-phase hyperfluorescence {384,1166,1392}. Ultrasonographic findings are nonspecific, and the utility of orbital MRI has not been established {203,1166}.

In immunocompetent individuals, optic nerve lymphomas are largely unknown; in immunocompromised patients, HIV/AIDS {688,693}, EBV infection {155}, HTLV-1 infection {1389}, and autoimmune disorders {1200} have all been implicated as possible etiological factors.

Histopathology

In most cases of secondary tumour involvement of the optic disc (74%) there is also adjacent juxtapapillary choroidal involvement {1166}. Patchy white areas or dome-shaped nodules and associated focal haemorrhages may be seen.

The histological features of secondary tumours in the optic disc are diverse, reflecting the various primary tumour types. As is the case in other locations, tumours may have infiltrative, perivascular, or nodular growth patterns, and they may be associated with necrosis or haemorrhage.

Optic nerve lymphomas can be localized within nerve fibre bundles, the leptomeninges, or both {606}. Virtually all primary CNS lymphomas extending into the optic nerve are diffuse large B-cell lymphomas with the characteristic proliferation of large atypical cells with prominent nucleoli and numerous mitoses and apoptotic bodies; they are immunopositive for CD20, CD19, CD79a, and BCL2 {606,773,801,1409}. In immunosuppressed patients, EBV-encoded small RNA (EBER) is often detectable by in situ hybridization. Prior steroid therapy may make diagnosis difficult, with treated tumours showing only apoptotic tumour cells and reactive T cells, gliosis, and macrophages {628}.

Histogenesis

Metastases most commonly originate from the breast and lung, followed (with equal frequencies) by the gastrointestinal tract and kidney {797,827,1166,1407}. Cutaneous melanoma only rarely spreads to the optic disc {922}. Other rare primaries include prostate carcinoma {1392}, multiple myeloma {1311}, medullary thyroid carcinoma {1398}, and adenoid cystic carcinoma {6}. In 20% of cases, the primary tumour is unknown {384,1166}. In

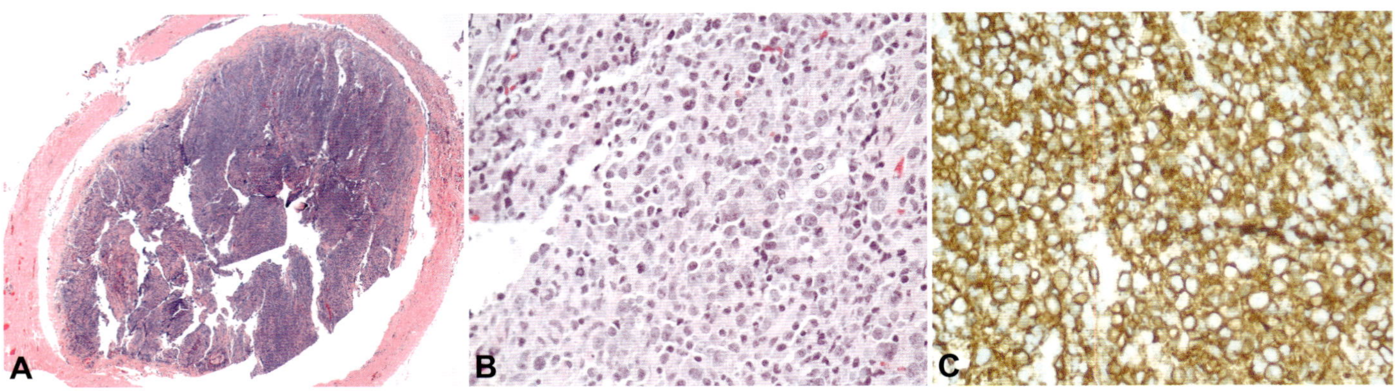

Fig. 4.12 Lymphomatous optic nerve infiltration. **A,B** The optic nerve parenchyma is diffusely infiltrated by large atypical cells with prominent nucleoli. **C** Immunohistochemical analysis reveals that these are CD20-positive B cells.

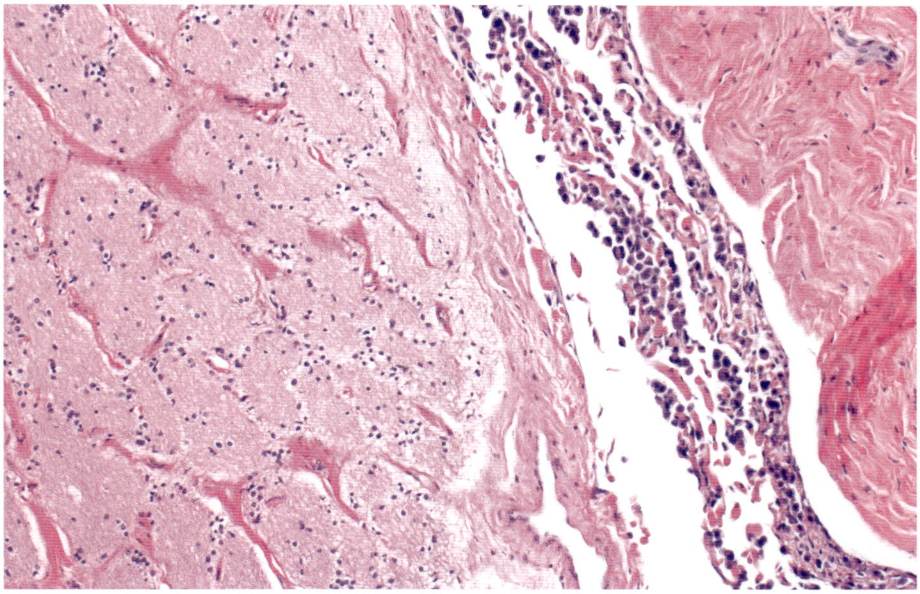

Fig. 4.13 Breast carcinoma metastatic to the optic nerve. The optic nerve leptomeninges are diffusely involved by discohesive carcinoma cells; the patient died from triple-negative breast cancer metastatic to the brain and optic nerve.

one study, involvement of the optic nerve was seen in 34% of patients who died of leukaemia {29}. Lymphoma of the optic nerve can occur as isolated disease or in association with primary CNS, primary intraocular, or systemic lymphoma.

Direct invasion by primary ocular tumours is most common with retinoblastoma and (less frequently) juxtapapillary or retinoinvasive uveal melanoma {1233}. Meningiomas and gliomas can also extend from the brain or its coverings into the optic nerve.

Genetic profile

The molecular characteristics of secondary tumours in the optic disc are diverse, reflecting the various primary tumour types. Diffuse large B-cell lymphoma typically shows monoclonal IG gene rearrangements {606} and characteristic expression of MYC, BCL2, and BCL6 {707}.

Prognosis and predictive factors

Prognosis is highly dependent on tumour stage and the primary site and tumour type. Optic nerve lymphomas often show an initial partial response to steroids, chemotherapy, and/or radiotherapy, but eventually relapse {520,906}.

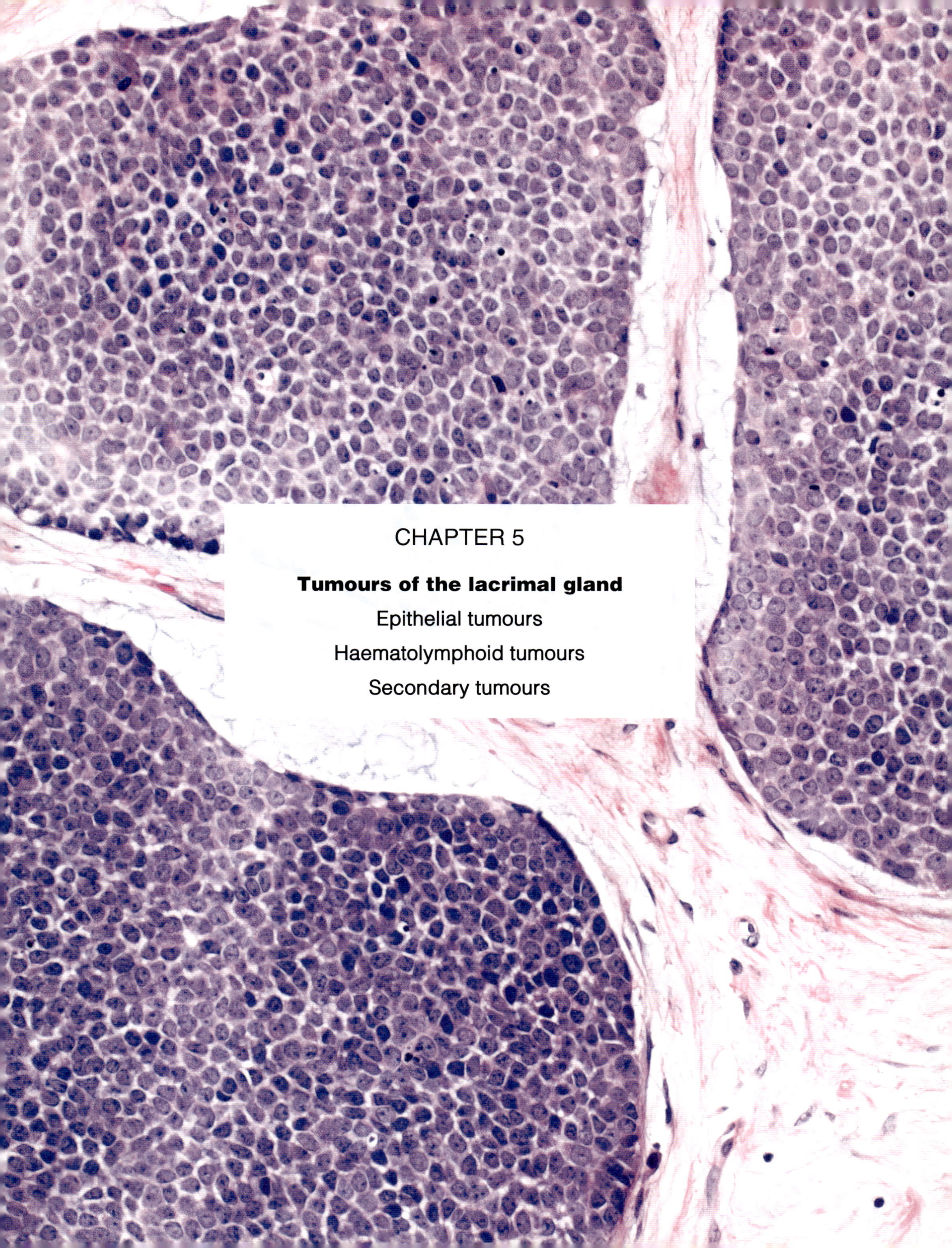

CHAPTER 5

Tumours of the lacrimal gland

Epithelial tumours

Haematolymphoid tumours

Secondary tumours

WHO classification of tumours of the lacrimal gland

Epithelial tumours	
Adenoid cystic carcinoma	8200/3
Mucoepidermoid carcinoma	8430/3
Adenosquamous carcinoma	8560/3
Carcinosarcoma	8980/3
Adenocarcinoma of the lacrimal gland	8140/3
Carcinoma ex pleomorphic adenoma	8941/3
Pleomorphic adenoma	8940/0
Myoepithelioma	8982/0
Myoepithelial carcinoma	8982/3
Oncocytoma	8290/0
Oncocytic carcinoma	8290/3
Epithelial–myoepithelial carcinoma	8562/3
Low-grade intraductal carcinoma	8500/2
Secretory carcinoma	8502/3
Hybrid neoplasms	See note[a]
Acinic cell carcinoma	8550/3
Adenolymphoma/Warthin tumour	8561/0
Haematolymphoid tumours	
Extranodal marginal zone lymphoma of mucosa-associated lymphoid tissue (MALT lymphoma)	9699/3
Follicular lymphoma	9690/3
Diffuse large B-cell lymphoma	9680/3
Reactive lymphoid hyperplasia	None
Secondary tumours	See note[b]

[a]Code hybrid neoplasms as both tumour types.

[b]Code secondary tumours according to the originating tumour type.

The morphology codes are from the International Classification of Diseases for Oncology (ICD-O) {381}. Behaviour is coded /0 for benign tumours; /1 for unspecified, borderline, or uncertain behaviour; /2 for carcinoma in situ and grade III intraepithelial neoplasia; and /3 for malignant tumours.

The classification is modified from the previous WHO classification, taking into account changes in our understanding of these lesions.

TNM classification of carcinoma of the lacrimal gland

Carcinoma of Lacrimal Gland

(ICD-O-3 C69.5)

TNM Clinical Classification

T – Primary Tumour

TX	Primary tumour cannot be assessed	
T0	No evidence of primary tumour	
T1	Tumour 2 cm or less in greatest dimension, with or without extraglandular extension into the orbital soft tissue	
	T1a	No periosteal or bone involvement
	T1b	Periosteal involvement without bone involvement
	T1c	Bone involvement
T2	Tumour more than 2 cm but not more than 4 cm in greatest dimension	
	T2a	No periosteal or bone involvement
	T2b	Periosteal involvement without bone involvement
	T2c	Bone involvement
T3	Tumour more than 4 cm or with extraglandular extension into orbital soft tissue, including optic nerve, or globe	
	T3a	No periosteal or bone involvement
	T3b	Periosteal involvement without bone involvement
	T3c	Bone involvement
T4	Tumour invades adjacent structures (sinuses, temporal fossa, pterygoid fossa, superior orbital fissure, cavernous sinus, and/or brain)	
	T4a	No more than 2 cm in greatest dimension
	T4b	More than 2 cm but no more than 4 cm in greatest dimension
	T4c	More than 4 cm in greatest dimension

N – Regional Lymph Nodes

NX	Regional lymph nodes cannot be assessed
N0	No regional lymph node metastasis
N1	Regional lymph node metastasis

M – Distant Metastasis

M0	No distant metastasis
M1	Distant metastasis

pTNM Pathological Classification

The pT and pN categories correspond to the T and N categories.

pM – Distant Metastasis*

pM1	Distant metastasis microscopically confirmed

Note

*pM0 and pMX are not valid categories.

Stage

No stage is at present recommended.

The information presented here has been excerpted from the 8th edition of the *TNM classification of malignant tumours* (2017) {132}.
A help desk for specific questions about the TNM classification is available at http://www.uicc.org/resources/tnm/helpdesk.

Tumours of the lacrimal gland: Introduction

Grossniklaus H.E.
Eberhart C.G.
Kivelä T.T.

The lacrimal gland is composed of lobules of glands with acini that drain via interlobular ducts into excretory ducts. The acini are lined internally by acinar epithelium and externally by myoepithelium. The ducts are lined internally by low cuboidal epithelium and externally by myoepithelium. It is also normal for there to be patches of lymphocytes and plasma cells present in the lacrimal gland. The most common causes of lacrimal gland enlargement are inflammatory processes, but neoplasms can also arise within the gland. Such neoplasms are generally classified as epithelial or haematolymphoid.

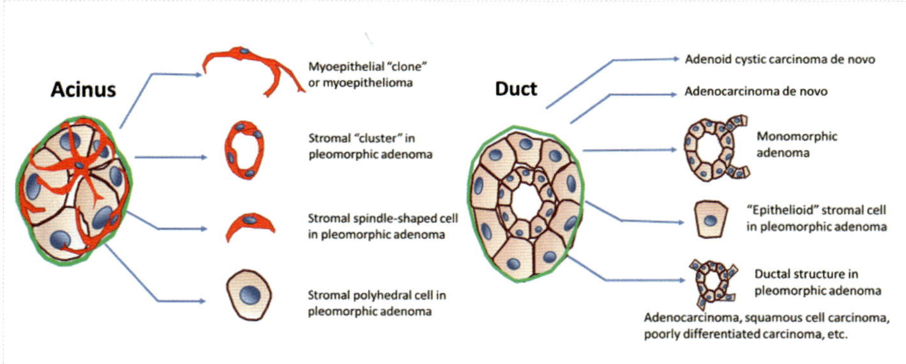

Fig. 5.01 Epithelial neoplasms of the lacrimal gland. At one end of the spectrum are acinic cell tumours, which arise from acinar epithelium; at the other end are monomorphic adenomas, which arise from the low cuboidal epithelium of the duct. Pleomorphic adenomas and carcinomas arise from the myoepithelium and ductal low cuboidal epithelium.

Epithelial neoplasms of the lacrimal gland are classified along a continuum on the basis of their origin in the gland. At one end of the continuum are acinic cell tumours, which arise in the inner epithelial layer of the acinus; at the other end are monomorphic adenomas, which arise from the inner layer of the duct. Pleomorphic adenomas contain two components: an epithelial component (probably arising from the inner layer of the duct) and a myoepithelial (stromal) component. The myoepithelial cells may form a clonal population that essentially takes over the tumour (myoepithelioma), or they may exist as clusters of cells, as spindle-shaped cells, or as polyhedral cells in the stroma of the pleomorphic adenoma. Carcinomas, such as squamous cell carcinoma, adenocarcinoma, and poorly differentiated carcinoma, can arise from the inner epithelial lining of the duct in pleomorphic adenoma (carcinoma ex pleomorphic adenoma). It is also possible for adenocarcinoma and adenoid cystic carcinoma to arise in the gland, also from the inner layer of the duct.

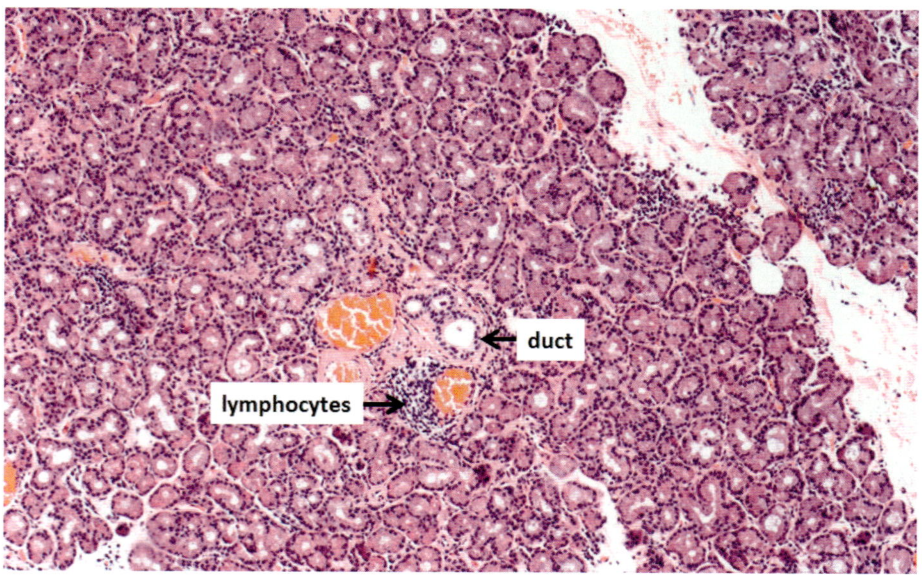

Fig. 5.02 Normal lacrimal gland. The lacrimal gland is composed of lobules of acini and occasional ducts; aggregates of lymphocytes and plasma cells are present.

Lymphoid aggregates in the gland may give rise to lymphomas; these are most commonly extranodal marginal zone lymphoma of mucosa-associated lymphoid tissue (MALT lymphoma), although other forms of lymphoma may also arise in the gland.

In general, when pleomorphic adenoma is the clinical diagnosis, it is advisable to excise the tumour in toto, including with an intact capsule. Rupture of the capsule can spread the tumour, and it may then recur and give rise to carcinoma ex pleomorphic adenoma. Tumours that appear nodular on imaging (CT or MRI) and do not mould to the adjacent bone are probably epithelial (pleomorphic adenoma), whereas tumours that mould to the adjacent bone are probably lymphoid (e.g. lymphoma). When a lymphoid lesion is clinically suspected, it is advisable to submit a portion of the biopsy specimen for flow cytometric immunophenotyping.

Epithelial tumours of the lacrimal gland

Adenoid cystic carcinoma of the lacrimal gland

Alkatan H.
Roberts F.
Thaung C.
White V.A.

Definition

Adenoid cystic carcinoma (ACC) of the lacrimal gland is a malignant neoplasm composed of epithelial and myoepithelial cells that form various patterns, including cribriform, tubular, and solid patterns.

ICD-O code

Adenoid cystic carcinoma 8200/3

Epidemiology

Epithelial lacrimal gland lesions constitute 10–12% of all orbital lesions {117,598} and 12–16% of biopsied lacrimal fossa lesions {317,1250}. ACC has been reported to account for 2–16% of all orbital malignancies {117,291,598}, 13% of all malignant lacrimal gland tumours including lymphomas, and 32% of malignant lacrimal gland tumours excluding lymphomas {743}. In combined data from several series, ACC was found to account for about 20% of epithelial lacrimal tumours and was the most common malignant tumour, accounting for approximately half or even more of all malignant epithelial lacrimal gland lesions {25,53,317}.

ACC has a wide age range (12–75 years) and a bimodal age distribution, with a small peak in the teenage years and a larger peak in adulthood (~40 years) {25,1332}. Unlike in ACC of the salivary glands, race, ethnicity, and geographical area do not seem to affect the prevalence of ACC of the lacrimal gland {1331}. Most reports describe no sex predilection.

Localization

At this anatomical site, ACC usually arises in the orbital lobe of the main lacrimal gland, although occasional cases have been reported in the palpebral lobe {1309} and in the accessory lacrimal glands {363}.

Clinical features

The clinical presentation, which is related to the growing tumour mass effect, includes globe displacement (typically downwards and medially) resulting in facial asymmetry; decreased eye motility, particularly in the upward gaze (with or without diplopia); a palpable lacrimal fossa swelling or mass; and ptosis {39,958,1332}. Proptosis was the most common clinical manifestation in some series {25,891}. Atypical cases of ACC with no superotemporal mass were recently reported {1414}. Pain (often with numbness), due to perineural and muscle invasion, is a presenting symptom in 80% of cases {39,891,958,1332}. The history is of short duration {958}, with a median duration of 7 months in ACC (vs 30 months in pleomorphic adenoma) in one report {25}. In another series, the mean duration of symptoms in ACC was found to be 10 months {291}.

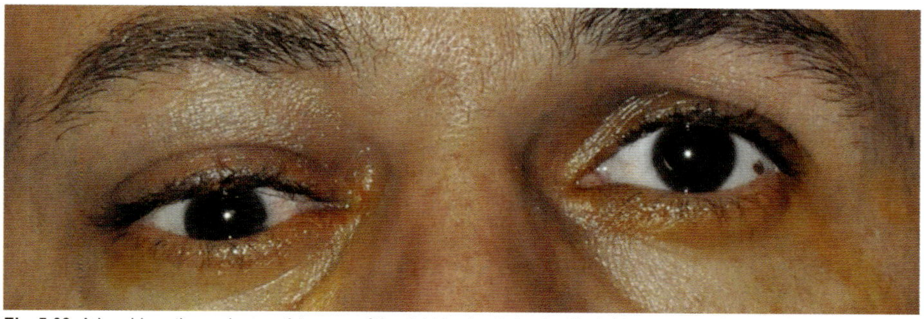

Fig. 5.03 Adenoid cystic carcinoma. A tumour of the right lacrimal gland, with right eye proptosis and globe displacement downwards.

Histopathology

ACC is an unencapsulated tumour that infiltrates the surrounding orbital soft tissue and includes proliferating myoepithelial cells and luminal ductal cells {1332,1355}. The tumour cells show small, angulated, hyperchromatic nuclei and scant cytoplasm. Depending on the cellular composition and cytomorphological features, the tumours can show several growth patterns, which are present either individually or together in variable combinations {891,1332}. The cribriform pattern, which is the most common, is described as a Swiss-cheese pattern because of the formation of cystic structures where the connective tissue stroma is filled with basophilic amorphous glycosaminoglycans and/or eosinophilic hyalinized basal lamina {25,891,1332}. The tubular pattern shows small glandular structures, whereas the solid pattern shows predominantly proliferating basaloid myoepithelial cells with few glycosaminoglycan deposits or cyst-like basal lamina glandular spaces. The sclerosing pattern is a variant of the tubular pattern. In most series, the solid pattern is the least common {25,958}; this pattern can be associated with higher numbers of mitotic figures, which may explain its worse prognosis {958,1355}. Histopathological documentation of perineural and bone invasion is essential. It is also important to document tumour size, extent, and margins histopathologically, according to the TNM classification system {1383}. The diagnosis can usually be rendered on the basis of light microscopic features.

Most ACCs express E-cadherin, KIT (CD117), and EGFR (HER1) {891}. The average Ki-67 proliferation index is about 30%, and tumour suppressor p53 staining is strongly positive, with an average positivity of 39% {788}. Unlike pleomorphic adenomas, most ACCs are MYB-positive, and all are PLAG1-negative {788,958}. High-grade transformation, previously referred to as dedifferentiation,

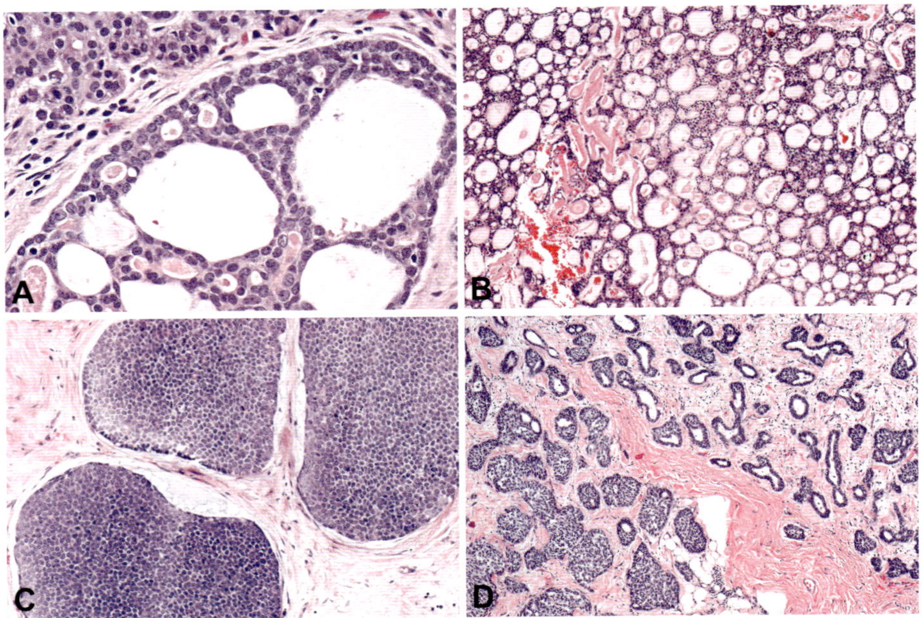

Fig. 5.04 Adenoid cystic carcinoma. **A** Cribriform pattern; tumour and adjacent lacrimal gland acini. **B** Cribriform pattern; the typical so-called Swiss-cheese appearance. **C** Solid pattern. **D** A combination of tubular and solid patterns.

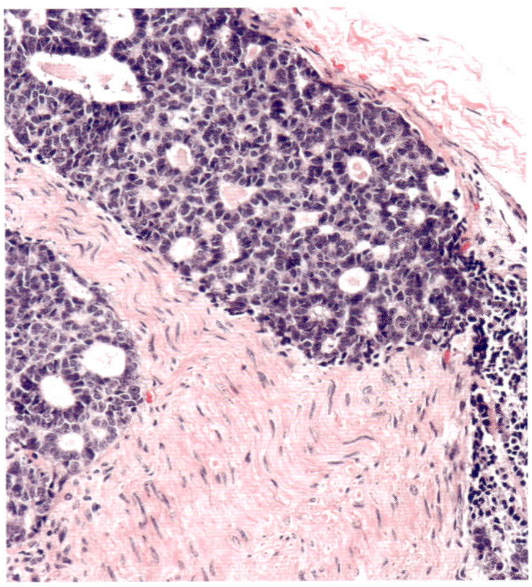

Fig. 5.05 Adenoid cystic carcinoma. Histopathological evidence of perineural invasion.

may occur; it shows a monophasic, mitotically active, pleomorphic carcinoma composed of areas consisting of ductal cells with loss of myoepithelial layers, adjacent to conventional ACC {1364}.

Differential diagnosis

The solid basaloid-looking ACC subtype (often with palisading), in which the glandular pattern is absent, must be differentiated from basal cell carcinoma; this differential can be particularly challenging in small biopsy specimens {958}. The hyaline areas seen in some fields of some ACCs can be confused with stromal areas of pleomorphic adenoma {958}. Other differential diagnoses include adenocarcinoma, myoepithelial carcinoma, epithelial–myoepithelial carcinoma, polymorphous adenocarcinoma, mucoepidermoid carcinoma, and basal cell adenoma/adenocarcinoma {53,1355}.

Histogenesis

Specialized myoepithelial cells, which are epithelial cells with contractile smooth muscle–like properties, may play a role in the histogenesis of salivary gland tumours and may similarly play a role in lacrimal gland tumours {956}.

Genetic profile

Loss of chromosome 6q is a frequent finding in ACC. This may be associated with t(6;9)(q22-23;p23-24), resulting in a *MYB-NFIB* fusion gene {194,1331,1364}. *KRAS*, *NRAS*, and *MET* mutations have been reported in lacrimal gland epithelial neoplasms, with the highest frequency (44%) in ACC {91}. Mutations of the Notch signalling pathway may play a role in ACC {891}. Expression of the anti-apoptosis protein BIRC5 (also called survivin) is high in ACC, and its inhibition is found to suppress ACC proliferation {861,886}.

Prognosis and predictive factors

Patient age at diagnosis, completeness of surgical resection, and tumour stage are important determinants of disease-specific survival for epithelial lacrimal gland tumours in general {743}. The reported 10-year survival rate for ACC is 10–51% {42,1418}. The histological features of ACC have prognostic implications: the solid pattern is associated with a worse prognosis, perineural invasion is associated with local recurrence and skull invasion, and bone invasion is associated with a fatal outcome in large tumours. Other prognostic factors include tumour size (per the TNM staging system; see p. 149) {25,39,1332,1383}. The recurrence rate of ACC can reach 75%. Distant metastasis, mainly to the lung, brain, and bone, and rarely to the liver and kidney, can result in death and can occur even after more than a decade {1023,1351}. ACC is one of the top 10 histopathological diagnoses of recurrent orbital lesions, accounting for 9% {1245}. Serial follow-up MRI is recommended to monitor disease progression, although CT is superior in detecting bony changes {205,1383}.

Mucoepidermoid carcinoma of the lacrimal gland

Roberts F.
Alkatan H.
White V.A.

Definition

Mucoepidermoid carcinoma (MEC) of the lacrimal gland is a malignant epithelial tumour characterized by squamous (epidermoid) cells, mucous cells, columnar cells, and intermediate cells.

ICD-O code

Mucoepidermoid carcinoma	8430/3
Adenosquamous carcinoma	8560/3

Synonyms

Mixed epidermoid and mucus-secreting carcinoma; mucoepidermoid tumour

Epidemiology

MEC is relatively rare, accounting for 1.5–4% of all epithelial tumours and about 7% of all malignant tumours in the lacrimal gland {25,191,1355}.

Etiology

Etiological factors have not been described for lacrimal gland carcinoma. MEC of the salivary gland is associated with radiation exposure.

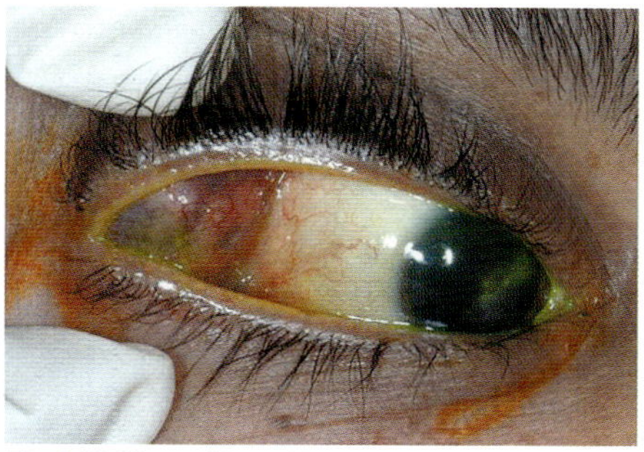

Fig. 5.06 Mucoepidermoid carcinoma. Tumour bulging from the superotemporal orbit.

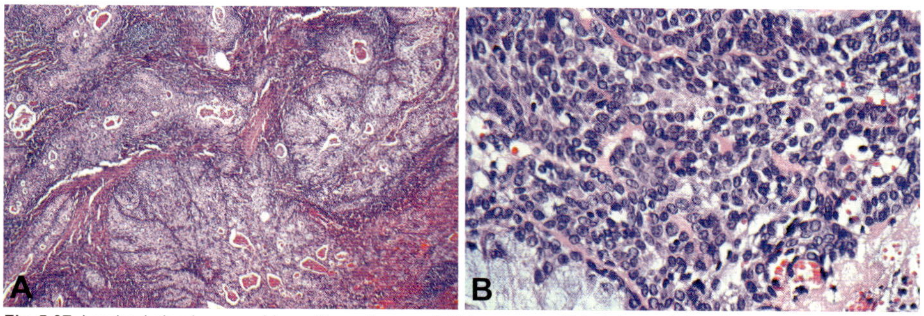

Fig. 5.07 Lacrimal gland mucoepidermoid carcinoma. **A** At low power. **B** An intermediate cell area.

Localization

MEC can arise throughout the main lacrimal gland and in accessory lacrimal glands

Clinical features

MEC usually presents as a slow-growing mass in the lacrimal gland region, clinically indistinguishable from more-common tumours such as pleomorphic adenoma {25,191}. Occasionally they may cause painful proptosis. These tumours usually appear circumscribed, with a greyish-white lobulated cut surface. Cystic areas may be evident depending on tumour grade. On CT, MEC is usually a well-circumscribed enhancing mass in the lacrimal gland region. Evidence of cystic change and calcification has been described.

Histopathology

MEC of the lacrimal gland is composed of variable proportions of four cell types. The squamous cells have medium to large nuclei with eosinophilic cytoplasm and intercellular bridges between cells, but without keratinization. Mucous cells and columnar cells form small glands, tubules, and cysts; the cysts contain inspissated mucin (which may calcify) and are lined by mucous cells, looking deceptively bland. The intermediate (or transitional) cells are oval, with a round nucleus and faintly eosinophilic cytoplasm. The stroma may be hyalinized with calcification and ossification. A granulomatous reaction to extravasated mucus may be seen.

There are several systems for grading salivary gland MEC, none of which is universally accepted. Most systems divide the tumours into three levels (low-grade, intermediate-grade, and high-grade) according to the proportions of cystic areas, mucous cells, intermediate cells, squamous cells, and solid areas {940}. Necrosis, perineural invasion, and mitotic counts are reported as prognostic factors of MEC in the major salivary glands.

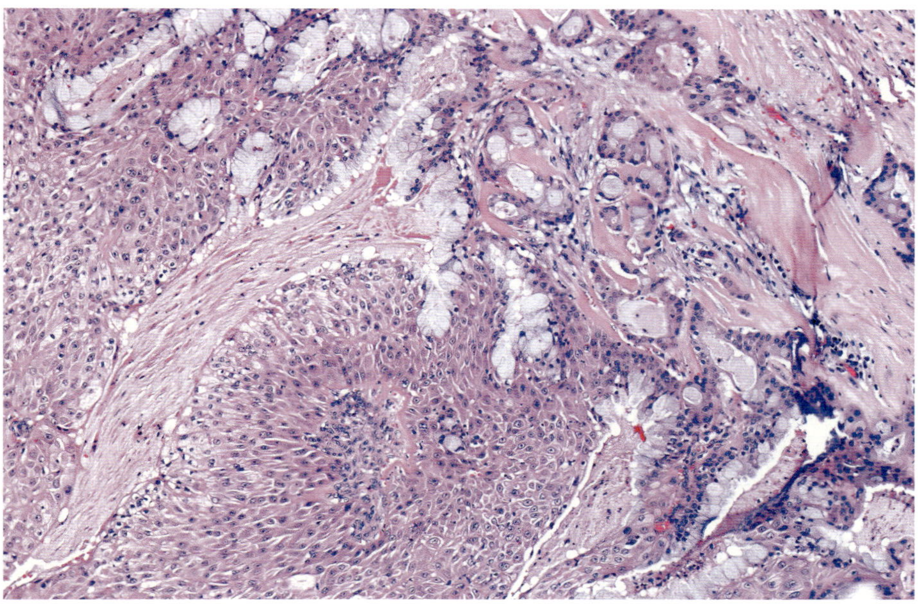

Fig. 5.08 Mucoepidermoid carcinoma. Solid sheets of intermediate cells juxtaposed with mucous cells.

Differential diagnosis

The differential diagnosis includes squamous cell carcinoma, sebaceous carcinoma, adenosquamous carcinoma, and pleomorphic adenoma.

Histogenesis

Lacrimal gland and salivary gland MECs share a common histogenesis; they are composed of varying proportions of luminal and myoepithelial cells. This is supported by reports describing MEC arising in pleomorphic adenoma {247}.

Genetic profile

A CRTC1-MAML2 fusion protein has been identified in some lacrimal gland MECs {1333}; this fusion, resulting from a t(11;19)(q21;p13.1) translocation, is also present in 80% of salivary gland MECs, where it is associated with a better prognosis.

Prognosis and predictive factors

Prognostic factors have not been formally reported for MEC of the lacrimal gland. In the salivary glands, the prognosis of MEC varies with tumour grade: grade 1 and 2 tumours show almost no recurrence, whereas grade 3 tumours are associated with a mortality rate of > 50%.

Carcinosarcoma of the lacrimal gland

Chan A.S.Y.
Salomao D.R.
White V.A.

Definition

Carcinosarcoma of the lacrimal gland is a biphasic malignancy with distinct carcinoma and heterologous sarcomatous components.

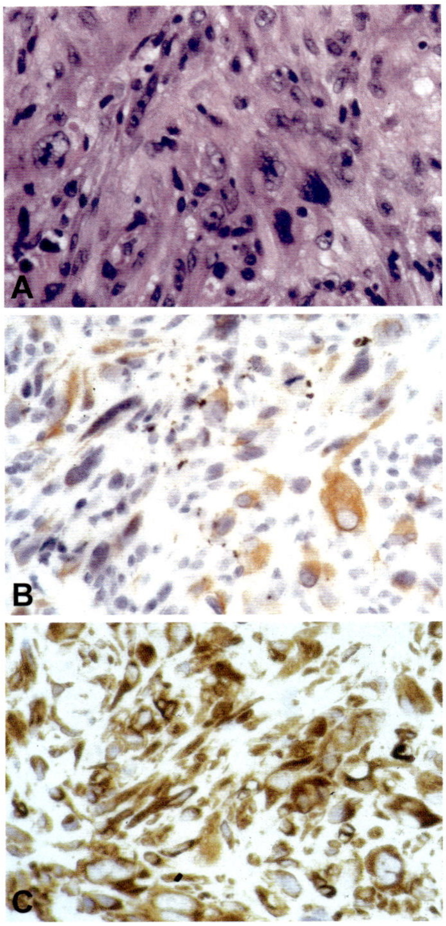

Fig. 5.09 Carcinosarcoma. **A** The tumour cell nuclei are vesicular and pleomorphic, with numerous nucleoli. **B** Pancytokeratin immunostaining (AE1/AE3) highlights the epithelial component of the tumour (peroxidase anti-peroxidase staining method). **C** Vimentin immunostaining highlights the sarcomatous component of the tumour (peroxidase anti-peroxidase staining method).

ICD-O code

Carcinosarcoma	8980/3

Synonym

True malignant mixed tumour

Epidemiology

Carcinosarcomas are extremely rare in the lacrimal gland, with only occasional cases reported in the literature {929,1230,1241}.

Etiology

Carcinosarcoma arises de novo, although some researchers believe that this tumour may arise from pleomorphic adenoma.

Localization

Carcinosarcoma can arise throughout the main lacrimal gland and probably in accessory lacrimal glands.

Clinical features

Patients present with a rapidly progressive orbital mass and symptoms related to mass effect, such as proptosis {1230}.

Histopathology

Carcinosarcomas are biphasic tumours, with malignant epithelial and high-grade sarcomatous components. The most common epithelial histological subtypes are adenocarcinoma and squamous cell carcinoma {1241}. The sarcomatous component can be fibrosarcoma, osteosarcoma, undifferentiated sarcoma, or (rarely) leiomyosarcoma {1230}. The sarcomatous elements are usually composed of pleomorphic spindle cells with high-grade nuclear features. Necrosis may be present. Cytokeratin immunohistochemistry is useful to highlight the epithelial malignancy. A variety of mesenchymal markers (e.g. vimentin and SMA) may be expressed in the sarcomatous component, depending on differentiation {929}.

Differential diagnosis

The sarcomatous spindle cell component may be mistaken for a spindle cell carcinoma (sarcomatoid carcinoma), pleomorphic carcinoma, or desmoplastic melanoma. Heterologous elements/osseous differentiation may be confused with a teratocarcinosarcoma or malignant teratoma {929}.

Histogenesis

The histogenesis is unknown. Salivary carcinosarcomas have been shown to be monoclonal in origin; they are postulated to originate from a pluripotent stem cell capable of differentiation into both epithelial and mesenchymal cells {1312}.

Genetic profile

The genetic profile is unknown. In salivary carcinosarcomas, gains of chromosomes 7 and 8q, as well as losses of chromosomes 10 and 9p, have been reported in both epithelial and sarcomatous components, with more chromosomal aberrations identified in the epithelial components. Recent studies have shown as much as 75% homology between the two components, supporting the theory of monoclonal tumour evolution from a single precursor cell {1312}.

Prognosis and predictive factors

Carcinosarcomas are aggressive tumours that are locally invasive, with high rates of recurrence, metastasis, and mortality {929}.

Adenocarcinoma of the lacrimal gland

Alkatan H.
Roberts F.
White V.A.

Definition

Adenocarcinoma of the lacrimal gland is a malignant epithelial tumour forming ductal and/or glandular structures (with or without cyst formation), exclusive of other known epithelial salivary gland carcinomas {1332}. Primary ductal adenocarcinoma (PDA) of the lacrimal gland is a rare high-grade adenocarcinoma and a counterpart of salivary duct carcinoma {591}; it also resembles invasive ductal carcinoma of the breast {808}.

ICD-O code

Adenocarcinoma of the lacrimal gland	8140/3

Synonyms

Unclassified adenocarcinoma; ductal carcinoma/adenocarcinoma; cystadenocarcinoma; mucinous cystadenocarcinoma; intestinal-type adenocarcinoma

Epidemiology

The relative prevalence of adenocarcinoma NOS is variable, ranging from 8.4% of all malignant epithelial tumours of the lacrimal gland in the USA to 23.1% in Egypt {317,743,1351}. Adenocarcinoma appears to occur more commonly in men, and patients are typically White (85%) {42}. PDA accounts for 2% of all epithelial lacrimal gland tumours {1355}. It appears to occur more commonly in men, with a patient age range of 34–78 years and a mean age of 58 years {661,686}.

Localization

Adenocarcinomas arise throughout the main lacrimal gland and (rarely) in accessory lacrimal glands.

Clinical features

Adenocarcinoma NOS and PDA share the typical clinical manifestations of lacrimal gland tumours, with mass effect causing proptosis, globe displacement, ptosis,

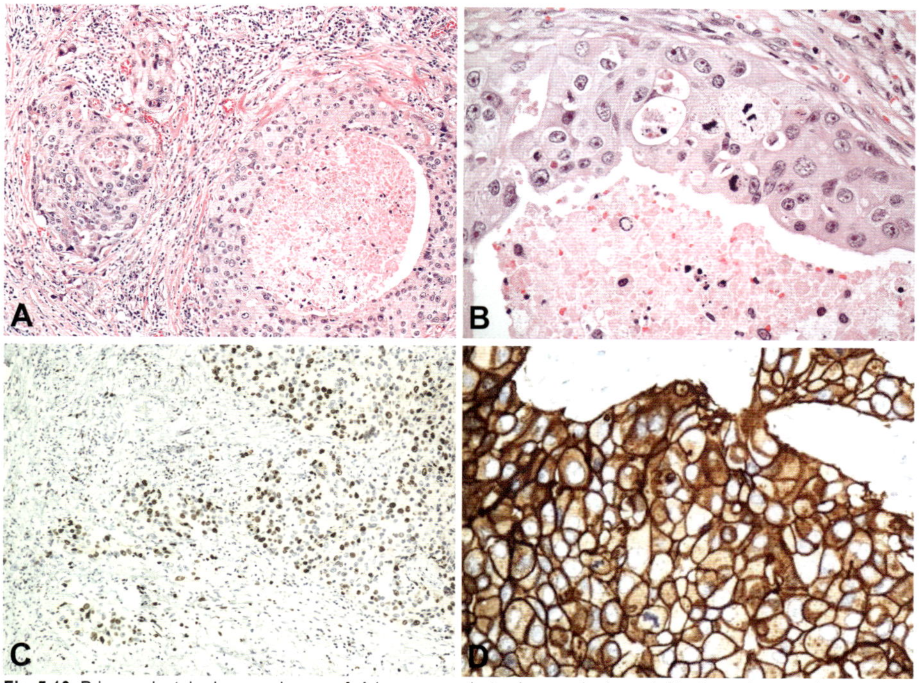

Fig. 5.10 Primary ductal adenocarcinoma. **A** A low-power photomicrograph shows infiltrating adenocarcinoma with a desmoplastic background and inflammatory cells. **B** A high-power photomicrograph shows large cells with abundant eosinophilic granular cytoplasm, numerous mitotic figures, and central comedo-necrosis. **C** The tumour shows a high Ki-67 proliferation index. **D** There is strong membranous immunostaining for ERBB2 (HER2), similar to that seen in ductal carcinoma of the breast.

restricted eye motility, visual disturbance, and diplopia {39,242,696,1332}. Pain is a cardinal symptom of adenoid cystic carcinoma, but it is also relatively common in adenocarcinoma {1332}. The duration of symptoms of PDA is 1–18 months {661,686}.

Histopathology

Adenocarcinoma NOS is a diagnosis of exclusion. It may show variable glandular formation with duct-like configuration, nests of clear cells, and possible solid areas resembling adenoid cystic carcinoma. It can show high-grade anaplastic proliferation with prominent glandular formation and extensive necrosis {1332,1355}. PDA is a rare and generally aggressive lacrimal gland tumour that has a striking histopathological resemblance to ductal carcinoma of the breast, with infiltrating ductal and intraductal elements. Extracellular mucin is uncommonly present {806}. The tumour cells in PDA show granular eosinophilic cytoplasm, large vesicular nuclei, frequent mitoses, and breast ductal carcinoma–like structures often demonstrating comedo-necrosis and/or cord-like infiltration {686,973,1419}. A scirrhous pattern of growth has recently been reported {40}. Perineural and lymphovascular invasion are common. The tumour cells are strongly immunoreactive for low-molecular-weight cytokeratins, CK7, CEA, epithelial membrane antigen, GCDFP-15, and androgen receptor {661,806}. Progesterone receptor and estrogen receptor are usually negative, and the Ki-67 proliferation index can reach 60% {40,661,1419}. PDA tumour cells do not express myoepithelial markers such as S100 protein, SMA, p63, and calponin {696,1419}. Ultrastructural studies of PDA show intracytoplasmic lumina containing homogeneous secretory granules, further demonstrating the similarity to malignant breast tumours {808}.

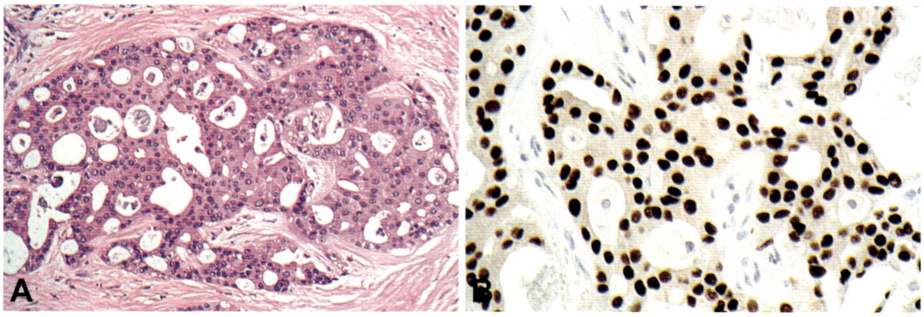

Fig. 5.11 Primary ductal adenocarcinoma. **A** Adenocarcinoma with apocrine features. **B** Positive nuclear staining for androgen receptor.

Differential diagnosis

PDA should be differentiated from adenocarcinoma NOS, adenocarcinoma ex pleomorphic adenoma, and mucoepidermoid carcinoma {696}. Other differential diagnoses include polymorphous low-grade adenocarcinoma and adenoid cystic carcinoma {808,973,1355}.

Histogenesis

Adenocarcinoma and PDA can arise de novo or in relation to a pleomorphic adenoma {25}. The exact nature of the PDA tumour cells and origin is unknown; however, the immunohistochemical staining patterns of the tumour cells indicate an acinar and/or ductal (but not myoepithelial) origin {668}.

Genetic profile

Amplification of the ERBB2 (HER2) signalling pathway, which is present in approximately 25% of salivary duct carcinomas, has also been reported in PDA of the lacrimal gland {40,1419}.

Prognosis and predictive factors

The previously reported average survival with adenocarcinoma was 1.5 years {1332,1355}. Early diagnosis and treatment improve the prognosis, with a reported 10-year overall survival rate of 28% and 10-year disease-specific survival rate of 51% {42}. The reported 5-year survival rate of patients with PDA is 44% (indicating a more aggressive course than that of adenoid cystic carcinoma), with a high rate of recurrence leading to fatal outcome {661,686}. Treatments include complete excision, lymph node dissection, orbital bone resection, and radiotherapy {668,686}. Poor prognosis of PDA may be associated with overexpression of ERBB2 (HER2) and p53 {661}. GCDFP-15, androgen receptor, and ERBB2 (HER2) have been proposed as biomarkers for treatment guidance and prognosis in PDA {1419}.

Carcinoma ex pleomorphic adenoma of the lacrimal gland

Salomao D.R.
White V.A.
Chan A.S.Y.

Definition
Carcinoma ex pleomorphic adenoma of the lacrimal gland is an epithelial malignancy arising from a primary or recurrent pleomorphic adenoma.

ICD-O code
Carcinoma ex pleomorphic adenoma 8941/3

Synonym
Malignant mixed tumour

Epidemiology
Carcinoma ex pleomorphic adenoma occurs in 6% of pleomorphic adenomas {1332}, and it accounts for 10% of all malignant lacrimal gland tumours {1335}.

Etiology
Multiple recurrences of pleomorphic adenoma and inadequate primary excision are thought to increase the risk of malignant transformation {1335}.

Localization
Carcinoma ex pleomorphic adenoma can occur in the main lacrimal gland, the accessory lacrimal glands, and ectopic lacrimal gland tissue.

Clinical features
Patients present with a previously long-standing, slow-growing lacrimal mass with or without associated inferior displacement of the eye or proptosis, or with a recurrent mass after previous pleomorphic adenoma excision. Pain, fixation, and/or rapidly progressing signs or symptoms may herald malignant transformation.

Histopathology
Macroscopic examination shows a heterogeneous mass. A residual pleomorphic adenoma component is usually seen.
Microscopically, only the epithelial elements have malignant features {39}. The malignant histological subtypes include adenocarcinoma (most common), mucoepidermoid carcinoma, myoepithelial carcinoma, and (rarely) adenoid cystic carcinoma {1332}. A transition between malignant and residual benign pleomorphic adenoma can usually be seen, and this helps with diagnosis.
Capsular extension in carcinoma ex pleomorphic adenoma may be difficult to assess in recurrent or multinodular pleomorphic adenoma. Intracapsular carcinomas are those confined to the capsule. Minimally invasive carcinomas are defined by minimal breach (< 4–6 mm) of the residual pleomorphic adenoma capsule; carcinomas with capsular breach beyond 6 mm are considered widely invasive according to the major salivary gland criteria {314}.

Differential diagnosis
The differential diagnosis includes pleomorphic adenoma, mucoepidermoid carcinoma, adenocarcinoma, carcinosarcoma, and adenoid cystic carcinoma.

Histogenesis
Carcinoma ex pleomorphic adenoma arises from the epithelial and/or myoepithelial components of a pleomorphic adenoma, where progressive transformation of the cells results in an intracapsular carcinoma.

Genetic profile
The *PLAG1* and *HMGA2* genetic alterations found in benign pleomorphic adenoma are also present in carcinoma ex pleomorphic adenoma. Other alterations associated with malignant change include mutations of *TP53*, amplifications of *ERBB2* (*HER2*) and 12q (*MDM2*), deletions of 5q23.2-31.2, gains of 8q12.1 (*PLAG1*) and 8q22.1-24.1 (*MYC*) {1335}, and recurrent gains involving *NFIB* and *PDGFB* {1334}.

Prognosis and predictive factors
The prognosis depends on the malignant histological subtype, grade, and degree of invasion {39}. Widely invasive carcinoma ex pleomorphic adenoma is considered to have a poor prognosis, with a mean survival of 36 months {1335}. Intracapsular and minimally invasive cases are considered to constitute early disease, and they have a more favourable prognosis. Recurrences may occur in 50% of cases, and 70% of cases may have local or distant metastases {1334}.

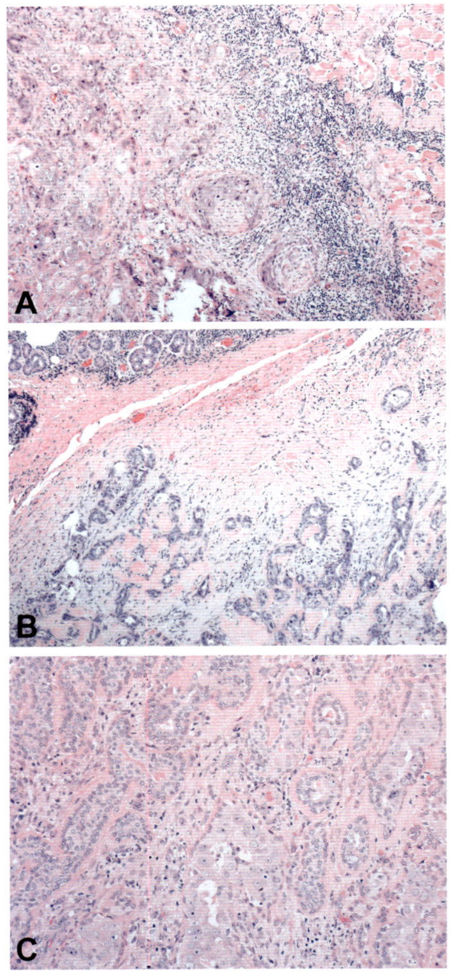

Fig. 5.12 Carcinoma ex pleomorphic adenoma. **A** A widely invasive example composed of infiltrating malignant glands invading into orbital skeletal muscle and showing perineural invasion; an increased lymphocytic response to invasive carcinoma is usually present and might be useful to highlight malignant change. **B** Malignant single glands abut the pleomorphic adenoma capsule. **C** Malignant glands are admixed with benign ductal glands within the pleomorphic adenoma and can be easily missed.

Pleomorphic adenoma of the lacrimal gland

Thaung C.
Iacob C.E.
White V.A.
Chan A.S.Y.

Definition
Pleomorphic adenoma of the lacrimal gland is a benign tumour composed of both epithelial and myoepithelial (stromal) elements, with considerable variation in the appearance and proportions of these components.

ICD-O code

Pleomorphic adenoma 8940/0

Synonyms

Mixed tumour; benign mixed tumour

Epidemiology

Pleomorphic adenomas constitute the majority of benign lacrimal gland epithelial tumours, and they account for approximately half of all lacrimal gland epithelial tumours overall {41,191,1331}. The mean patient age at presentation is 40 years, although the range is wide, from childhood to the ninth decade of life {1331}. No particular race or geographical location has been identified as a predisposing factor.

Localization

Nearly all cases at this anatomical site occur within the lacrimal gland proper, with about 90% occurring in the orbital lobe and the rest in the palpebral lobe {927,1352}. Very rare cases have occurred in other locations containing accessory or ectopic lacrimal gland tissue, including the eyebrow, the eyelids away from the palpebral lobe, and even intraocularly {869}.

Clinical features

Patients typically present with symptoms of a slow-growing painless mass, such as non-axial proptosis, diplopia, mechanical ptosis, and reduced vision {41,1331,1334}, with an average symptom duration of 2 years. Pain and inflammation are uncommon {191,920}.

Contrast-enhanced CT usually demonstrates a solid, well-defined oval or round soft tissue mass. There may be remodelling of the adjacent bone, with expansion of the lacrimal fossa, and occasionally calcification or cystic change {937,1199,1331,1352}. The internal architecture is often homogeneous on CT and heterogeneous on MRI {937,1352}.

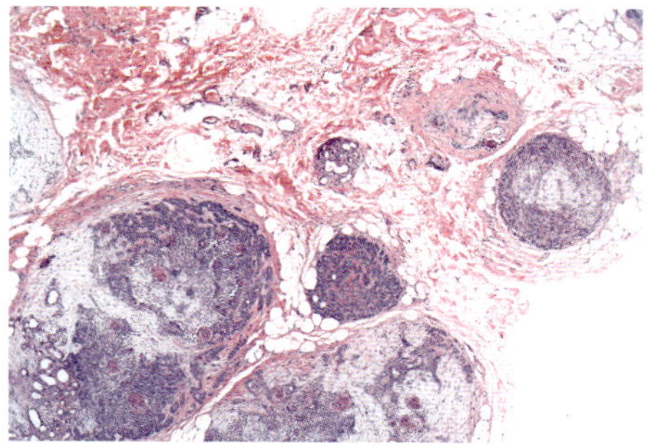

Fig. 5.14 Recurrent pleomorphic adenoma. Orbital fat with several separate nodules of recurrent tumour.

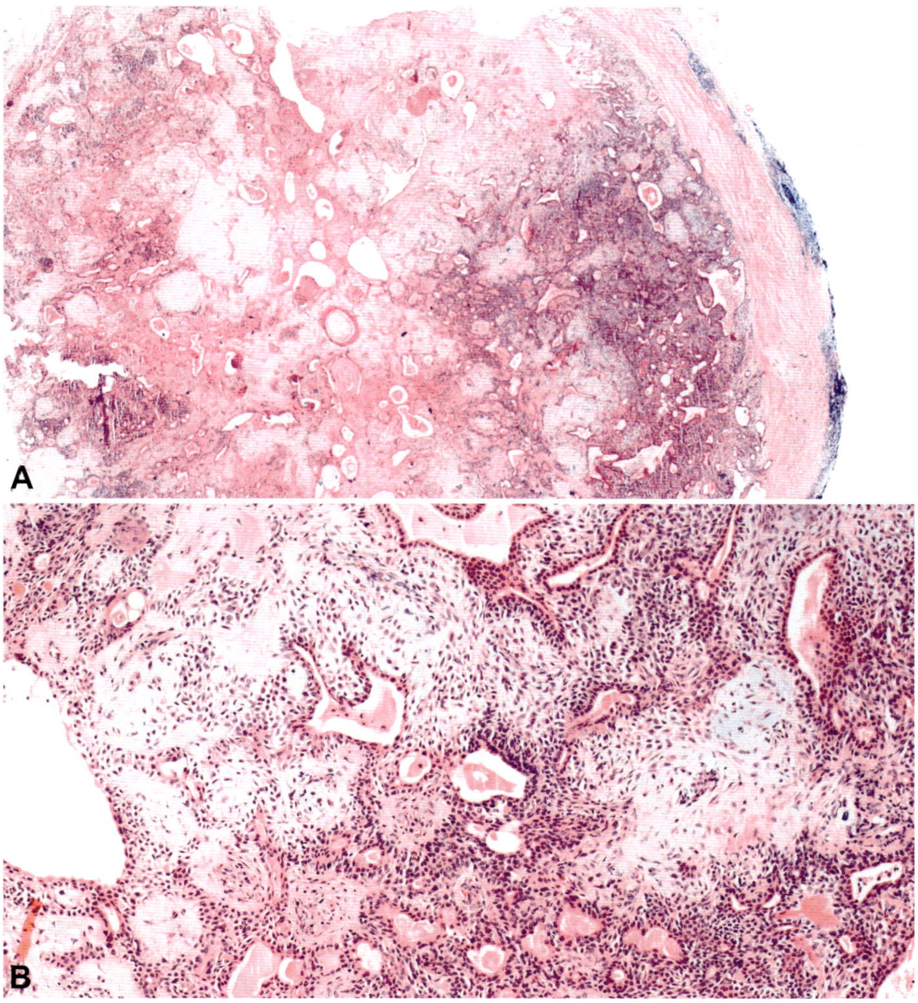

Fig. 5.13 Pleomorphic adenoma. **A** This example is encapsulated. **B** At higher magnification, the tumour's two components – epithelial and myoepithelial (stromal) – are apparent.

Histopathology

On macroscopic examination, pleomorphic adenoma is typically a well-defined nodule with a tan or pale cut surface, which may be soft and glistening or firm {191,1362}; 10% of cases show cysts macroscopically {191}.

The microscopic appearance varies depending on the relative proportions of the components. The epithelial areas generally have ductal structures with double-layered lumina and (variably) non-ductal epithelial cells including squamous, clear, round, and plasmacytoid cells {788,1331}. The stromal areas, derived from myoepithelial cells, may be fibrous, hyaline, myxoid, chondroid, or occasionally even osseous or adipose. There may be cystic degeneration, calcification, or ossification {191}. The cytology is generally bland, but occasional cases manifest focal mitoses or some cytological atypia (not enough to qualify as carcinoma ex pleomorphic adenoma) {1355}.

Pleomorphic adenomas have a pseudocapsule, which may be absent in areas with protrusion of satellite nodules {1362,1374}. The secretory material in the lumina may give a positive periodic acid–Schiff (PAS) reaction and be positive for mucicarmine {788}.

Immunohistochemistry is not usually necessary for diagnosis. In lacrimal gland pleomorphic adenomas, luminal epithelial cells may be positive for CK7 and CK8/18, and stromal cells can be positive for CK5/6, CK14, calponin, S100 protein, vimentin, and SMA {534}. The Ki-67 proliferation index is typically low {534,788}.

PLAG1 has been suggested as a useful immunohistochemical marker for pleomorphic adenoma of the salivary gland; it is expressed more strongly in the myoepithelial cells {254,772,999}. More recently, it has also been used as a marker for lacrimal gland pleomorphic adenoma, although the evidence base is still relatively small {788,1334}.

Differential diagnosis

The differential diagnosis includes myoepithelioma {772,1362}, adenoid cystic carcinoma, and carcinoma ex pleomorphic adenoma.

Histogenesis

To date, the evidence regarding the histogenesis of pleomorphic adenomas (from studies on salivary gland tumours) is inconclusive. Some studies suggest that this biphasic tumour originates from different cell types; others suggest an origin from a single cell type, possibly ductal epithelial, modified myoepithelial, or mesenchymal {41,324,900}. Epithelial–mesenchymal transition may be a key process {324}.

Genetic profile

The literature on lacrimal gland pleomorphic adenoma is limited. The following information relates predominantly to salivary gland pleomorphic adenoma.

In a substantial proportion of cases, salivary gland pleomorphic adenomas have specific chromosomal aberrations, including 8q12 rearrangements (found in 50% of cases) and 12q14-15 rearrangements (found in 10–15%) {1216}. Such rearrangements commonly affect *PLAG1* (on chromosome 8q12.1) and *HMGA2* (on chromosome 12q14.3). *PLAG1* rearrangements can give rise to fusion proteins, with partners including *CTNNB1*, *CHCHD7*, *LIFR*, and *TCEA1*. *HMGA2* rearrangements, which are less frequent, can also give rise to fusion proteins, with partners including *NFIB* and *WIF1* {772}.

PLAG1, a DNA-binding transcription factor, is frequently upregulated as a result of the above-described genetic changes {772}. In tumorigenesis, it may play a dual role of upregulating growth factor genes and downregulating genes that inhibit cell proliferation {253}. HMGA2, which is involved in cell proliferation and growth regulation, is overexpressed in several tumour types, including pleomorphic adenoma {1334}.

The genetic profile of lacrimal gland pleomorphic adenomas is less well characterized than that of salivary gland cases, but early evidence suggests that tumours in these two sites have similar profiles {1334}.

Prognosis and predictive factors

Pleomorphic adenoma is benign. However, it can recur (or rather, persist) if incompletely excised. A small number of cases may give rise to carcinoma (see *Carcinoma ex pleomorphic adenoma of the lacrimal gland*, p. 156). The incidence of recurrent tumour is difficult to assess because it depends on the surgical technique and length of follow-up; in one recent series, the rate was reported to be 25% {1334}.

Risk factors for recurrence (determined mainly on the basis of salivary gland studies) include incomplete surgical excision (in particular for tumours with an irregular outline or multinodular growth pattern) and preoperative or intraoperative tumour rupture (including rupture of the capsule) {893,1352,1375}. Recurrent tumours are often multifocal and therefore more difficult to excise than the original defined single nodule {1375}.

Malignant change has been described in as many as 5% of pleomorphic adenomas of the salivary gland {1360}; in recurrent tumours, the risk may be as high as 23% {1374}. Malignant change is associated with increasing length of history and number of recurrences {1374}.

Myoepithelial tumours of the lacrimal gland

Iacob C.E.
White V.A.
Croxatto J.O.
Thaung C.

Definition

Myoepithelial tumours of the lacrimal gland comprise myoepitheliomas and myoepithelial carcinomas. Myoepithelioma of the lacrimal gland is a benign lacrimal gland tumour composed of cells with myoepithelial differentiation. Myoepithelial carcinoma is the malignant counterpart of myoepithelioma, with invasive biological behaviour.

ICD-O codes

Myoepithelioma	8982/0
Myoepithelial carcinoma	8982/3

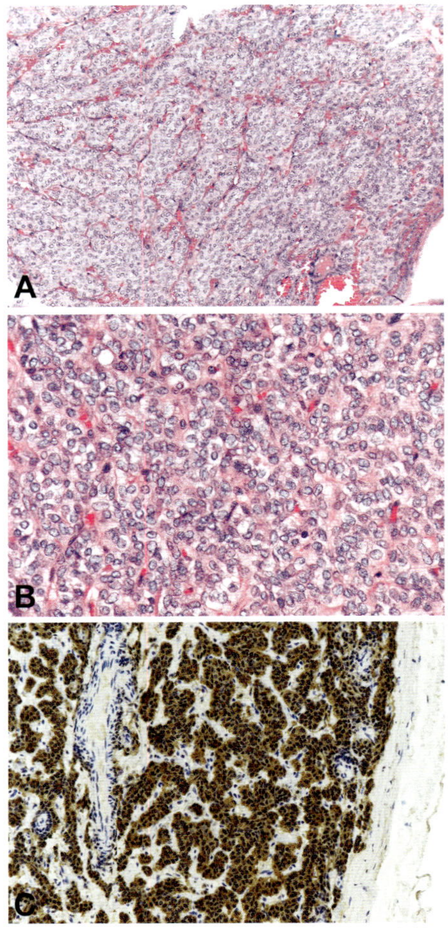

Fig. 5.15 Myoepithelioma of the lacrimal gland. **A** Trabecular growth pattern. **B** Sheets of cells with monotonous oval nuclei and variable pink cytoplasm. **C** A well-delineated neoplasm with consistently S100-positive myoepithelial cells.

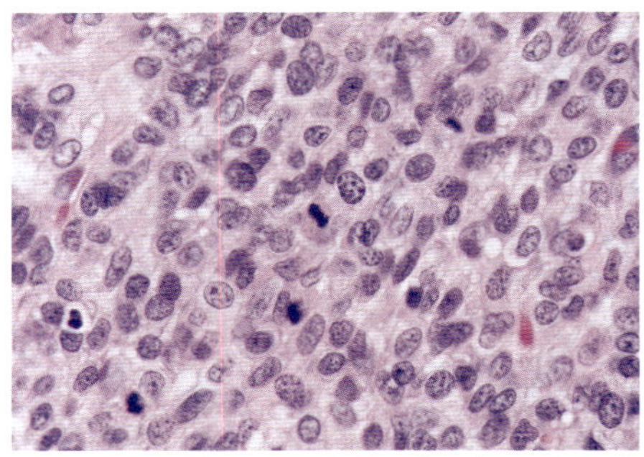

Fig. 5.16 Myoepithelial carcinoma of the lacrimal gland. Pleomorphic nuclei with mitoses (oil immersion).

Synonyms

Myoepithelioma: myoepithelial adenoma
Myoepithelial carcinoma: malignant myoepithelioma

Epidemiology

Myoepithelial tumours account for < 1% of lacrimal gland neoplasms. Patient age at presentation varies widely, and males and females are equally affected {116}.

Localization

Orbital myoepithelial neoplasms arise in the main lacrimal gland. Myoepithelial carcinomas of the lacrimal gland invade widely, including to the posterior cranial fossa or neighbouring bone structures of the orbit {466}.

Clinical features

Myoepitheliomas and myoepithelial carcinomas are usually non-tender, slow-growing, well-circumscribed orbital masses. They can arise de novo or as a clonal expansion in other tumours, such as pleomorphic adenomas {101}.

Histopathology

Myoepitheliomas are usually well delineated, and they are sometimes surrounded by a variably thick fibrous capsule. They are densely cellular and harbour spindle, plasmacytoid, epithelioid, or clear cells, proliferating in trabeculae or sheets. Occasional rudiments of ducts or microcysts can be encountered, and intracellular mucin production can be rarely seen. Interlacing fibrous fascicles can be present; tumours with hyalinized areas have also been described. The nuclei are usually normochromatic, smoothly bordered, and round to oval, without mitotic activity. Pink cytoplasm is present in a variable amount, with more-abundant cytoplasm in the plasmacytoid variant. The neoplastic cells are positive for cytokeratins (CK7 and CK14) and for myoepithelial markers (S100 protein, SMA, MSA, calponin, p63, and rarely GFAP) {431}.

Myoepithelial carcinomas can show cytologically bland cells or can be composed of cells with nuclear atypia and mitoses; in both cases, the tumours are characterized by invasion into neighbouring structures (e.g. the lacrimal gland parenchyma, orbital soft tissue, and perineural or vascular spaces) {411}. Myoepithelial carcinomas can arise from pleomorphic adenomas.

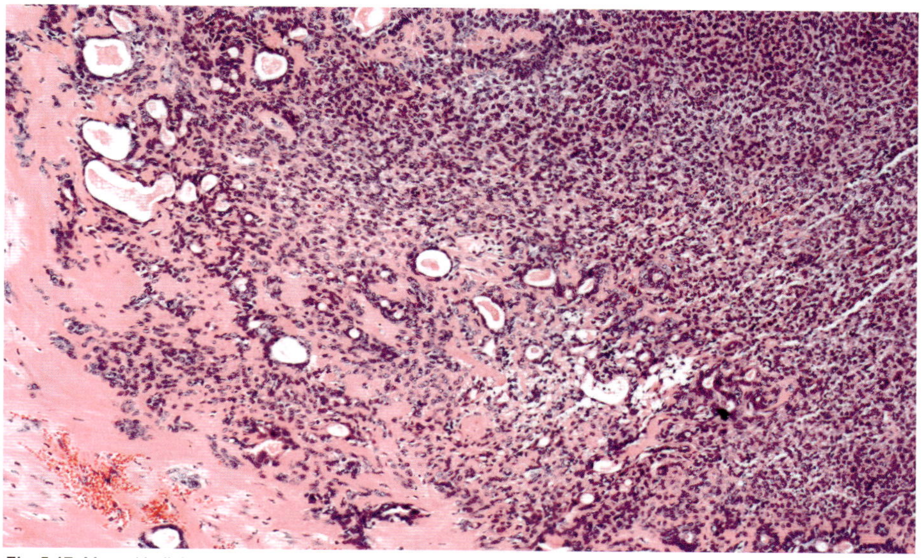

Fig. 5.17 Myoepithelial carcinoma of the lacrimal gland arising in pleomorphic adenoma. A lacrimal gland pleomorphic adenoma on the left gives rise to a myoepithelial carcinoma on the right; the carcinoma is cellular.

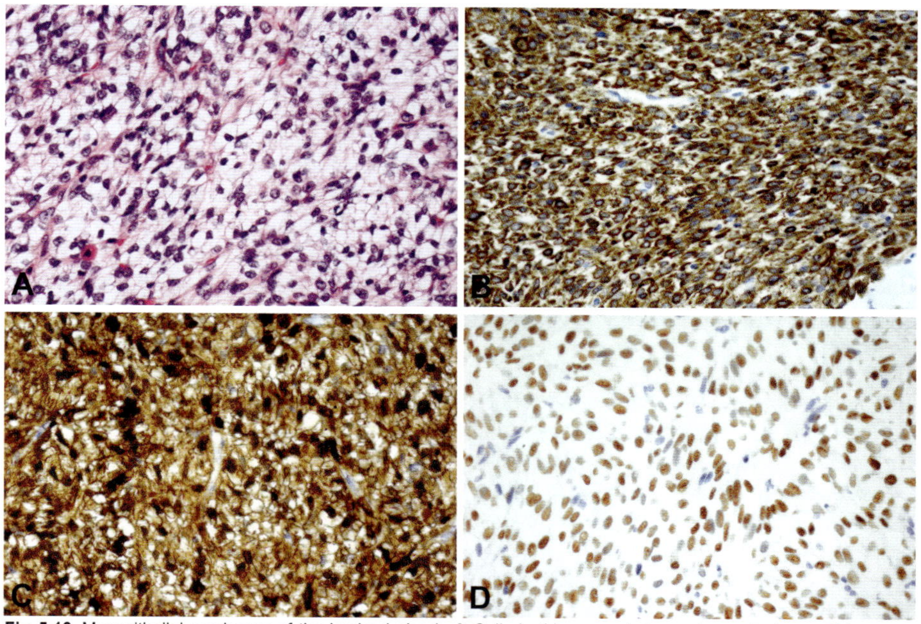

Fig. 5.18 Myoepithelial carcinoma of the lacrimal gland. **A** Cells in this example have clear cytoplasm. **B** Immunohistochemical staining (AE1/AE3) is positive for cytokeratins. **C** The tumour cells express S100 protein. **D** The nuclei express p63.

Differential diagnosis

Myoepithelial tumours can be distinguished from pleomorphic adenomas by their lack of mesenchymal proliferation and absence of ubiquitous ductal differentiation. Myoepithelial tumours with spindle cells must be distinguished from mesenchymal neoplasms; their cytokeratin reaction is essential in this regard. Clear cell myoepithelial tumours show some morphological similarities to clear cell adenocarcinoma, but the latter fails to show immunoreaction for myoepithelial markers.

Histogenesis

At this site, myoepithelial tumours arise from the myoepithelial cells of the lacrimal gland ducts.

Genetic profile

No specific genetic alterations have been described in myoepithelioma. In myoepithelial carcinoma, in particular the clear cell variant, *EWSR1* gene rearrangement has been reported {466,1198}. An immunohistochemical study conducted on a sizable cohort of salivary gland myoepitheliomas and myoepithelial carcinomas found that the benign tumours showed significantly increased expression of positive regulators of the cell cycle (cyclin D1 and E2F1); the malignant tumours additionally showed prominent accumulation of p53 protein {1313}. These findings have not yet been validated in lacrimal gland tumours.

Prognosis and predictive factors

Local complete excision is usually curative for myoepitheliomas. Myoepithelial carcinomas have a recurrence rate of > 20% {116}, and late metastasis may occur.

Oncocytic tumours of the lacrimal gland

Iacob C.E.
White V.A.
Croxatto J.O.
Thaung C.

Definition

Oncocytic tumours of the lacrimal gland are neoplasms (oncocytomas and oncocytic carcinomas) composed of epithelial cells with a large amount of granular eosinophilic cytoplasm rich in mitochondria.

ICD-O codes

Oncocytoma	8290/0
Oncocytic carcinoma	8290/3

Synonyms

Oncocytoma: oncocytic adenoma; oxyphilic adenoma
Oncocytic carcinoma: oncocytic adenocarcinoma; malignant oncocytoma

Epidemiology

Oncocytomas are uncommon, accounting for < 1% of lacrimal gland neoplasms. They are tumours of adulthood, with incidence peaking in the sixth and eight decades of life, and they tend to have a slight female predominance {879}. Oncocytic carcinomas are extremely rare at this site; one case arising in the setting of neurofibromatosis has been described {98}.

Etiology

A study of oncocytic thyroid tumours suggested that a defect in the oxidative phosphorylation chain resulted in low ATP levels triggering excessive stimulation of mitochondrial development. Such a mechanism might be responsible for oncocytic metaplasia, hyperplasia, or neoplasia {1038}, but has not yet been validated for periocular oncocytic lesions.

Localization

Periocular oncocytic neoplasms arise in the ducts of the accessory and main lacrimal glands. In accessory lacrimal glands, the caruncle is the most frequent location, followed by the conjunctiva, lacrimal sac, plica semilunaris, and eyelid (peripunctal). Periocular oncocytic neoplasms arising in the ducts of the main lacrimal gland include orbital oncocytic tumours {555,879}.

Clinical features

Oncocytomas are well-delineated masses with pushing borders causing compressive phenomena according to their location (e.g. obstruction of the lacrimal passage and swelling of eyelid). Orbital tumours can cause fullness of the temporal aspect of the orbit, proptosis, nasal deviation of the eye, and eyelid ptosis. Early-stage oncocytic carcinomas can also be well delineated.

Histopathology

Oncocytomas are well delineated and display solid or papillary architecture, with a proliferation of polygonal epithelial cells showing a low N:C ratio and bland nuclear features. Abundant eosinophilic granular cytoplasm due to massive mitochondrial accumulation is characteristic. Phosphotungstic acid haematoxylin staining may be helpful in discerning these cytoplasmic details by optical microscopy. Ultrastructural analysis reveals a plethora of cytoplasmic mitochondria {152}. Immunohistochemical staining with antimitochondrial antibodies (e.g. MU213-UC) may also be helpful. The immunohistochemical profile of oncocytomas is similar to that of lacrimal gland ducts: they are positive for CK4, CK5/6, CK7, CK8, CK17, and CK18 but show no labelling for CK20 or for markers of keratinizing epithelium {879}.

Oncocytic carcinomas display nuclear atypia, mitoses, and infiltrative features, with invasion of neighbouring soft tissues or bony structures {98,560,1263}.

Differential diagnosis

Warthin tumour is easily distinguished from oncocytoma by its accompanying lymphoid hyperplasia. Differentiation from oncocytic hyperplasia usually relies on the nodular, well-circumscribed appearance of oncocytoma

Histogenesis

Oncocytic transformation in the ducts of the lacrimal glands (accessory or main) forms an almost indistinguishable continuum between oncocytic metaplasia, hyperplasia, and neoplasia. Similar oncocytic transformation is seen in the epithelia of other anatomical sites, such as the thyroid, salivary gland, kidney, parathyroid, pituitary, breast, and sinonasal tract {152}.

Genetic profile

Salivary gland oncocytoma has been found to have several-fold increased cytoplasmic mitochondrial DNA, as well as mitochondrial DNA transcripts coupled with substantial upregulation of nuclear

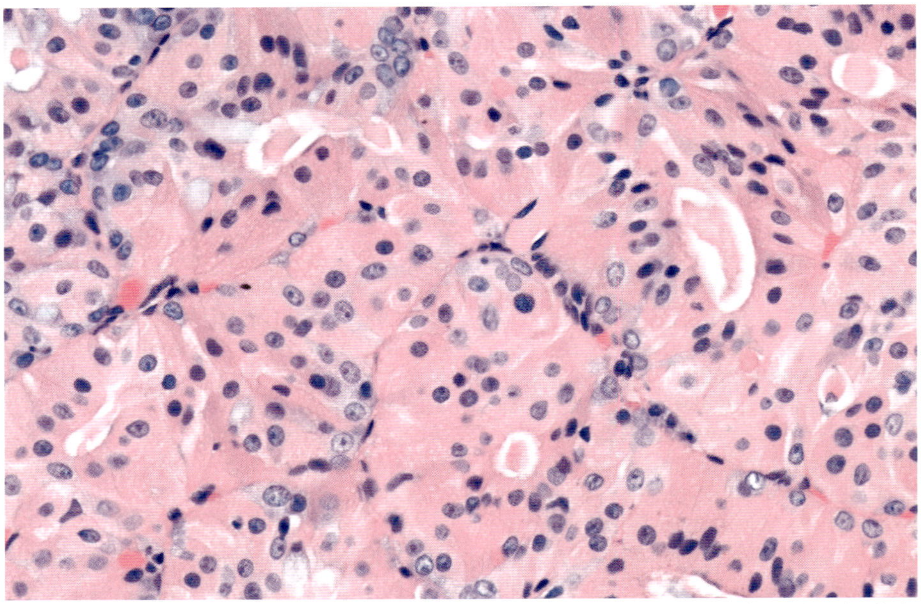

Fig. 5.19 Oncocytoma of the lacrimal gland. Eccentric smoothly bordered nuclei with vesicular chromatin and a single conspicuous nucleolus, accompanied by abundant granular cytoplasm.

genes involved in oxidative phosphorylation; these findings suggest a coordinated regulation of nuclear and mitochondrial DNA {469}, but such findings have not been validated in the lacrimal gland.

Prognosis and predictive factors

Complete surgical excision is the treatment of choice for oncocytomas and oncocytic carcinomas.

Rare neoplasms of the lacrimal gland

White V.A.
Chan A.S.Y.
Croxatto J.O.
Iacob C.E.
Salomao D.R.
Thaung C.

Epithelial–myoepithelial carcinoma of the lacrimal gland

Definition

Epithelial–myoepithelial carcinoma of the lacrimal gland is a low-grade malignant salivary-type carcinoma characterized by a biphasic arrangement of inner luminal ductal cells and outer myoepithelial cells {1059,1060}.

ICD-O code

Epithelial–myoepithelial carcinoma 8562/3

Synonym

Adenomyoepithelioma

Epidemiology

Epithelial–myoepithelial carcinoma is an uncommon neoplasm; only 6 cases have been reported in the lacrimal gland, some of which arose in a pleomorphic adenoma {63,177,411,1189,1316,1376}.

Localization

Epithelial–myoepithelial carcinoma occurs in the orbital lobe of the lacrimal gland.

Clinical features

Patients present with a slow-growing mass lesion confined to the gland.

Histopathology

Epithelial–myoepithelial carcinoma displays a pattern of simple glands with a distinctive biphasic morphology visible on H&E staining, with inner cuboidal, densely eosinophilic luminal cells and outer lining myoepithelial cells, which frequently have clear or vacuolated cytoplasm. Myoepithelial overgrowth is common. High-grade transformation has been described. Staining for low-molecular-weight cytokeratins highlights the inner luminal layer, whereas staining for myoepithelial markers, such as SMA, p63, and S100 protein, highlights the outer layer. High-grade transformation is characterized by anaplasia and an increased mitotic rate, with loss of the bilayered pattern.

Differential diagnosis

The differential diagnosis includes other biphasic neoplasms of salivary gland type, including pleomorphic adenoma and adenoid cystic carcinoma.

Genetic profile

Approximately one quarter of salivary cases have shown *HRAS* mutations {1061}.

Prognosis and predictive factors

Too few cases have been reported for an adequate assessment of prognostic and predictive factors. In the salivary gland, most cases are indolent, but poor outcome is more common with larger tumours, extension to resection margins,

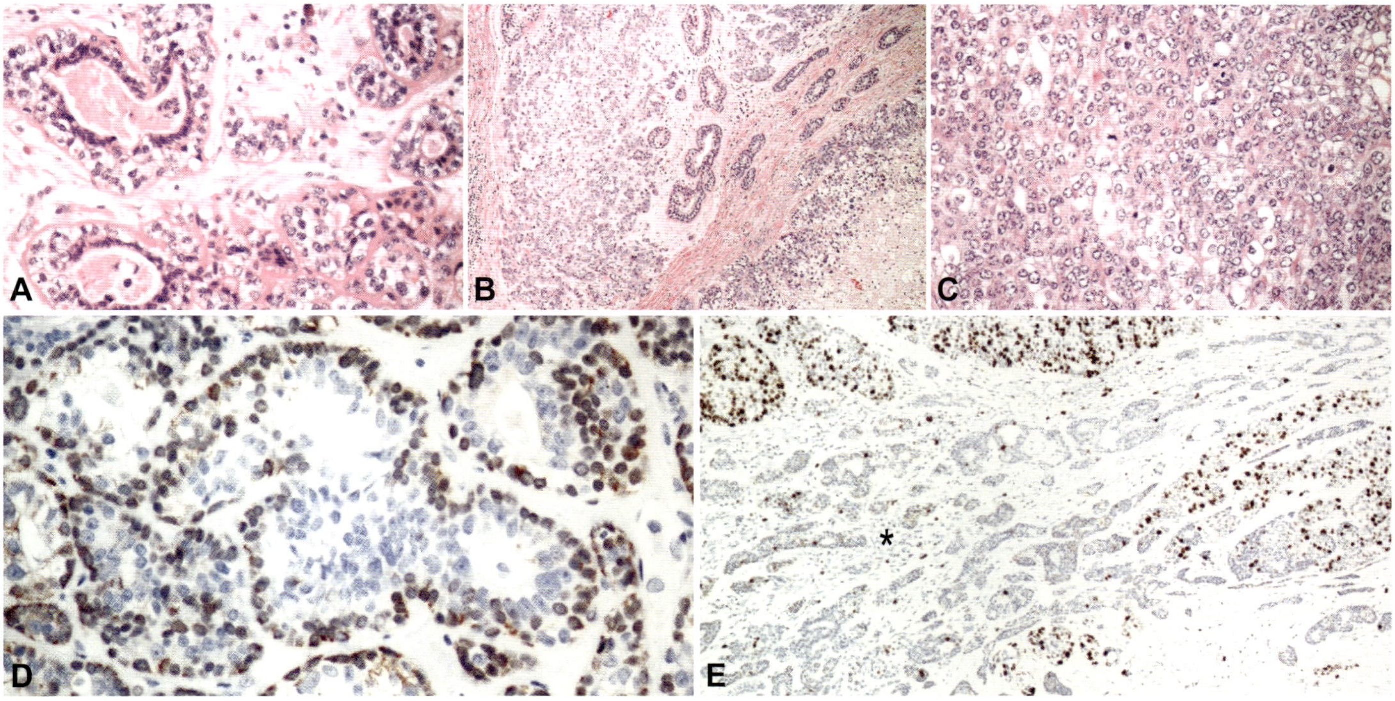

Fig. 5.20 Epithelial–myoepithelial carcinoma. **A** The typical biphasic pattern, with an inner cuboidal layer and an outer layer of myoepithelial cells, which are often clear. **B** This tumour showed areas of high-grade transformation (dedifferentiation) with loss of the biphasic pattern. **C** The areas of high-grade transformation (dedifferentiation) showed solid areas with loss of the biphasic pattern, increased pleomorphism, and mitoses. **D** p63 staining highlights the outer layer of myoepithelial cells, demonstrating the biphasic pattern. **E** Ki-67 staining shows the difference in proliferative activity between the typical epithelial–myoepithelial carcinoma pattern (asterisk) and the high-grade area (top and bottom).

myoepithelial anaplasia, high-grade transformation, necrosis, and lymphovascular invasion.

Low-grade intraductal carcinoma of the lacrimal gland

Definition
Low-grade intraductal carcinoma of the lacrimal gland is a non-invasive neoplasm characterized by intracystic/intraductal proliferation of neoplastic epithelial cells; it is similar to intraductal carcinoma of the breast {1062}.

ICD-O code
Low-grade intraductal carcinoma	8500/2

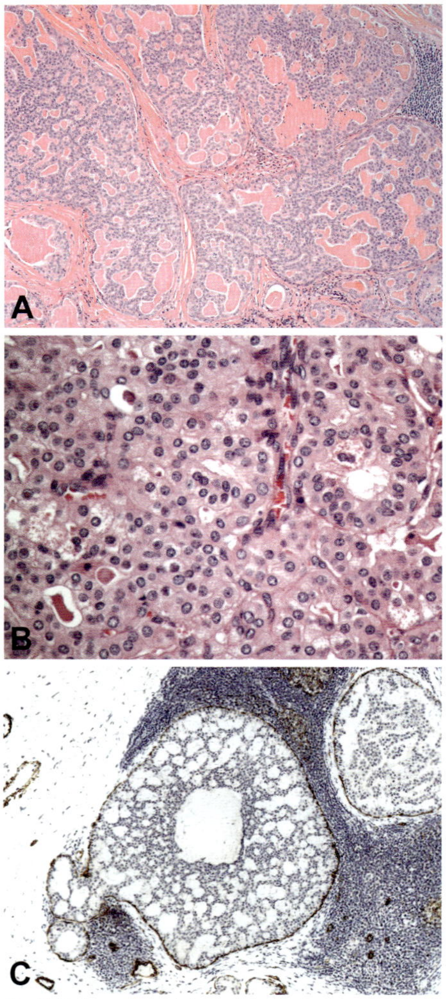

Fig. 5.21 Low-grade intraductal carcinoma. **A** Closely packed areas of intraductal carcinoma. **B** Minimally pleomorphic cells bearing a resemblance to low-grade ductal carcinoma in situ of breast. **C** A rim of myoepithelial cells surrounding intraductal carcinoma (smooth muscle myosin heavy chain staining).

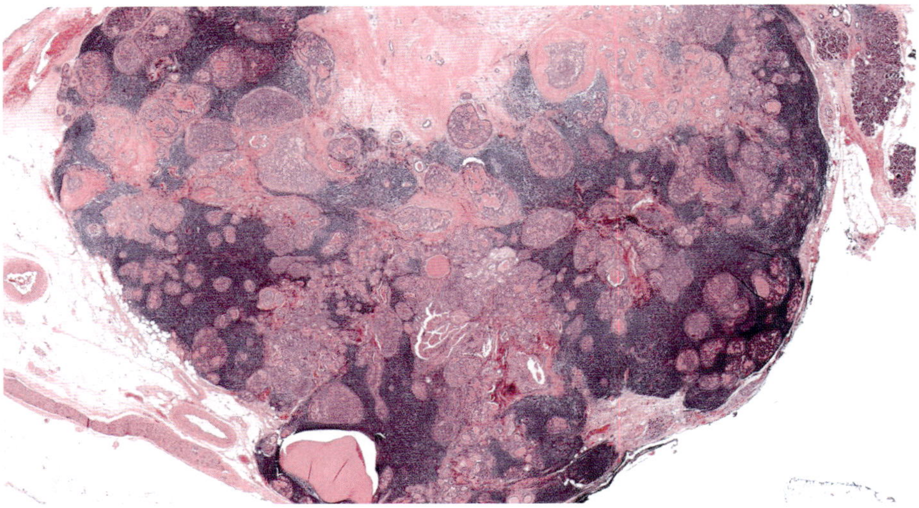

Fig. 5.22 Low-grade intraductal carcinoma. A low-power view showing the circumscribed nature of the tumour, with involved ducts scattered throughout the lacrimal gland, intense lymphoid infiltrate, sclerotic areas, and a small amount of remaining glandular tissue visible at the upper right.

Synonyms
Cribriform cystadenocarcinoma; low-grade salivary duct carcinoma

Epidemiology
Only one case has been reported in the lacrimal gland {151} and only a small number of cases in the salivary glands {128,1354}.

Clinical features
Patients present with a slow-growing mass lesion confined to the gland.

Histopathology
Histopathology shows a proliferation of variously sized cysts and lobules of malignant cells, all surrounded by a layer of myoepithelial cells, similar to the histopathology of intraductal carcinoma of breast. The lining of myoepithelial cells should be highlighted by staining with p63, S100 protein, or smooth muscle myosin heavy chain to confirm the in situ status. The cells do not stain for estrogen receptor, progesterone receptor, or ERBB2 (HER2).

Differential diagnosis
The presence of invasion as seen in high-grade ductal carcinoma should be excluded.

Prognosis and predictive factors
Because this is an in situ neoplasm, complete excision should be curative; incomplete excision could result in recurrence.

Secretory carcinoma of the lacrimal gland

Definition
Secretory carcinoma of the lacrimal gland is a low-grade carcinoma (with a resemblance to secretory carcinoma of the breast) that contains the *ETV6-NTRK3* gene fusion {1062}.

ICD-O code
Secretory carcinoma	8502/3

Synonym
Mammary analogue secretory carcinoma

Epidemiology
Secretory carcinoma in the salivary glands was first described in 2010 {1197}. Most cases of secretory carcinoma were previously classified as the papillary–cystic type of acinic cell carcinoma, which is now known to be rare. Secretory carcinoma of the salivary glands, which is similar to juvenile secretory carcinoma of the breast, is common in the minor salivary glands. One case in the lacrimal gland was initially diagnosed as acinic cell carcinoma.

Localization
Secretory carcinoma occurs in the orbital lobe of the lacrimal gland.

Clinical features
Patients present with a slow-growing mass in the lacrimal gland.

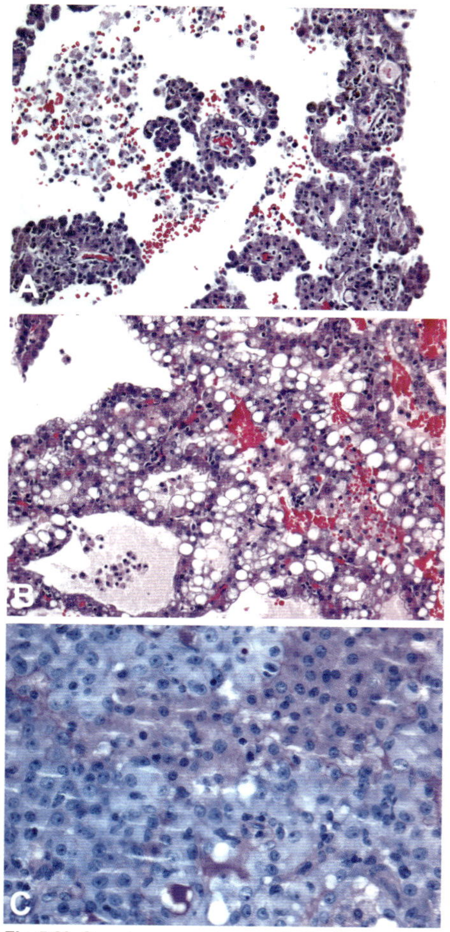

Fig. 5.23 Secretory carcinoma. **A** Papillary structures. **B** Macrocystic and microcystic areas. **C** Periodic acid–Schiff (PAS) staining reveals a faint cytoplasmic blush and extracellular mucin, but does not reveal the true secretory granules seen in acinic cell carcinoma.

Histopathology

Secretory carcinoma bears a superficial resemblance to the papillary–cystic type of acinic cell carcinoma, but it is analogous to secretory carcinoma of the breast. It is circumscribed, but may be infiltrative with perineural invasion. It shows cysts lined by papillary structures, microcystic areas, and solid areas. The cells have abundant granular eosinophilic cytoplasm, but true zymogen granules (as seen in acinic cell carcinoma) are not present, as demonstrated by periodic acid–Schiff (PAS) staining, although there are prominent extracellular PAS-positive secretions. The carcinoma stains strongly for S100 protein and mammaglobin, which are defining features.

Differential diagnosis

The differential diagnosis includes acinic cell carcinoma. FISH analysis for the

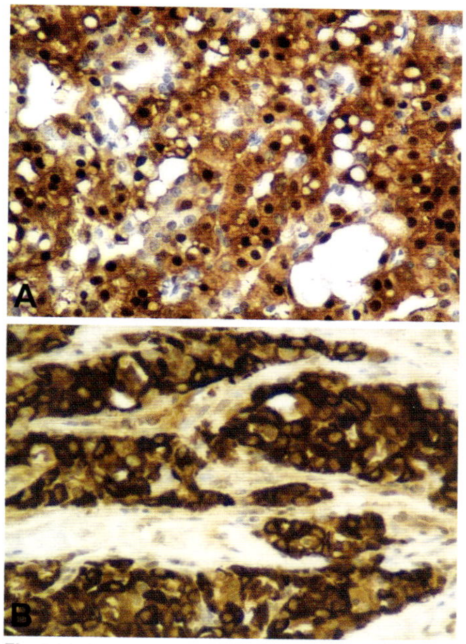

Fig. 5.24 Secretory carcinoma. Strong staining for S100 protein (**A**) and mammaglobin (**B**).

ETV6-NTRK3 translocation should be performed to confirm the diagnosis.

Genetic profile

The tumour contains the translocation t(12;15)(p13;q25), which fuses the *ETV6* gene on chromosome 12 with the *NTRK3* gene on chromosome 15 {1059,1061}.

Prognosis and predictive factors

In the salivary glands, this is a low-grade malignancy, despite the presence of local metastases in 25% of cases. High-grade transformation has been reported in the salivary glands; this and high clinical stage are adverse prognostic factors.

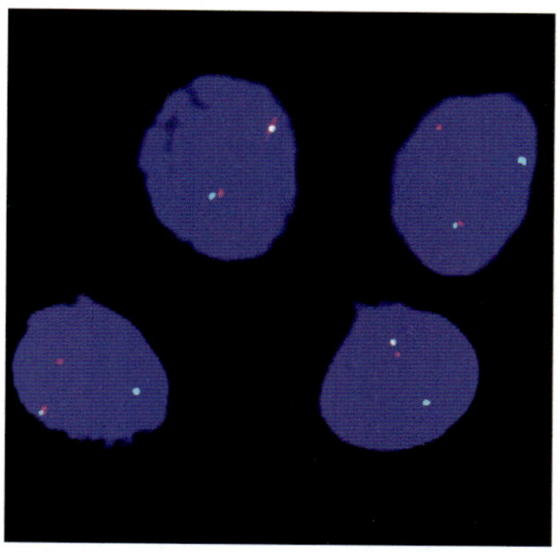

Fig. 5.25 Secretory carcinoma. *ETV6* break-apart dual-colour FISH confirms the specific translocation present in secretory carcinoma (with DAPI counterstaining).

Hybrid neoplasms of the lacrimal gland

Definition

Hybrid neoplasms are defined as being composed of two distinct types of salivary adenoma or (usually) carcinoma that are present in the same area, producing a single mass lesion.

ICD-O codes

Code as both tumour types.

Epidemiology

At the time of a recent review, 38 cases had been described in the literature; most occurred in the parotid gland, but 1 case was described in the lacrimal gland {475}. The male-to-female ratio was 1.6:1, and patient age at diagnosis was 26–81 years.

Localization

Hybrid neoplasms arise as a unilateral mass within the lacrimal gland.

Clinical features

Patients present with a mass lesion of the lacrimal gland, which can be slow-growing or fast-growing.

Histopathology

In 10 of the 38 cases described, the tumour combination consisted of adenoid cystic carcinoma and epithelial–myoepithelial carcinoma. In another 11 cases, adenoid cystic carcinoma was one of the components, and in another 7 cases, epithelial–myoepithelial carcinoma was a component. The reported lacrimal case consisted of squamous cell carcinoma and salivary duct carcinoma. A lacrimal case composed of squamous cell carcinoma and epithelial–myoepithelial carcinoma has also been seen.

Differential diagnosis

The question has been raised as to whether most hybrid carcinomas actually constitute a lower-grade carcinoma with high-grade transformation {1062,1355}. To date, there is no conclusive evidence for either hypothesis. In order for a diagnosis of hybrid carcinoma or carcinoma with high-grade transformation to be made, it is crucial that the entire neoplasm be examined, because the secondary component may constitute only a small proportion of the mass.

Prognosis and predictive factors

The prognosis depends on the higher-grade component.

Acinic cell carcinoma of the lacrimal gland

Definition

Acinic cell carcinoma of the lacrimal gland is a malignant salivary gland–type neoplasm with acinar differentiation and zymogen secretory granules {260}. It should not be mistaken for a mammary analogue secretory carcinoma {722}.

ICD-O code

Acinic cell carcinoma 8550/3

Synonyms

Acinic cell adenocarcinoma; acinar cell carcinoma

Epidemiology

Acinic cell carcinoma is an extremely rare lacrimal gland tumour, with a slight female predominance. It is more common in White populations (accounting for 85% of all cases), and it has a bimodal age presentation, with incidence peaks among individuals aged > 60 years and < 20 years {75,899}.

Localization

Acinic cell carcinoma in the lacrimal gland may extend into the orbit and intracranially. Orbital extension from a sinonasal acinic cell carcinoma may also occur {75,847}.

Clinical features

Patients present with a slow-growing, painless lacrimal gland mass associated with inferior displacement of the eye or proptosis {1308}. Lymph node metastases are rare and usually associated with high-grade transformation.

Histopathology

Macroscopically, the tumours are circumscribed and encapsulated, with firm greyish-white solid areas and/or cystic areas. Infiltrative borders and multinodularity are uncommon in primary tumours but may be present in recurrences {1308}.

Microscopically, the tumour cells are round polygonal cells with abundant basophilic granular cytoplasm, central/eccentric vesicular nuclei, and distinct nucleoli {260,545}. The cytoplasmic granules give a diastase-resistant positive periodic acid–Schiff (PAS) reaction. Occasionally, clear cells may be present. The growth patterns include solid (seen in 25% of cases), microcystic, follicular, papillary, and cystic. The solid growth pattern is composed of sheets of tumour cells with a trabecular or acinar arrangement. The microcystic pattern is lattice-like, with interspersed small lumina. The rarer papillary–cystic variant is characterized by macrocystic spaces and papillary proliferations {75}. Occasionally, stromal lymphoid aggregates may be substantial. Necrosis, mitoses, nuclear pleomorphism, and perineural invasion are present when tumours show high-grade transformation or so-called dedifferentiation to a form resembling high-grade adenocarcinoma or undifferentiated carcinoma.

DOG1 and SOX10 are immunopositive (but not diagnostic) in tumours with acinar cell and intercalated duct cell features {847,1308}. Acinic cell carcinomas are usually negative for p63, S100 protein, and mammaglobin, which are useful markers for excluding mammary analogue secretory carcinoma.

Differential diagnosis

Acinic cell carcinomas with clear cells and the microcystic and follicular variants may resemble mucoepidermoid carcinoma. Papillary–cystic cases with stromal lymphoid aggregates may be mistaken for papillary cystadenoma. Mammary analogue secretory carcinoma positive for the *ETV6-NTRK3* translocation should also be excluded, in particular as a differential diagnosis of the papillary–cystic variant {1308}.

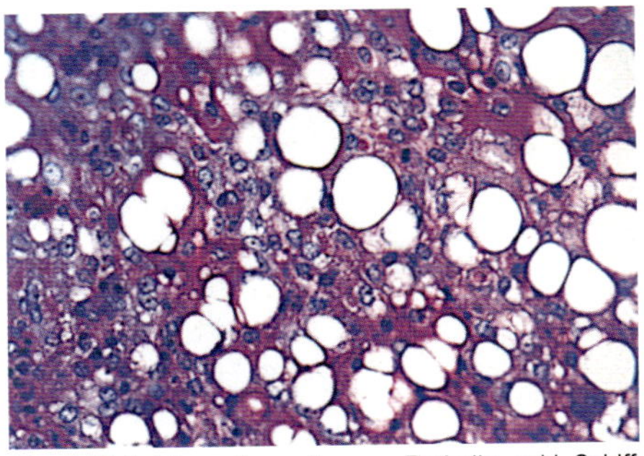

Fig. 5.27 Acinic cell carcinoma. Periodic acid–Schiff (PAS) staining showing the cytoplasmic granularity as PAS-positive secretions {996}.

Histogenesis

These tumours are thought to arise from stem cells located at the acinar–intercalated ductal region of the salivary or lacrimal gland {1308}.

Genetic profile

Genetic events that have been implicated in acinic cell carcinoma (with unknown clinical significance) include alterations in the PI3K pathway and the PTEN-activated mTOR signalling pathway, as well as mutations in the tumour suppressor gene *CDKN2A*, the p53-binding gene *PPP1R13B*, and the cell growth regulator gene *EP300* {1308}.

Genetic susceptibility

Familial cases of acinic cell carcinomas in the setting of Cowden syndrome suggest a role for germline *PTEN* mutations {1308}.

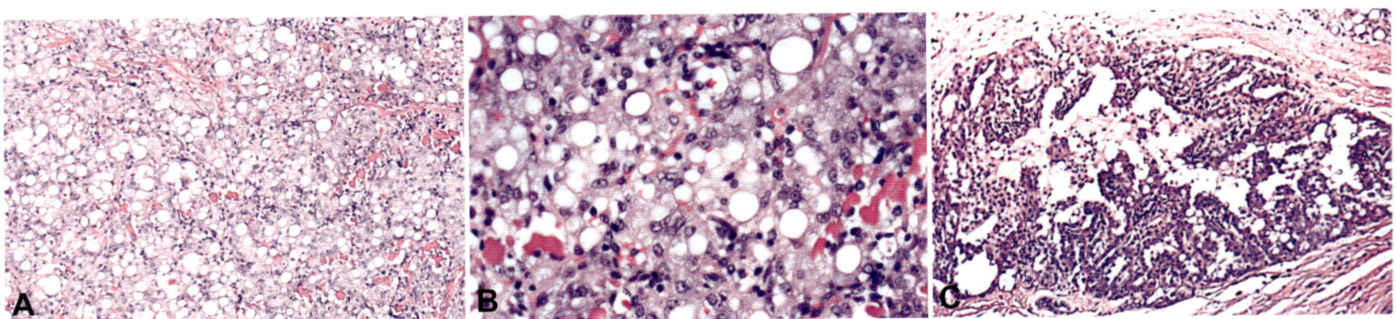

Fig. 5.26 Acinic cell carcinoma. **A** The carcinoma is composed of sheets of cells similar to glandular acini. **B** There are scattered lumina of glandular acini present within sheets of tumour cells with round vesicular nuclei, prominent nucleoli, and numerous microcystic vacuoles. **C** Papillary–cystic architecture is seen when microcystic spaces coalesce {996}.

Prognosis and predictive factors

Acinic cell carcinomas are low-grade malignancies, with a 20-year disease-specific survival rate of nearly 90%. Poor prognostic factors include older age, pain and fixation at presentation, male sex, non-White race, and more extensive disease {899}. Histological features associated with poor prognosis include extracapsular extension, increased mitoses, a desmoplastic and lymphoid stromal reaction, perineural and vascular invasion, and high-grade features {722,1308}.

Warthin tumour of the lacrimal gland

Definition

Warthin tumour is a benign neoplasm of the lacrimal and salivary glands. It is composed of oncocytic epithelium arranged in cystic, ductal, and papillary structures surrounded by a dense lymphoid stroma {1412}.

ICD-O code

Adenolymphoma/ Warthin tumour 8561/0

Synonyms

Adenolymphoma; papillary cystadenoma lymphomatosum; cystadenolymphoma

Epidemiology

This is the second most common benign neoplasm of the salivary glands, but it is rare in the lacrimal gland, with only one seemingly definite case reported to date {118}. Warthin tumours occur in older individuals (in the sixth and seventh decades of life), with a slight male predominance.

Etiology

In the salivary glands, Warthin tumour has been linked to cigarette smoking, irradiation, autoimmune diseases, and EBV infection, but not all of these associations have been substantiated. In the lacrimal gland, no definite etiological factors are known.

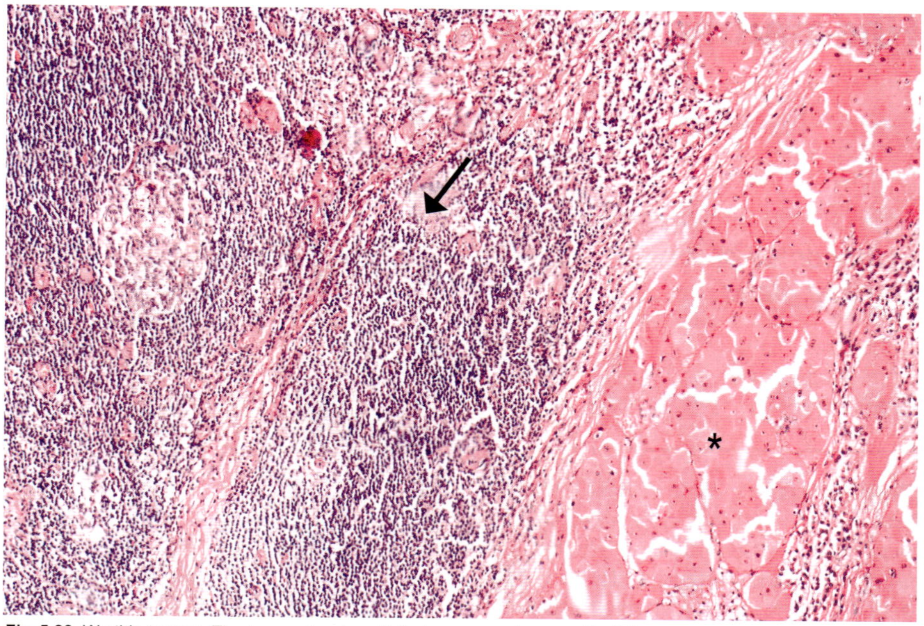

Fig. 5.28 Warthin tumour. The tumour has two distinct components: an epithelial component with oncocytic changes (asterisk) and a lymphocytic component with a germinal centre (arrow).

Localization

The single reported lacrimal gland case occurred in the orbital lobe of the gland.

Clinical features

The tumour presents as a slow-growing mass lesion indistinguishable from other benign lacrimal gland tumours.

Histopathology

The tumour shows two distinct morphological components: an epithelial component and a lymphocytic component. There are strips of regular, bilayered, markedly oncocytic epithelium with inner columnar cells and outer cuboidal cells. Oncocytic cells have granular eosinophilic cytoplasm and round nuclei with prominent nucleoli. The ductal and papillary structures are surrounded by a dense infiltrate of small benign lymphocytes, with occasional germinal centres. The tumours are well circumscribed, are surrounded by a thin capsule, and do not invade the surrounding gland.

Differential diagnosis

The differential diagnosis includes lymphoma and oncocytoma.

Histogenesis

In the parotid gland, Warthin tumours are postulated to arise within salivary gland tissue entrapped within intraparotid lymph nodes. However, the same assumption cannot be made for cases occurring in the lacrimal gland or in other salivary glands.

Genetic profile

A subset of Warthin tumours have the same specific translocation as a subset of mucoepidermoid carcinomas: a t(11;19)(q21-22;p13) translocation producing the CRTC1-MAML2 fusion protein {1412}.

Prognosis and predictive factors

As is the case for other benign lacrimal tumours, complete excision with a rim of normal tissue is the standard treatment for Warthin tumour, and this treatment is usually curative.

Haematolymphoid tumours of the lacrimal gland

Lymphomas of the lacrimal gland

Coupland S.E.
Bermúdez Magner A.
Chan A.S.Y.

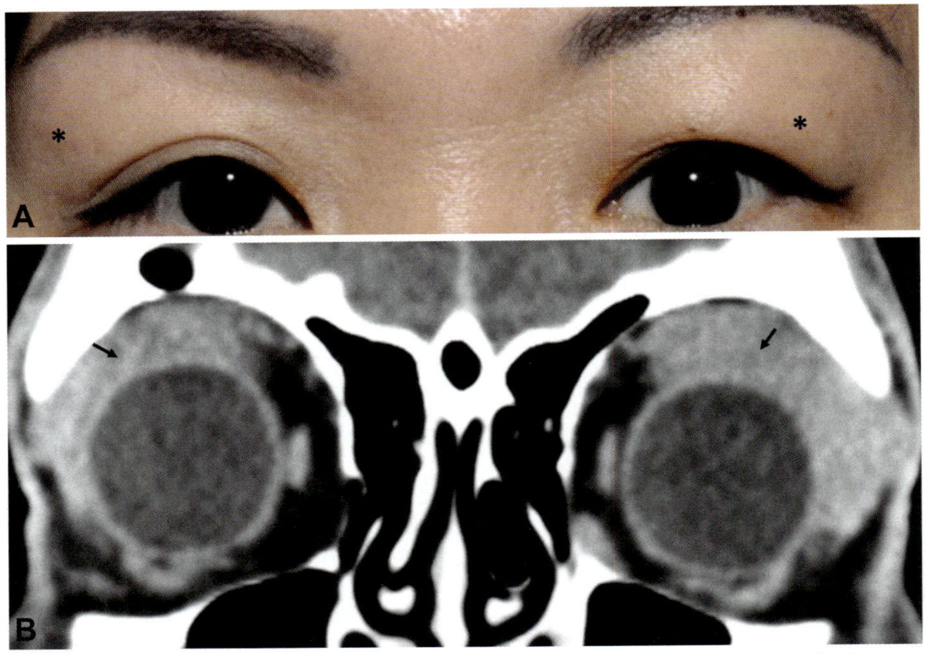

Fig. 5.29 Lacrimal gland lymphoma. **A** Bilateral superotemporal eyelid fullness (asterisks) due to bilateral lacrimal swelling. **B** CT coronal view showing bilateral lacrimal gland enlargement in the superotemporal orbit (arrows); note the tumour's moulding around the globe without causing globe deformity.

Definition

Primary lacrimal gland lymphomas are malignant proliferations of lymphocytes arising in the lacrimal gland without evidence of concurrent systemic lymphoma. Secondary lacrimal gland lymphomas occur in patients as part of disseminated non-Hodgkin lymphoma {233}.

ICD-O codes

MALT lymphoma	9699/3
Follicular lymphoma	9690/3
Diffuse large B-cell lymphoma	9680/3

Synonyms

Lymphomas of the lacrimal gland; lacrimal gland non-Hodgkin lymphomas; lacrimal gland extranodal marginal zone lymphomas of mucosa-associated lymphoid tissue (MALT lymphoma)

Epidemiology

Lacrimal gland lymphomas are rare, accounting for about 9% of all ocular adnexal lymphomas, which in turn constitute 2% of all extranodal lymphomas {43,231,340,350,959}. They occur most commonly in elderly women, particularly in the setting of Sjögren syndrome. There is no race predilection.

Etiology

The etiology is unknown, but lacrimal gland lymphomas are presumed to be caused by chronic antigen stimulation leading to chronic dacryoadenitis, reactive lymphoid hyperplasia, and ultimately lymphoma {43,231,340,350,959}.

Localization

Lacrimal gland lymphomas occur in the superolateral aspects of the orbits.

Clinical features

These lymphomas usually present as painless palpable masses causing displacement of the eyeball, decreased motility, diplopia, and ptosis {391,1335}. They tend to involve both the orbital and palpebral lobes, but only as limited disease (i.e. Ann Arbor stage IE or TNM stage T2) {233,959}. Low-grade lymphomas usually mould around the globe (which is apparent on imaging), whereas high-grade non-Hodgkin lymphomas can infiltrate

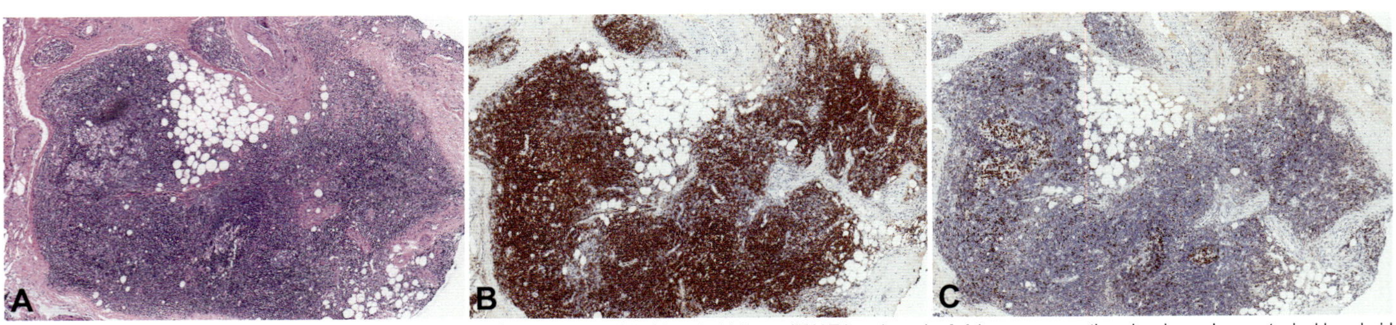

Fig. 5.30 Lacrimal gland extranodal marginal zone lymphoma of mucosa-associated lymphoid tissue (MALT lymphoma). **A** A low-power section showing a dense atypical lymphoid infiltrate within the connective and adipose tissues adjacent to the lacrimal gland. **B** CD20 immunostaining of the same lesion highlights the vaguely nodular pattern and extensive nature of the infiltrate of B cells. **C** Ki-67 staining highlights the residual reactive germinal centres and the low-growth fraction of the tumour cells within the marginal zone.

bone {43,391,1335}. Tissue biopsy is required in all cases.

Histopathology

Most lacrimal gland non-Hodgkin lymphomas are of B-cell type and are usually low-grade, although high-grade transformation can occur {43,231,340,350,959}. The most common subtype is MALT lymphoma, followed by follicular lymphoma and diffuse large B-cell lymphoma {959}. Histologically, MALT lymphomas show a nodular to diffuse heterogeneous B-cell infiltrate surrounding scattered reactive germinal centres and effacing the normal glandular architecture. They are variably composed of atypical small lymphocytes, centrocyte-like cells, monocytoid B cells, immunoblasts, lymphoplasmacytic cells, and plasma cells. Plasmacellular differentiation, including Dutcher bodies, may be striking. Lymphoepithelial lesions, resulting from infiltration of the ductal and epithelial structures by neoplastic B cells, can be seen. MALT lymphoma cells show reactivity for B-cell markers (CD20, CD79a, and PAX5), BCL2, and surface immunoglobulin. They are negative for CD5, CD10, CD23, and cyclin D1. Cytokeratin staining highlights epithelial remnants in the lymphoepithelial lesions. The Ki-67 proliferation index is low (~5%). Molecular testing using IGH PCR demonstrates clonal rearrangement of the immunoglobulin chains.

Differential diagnosis

The differential diagnosis includes chronic autoimmune dacryoadenitis, lacrimal gland IgG4-related disease, and sarcoidosis {43,391}.

Histogenesis

The histogenesis depends on the B-cell lymphoma subtype and its associated neoplastic clone in the B-cell differentiation pathway {1231}.

Genetic profile

The genetic profile depends on the lymphoma subtype.

Prognosis and predictive factors

Most patients with stage I or II lymphoma are treated with low-dose radiotherapy, with or without chemotherapy {959}. Patients presenting with stage > III lymphoma are treated with chemotherapy alone. The 5-year overall survival rate for lacrimal gland lymphomas is 70%, but the prognosis for individuals cases depends on the histological type and clinical stage {231,340,350,959}.

Reactive lymphoid hyperplasia of the lacrimal gland

Coupland S.E.
Bermúdez Magner A.
Biswas J.

Definition

Reactive lymphoid hyperplasia (RLH) of the lacrimal gland is a polyclonal proliferation of lymphocytes arising from intrinsic lacrimal lymphoid tissues.

ICD-O code

None

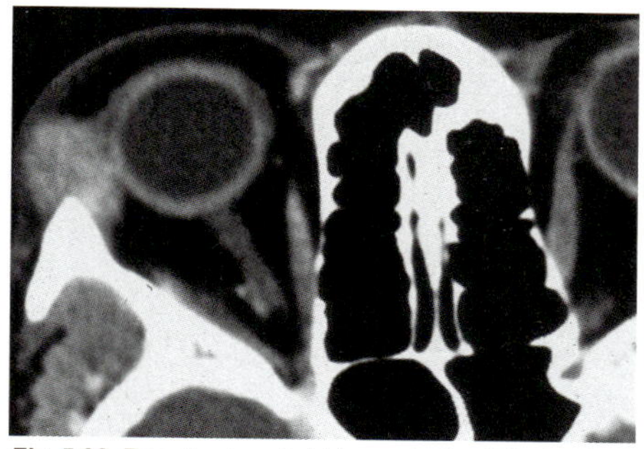

Fig. 5.32 Reactive lymphoid hyperplasia of the lacrimal gland. This CT image shows uniform enlargement of a lacrimal gland with reactive lymphoid hyperplasia.

Synonyms

Benign lymphoid hyperplasia; lacrimal gland lymphoid hyperplasia

Epidemiology

There is a higher incidence in females and in the setting of autoimmune disease.

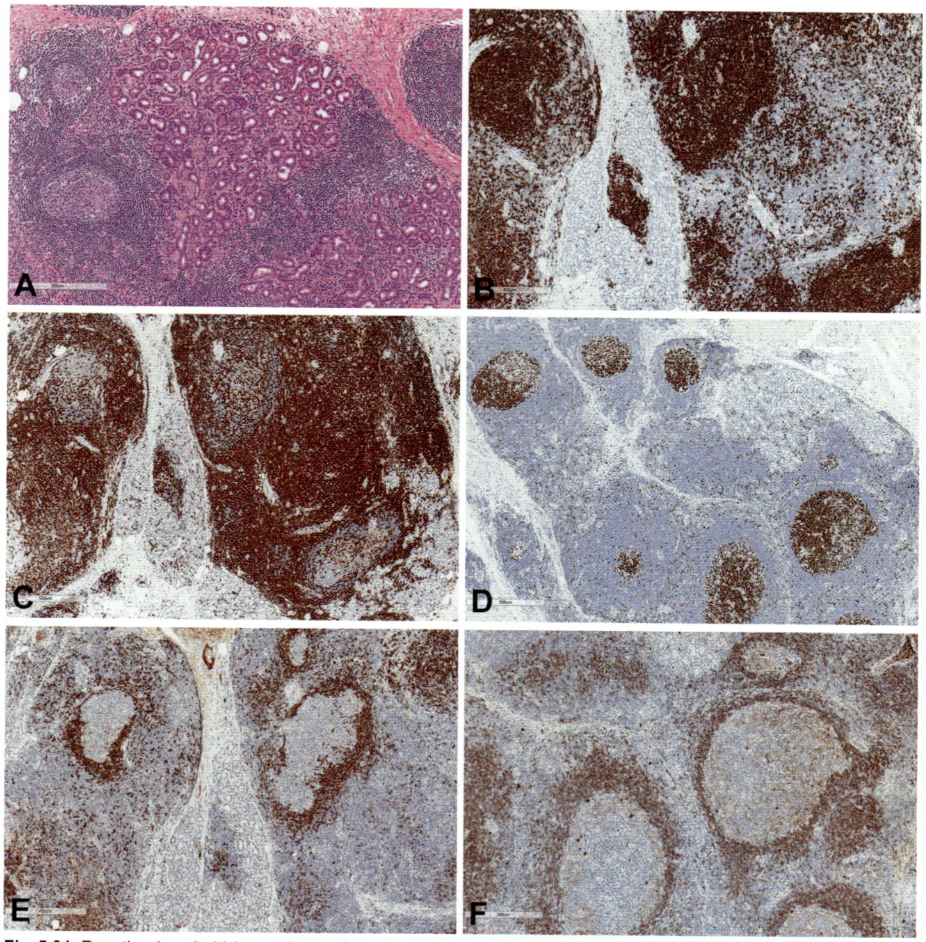

Fig. 5.31 Reactive lymphoid hyperplasia of the lacrimal gland. **A** Lymphocytic inflammation with lymphoid follicles containing germinal centres infiltrates between the lacrimal gland acini. **B** CD20 staining predominantly highlights the lymphoid follicles. **C** CD3 staining shows that numerous T cells are present. **D** Ki-67 staining shows that there is a high proliferation rate in the germinal centres. **E** IgD staining highlights a regular mantle zone surrounding reactive germinal centres and occasional cells in the interfollicular zone. **F** IgM positivity is restricted predominantly to the mantle zone, but it also highlights a very narrow marginal zone, indicating that the marginal zone is not expanded, which is further evidence of the non-neoplastic nature of the lesion. The lesion was shown to be polyclonal on IGH PCR.

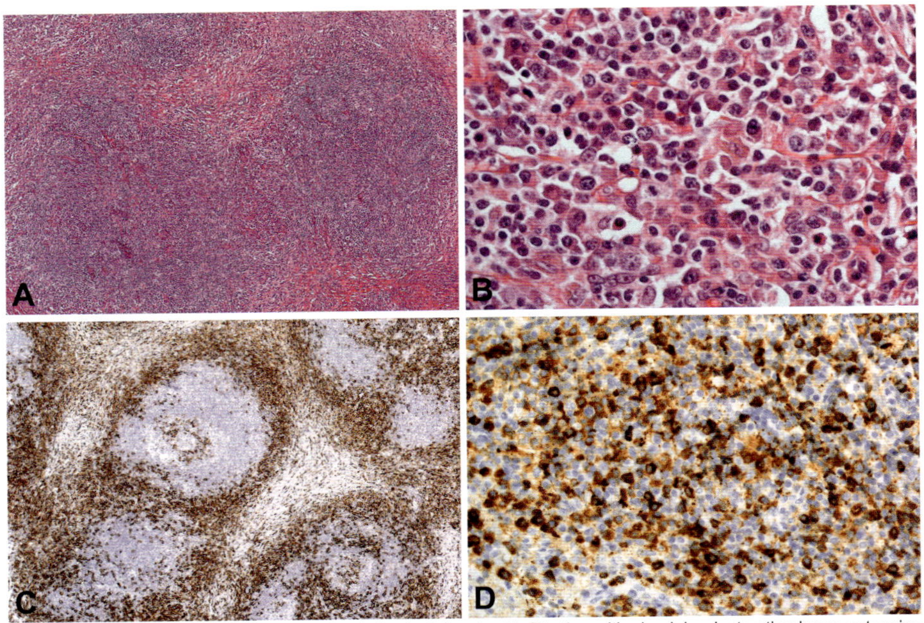

Fig. 5.33 IgG4-related disease of the lacrimal gland. **A** Lacrimal infiltration with glandular destruction by an extensive sclerosing lymphoplasmacytic infiltrate. **B** Higher magnification reveals that a substantial proportion of the infiltrating cells are plasma cells. **C** Immunostaining for the plasma cell marker CD138 highlights the extent of the plasma cells' infiltration surrounding secondary lymphoid follicles (DAB). **D** The vast majority of the plasma cells are immunopositive for IgG4 (DAB).

The incidence is increasing. There is no race predilection {43,231,340,350,1335}.

Etiology

The etiology is unknown, but lacrimal gland RLH is probably caused by chronic antigen stimulation (by either exogenous or endogenous antigens) leading to chronic dacryoadenitis and ultimately RLH {43,660}.

Localization

Lacrimal gland RLH occurs in the superolateral orbit.

Clinical features

RLH usually presents as painless palpable masses leading to globe displacement, decreased motility, diplopia, and ptosis. It has a tendency to involve bilateral lacrimal glands and is typically diffuse, involving both the orbital and palpebral lobes. RLH usually moulds to the globe, with a heterogeneous density on CT. Tissue biopsy is required in all cases {340,1335}.

Histopathology

This diagnosis requires histopathological evaluation, immunophenotyping, and molecular studies to exclude low-grade lymphoma. RLH shows a focal or diffuse infiltrate of mature lymphocytes within the lacrimal gland, splaying but not destroying the acini. The infiltrate comprises a mixture of B cells and T cells arranged physiologically within and around scattered secondary follicles. Areas of fibrosis and sclerosis may be seen. Molecular studies show a polyclonal or oligoclonal amplification product {231,340,350}.

Differential diagnosis

The differential diagnosis includes chronic autoimmune dacryoadenitis, lacrimal gland IgG4-related disease, sarcoidosis, extranodal marginal zone lymphoma of mucosa-associated lymphoid tissue (MALT lymphoma), and follicular lymphoma {340,1335}.

IgG4-related disease merits special consideration, because it may occur in the setting of RLH. IgG4-related disease is a novel clinical entity characterized by infiltration by IgG4-immunopositive plasma cells, an elevated serum IgG4 concentration, and enlargement/masses in various organs (including the lacrimal gland, salivary glands, and pancreas) {414}. In one study, IgG4-related disease was identified in approximately 5–25% of cases originally diagnosed as idiopathic orbital inflammation and 40–50% of cases originally diagnosed as RLH {44}. However, IgG4-positive plasma cells are also common in other orbital conditions, such as sarcoidosis, granulomatosis with polyangiitis, and nonspecific orbital inflammation {1381}. Histological features suggestive of IgG4-related disease include sclerosis (formerly known as sclerosing pseudotumour) and RLH with associated increased numbers of IgG4-positive plasma cells in the tissue.

Histogenesis

Chronic antigen stimulation leads to polyclonal expansion of B cells and T cells {510}.

Prognosis and predictive factors

RLH of the lacrimal gland can be treated medically (e.g. with steroids), by surgical excision, and/or with low-dose external beam radiation therapy. Most cases have a favourable outcome, but recurrence and malignant transformation with time can rarely occur {231,350}.

Secondary tumours of the lacrimal gland

Verdijk R.M.

Definition

Secondary tumours of the lacrimal gland are metastatic tumours involving the lacrimal gland that originate in a distant site or are discontinuous from a primary tumour elsewhere in the periorbital area.

ICD-O codes

Code according to the originating tumour type.

Epidemiology

Secondary tumours are rare at this anatomical site, accounting for far less than 1% of all malignant tumours of the lacrimal gland {1319,1336}. Reports of lacrimal gland metastatic disease are mainly anecdotal case reports; no comprehensive series have been published {99,192,274,613,882}. The true incidence of tumours metastatic to the lacrimal gland is probably higher than suggested in the literature. Series reports on the tissue specificity of metastasis to the orbit often mention fat, muscle, and bone, but rarely mention the lacrimal gland {11,408}. Orbital metastatic presentation as a lacrimal gland tumour is unusual {408}. In the series of orbital metastases described by Font and Ferry in 1976 {364}, only one case was clinically suspected to be pleomorphic adenoma of the lacrimal gland. Several factors may result in underestimation of the true incidence; for example, patients with small lesions may remain asymptomatic, and the orbit and lacrimal gland are not part of standard autopsy protocols.

Clinical features

The signs and symptoms are comparable to those of a primary malignant lacrimal gland tumour: ptosis, increased retrobulbar resistance, diplopia, reduced eye movement, and proptosis.

CT and MRI show a soft tissue mass in the lacrimal fossa, which may show bony erosion. Almost all orbital metastases evaluated by MRI show some degree of enhancement with contrast agents.

The diagnosis is made on the basis of a thorough history, ocular examination, general physical assessment looking for a primary neoplasm and other metastases, orbital CT or MRI, and lacrimal gland open biopsy or fine-needle aspiration biopsy. Biopsy is necessary to confirm that the lesion is a metastatic tumour and not a simulating lesion such as idiopathic orbital inflammation.

Histopathology

The macroscopic appearance depends on the origin of the metastasis; it may be fibrous with metastatic breast carcinoma or fleshy with haemorrhage in renal cell carcinoma and neuroendocrine tumours (carcinoids).

Generally, metastases retain (to some extent) the histological pattern and cytological characteristics of the primary tumour.

Immunohistochemistry is a valuable tool for distinguishing between primary and metastatic lacrimal gland neoplasms. No marker is entirely specific; therefore, the use of a carefully constructed panel of markers is important {464,654}. Breast carcinoma, the most important primary tumour metastasizing to the lacrimal gland, is especially problematic. Breast carcinoma can exhibit nuclear immunoreactivity for estrogen receptor, a finding that may also be present in primary lacrimal gland neoplasms, such as secretory carcinoma. Breast-specific markers such as GCDFP-15 and mammaglobin are expressed in cells with apocrine features, including those present in the breast, axillary and anogenital skin apocrine glands, salivary glands, and lacrimal glands {654}.

Neuroendocrine markers such as synaptophysin and chromogranin are useful for the identification of neuroendocrine tumours. The addition of TTF1 and CDX2 may further reveal lung or gastrointestinal origin. Anti-TTF1 antibody may also stain small cell carcinomas from other sites, including the prostate, urinary bladder, and uterine cervix. Dot-like staining for CK20 may identify Merkel cell carcinoma. Renal cell carcinomas usually stain weakly for pancytokeratin (AE1/AE3) and CK7 and exhibit strong cytoplasmic immunoreactivity for vimentin and CD10. The renal cell carcinoma marker antibody is directed against a normal proximal tubular brush border glycoprotein. It stains most clear cell and papillary renal cell carcinomas, but the sensitivity is lower for high-grade carcinomas and metastatic carcinomas {654}.

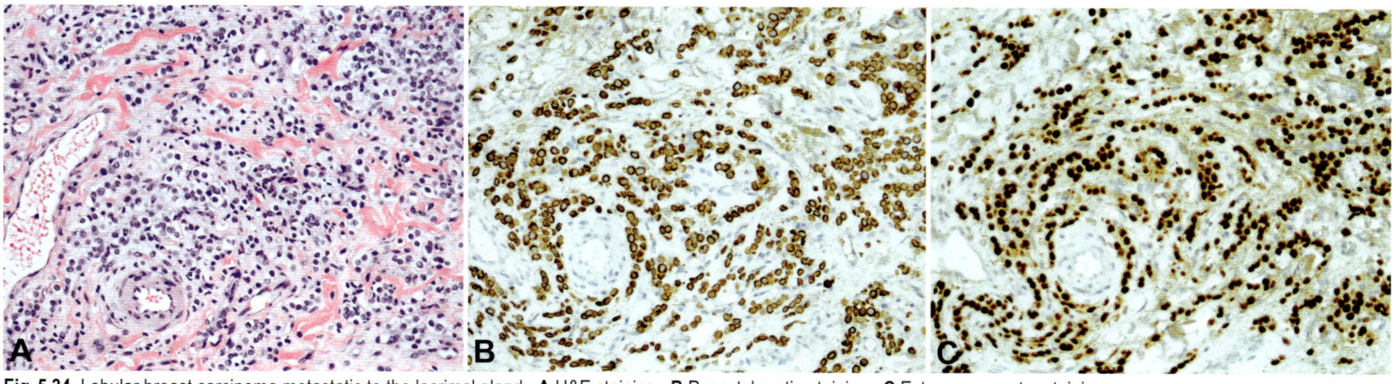

Fig. 5.34 Lobular breast carcinoma metastatic to the lacrimal gland. **A** H&E staining. **B** Pancytokeratin staining. **C** Estrogen receptor staining.

Histogenesis

The primary origins of tumours metastatic to the lacrimal gland as reported in the literature are summarized in Table 5.01 {10,11,99,192,274,281,287,364,366,452, 459,517,613,857,882,955,1012,1160, 1261}. These findings are generally consistent with the frequencies observed in tumours metastatic to the orbit {187,348, 443,1154,1262}; however, lung carcinoma and prostate carcinoma are almost absent from this list of 23 lacrimal gland cases reported worldwide, with the exception of one small cell lung carcinoma in a 65-year-old woman {1261}.

Genetic profile

For poorly differentiated secondary neoplasms of unknown primary site in which conventional light microscopic and immunohistochemical techniques fail to yield a specific diagnosis, cytogenetic analysis promises to increase diagnostic acuity. However, the information on nonrandom (recurrent) chromosomal aberrations in solid tumours is currently limited. Many of the same molecular genetic alterations of tumour suppressor genes and oncogenes can be found in widely disparate tumour types. Only alterations that are specific for (or relatively restricted to) certain malignancies are candidates as markers for diagnosis of a metastasis with identification of the primary site. DNA methylation profiling {822} and RNA expression profiling {453} are promising potential tools for the identification of primary tumour origin in the future.

Prognosis and predictive factors

The prognosis of metastatic disease is highly dependent on tumour stage, primary site, and the exact tumour type. The decision to treat with irradiation, chemotherapy, and/or adjuvant targeted therapies may be facilitated by specific immunohistochemical and molecular findings, such as hormone receptor expression and *ERBB2* (*HER2/neu*) amplification status in breast carcinoma.

Table 5.01 Reported cases of tumours metastatic to the lacrimal gland

Tumour type	Sex	Age (years)	Primary site	Reference
Breast carcinoma	NS	NS	Breast	{366}
Breast carcinoma	NS	NS	Breast	{366}
Breast carcinoma	F	77	Breast	{857}
Breast carcinoma	F	69	Breast	{857}
Breast carcinoma	F	61	Breast	{517}
Breast carcinoma	F	56	Breast	{517}
Breast carcinoma	F	80+	Breast	{955}
Breast carcinoma	F	72	Breast	{281}
Breast carcinoma	F	58	Breast	{11}
Neuroendocrine tumour	NS	NS	NS	{287}
Neuroendocrine tumour	M	82	Mediastinum	{459}
Neuroendocrine tumour	M	57	Kidney	{613}
Neuroendocrine tumour	M	51	Ileum	{364}
Renal cell carcinoma	M	59	Kidney	{1160}
Renal cell carcinoma	M	65	Kidney	{274}
Renal cell carcinoma	F	61	Kidney	{1012}
Small cell carcinoma	F	65	Lung	{1261}
Oesophageal squamous cell carcinoma	M	64	Oesophagus	{882}
Thyroid carcinoma	F	56	Thyroid	{99}
Hepatocellular carcinoma	M	56	Liver	{192}
Malignant pleural mesothelioma	F	55	Pleura	{452}
Choriocarcinoma	F	21	Uterus	{10}
Mucus-secreting carcinoma	NS	NS	Unknown	{366}

F, female; M, male; NS, not specified.

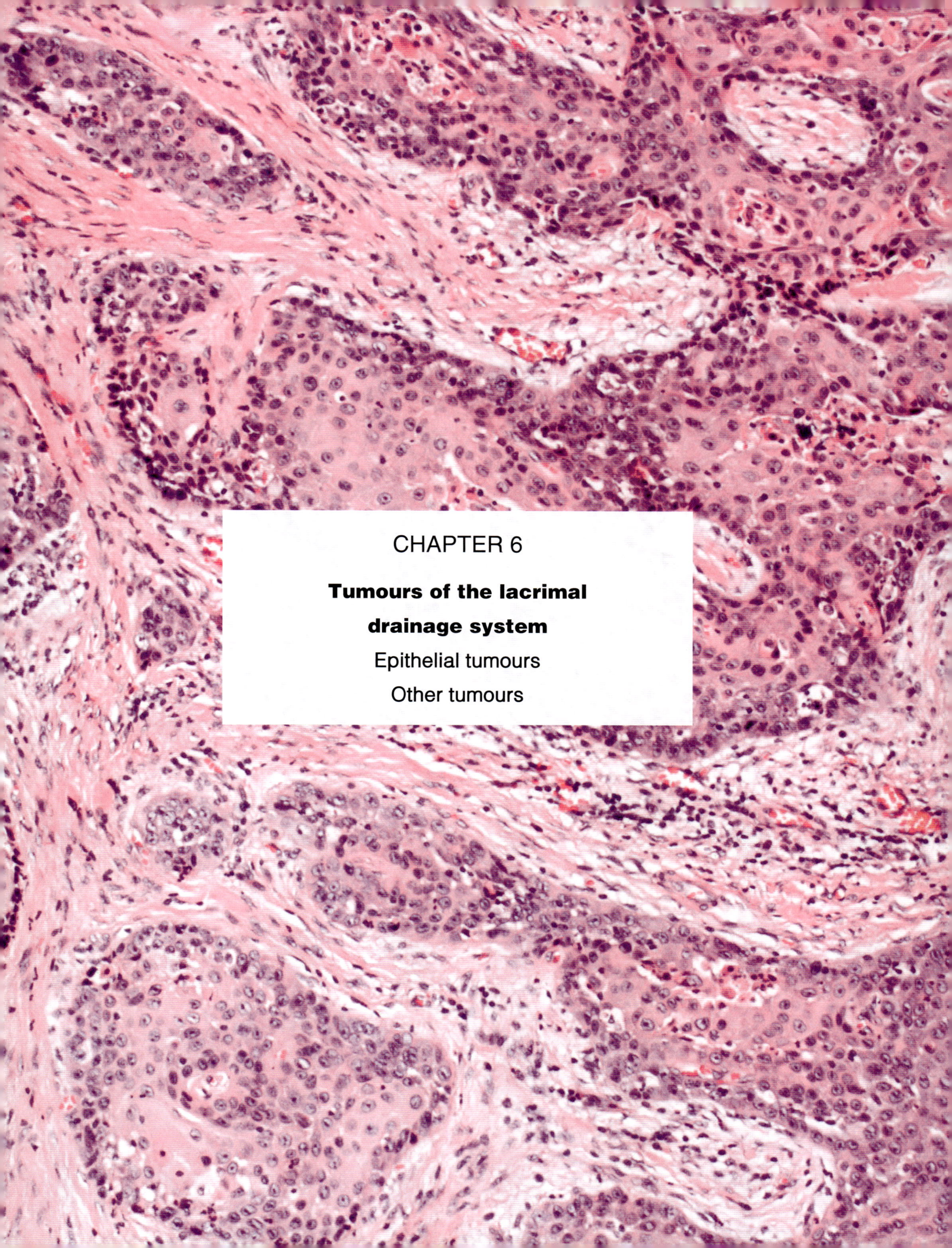

CHAPTER 6

Tumours of the lacrimal drainage system

Epithelial tumours

Other tumours

WHO classification of tumours of the lacrimal drainage system

Epithelial tumours	
Squamous cell carcinoma NOS	8070/3
Non-keratinizing squamous cell carcinoma	8072/3
Adenocarcinoma NOS	8140/3
Mucoepidermoid carcinoma	8430/3
Adenosquamous carcinoma	8560/3
Adenoid cystic carcinoma	8200/3
Lymphoepithelial carcinoma	8082/3
Sinonasal papilloma, exophytic type	8121/0
Sinonasal papilloma, inverted type	8121/1
Other tumours	
Melanoma NOS	8720/3
Extranodal marginal zone lymphoma of mucosa-associated lymphoid tissue (MALT lymphoma)	9699/3
Secondary tumours	See note[a]

[a]Code secondary tumours according to the originating tumour type.

The morphology codes are from the International Classification of Diseases for Oncology (ICD-O) {381}. Behaviour is coded /0 for benign tumours; /1 for unspecified, borderline, or uncertain behaviour; /2 for carcinoma in situ and grade III intraepithelial neoplasia; and /3 for malignant tumours.

The classification is modified from the previous WHO classification, taking into account changes in our understanding of these lesions.

Tumours of the lacrimal drainage system: Introduction

Eberhart C.G.
Grossniklaus H.E.
Kivelä T.T.

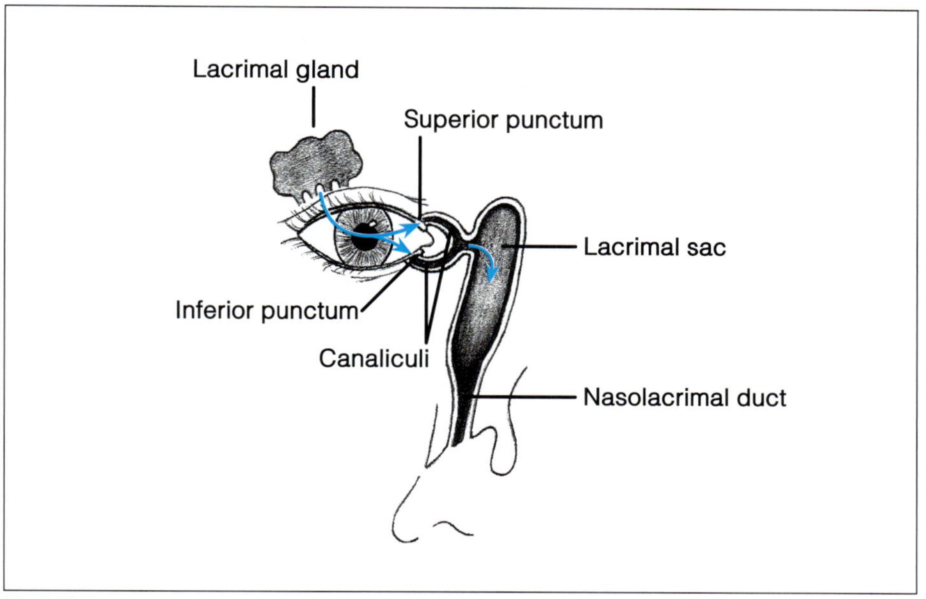

Fig. 6.01 The normal anatomy of the lacrimal drainage system.

The lacrimal drainage system serves as a conduit for the exit of tears from the eye into the nasal cavity. Tears on the ocular surface enter the canaliculi through puncta on the medial aspects of the upper and lower eyelids; both the puncta and canaliculi are lined by stratified, non-keratinized epithelium, which is generally 5–10 cells thick. The tears then drain into the lacrimal sac, which is lined by stratified columnar epithelium containing mucus-secreting goblet cells, and exit via the similarly lined nasolacrimal duct into the nasal cavity.

Disorders of the lacrimal drainage system are relatively common, accounting for approximately 3% of clinical visits in some series {634}. Most cases are associated with chronic inflammation and fibrosis of the lacrimal sac wall. Infectious organisms are identified in some cases of chronic dacryocystitis, but many cases represent nonspecific processes. A discrete dacryolith composed of variably mineralized inflammatory and shed epithelial cells, often containing bacteria or other infectious organisms, is sometimes removed and sent for microscopic evaluation.

Although neoplasms of the lacrimal drainage system are relatively rare, they must be considered whenever patients present with obstructive lesions. Epithelial neoplasms are the most common tumours of the lacrimal drainage system {473}. Papillomas can be covered with squamous or so-called transitional epithelium, and they display exophytic or inverted/endophytic growth patterns; inverted papillomas are more likely to recur and progress to carcinoma. Conventional squamous cell carcinoma and non-keratinizing squamous cell carcinoma are the most common malignant lesions at this anatomical site. HPV infection has been identified in both benign/papillomatous and malignant (squamous or non-keratinizing squamous) lesions {9,1196}. Less common primary epithelial neoplasms at this site include adenocarcinoma, mucoepidermoid carcinoma, adenoid cystic carcinoma, and lymphoepithelial carcinoma.

Haematolymphoid malignancies, including large B-cell lymphomas, also present at this site and must be differentiated from reactive lymphoid hyperplasia. Metastatic lesions, which are seen in the lacrimal drainage system only rarely, generally also involve orbital soft tissue or other surrounding structures {473}.

Epithelial tumours of the lacrimal drainage system

Squamous cell carcinoma of the lacrimal drainage system

Heegaard S.
Rašić D.M.
Bermúdez Magner A.

Definition

Squamous cell carcinoma (SCC) of the lacrimal drainage system is a malignant tumour of squamous epithelium that arises de novo or from a pre-existing benign neoplasm.

ICD-O code

Squamous cell carcinoma NOS 8070/3

Synonym

Epidermoid carcinoma

Epidemiology

SCC is the most common malignant epithelial neoplasm, accounting for > 60% of all malignant epithelial tumours {105,655} and 14% of all lacrimal sac neoplasms {854,946,1009}. It is typically diagnosed in the fifth to eighth decade of life, with a mean patient age at diagnosis of 60 years (range: 34–75 years) and no significant sex or race predilection {9,119,946,1217}.

Etiology

HPV infection has been implicated in the etiology {738,841,1196}. Nearly 90% of all lacrimal sac SCCs are positive for a high-risk HPV type (HPV16, 18, or 33) {9,655}. There is also a strong association between inverted papilloma and papillary SCC {1024}; about 10% of patients with inverted papilloma may develop invasive or in situ SCC, either de novo or in association with a recurrence {1024}. Chronic inflammation affecting the lacrimal sac epithelium is also thought to play a role in inducing malignant transformation {1024}.

Localization

At this anatomical site, SCC arises mainly in the lacrimal sac and/or canaliculi {119,639,946,1217}; it is exceedingly rare in the nasolacrimal duct {1021}.

Clinical features

The early symptoms are often nonspecific. In some cases, clinical suspicion of a neoplasm arises intraoperatively during routine dacryocystorhinostomy; in particular, the in situ variant of SCC has been described in lacrimal sac incisional biopsy specimens {315,473,634,1217}. Unilateral epiphora and a painless, incompressible mass over the medial canthus are the typical presenting features, sometimes erroneously diagnosed as recurrent dacryocystitis {119,315,589,1217}. Low signal intensity on T2-weighted MRI is also suggestive {655,946}. Other signs include blood-stained ocular discharge and skin ulceration or telangiectasia over the lacrimal sac area. Involvement of the orbit, paranasal sinuses, and cranium (mainly by direct invasion) and regional lymphadenopathy (affecting the preauricular, submandibular, jugulodigastric, cervical, and supraclavicular nodes) have been described {119,315,946,1217}. Lymph node metastases are late occurrences {100,655,819,1337}. Only one case report of bilateral lacrimal sac SCC was found in the literature {486}.

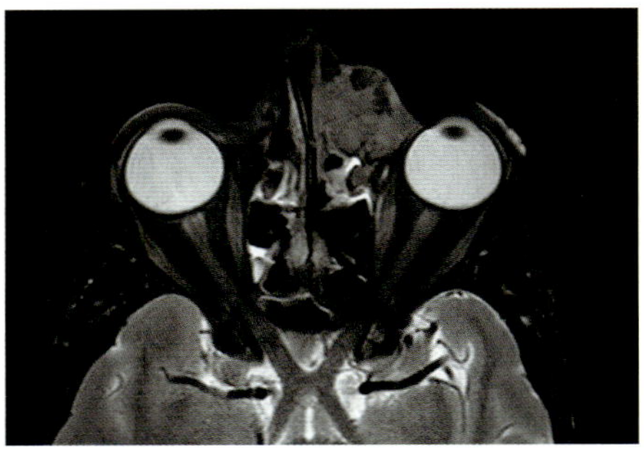

Fig. 6.02 Lacrimal drainage system squamous cell carcinoma. T2-weighted fat-suppressed axial MRI shows a tumour in the left lacrimal sac area, with ethmoid sinus and nasal cavity involvement.

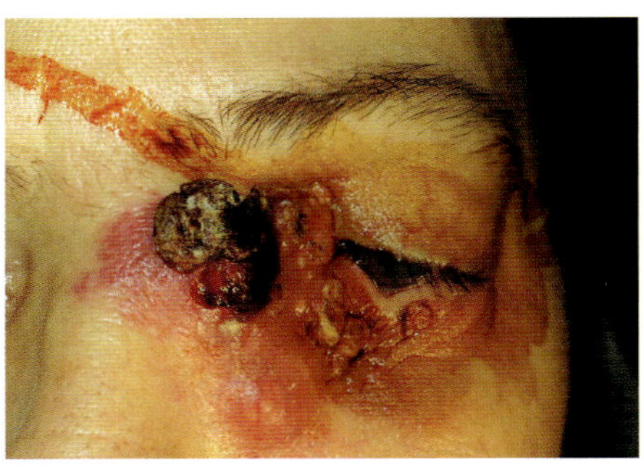

Fig. 6.03 Lacrimal drainage system squamous cell carcinoma. An example presenting as a large ulcerating mass over and below the left medial canthal ligament in a middle-aged woman.

Histopathology

The tumour is composed of nests and strands of hexagonal to polygonal epithelial tumour cells of various sizes. The cells have eosinophilic cytoplasm, large hyperchromatic nuclei, and a moderately high mitotic index, and there is focal koilocytosis. Occasionally, extracellular or intracellular keratinization with intercellular bridging and squamous eddies are seen {9,119,639}. A lobular growth pattern, foci of comedo-necrosis, desmoplastic stromal reaction, and a dense inflammatory background can be seen {9}. The tumour can be in situ or invasive and can be well, moderately, or poorly differentiated. The tumour can be non-keratinizing, partially keratinizing, or predominantly keratinizing {486,589,1024,1400}. Vascular and lymphatic spread can be present even in well-differentiated tumours {119}. Perineural invasion has been noted in predominantly keratinizing neoplasms {9}. The papillary and basaloid morphological variants are the most common {486,639,1024,1244}. The presence of a high-risk HPV type seems to be strongly associated with a non-keratinizing or only partially keratinizing histomorphology {9}.

Differential diagnosis

The differential diagnosis includes other malignant epithelial neoplasms of the lacrimal sac, as well as inverted papilloma.

Histogenesis

At this anatomical site, SCC derives from the lacrimal sac epithelium {100, 473,655,819}.

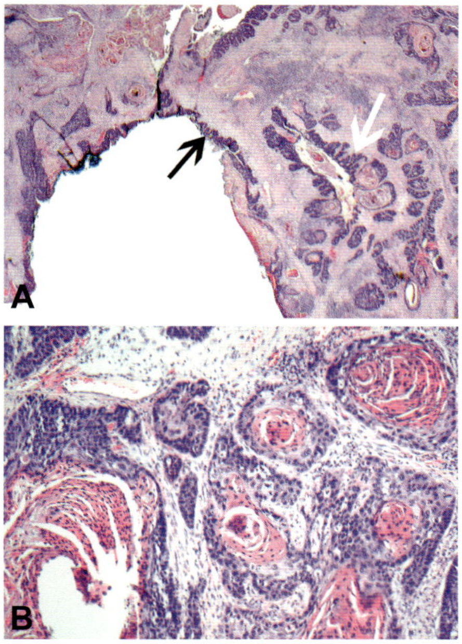

Fig. 6.04 Lacrimal sac keratinizing squamous cell carcinoma (SCC). **A** A low-power view showing the inner lining of the lacrimal sac (black arrow) and invasive lobules of keratinizing SCC (white arrow). **B** At higher power, keratin can be seen among the invasive SCC islands.

Prognosis and predictive factors

For lacrimal sac carcinomas in general, the reported 5-year survival rates in larger series range from 38% to 93% {355,639,854,1009}. Long-term follow-up is essential, because recurrence (seen in ~50% of cases) and metastasis are relatively common {315,655}. The mortality rate is 37.5–43.7% among all patients with lacrimal sac carcinomas {315,655,854} and nearly 50% in the subset of patients with large and invasive tumours {315}.

Non-keratinizing squamous cell carcinoma of the lacrimal drainage system

Heegaard S.
Rašić D.M.
Bermúdez Magner A.

Definition

Non-keratinizing squamous cell carcinoma (SCC) of the lacrimal drainage system is a variant of SCC characterized by a distinctive ribbon-like growth pattern with absent to limited maturation.

ICD-O code

Non-keratinizing SCC 8072/3

Synonyms

Transitional cell carcinoma; poorly differentiated SCC

Epidemiology

Non-keratinizing SCC is the second most common malignancy of the lacrimal drainage system (after conventional SCC), accounting for 13–15% of all tumours at this anatomical site. The mean patient age at presentation is about 50 years, with no significant sex predilection {69,325,467,854}. There may be a predilection for White individuals, given that non-keratinizing SCCs accounted for only 1.1% of cases reported in a Chinese series of lacrimal sac tumours {105}.

Etiology

HPV infection has been implicated in the etiology, with studies demonstrating the presence of HPV DNA (HPV6, 11, and 16) in some cases {69,738,1196,1326}.

Localization

At this anatomical site, non-keratinizing SCC arises mainly in the lacrimal sac, but the canaliculi and nasolacrimal duct may also be affected {20,325,333,467}.

Clinical features

Non-keratinizing SCC is characterized by unilateral, relatively rapidly appearing, usually painless, palpable, irreducible swelling above and below the medial canthal area. Bloody epiphora has also been described. In later stages, the tumour may produce non-axial displacement of the globe, accompanied by telangiectasias, fistulae, and ulceration of the overlying skin {20,69,325,888}.

Histopathology

The tumour is characterized by a mixed (exophytic and inverted/endophytic) papillary architecture, with atypical transitional epithelium overlying branching fibrovascular cores. Invasive acanthosis growing inwards towards the underlying stroma is typical. The multilayered epithelium shows full-thickness loss of maturational sequencing and disturbed cell polarity {20,325,513,888}. The tumour cells are spindled and elongated. Areas containing goblet cells and conspicuous squamous metaplasia (or with an admixed component of SCC {894}) have been described. Foci with increased cellularity, nuclear pleomorphism, prominent nucleoli, and conspicuous mitotic figures are also common {38,69,888,1009}. The tumour can be in situ or invasive and can be well, moderately, or poorly differentiated. Immunohistochemical staining shows positivity for CK7 and positivity or negativity for CK20 {20,325}.

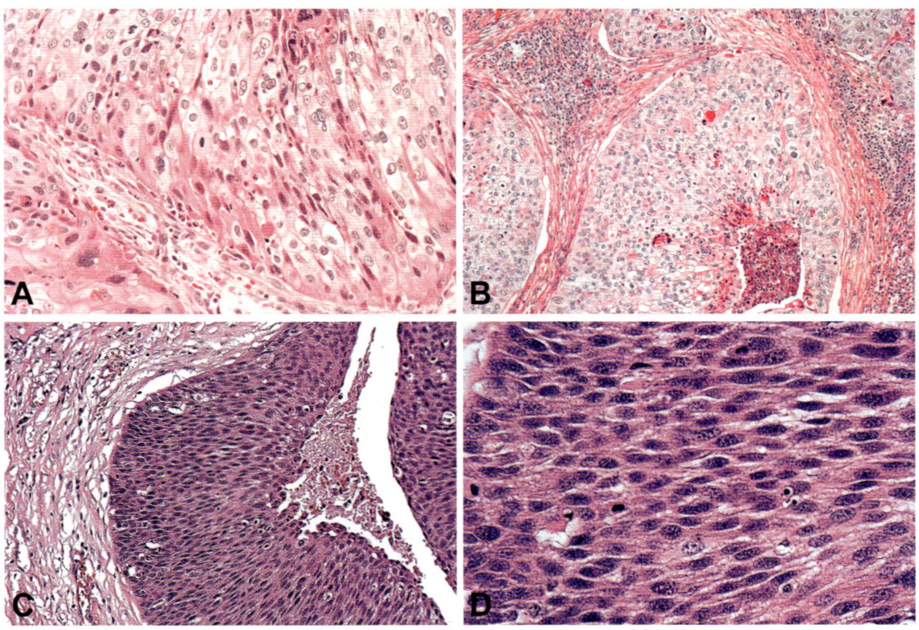

Fig. 6.05 Non-keratinizing squamous cell carcinoma (SCC). **A** Non-keratinizing SCC of the lacrimal drainage system; atypical transitional epithelium with spindled and elongated tumour cells with prominent nucleoli. **B** Non-keratinizing SCC of the lacrimal drainage system; invasive tumour islands showing acanthosis, increased cellularity, nuclear pleomorphism, and prominent nucleoli. **C,D** Invasive non-keratinizing SCC (also called transitional cell carcinoma) of the lacrimal sac; higher magnification showing cell morphology.

Differential diagnosis
The differential diagnosis includes papilloma and conventional SCC {38,325, 467,582}.

Histogenesis
At this anatomical site, non-keratinizing SCC derives from the lacrimal sac epithelium {100,473,655,1337}.

Prognosis and predictive factors
Non-keratinizing SCCs have the worst prognosis of all lacrimal drainage system malignant epithelial neoplasms {655,888,930,1214}. A relatively small number of cases show high postoperative recurrence and mortality rates (as high as 100%), with metastatic spread affecting the regional lymph nodes, lungs, oesophagus, liver, and bone {325,513,655,819}. Delayed presentation and inadequate or prolonged initial and additional treatments are common. Orbital and/or sinonasal invasion in later stages is associated with recurrent disease. These factors are the main causes of mortality in patients with these tumours {513,655}. Well-differentiated in situ tumours with rare mitotic figures are associated with a better prognosis. Poorly differentiated invasive tumours with marked cellular pleomorphism, conspicuous squamous metaplasia, and numerous mitotic figures have high rates of recurrence and a worse prognosis {888}.

Adenocarcinoma of the lacrimal drainage system

Heegaard S.
Rašić D.M.
Bermúdez Magner A.

Definition
Adenocarcinoma of the lacrimal drainage system is a primary malignant epithelial tumour with glandular differentiation.

ICD-O code
Adenocarcinoma NOS 8140/3

Epidemiology
Adenocarcinoma accounts for < 5% of all malignant lacrimal drainage system epithelial neoplasms {105,129,655,1337}. It is typically diagnosed in the fifth to sixth decade of life and shows no significant sex or race predilection {655,903}.

Etiology
At this anatomical site, adenocarcinoma is thought to develop in serous, mucous, or mixed glands in the walls of the lacrimal sac and/or nasolacrimal duct {102,903}.

Localization
At this anatomical site, adenocarcinoma is almost always localized to the lacrimal sac and/or nasolacrimal duct, but it can extend into the canaliculi {79,473,655}.

Clinical features
The typical presenting features are unilateral epiphora and a slow-growing, palpable, non-tender, immobile, firm, incompressible mass over the medial canthus {76,129,473,655}. These tumours are sometimes erroneously diagnosed as recurrent dacryocystitis. Diagnostic signs that suggest malignancy include bloody tears, skin ulceration or telangiectasia overlying the lacrimal sac area, non-axial proptosis with or without diplopia, blepharoptosis, periorbital oedema, and regional lymphadenopathy {79,129,473,1337}. Pain is absent in the vast majority of cases {511,819,1299,1413}.

Histopathology
Adenocarcinoma of the lacrimal drainage system is composed of pleomorphic cells with glandular differentiation manifesting lumen formation and displaying mucin production. The tumour cells are arranged in sheets (multistratified), cords, and nests. Irregularly shaped small glands or single cells can also be seen, in an infiltrative papillary or nonpapillary, glandular, or pseudoglandular growth pattern {129,511,903,1214}. Cribriform or tubular structures with or without comedo-necrosis, as well as histiocytoid cells with relatively rich, slightly eosinophilic to clear cytoplasm, are sometimes observed. Cuboidal epithelial cells with eosinophilic granular cytoplasm and uniform nuclei can also be present {511,655}. Histomorphological signs of malignancy, such as pleomorphic hyperchromatic nuclei, prominent nucleoli, mitotic figures, an inflammatory cell infiltrate, invasion through the basement membrane into the lacrimal sac wall collagenous stroma, lymphatic invasion, and vascular and perineural invasion, are mandatory for the diagnosis {129,511,903,1009}.

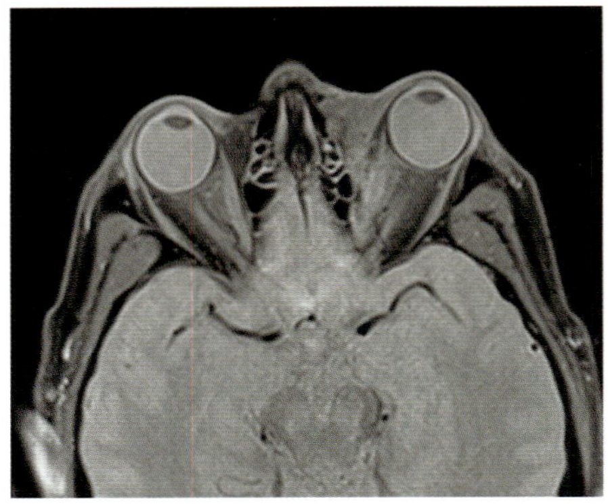

Fig. 6.06 Lacrimal drainage system adenocarcinoma. T2-weighted fat-suppressed axial MRI shows a tumour in the left lacrimal sac area, with medial rectus muscle invasion.

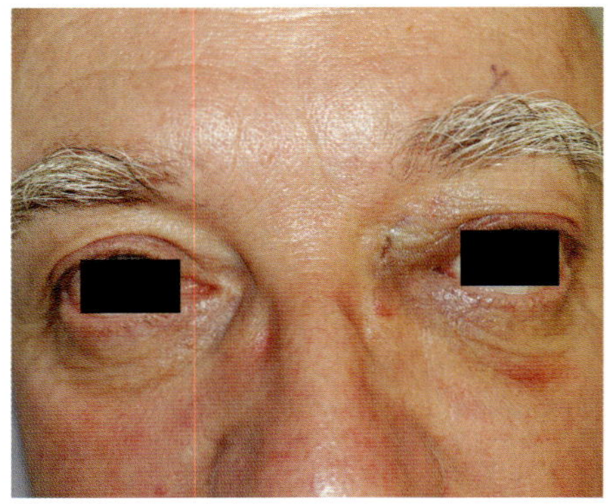

Fig. 6.07 Lacrimal drainage system adenocarcinoma. A tumour mass over the left medial canthus area, with overlying skin ulceration and telangiectasia.

Adenocarcinomas can be classified as low-grade or high-grade; as well differentiated or poorly differentiated; and as classic, oncocytic, mucus-secreting, ductal, or polymorphous low-grade. Adenocarcinoma is immunoreactive for pancytokeratin (AE1/AE3), CK7, androgen receptor, epithelial membrane antigen, GCDFP-15, mTOR, 4E-BP1, and phosphorylated 4E-BP1. The Ki-67 proliferation index is usually 20–30%. Adenocarcinoma is negative for CK20, estrogen receptor, progesterone receptor, chromogranin A, synaptophysin, and ERBB2 (HER2) {76,511,1299}.

Differential diagnosis
The differential diagnosis includes other malignant epithelial neoplasms of the lacrimal sac {473,655,819}.

Histogenesis
At this anatomical site, adenocarcinoma derives from lacrimal sac and/or nasolacrimal duct glandular cells (interspersed within the epithelium) {76,102,655,819}.

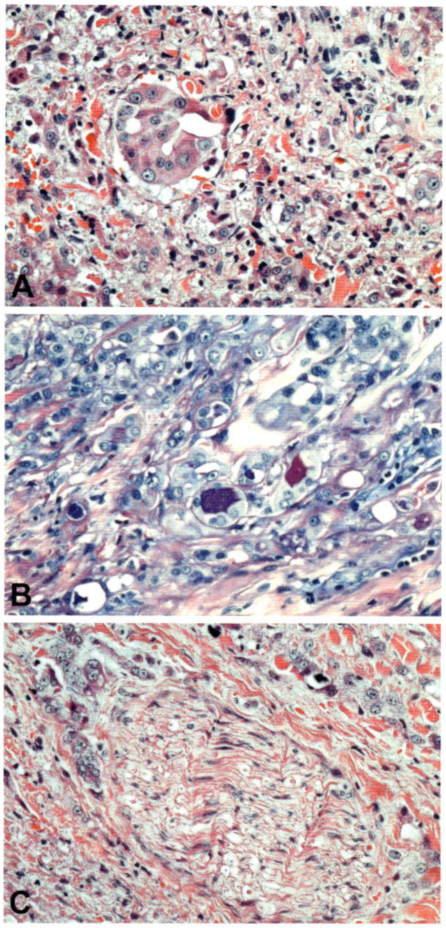

Fig. 6.08 Lacrimal drainage system adenocarcinoma. **A** Cuboidal epithelial cells with eosinophilic granular cytoplasm and uniform nuclei. **B** Malignant cells with marked nuclear pleomorphism, a single central prominent nucleolus, mitotic figures, and mucin production, highlighted by periodic acid–Schiff (PAS) staining. **C** Perineural invasion of adenocarcinoma cells.

Prognosis and predictive factors

Significant data on the prognosis and predictive factors of adenocarcinoma from large clinical studies are not available {473,655,819,1337}. Current practices are based on information from a few case series {854,1009,1214} and a small number of isolated case reports. Long-term follow-up is essential, because recurrence and metastasis are relatively common {473,655,819,894}. Local destruction occurs more commonly than metastasis {129}.

Mucoepidermoid carcinoma of the lacrimal drainage system

Heegaard S.
Rašić D.M.
Bermúdez Magner A.

Definition

Mucoepidermoid carcinoma (MEC) of the lacrimal drainage system is a malignant glandular epithelial neoplasm characterized by squamous (epidermoid) cells, intermediate cells, and mucous cells.

ICD-O code

Mucoepidermoid carcinoma	8430/3
Adenosquamous carcinoma	8560/3

Synonym

Mixed epidermoid and mucus-secreting carcinoma

Epidemiology

MEC occurs in adults. The 14 cases that have been reported in the lacrimal sac {544} presented in the third to seventh decades of life.

Etiology

A possible association with papillomavirus has been reported {508}, and a causal link with cytomegalovirus has also been suggested. MEC is the most common radiation-induced neoplasm.

Localization

At this anatomical site, MEC arises in the lacrimal sac.

Clinical features

Sanguineous discharge or tearing is indicative of a tumour, as are swelling and a mass in the medial canthal area. MEC presents as a firm, solid, non-inflamed, and painless palpable mass. The extension of a lump above the medial canthal tendon is highly suggestive of a tumour {894}. Bloody reflux upon irrigation can also be observed.

Histopathology

The characteristic histological feature of this tumour is mucin production. MEC cells form sheets, islands, duct-like structures, and occasionally microcystic glandular structures of various sizes. MEC is composed of a mixture of three types of epithelial cells: intermediate cells, with scant cytoplasm and large polygonal hyperchromatic pleomorphic nuclei; squamous cells, with abundant eosinophilic cytoplasm; and mucous cells, with eccentric nuclei and intracytoplasmic mucin, which gives a positive periodic acid–Schiff (PAS) reaction. The squamous cells may form focal keratin pearls and intracellular keratinization, and the epithelial islands are scattered in a fibrohyalinized stroma. MECs can be high-grade, intermediate-grade, or low-grade tumours. High-grade tumours are composed mainly of squamous cells, with sparse mucous cells. These tumours are associated with a poor prognosis. Intermediate-grade MECs are solid tumours with no cyst formation. They are composed predominantly of solid sheets and clusters of squamous cells and intermediate cells with cytological atypia. They have prominent nucleoli and show brisk mitotic activity. Low-grade tumours have a large number of mucous cells, with sparse squamous cells. These tumours tend not to be infiltrative, and they have a good prognosis. Low-grade tumours show prominent cystic structures lined by a variety of cells, usually 1–3 layers thick; the predominant cell type is the mucous cell. There is no perineural invasion, and mitotic figures are rare or absent.

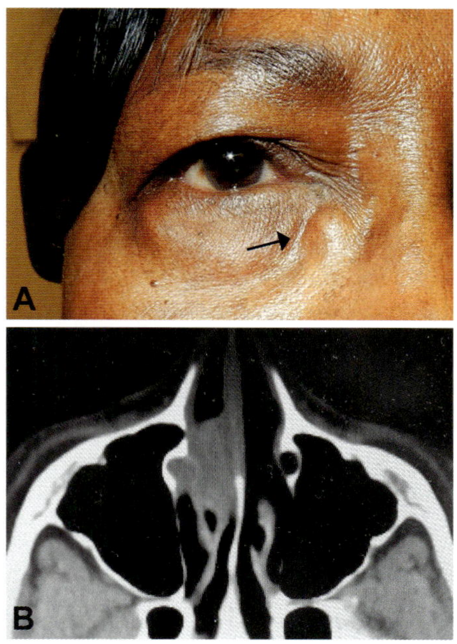

Fig. 6.09 Mucoepidermoid carcinoma. **A** An example presenting as a mass in the medial canthal area; the tumour (arrow) is firm, solid, non-inflamed, and painless. **B** CT shows a tumour in the right lacrimal sac, as well as signs of bone invasion.

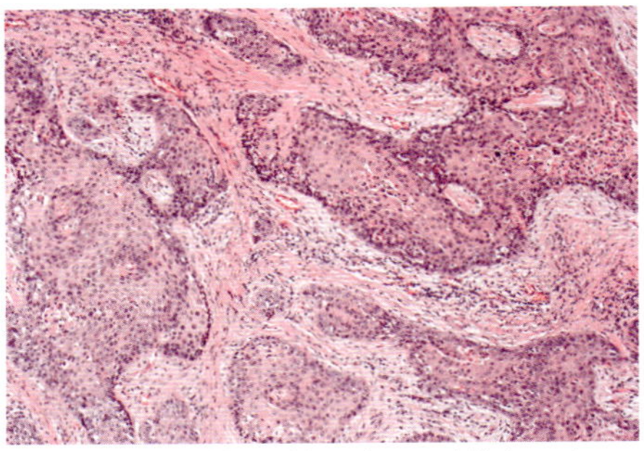

Fig. 6.10 Mucoepidermoid carcinoma. A high-grade example composed of a mixture of intermediate cells, with scant cytoplasm and large polygonal hyperchromatic pleomorphic nuclei, and squamous (epidermoid) cells, with abundant eosinophilic cytoplasm; very few mucous cells are seen.

The mucins expressed by MECs include epithelial membrane antigen (common in high-grade tumours), MUC2, MUC4 (common in low-grade tumours), MUC5AC, and MUC5B. MECs are usually positive for CK5/6, CK7, CK14, and BerEP4, and negative for CK20. The tumour cells can be focally positive for vimentin, CEA, and p63 {508}. Myoepithelial markers are negative.

Differential diagnosis

The differential diagnosis includes chronic dacryocystitis, cystadenoma, cystadenocarcinoma, squamous cell carcinoma, epithelial–myoepithelial carcinoma, clear cell carcinoma NOS, and metastatic tumours.

Histogenesis

At this anatomical site, MEC may arise from the lacrimal sac epithelium or submucosal glands {856}.

Prognosis and predictive factors

The prognosis of MEC depends on the ratio of its cellular components, its differentiation, and its organ of origin. Low-grade MECs rarely metastasize; however, local recurrence is common when the tumour is not completely excised. p53 positivity indicates a good prognosis. Poor prognostic factors include older age, male sex, local spread, vascular invasion, necrosis, high mitotic rate, and high histological grade.

Adenoid cystic carcinoma of the lacrimal drainage system

Heegaard S.
Rašić D.M.
Bermúdez Magner A.

Definition

Adenoid cystic carcinoma (ACC) of the lacrimal drainage system is a malignant neoplasm composed of epithelial and myoepithelial cells that form various patterns, including cribriform, tubular, and solid patterns.

ICD-O code

Adenoid cystic carcinoma 8200/3

Synonym

Cribriform carcinoma

Epidemiology

Only 11 cases of ACC of the lacrimal sac have been described in the literature {951}, in men (4 cases) and women (7 cases) aged 38–74 years. The disease is typically diagnosed in the fourth to sixth decade of life. The median patient age at diagnosis of ACC is a decade younger than that of cancer overall {951}.

Localization

At this anatomical site, ACC arises in the lacrimal sac.

Clinical features

Sanguineous discharge and tearing have been described. Swelling of the lacrimal sac area and the presence of a painful, sometimes ulcerating mass in the medial canthal area are also characteristic {611,903}. The extension of a lump above the medial canthal tendon is highly suggestive of a tumour {894}.

Histopathology

Macroscopically, ACC is fleshy and white. Microscopically, the tumour is characterized by a mixture of cribriform, tubular, and solid patterns {611}. The cribriform subtype is the most common. It is composed of islands of basaloid (cuboidal) epithelial cells surrounding variably sized cyst-like spaces forming a so-called Swiss-cheese or sieve-like pattern. These basaloid cells have large ovoid nuclei and scant eosinophilic cytoplasm. The cyst-like spaces are referred to as pseudocysts because they do not constitute true glandular lumina. The pseudocysts contain basophilic glycosaminoglycans (which stain with Alcian blue) or eosinophilic basement membrane material that gives a positive periodic acid–Schiff (PAS) reaction {611,1342}. The tubular subtype shows similar cytology, with the tumour cells arranged in nests surrounded by variable amounts of eosinophilic, often hyalinized stroma. Occasionally, the stromal component is increased, compressing the tumour cells into thin strands, forming a so-called trabecular pattern. Well-formed ducts with recognizable inner epithelial and outer myoepithelial layers may also be seen. The solid subtype contains aggregates of basaloid cells, without tubular or cystic formation. Although the basaloid cytology of the tumour cells is retained, they

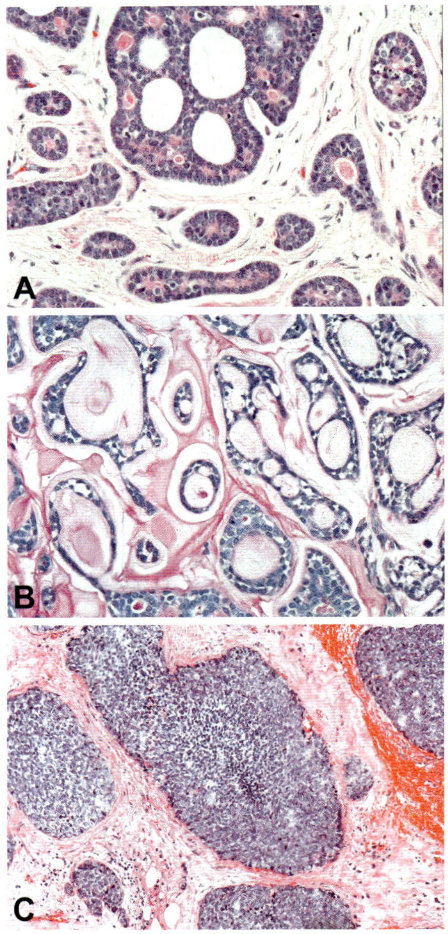

Fig. 6.11 Adenoid cystic carcinoma. **A** Cribriform pattern; islands of basaloid (cuboidal) epithelial cells surrounding variably sized cyst-like spaces, forming a so-called Swiss-cheese or sieve-like pattern. **B** Tubular pattern; the tumour cells completely surround pseudocystic spaces containing eosinophilic material; an area of cribriform pattern is visible to the right. **C** Solid pattern; there are variably sized and shaped nests of tumour cells, without pseudocystic spaces.

may be larger, and nuclear pleomorphism may be more pronounced. The solid pattern is associated with a poor prognosis. Perineural infiltration, which often results in local recurrences, can be seen with infiltrative growing tumours.
ACCs are immunoreactive for CK7, CK14, CK17, and CK19. Myoepithelial differentiation surrounding the pseudocysts can be demonstrated by SMA and S100 protein staining. Ki-67 and p53 may show increased staining in areas of high-grade transformation – an indicator of poor prognosis.

Differential diagnosis
The differential diagnosis includes other tumours that exhibit tubular and cribriform structures (e.g. polymorphous low-grade adenocarcinoma), tumours with basaloid cellular morphology (e.g. basal cell adenoma and basal cell adenocarcinoma), and tumours with a dual population of ductal and myoepithelial cells (e.g. pleomorphic adenoma).

Histogenesis
ACC is a rare form of adenocarcinoma that arises within secretory glands.

Genetic susceptibility
There is some evidence that the *TP53* tumour suppressor gene is somehow inactivated in advanced and aggressive forms of ACC.

Prognosis and predictive factors
ACC is known for its relentless and prolonged course; life-long follow-up is essential, especially for younger patients {903}. Tumour size is known to influence survival. Other factors that influence survival include histological patterns, clinical stage, bone involvement, and status of surgical margins {611,1234}.

Lymphoepithelial carcinoma of the lacrimal drainage system

Heegaard S.
Rašić D.M.
Bermúdez Magner A.

Definition
Lymphoepithelial carcinoma of the lacrimal drainage system is a poorly differentiated/undifferentiated squamous cell carcinoma accompanied by reactive lymphoplasmacytic infiltration.

ICD-O code
Lymphoepithelial carcinoma 8082/3

Synonyms
Non-keratinizing undifferentiated nasopharyngeal-type carcinoma; undifferentiated carcinoma with lymphocytic stroma; lymphoepithelioma-like carcinoma; lymphoepithelioma

Epidemiology
Lymphoepithelial carcinoma is rare in the lacrimal drainage system, with only 11 reported cases {276}, in women (9 cases) and men (2 cases) aged 20–82 years; 9 of these patients were Asian, 1 was African-American, and 1 was White {276}.

Etiology
Nearly all lymphoepithelial carcinoma cases are strongly associated with EBV infection; 78% of cases in the lacrimal sac were found to be EBV-positive {276}.

Localization
At this anatomical site, lymphoepithelial carcinomas present in the lacrimal sac and nasolacrimal duct.

Clinical features
The duration of symptoms is 1–24 months. Epiphora and swelling over the lacrimal sac are common, and a hard, non-tender, immobile mass above the medial tendon is characteristic {536,732}.

Histopathology
Macroscopically, the tumour is polypoid, whitish, and firm. Microscopically, it is characterized by polygonal, undifferentiated malignant epithelial cells occurring in sheets, in clusters, and as isolated cells, mixed with an intense lymphoid infiltrate. The malignant cells have round vesicular nuclei and a single large central nucleolus. The background lymphoid infiltrate is composed of a mixture of B lymphocytes, T lymphocytes, plasma cells, and macrophages. Immunohistochemically, the epithelial tumour cells are positive for CK5/6, CK14, and CK19 {276}. There are both CD20+ B lymphocytes and CD3+ T lymphocytes, indicating a polyclonal composition. Tumour cells are also positive for epithelial membrane antigen and p63 {536}.

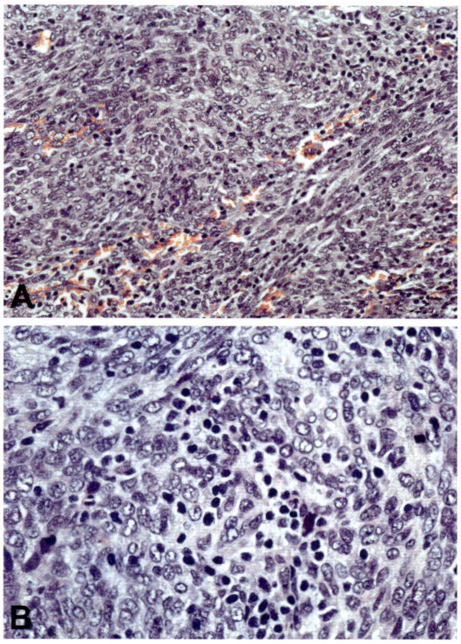

Fig. 6.12 Lymphoepithelial carcinoma. **A** Clusters of undifferentiated malignant epithelial cells associated with a lymphoid infiltrate. **B** The malignant epithelial cells have round vesicular nuclei and a single large central nucleolus; lymphocytes and plasma cells are scattered between the tumour cells.

Differential diagnosis
Lymphoepithelial carcinoma must be distinguished from the vastly more aggressive sinonasal undifferentiated carcinoma, which is EBV-negative. Other important differential diagnoses are melanoma and non-Hodgkin lymphoma.

Prognosis and predictive factors
The reported disease-free survival is 15–33 months. Three patients developed locoregional relapses or metastases despite treatment. Lymphoepithelial carcinoma can be life-threatening if diagnosed late, with a mortality rate of about 50% {276}.

Exophytic papilloma of the lacrimal drainage system

Heegaard S.
Heathcote G.
Mittal R.
Rašić D.M.

Definition
Exophytic papilloma of the lacrimal drainage system is a benign neoplasm characterized by outward growth of

papillomatous epithelium with delicate fibrovascular cores.

ICD-O code
Sinonasal papilloma, exophytic type 8121/0

Synonyms
Schneiderian papilloma (not recommended); everted papilloma; fungiform papilloma; transitional (cell) papilloma; squamous papilloma

Epidemiology
Exophytic papilloma primarily arises in the fourth to fifth decade of life, but it can occur in people of any age (reported range: 9–88 years). It is more common in males, with a male-to-female ratio of 1.3:1 to 2.3:1 {854,1009,1214}.

Etiology
Papillomas of the nasolacrimal drainage system are relatively rare and are histologically diverse. Small case studies that have included papillomas of various histological types (transitional, squamous, or mixed), grades (with or without dysplasia), and architecture (exophytic, inverted/endophytic, or mixed) have reported a variable association with HPV infection (in > 50% of cases), as determined using consensus and type-specific PCR primers. DNA and RNA in situ hybridization techniques have also demonstrated an association with HPV infection in > 50% of cases {738,841,1196}.

Localization
At this anatomical site, exophytic papillomas usually arise in the lacrimal sac. As they enlarge, they may secondarily involve the nasolacrimal duct and nasal cavity {546}.

Clinical features
Persistent and chronic epiphora and/or a non-tender mass above the medial tendon are the typical presenting features. Punctal bleeding, epistaxis, and pain are rare. The duration of clinical symptoms may vary from a month to several years. About 30–40% of cases have been discovered as an incidental finding during dacryocystorhinostomy or dacryocystectomy {333,492,894,1009,1301}.

Histopathology
Grossly, exophytic papilloma may present as a single polypoid or confluent firm to fleshy mass. Microscopically, as the name "exophytic papilloma" implies, the neoplasm shows outward proliferation or finger-like projections of epithelial cell masses, with a branching fibrovascular core. The epithelium may vary from non-keratinized stratified squamous in appearance (with scattered dyskeratotic cells) to stratified columnar in appearance (with scattered goblet cells with or without fine cilia); in mixed papillomas, both epithelial cell types are present. In addition to mucocytes, small mucin cysts may also be observed. Scattered typical mitotic figures may be present. Some cases show koilocytic change and/or various grades of dysplasia, the incidence of which is variable.
Malignant transformation of exophytic papilloma is distinctly uncommon {1009}; however, Stefanyszyn et al. reported an equal incidence of malignant change in exophytic and inverted (endophytic) papillomas {1214}.
Exophytic papillomas are immunoreactive for pancytokeratin and epithelial membrane antigen, and they show strong diffuse cytoplasmic expression of CK18. The basilar cells predominantly express CK17 and the suprabasal cells, CK7.

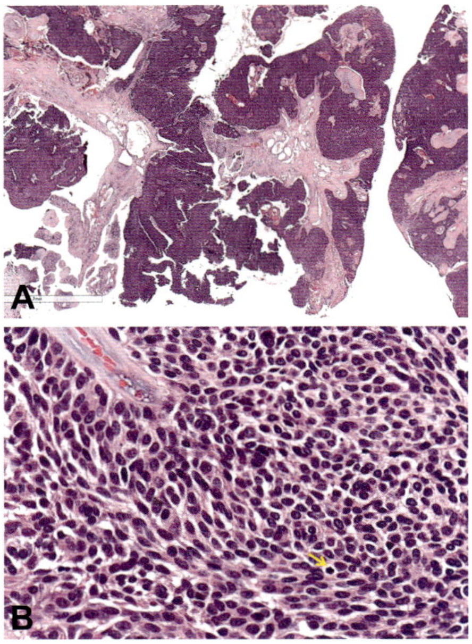

Fig. 6.13 Exophytic papilloma. **A** Outward growth of papillary fronds with branching fibrovascular cores. **B** Higher magnification shows the hyperplastic epithelium, predominantly lined by transitional cells; a typical mitotic figure is present (arrow).

Differential diagnosis
The differential diagnosis includes chronic dacryocystitis, papillary cystadenoma, mucoepidermoid carcinoma, conventional squamous cell carcinoma, and non-keratinizing squamous cell carcinoma.

Histogenesis
The Schneiderian membrane is an embryologically unique membrane, being ectodermal in origin. It develops into the mucosa of the sinonasal tract and lacrimal apparatus; however, it is unclear how papillomas of varying histology and architecture develop from the membrane. There is evidence that chronic inflammation and viral infection may play a role in tumorigenesis.

Prognosis and predictive factors
Complete surgical excision is the treatment of choice. With complete excision, recurrence and progression to malignancy are distinctly uncommon in exophytic papilloma.

Inverted papilloma of the lacrimal drainage system

Heegaard S.
Heathcote G.
Mittal R.
Rašić D.M.

Definition
Inverted papilloma of the lacrimal drainage system is a benign neoplasm characterized by an inverted/endophytic or mixed growth pattern.

ICD-O code
Sinonasal papilloma, inverted type 8121/1

Synonyms
Endophytic papilloma; transitional (cell) papilloma, endophytic; inverting papilloma; squamous papilloma; Schneiderian papilloma

Epidemiology
Inverted papilloma is the most common epithelial neoplasm of the lacrimal drainage system. It occurs in adults of both sexes.

Etiology
A possible association with HPV infection has been reported {840}.

Localization
At this anatomical site, inverted papilloma usually arises in the lacrimal sac, where the tumour grows from the surface epithelium, but it has also been reported to arise from the nasolacrimal duct {1343}.

Clinical features
Inverted papilloma usually presents as a swelling in the medial canthal area, associated with tearing. Patients often have a history of a coexisting or previous inverted papilloma of the sinonasal tract.

Histopathology
The lumen of the lacrimal sac is obliterated by a mass, on the cut surface of which can be seen ribbons of thickened and folded epithelium {467}.
Although there is no actual transitional cell, transitional epithelium is recognizable because of the coexistence of features of squamous and glandular differentiation. Transitional epithelium is characterized by stratification, tonofibrils (identifiable on electron microscopy), goblet cells, microcysts containing mucin and neutrophils, a surface layer of columnar (possibly ciliated) cells, a lack of substantial surface keratin, and the absence of intercellular bridges.
The epithelium may undergo focal surface keratinization {467}. Areas of squamous metaplasia may show koilocytic atypia. The terms "inverted" and "endophytic" refer to the downward displacement of the thickened neoplastic surface epithelium into the underlying stroma, but this is not always seen in mixed exophytic/inverted tumours {546}.
Inverted papillomas show positivity for pancytokeratin, but specific biomarkers have not been identified.

Differential diagnosis
The differential diagnosis includes squamous papilloma, conventional squamous cell carcinoma (SCC), and non-keratinizing SCC.

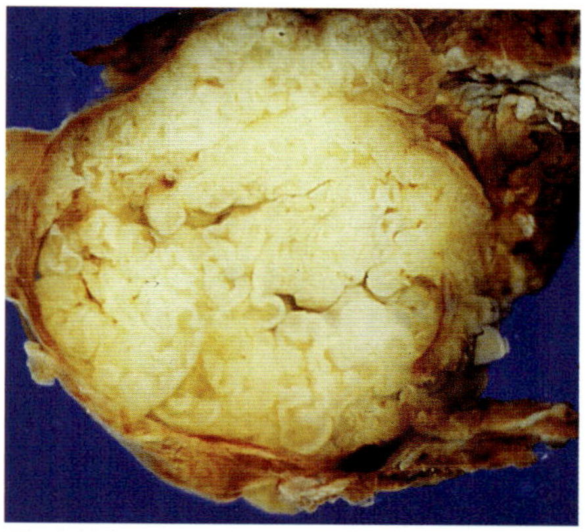

Fig. 6.14 Inverted papilloma. A dacryocystectomy specimen with inverted papilloma filling the lumen of the lacrimal sac; ribbons of thickened epithelium can be identified within the mass.

Histogenesis
The first step in the histogenesis of a papilloma is transitional metaplasia of the normal surface epithelium, which is followed by the development of a hyperplastic ribbon of transitional epithelium. As the surface epithelium thickens, it expands inwards, outwards, or both.

Prognosis and predictive factors
If not completely excised, inverted papillomas may recur and may undergo malignant transformation to non-keratinizing SCC, conventional SCC, mucoepidermoid carcinoma, or adenocarcinoma. A recurrence of a transitional inverted papilloma is likely to show more squamous metaplasia, as well as cytological atypia and increased mitotic activity {467}; this may in part explain why conventional SCC is more common in the lacrimal sac than non-keratinizing SCC {1214}. Extension of the papilloma along the nasolacrimal duct appears to increase the risk of recurrence, but recurrence itself does not seem to increase the risk of malignant transformation, despite the cellular atypia seen in recurrences {1009}. The tumour may also extend into the nose and/or orbit through bone that has eroded under pressure; imaging studies may therefore lead to an erroneous diagnosis of malignancy.

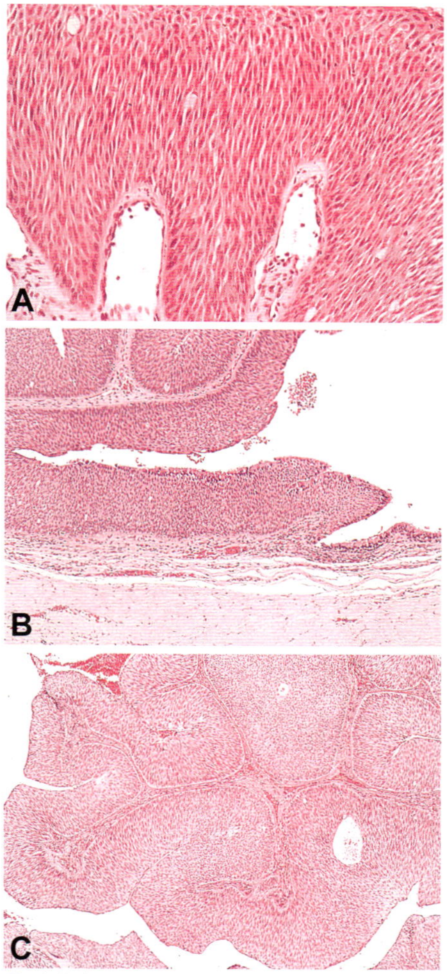

Fig. 6.15 Inverted papilloma. **A** An example with thickened surface epithelium composed of closely packed, vertically aligned, spindle-shaped cells with scattered goblet cells; intercellular bridges cannot be identified, although there is slight surface keratinization. **B** Adjacent to the papilloma, the junction between normal lacrimal sac epithelium and transitional epithelium is seen. **C** An example with thickened surface epithelium in which there are two microcysts.

Other tumours of the lacrimal drainage system

Melanoma of the lacrimal drainage system

Heegaard S.
Vemuganti G.
Eberhart C.G.

Definition
Melanoma of the lacrimal drainage system is an invasive melanocytic neoplasm.

ICD-O code
Melanoma NOS 8720/3

Synonym
Lacrimal sac melanoma

Epidemiology
Melanomas of the lacrimal drainage system are extremely rare. In a meta-analysis of lacrimal sac neoplasms, melanoma accounted for 4% of the tumours {473}.

Etiology
The etiology is unknown, but it is probably similar to that of melanomas occurring at other mucosal sites not exposed to sun.

Localization
At this anatomical site, the lacrimal sac is the most common location, but tumours can invade other parts of the lacrimal drainage system or adjacent soft tissue and bone (e.g. the lacrimal crest) {932}. Rare cases arising in the nasolacrimal duct have also been reported {331}.

Clinical features
Mass lesions in the medial canthal area or lacrimal sac are associated with epiphora, bloody discharge, and (rarely) pain. They can mimic dacryocystitis, and repeated biopsies are sometimes necessary for diagnosis {739,971}.

Histopathology
The mucosal linings of the lacrimal sac and surrounding soft tissues are infiltrated by variably pigmented spindled or epithelioid melanocytes with moderate to abundant pigmented granular cytoplasm, often showing large vesicular nuclei with prominent nucleoli. Nuclear pleomorphism and variable numbers of mitotic figures are present. Tumour cells are immunoreactive for HMB45 antigen and melan-A.

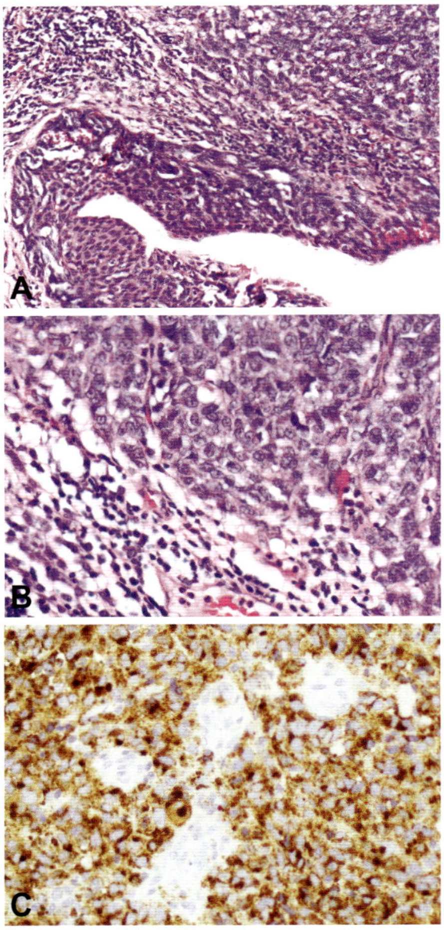

Fig. 6.16 Melanoma of the lacrimal sac. **A,B** An invasive melanoma arising in the lacrimal sac of a White, 52-year-old man, who presented with increased tearing but no pain or bleeding. **C** The melanoma was centred in the lacrimal sac but diffusely invaded the orbit and the extraocular muscles (HMB45 staining).

Differential diagnosis
Primary melanoma of the lacrimal sac should be distinguished from conjunctival melanoma with secondary lacrimal drainage system involvement or metastasis {1036}.

Histogenesis
Melanomas of the lacrimal sac and nasolacrimal duct are believed to originate from melanocytes derived from the neural crest, but it is not entirely clear whether intraepithelial or subepithelial cells are transformed {537}.

Prognosis and predictive factors
The primary treatment modality is surgery (i.e. dacryocystectomy). Poor prognostic factors include positive surgical margins, large tumour size, and dissemination of the tumour {1224}. Local recurrence is common. For advanced cases, treatment may range from wide en bloc resection to postoperative radiotherapy, chemotherapy, and immunotherapy in a variety of combinations.

Lymphomas of the lacrimal drainage system

Bermúdez Magner A.
Eberhart C.G.
Heegaard S.
Vemuganti G.
Biswas J.

Definition
Primary lacrimal drainage system lymphomas are malignant proliferations of lymphocytes arising in the lacrimal drainage system without evidence of concurrent systemic lymphoma. Secondary lacrimal drainage system lymphomas occur in patients as part of disseminated disease.

ICD-O code
MALT lymphoma 9699/3

Synonym
Lacrimal sac lymphomas

Epidemiology

The proportion of lacrimal drainage system tumours diagnosed as lymphoma varies widely across studies, but a review of 420 cases at this site found that 11% were lymphoid {473}. The patient age at presentation varies, but primary lymphomas most commonly arise in elderly individuals and are of B-cell origin {1193,1401}. There is no known race predilection.

Etiology

These lymphomas are presumed to be caused by chronic antigen stimulation leading to chronic inflammation, reactive lymphoid hyperplasia (RLH), and ultimately lymphoma {43,231,340,350,959}. A case of diffuse large B-cell lymphoma of the lacrimal sac was reported to have arisen in a patient with IgG4-related disease {762}.

Localization

At this anatomical site, lymphoma can arise in the lacrimal sac, nasolacrimal duct, and canaliculi. Most cases affect only one side, but bilateral lacrimal sac lymphomas have also been reported {1293}. Nasal spread of a conjunctival extranodal marginal zone lymphoma of mucosa-associated lymphoid tissue (MALT lymphoma) through the nasolacrimal duct can also occur {495}.

Clinical features

Common presenting clinical symptoms include epiphora, swelling, dacryocystitis, and secondary acquired nasolacrimal obstruction {1193}. Imaging studies of lacrimal sac lymphoma have revealed mild to moderate enhancement and remodelling of the lacrimal duct, with bone compression {441}.

Histopathology

The histopathology of lymphoid neoplasms in the lacrimal drainage system reflects the specific type of lymphoma. Both primary MALT lymphomas and primary diffuse large B-cell lymphomas are common at this site, and the former can transition to the latter {473,1193}; together, they account for the majority of cases. Chronic lymphocytic leukaemia/small lymphocytic lymphoma and extranodal NK/T-cell lymphoma have also been described in the lacrimal sac, but they are much rarer {656,798}.

Differential diagnosis

Lymphoma at this site must be differentiated from chronic dacryocystitis and RLH; this differentiation can be difficult with low-grade B-cell neoplasms (e.g. MALT lymphoma) if only limited material is available for immunophenotypic or molecular analysis. Rare lymphomas can have a microscopic appearance resembling that of a sclerosing inflammatory process or a desmoplastic metastatic carcinoma {535}. In a meta-analysis of specimens from 3865 lacrimal sac wall biopsies, 55 biopsies (1.4%) revealed neoplasms, comprising lymphoma (most commonly) and several very rare tumour-like pathologies: dacryoliths, pyogenic granuloma/granulation tissue, RLH, granulomatosis with polyangiitis (Wegener granulomatosis), and sarcoidosis {649}.

Chronic dacryocystitis accounts for approximately 3% of ophthalmology clinic visits; it occurs most often in adults and is more common in women than in men {22,649,1025}. Inflammatory narrowing of the nasolacrimal duct can lead to obstructive symptoms {813}. The underlying cause of the inflammation is often unclear, but infectious, traumatic/mechanical, autoimmune, and neoplastic etiologies should be considered. Lacrimal sac infections can be caused by bacteria, including the bacteria that cause tuberculosis (*Mycobacterium tuberculosis*), leprosy and syphilis; they can also be caused by fungi and the organism that causes rhinosporidiosis. *Staphylococcus* and *Pseudomonas* species were the most common infectious agents in one study {34}. IgG4-related disease, RLH, and graft-versus-host disease have also been associated with chronic dacryocystitis {86,153,1240,1380}. Medial canthal swelling with epiphora and punctal discharge are the most common symptoms of chronic dacryocystitis. On gross examination, the lacrimal sac is often seen to be thickened. On cut section, purulent material can sometimes be seen within the lumen. In large studies of dacryocystorhinostomy specimens, the main finding was chronic inflammation of the lacrimal sac (found in > 94% of cases), with prominent associated fibrosis noted in only a minority of cases {22,649,1025}.

Histogenesis

The histogenesis depends on the lymphoma subtype and its associated neoplastic clone in the B-cell or other differentiation pathway.

Genetic profile

The genetic profile depends on the lymphoma subtype.

Prognosis and predictive factors

In one multi-institution study of primary lacrimal sac lymphoma, systemic spread occurred in 33% of cases, and the 5-year overall survival rate was 65% {1193}.

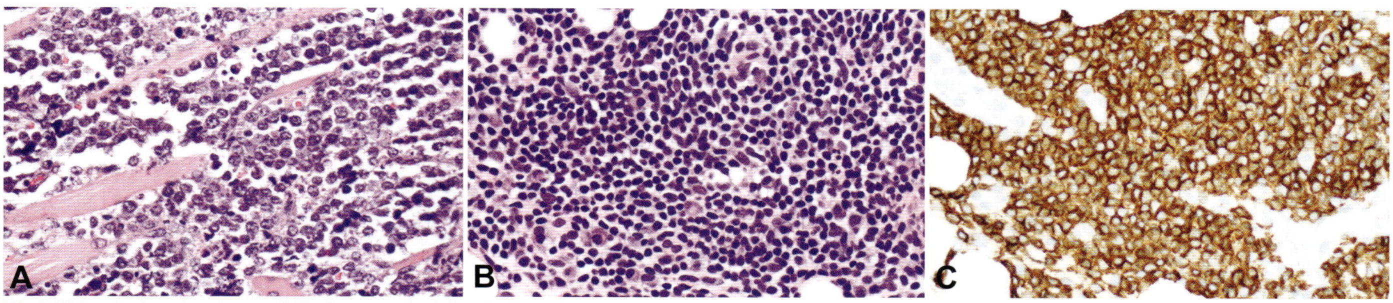

Fig. 6.17 Lacrimal sac lymphoma. **A** The large, atypical, discohesive cells with prominent nucleoli infiltrating the lacrimal sac wall are typical of diffuse large B-cell lymphoma. **B** This inflammatory mass arising in the lacrimal sac is composed of relatively bland lymphoid cells, but the predominance of monocytoid B cells and molecular evidence of B-cell clonality was sufficient to establish a diagnosis of extranodal marginal zone lymphoma of mucosa-associated lymphoid tissue (MALT lymphoma). **C** CD20 immunostaining of this MALT lymphoma reveals that the majority of the lymphoid infiltrate comprises B cells.

Secondary tumours of the lacrimal drainage system

Bermúdez Magner A.
Eberhart C.G.
Heegaard S.

Definition

Secondary tumours of the lacrimal drainage system are tumours that originate elsewhere and involve the lacrimal drainage system by extension from neighbouring structures or by metastasis from another site.

ICD-O codes

Code according to the originating tumour type.

Epidemiology

Secondary tumours of the lacrimal drainage system generally occur in older individuals and are quite rare.

Clinical features

Like other tumours at this site, the majority of secondary neoplasms present with symptoms typical of acquired nasolacrimal obstruction, including epiphora, epistaxis, and a palpable mass with or without pain. They are typically initially diagnosed clinically as either chronic dacryocystitis or a primary malignancy.

Histopathology

These tumours can grow into bulky masses that fill the nasolacrimal drainage system and invade into adjacent orbit and bone. The microscopic appearance generally corresponds to that of the primary tumour.

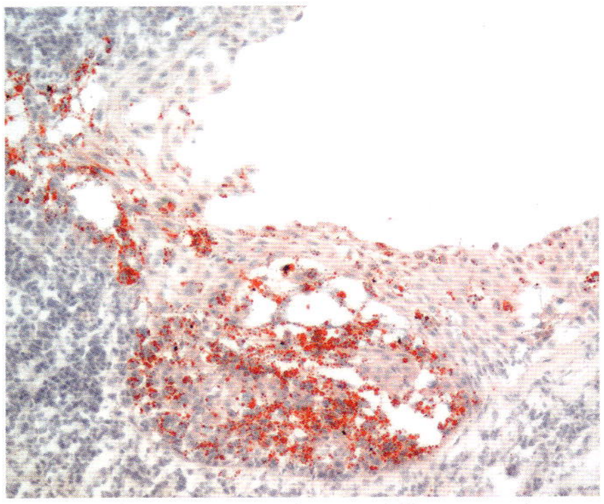

Fig. 6.18 Sebaceous carcinoma. This example extended from the eyelid down the canaliculus, as demonstrated on an intraoperative frozen section stained with Oil Red O.

Histogenesis

Lacrimal drainage system metastases have been reported from renal cell carcinoma, hepatocellular carcinoma, and cutaneous melanoma {418,1340,1378}. Nasopharyngeal carcinoma can spread directly into the lacrimal drainage system {1176}. Conjunctival melanoma and sebaceous carcinoma can recur in the nasolacrimal system, often several years after initial treatment {758,811,963}; it is sometimes unclear whether such recurrence results from direct extension or metastatic seeding.

Genetic profile

The genetic profile depends on the tumour type.

Prognosis and predictive factors

The outcomes for patients with tumours that metastasize to the lacrimal drainage system from distant sites are generally poor; death from disease is common.

Contributors

Dr Maysa AL HUSSAINI
Dept of Pathology and Laboratory Medicine
King Hussein Cancer Center
202 Queen Rania Al Abdullah Street
Amman 11941
JORDAN
Tel. +962 79 560 2694
Fax +962 6 530 0460
mhussaini@khcc.jo

Dr Daniel ALBERT
Department of Ophthalmology
Oregon Health & Science University
1603 South-East River Ridge Drive
Portland OR 97222
USA
Tel. +1 503 494 7896
albedan@ohsu.edu

Dr Hind ALKATAN
Departments of Ophthalmology & Pathology
Post Graduate Medical Education
College of Medicine
King Saud University Medical City
PO Box 18097
Riyadh 11415
SAUDI ARABIA
Tel. +966 50 449 2399
Fax +966 11 205 2740
hindkatan@yahoo.com

Dr Claudia AUW-HAEDRICH
Eye Center Freiburg
Killianstraße 5
79106 Freiburg
GERMANY
Tel. +49 761 270 40010
Fax +49 761 270 41090
claudia.auw-haedrich@uniklinik-freiburg.de

Dr Nikolaos E. BECHRAKIS
Department of Ophthalmology
Essen University Hospital
Hufelandstraße 55
45147 Essen
GERMANY
Tel. +49 201 723 3568
nikolaos.bechrakis@uk-essen.de

Dr Antonio BERMÚDEZ MAGNER
Department of Pathology
Instituto de Oftalmología
Conde de Valenciana
Chimalpopoca
06800 Mexico City
MEXICO
Tel. +52 1 55 54 54 22 69
Fax +52 5 55 52 59 74 23
antoniobermudez@gmail.com

Dr Jyotirmay BISWAS
Ophthalmic Pathology
Medical Research Foundation
18 College Road
600006 Chennai
INDIA
Tel. +91 98 4142 8151
Fax +91 44 2825 4180
drjb@snmail.org

Dr Fred T. BOSMAN*
Department of Pathology
University of Lausanne Medical Center
Rue du Bugnon 25
1011 Lausanne
SWITZERLAND
Tel. +41 21 731 10 30
Fax +41 21 314 72 05
fred.bosman@chuv.ch

Dr Anita Sook Yee CHAN
Ophthalmic Pathology Service
Singapore National Eye Center
Singapore General Hospital
11 Third Hospital Avenue
Singapore 168751
SINGAPORE
Tel. +65 8121 8507
Fax +65 6227 7255
anita.chan.s.y@snec.com.sg

Dr Svetlana CHEREPANOFF
Department of Pathology
St Vincent's Hospital Sydney
390 Victoria Street
Darlinghurst NSW 2010
AUSTRALIA
Tel. +61 2 8382 9168
Fax +61 2 8382 2888
svetlana.cherepanoff@gmail.com

Dr Patricia CHÉVEZ-BARRIOS
Department of Pathology
Houston Methodist Hospital
6565 Fannin Street, M227
Houston TX 77030
USA
Tel. +1 713 441 6484
Fax +1 713 793 1178
pchevez-barrios@houstonmethodist.org

Dr Sarah E. COUPLAND*
Department of Molecular and Clinical
Cancer Medicine
Institute of Translational Medicine
University of Liverpool
William Henry Duncan Building, 3rd Floor
Liverpool L7 8TX
UNITED KINGDOM
Tel. +44 151 706 5885
Fax +44 151 706 5859
s.e.coupland@liverpool.ac.uk

Dr J. Oscar CROXATTO
Departamento de Patología Ocular
Fundación Oftalmológica Argentina
Jorge Malbran
Viamonte 1181 6 Piso, C1053ABW
1014 Buenos Aires
ARGENTINA
Tel. +54 11 4519 8685
juan.croxatto@gmail.com

Dr Thomas CUMMINGS*
Department of Pathology
Duke University Medical Center
DUMC Box 3712
Durham NC 27710
USA
Tel. +1 919 684 6592
Fax +1 919 613 2381
thomas.cummings@duke.edu

Dr Sander DUBOVY*
Department of Ophthalmology
Bascom Palmer Eye Institute
900 North-West 17th Street
Miami FL 33136
USA
Tel. +1 305 326 6357
Fax +1 305 547 3674
sdubovy@med.miami.edu

---

* Indicates participation in the Working Group Meeting on the WHO Classification of Tumours of the Eye that was held in Lyon, France, 11–13 January 2018.
# Indicates disclosure of interests (see p. 189).

Dr Ralph C. EAGLE Jr*
Department of Pathology
Wills Eye Hospital
840 Walnut Street, Suite 1410
Philadelphia PA 19107
USA
reagle@willseye.org

Dr Charles G. EBERHART*
Ophthalmic Pathology Division
Wilmer Eye Institute
Johns Hopkins University
600 North Wolfe Street
Baltimore MD 21287
USA
Tel. +1 410 502 5185
ceberha@jhmi.edu

Dr Deepak P. EDWARD
University of Illinois Eye and Ear Infirmary
1855 West Taylor Street
Chicago IL 60612
USA
deepedwa@uic.edu

Dr Robert FOLBERG
William Beaumont Hospital
O'Dowd Hall, Room 428
586 Pioneer Drive
Rochester MI 48309
USA
Tel. +1 248 370 2452
Fax +1 248 370 3638
rfolberg@oakland.edu

Dr Hans E. GROSSNIKLAUS*
Emory Eye Center
1365 Clifton Road, BT 428
Atlanta GA 30322
USA
ophtheg@emory.edu

Dr J. William HARBOUR#
Ophthalmology
Bascom Palmer Eye Institute
900 North-West 17th Street, Room 271
Miami FL 33136
USA
Tel. +1 305 326 6166
harbour@med.miami.edu

Dr George HAROCOPOS
Department of Ophthalmology
Washington University School of Medicine
660 South Euclid Avenue, Campus Box 8096
St Louis MO 63110
USA
harocopos@vision.wustl.edu

Dr Godfrey HEATHCOTE
Department of Pathology
Dalhousie University
Sir Charles Tupper Medical Building, 11 B2
Halifax NS B3H 4H7
CANADA
Tel. +1 902 494 2502
Fax +1 902 494 2519
godfrey.heathcote@dal.ca

Dr Steffen HEEGAARD*
Dept of Ophthalmology and Pathology
Rigshospitalet
University of Copenhagen
Frederik d. V's Vej 11
2100 Copenhagen
DENMARK
Tel. +45 35 32 60 75
sthe@sund.ku.dk

Dr Martina C. HERWIG-CARL
Department of Ophthalmology
University of Bonn
Ernst-Abbe-Straße 2
53127 Bonn
GERMANY
Tel. +49 228 2871 5505
martina.herwig@ukbonn.de

Dr Codrin E. IACOB
Department of Pathology
New York Eye and Ear Infirmary
of Mount Sinai
310 East 14th Street, 3rd Floor
New York NY 10003
USA
Tel. +1 212 979 4156
Fax +1 212 677 1284
ciacob@nyee.edu

Dr Satoru KASE
Department of Ophthalmology
Teine Keijinkai Hospital
Maeda 1-12, Teine-ku
Sapporo 006-0811
JAPAN
kaseron@med.hokudai.ac.jp

Dr Tero T. KIVELÄ*
Ophthalmic Pathology Laboratory
Helsinki University Central Hospital
Haartmaninkatu 4 C PL220
00029 Helsinki
FINLAND
tero.kivela@helsinki.fi

Dr Nora LAVER
Ocular Pathology Laboratory
Tufts Medical Center
800 Washington Street, Box 6700
Boston MA 02111
USA
nlaver@tuftsmedicalcenter.org

Dr Alexander J. LAZAR*
Departments of Pathology
and Genomic Medicine
University of Texas MD Anderson Cancer
1515 Holcombe Boulevard, Unit 85
Houston TX 77030
USA
alazar@mdanderson.org

Dr Bin LI
Beijing Institute of Ophthalmology
Beijing Tongren Hospital
Capital Medical University
Chong Wen Men
Beijing 100005
CHINA
Tel. +86 10 5826 8264
Fax +86 10 6512 5617
libin43_99@163.com

Dr Karin U. LOEFFLER
Universitäts-Augenklinik Bonn
Ernst-Abbe-Straße 2
53127 Bonn
GERMANY
Tel. +49 228 2871 9839
karinloeffler@uni-bonn.de

Dr Curtis MARGO
Departments of Ophthalmology and
Pathology & Cell Biology
Morsani College of Medicine
University of South Florida, Eye Pathology
13330 USF Laurel Drive, 4th Floor
Tampa FL 33612
USA
Tel. +1 813 974 3744
Fax +1 813 974 0337
cmargo@health.usf.edu

Dr Miguel A. MATERIN
Department of Ophthalmology
Duke University Medical Center
2351 Erwin Road
Durham NC 27705
USA
Tel. +1 919 684 8434
miguel.materin@duke.edu

Dr Pia MENDOZA
Department of Pathology
Emory University School of Medicine
1365 Clifton Road North-East
Atlanta GA 30322
USA
Tel. +1 404 712 8210
pia.mendoza@emory.edu

Dr Peter MEYER
University Eye Clinic Basel
Mittlere Strasse 91
4056 Basel
SWITZERLAND
meyerpe@uhbs.ch

Dr Daniela MIHIC-PROBST
Dept of Pathology and Molecular Pathology
University Hospital Zurich
Schmelzbergstrasse 12
8091 Zurich
SWITZERLAND
Tel. +41 44 255 25 95
Fax +41 44 255 44 16
daniela.mihic@usz.ch

Dr Tatyana MILMAN
Department of Ophthalmology
Wills Eye Hospital
840 Walnut Street, Suite 1410
Philadelphia PA 19107
USA
Tel. +1 215 928 3280
Fax +1 215 825 4703
tatyana.milman@gmail.com

Dr Ruchi MITTAL
Dalmia Ophthalmic Pathology Services
L.V. Prasad Eye Institute
Patia, Bhubaneswar
751024 Odisha
INDIA
Tel. +91 674 3987 179
Fax +91 674 3987 130
drruchimittal@lvpei.org

Dr Alexandre MOULIN
Department of Ophthalmology
University of Lausanne
Jules Gonin Eye Hospital
Avenue de France 15
1004 Lausanne
SWITZERLAND
Tel. +41 21 626 85 41
Fax +41 21 626 81 38
alexandre.moulin@fa2.ch

Dr Hardeep Singh MUDHAR*
National Specialist Ophthalmic Pathology Service, Dept of Histopathology
Royal Hallamshire Hospital, E-Floor
Glossop Road
Sheffield S10 2JF
UNITED KINGDOM
Tel. +44 114 226 8967
Fax +44 114 271 2200
hardeep.mudhar@sth.nhs.uk

Dr Hiroko OHGAKI*
Department of Neuropathology
Charité – Universitätsmedizin Berlin
Campus Charité Mitte
Charitéplatz 1
Virchowweg 15
10117 Berlin
GERMANY
hiroko.ohgaki@charite.de

Dr Jacob PE'ER
Division of Ophthalmology
Hadassah - Hebrew University Medical Center
PO Box 12,000
91120 Jerusalem
ISRAEL
peer@hadassah.org.il

Dr Narsing RAO
USC Roski Eye Institute
1450 San Pablo Street
Los Angeles CA 90033
USA
Tel. +1 323 442 5551
Fax +1 323 442 5574
nrao@usc.edu

Dr Dejan M. RAŠIĆ
Dept of Ophthalmology and Pathology
Clinic for Eye Diseases
Clinical Centre of Serbia
Pasterova 2
Belgrade 11000
SERBIA
Tel. +381 64 276 35 55
Fax +381 11 268 81 64
drnajed@gmail.com

Dr Fiona ROBERTS
Department of Pathology
Queen Elizabeth University Hospital
Govan Road
Glasgow G51 4TF
UNITED KINGDOM
Tel. +44 141 354 9512
f.roberts@nhs.net

Dr Fausto RODRIGUEZ
Department of Pathology
Johns Hopkins Hospital
Sheikh Zayed Tower
Room M2101
1800 Orleans Street
Baltimore MD 21231
USA
frodrig4@jhmi.edu

Dr Elisabeth J. RUSHING
Institute of Neuropathology
UniversitätsSpital Zürich
Schmelzbergstrasse 12
8091 Zurich
SWITZERLAND
Tel. +41 44 255 43 81
Fax +41 44 255 44 02
elisabethjane.rushing@usz.ch

Dr Diva R. SALOMAO*
Department of Pathology
Mayo Clinic College of Medicine
200 First Street South-West
Rochester MN 55905
USA
salomao.diva@mayo.edu

Dr Maria A. SAORNIL
Department of Ophthalmology
Hospital Clínico Universitario de Valladolid
Ramón y Cajal 3
47005 Valladolid
SPAIN
saornil@ono.com

Dr Lynn SCHOENFIELD
Department of Pathology
Ohio State University Wexner Medical Center
337 North Doan Hall
410 West 10th Avenue
Columbus OH 43210
USA
Tel. +1 614 688 8698
lynn.schoenfield@osumc.edu

Dr Arun SINGH
Cole Eye Institute
Cleveland Clinic
9500 Euclid Avenue
Cleveland OH 44195
USA
Tel. +1 216 445 9479
Fax +1 216 445 2226
singha@ccf.org

Dr Charles S. SPECHT
Department of Pathology (Neuropathology)
Penn State Health Hershey Medical Center
500 University Drive
Hershey PA 17033-0850
USA
Tel. +1 717 531 1305
Fax +1 717 531 7741
cspecht@pennstatehealth.psu.edu

Dr Anat O. STEMMER-RACHAMIMOV
Pathology, Neuropathology Division
Massachusetts General Hospital
55 Fruit Street, Warren Building, 333A
Boston MA 02114
USA
Tel. +1 617 726 5156
Fax +1 617 724 1813
astemmerrachamimov@partners.org

Dr Nasreen SYED
F.C. Blodi Eye Pathology Laboratory
University of Iowa
233 Medical Research Center
Iowa City IA 52242
USA
Tel. +1 319 335 7192
nasreen-syed@uiowa.edu

Dr Caroline THAUNG
Department of Eye Pathology
UCL Institute of Ophthalmology
11-43 Bath Street
London EC1V 9EL
UNITED KINGDOM
Tel. +44 207 608 6890
Fax +44 207 608 6862
c.thaung@ucl.ac.uk

Dr Mark O.M. TSO
Wilmer Eye Institute
Johns Hopkins University SOM
4035 Smith Building
400 North Broadway Street
Baltimore MD 21287-9142
USA
Tel. +1 410 614 0229
Fax +1 410 614 1114
matso@jhmi.edu

Dr Paul VAN DER VALK
Afd. Pathologie
VU University Medical Center
Postbus 7057
1007 MB Amsterdam
NETHERLANDS
Tel. +31 20 444 4977
p.vandervalk@vumc.nl

Dr Rita VAN GINDERDEUREN
Ophthalmology and Pathology
University Clinics Leuven, UZ Leuven
Herestraat 49
3000 Leuven
BELGIUM
Tel. +32 495 218413
Fax +32 16 332367
rita.vanginderdeuren@uzleuven.be

Dr Geeta VEMUGANTI*
School of Medical Sciences
University of Hyderabad
Prof. C.R. Rao Road
Gachibowli
500046 Hyderabad
INDIA
Tel. +91 40 2313 5472
gkvemuganti@gmail.com

Dr Robert M. VERDIJK#
Department of Pathology,
Section Ophthalmic Pathology
Erasmus MC Cancer Institute
Erasmus MC University Medical Center
Rotterdam
PO Box 2040
3000 CA Rotterdam
NETHERLANDS
Tel. +31 10 704 3960
r.verdijk@erasmusmc.nl

Dr Valerie A. WHITE*
WHO Classification of Tumours Group
International Agency for Research on Cancer
150 Cours Albert Thomas
69372 Lyon
FRANCE
Tel. +33 4 72 73 86 77
Fax +33 4 72 73 86 98
whitev@iarc.fr

Dr David WILSON
Department of Ophthalmology
Casey Eye Institute
3375 South-West Terwilliger Boulevard
Portland OR 97239
USA
Tel. +1 503 494 3051
Fax +1 503 494 5446
wilsonda@ohsu.edu

Dr Matthew WILSON
Hamilton Eye Institute
930 Madison Avenue
Suite #200
Room 476
Memphis TN 38103
USA
mwilson5@uthsc.edu

Declaration of interests

Dr Harbour reports receiving personal consulting fees from and holding intellectual property in Castle Biosciences, Inc.

Dr Verdijk reports receiving research support from Stichting Nederlands Oogheelkundig Onderzoek (SNOO), Stichting Wetenschappelijk Onderzoek Het Oogziekenhuis (SWOO), and Henkes Stichting.

IARC/WHO Committee for the International Classification of Diseases for Oncology (ICD-O)

Dr Ian A. CREE
WHO Classification of Tumours Group
International Agency for Research on Cancer
150 Cours Albert Thomas
69372 Lyon
FRANCE
Tel. +33 4 72 73 85 34
Fax +33 4 72 73 86 98
creei@iarc.fr

Dr Robert JAKOB
Data Standards and Informatics
World Health Organization (WHO)
20 Avenue Appia
1211 Geneva 27
SWITZERLAND
Tel. +41 22 791 58 77
Fax +41 22 791 48 94
jakobr@who.int

Dr Brian ROUS
National Cancer Registration Service
Victoria House, Capital Park
Fulbourn CB21 5XA
UNITED KINGDOM
Tel. +44 1223 213 625
Fax +44 1223 213 571
brian.rous@phe.gov.uk

Dr Ariana ZNAOR
Section of Cancer Surveillance
International Agency for Research on Cancer
150 Cours Albert Thomas
69372 Lyon
FRANCE
Tel. +33 4 72 73 83 52
Fax +33 4 72 73 86 96
znaora@iarc.fr

Sources of figures and tables

Sources of figures

1.01	White V.A.
1.02	Gichuhi S, Sagoo MS, Weiss HA, Burton MJ (2013). Epidemiology of ocular surface squamous neoplasia in Africa. Trop Med Int Health. 18(12):1424–43. PMID:24237784. https://creativecommons.org/licenses/by/4.0/
1.03 A–D	Eagle R.C. Jr
1.03 E,F	Dr Christopher W. Toon Northern Clinical School University of Sydney St Leonards AUSTRALIA
1.04	Alkatan H.
1.05	Mudhar H.S.
1.06	Reproduced from Oellers P, Karp CL, Shah RR, Winnick M, Matthews J, Dubovy S (2014). Conjunctival keratoacanthoma. Br J Ophthalmol. 98(2):275–6,285. PMID:24288390. Copyright 2014. With permission from BMJ Publishing Group Ltd.
1.07	Grossniklaus H.E.
1.08	Cummings T.
1.09 A	Li B.
1.09 B–D	Grossniklaus H.E.
1.10 A,B	Mudhar H.S.
1.10 C,D	Grossniklaus H.E.
1.11	Grossniklaus H.E.
1.12	White V.A.
1.13	Eberhart C.G.
1.14	Grossniklaus H.E.
1.15	Mudhar H.S.
1.16–1.17	Auw-Haedrich C.
1.18	Iacob C.E.
1.19	Reprinted, with permission, from Margo CE, Grossniklaus HE (2001). Pseudoadenomatous hyperplasia of the conjunctiva. Ophthalmology. 108(1):135–8. PMID:11150278
1.20–1.23	Margo C.
1.24	Coupland S.E.
1.25	Rašić D.M.
1.26–1.27	Elder DE, Massi D, Scolyer RA, Willemze R, editors (2018). WHO classification of skin tumours. 4th ed. Lyon: International Agency for Research on Cancer; p. 143. Available from: http://publications.iarc.fr/560.
1.28–1.29	Pe'er J.
1.30	Mudhar H.S.
1.31	Dr Carol Shields and Dr Jerry Shields Ocular Oncology Service Wills Eye Hospital Philadelphia PA USA
1.32	Eagle R.C. Jr
1.33–1.34	Van Ginderdeuren R.
1.35 A	Kivelä T.T.
1.35 B,C	Chan A.S.Y.
1.36–1.38	Coupland S.E.
1.39	White V.A.
1.40	Reprinted, with permission from Taylor and Francis, from Nair AG, Kaliki S, Kamal S, Mishra DK, Vemuganti GK (2015). Conjunctival leiomyosarcoma: a report of two cases. Orbit. 34(5):274–8. PMID:26214581
1.41 A	Mendez Mdel C, Muiños Y, Blanco G, Saornil MA, García-Alvarez C, Sarasa JL, et al. (2012). Embryonal rhabdomyosarcoma of the caruncle in a 4 year-old boy: case report. Arq Bras Oftalmol. 75(3):207-9. PMID:22872206
1.41 B,C	Saornil M.A.
1.42	Grossniklaus H.E.
1.43–1.44	Mudhar H.S.
1.45–1.46	Grossniklaus H.E.
1.47	Alkatan H.
1.48	Laver N.
1.49	Li B.
1.50 A	Harocopos G.
1.50 B,C	Li B.
1.51	Dr Philip L. Custer Department of Ophthalmology and Visual Sciences Washington University School of Medicine in St. Louis St. Louis MO USA
1.52 A	Alkatan H.
1.52 B	Harocopos G.
1.53	Cummings T.
1.54	Verdijk R.M.
1.55 A	Cummings T.
1.55 B	Stemmer-Rachamimov A.O.
1.56	Alkatan H.
1.57–1.58	Herwig-Carl M.C.
1.59	Verdijk R.M.
1.60	Moulin A.
1.61–1.62	Eagle R.C. Jr
1.63	Mudhar H.S.
2.01	Brierly JD, Gospodarowicz MK, Wittekind C, editors (2017). TNM classification of malignant tumours. 8th ed. Oxford: Wiley Blackwell.
2.02	Grossniklaus H.E.
2.03	With permission, from Brown HH, Wells JR, Grossniklaus HE (2013). Tissue preparation for pathological examination. In: Grossniklaus HE, editor. Pocket guide to ocular oncology and pathology. Berlin: Springer-Verlag; pp. 61–8. With permission of Springer Nature.
2.04	Bechrakis N.E.
2.05	Eagle R.C. Jr
2.06–2.07	Bechrakis N.E.
2.08 A	Grossniklaus H.E.
2.08 B	Eagle R.C. Jr
2.08 C	Bechrakis N.E.
2.08 D	Mudhar H.S.
2.09	Mudhar H.S.
2.10	Grossniklaus H.E.
2.11 A	Pe'er J.
2.11 B	Grossniklaus H.E.
2.12	Mudhar H.S.
2.13	Grossniklaus H.E.
2.14	Bechrakis N.E.
2.15	Eagle R.C. Jr
2.16	Mudhar H.S.
2.17–2.18	Grossniklaus H.E.
2.19	Iacob C.E.
2.20	Meyer P.
2.21	Kivelä T.T.
2.22 A,B	Grossniklaus H.E.
2.22 C	Pe'er J.
2.23	Salomao D.R.
2.24	Kivelä T.T.
2.25–2.26	Moulin A.
2.27	Eagle R.C. Jr
2.28	Li B.
2.29 A,B	Li B.
2.29 C	Rao N.
2.30–2.32	Roberts F.
2.33 A	Roberts F.
2.33 B	Kivelä T.T.
2.34–2.37	Eagle R.C. Jr
2.38	Mudhar H.S.
2.39 A,C	Rao N.
2.39 B	Mudhar H.S.
2.40–2.43	Mudhar H.S.
2.44	Eagle R.C. Jr
2.45 A	Eagle R.C. Jr
2.45 B,C	Grossniklaus H.E.
2.46–2.47	Grossniklaus H.E.
2.48	Salomao D.R.
2.49 A	Grossniklaus H.E.
2.49 B	Eagle R.C. Jr
2.49 C	White V.A.
2.50	Eagle R.C. Jr
2.51	Mudhar H.S.
2.52–2.53	Grossniklaus H.E.
2.54	Salomao D.R.
2.55	Eagle R.C. Jr
2.56	Mudhar H.S.
2.57	Eagle R.C. Jr
2.58 A	Eagle R.C. Jr

2.58 B	Rodriguez F.
2.59 A	Dr Michele M. Bloomer Department of Ophthalmology University of California, San Francisco San Francisco CA USA
2.59 B,C	Mudhar H.S.
2.60–2.63	Eagle R.C. Jr
2.64	Materin M.A.
2.65	Reprinted, with permission, from Williams AT, Font RL, Van Dyk HJ, Riekhof FT (1978). Osseous choristoma of the choroid simulating a choroidal melanoma. Association with a positive 32P test. Arch Ophthalmol. 96(10):1874–7. PMID:697626
2.66–2.67	Grossniklaus H.E.
2.68–2.69	Modified, with permission, from O'Keefe JS, Sippy BD, Martin DF, Holden JT, Grossniklaus HE (2002). Anterior chamber infiltrates associated with systemic lymphoma: report of two cases and review of the literature. Ophthalmology. 109(2):253–7. PMID:11825804
2.70	Coupland S.E.
2.71 A	Dr Bertil Damato Department of Ophthalmology University of California, San Francisco San Francisco CA USA
2.71 B	Dr Jay S. Duker Department of Ophthalmology and New England Eye Center Tufts University School of Medicine Boston MA USA
2.71 C,D	Coupland S.E.
2.72–2.73	Meyer P.
3.01 left	Eagle R.C. Jr
3.01 right	Kivelä T.T.
3.02 A,B,D	Eagle R.C. Jr
3.02 C	Reprinted, with permission, from Zimmerman LE (1969). Retinoblastoma, including a report of illustrative cases. Med Ann Dist Columbia. 38(7):366–74. PMID:5255154
3.03–3.08	Eagle R.C. Jr
3.09–3.10	Margo C.
3.11	Eberhart C.G.
3.12	Mudhar H.S.
3.13	Eberhart C.G.
3.14	Reprinted, with permission, from Hudson LE, Mendoza PR, Yan J, Grossniklaus HE (2017). Reactive retinal astrocytic tumor (focal nodular gliosis): a case report. Ocul Oncol Pathol. 3(1):1–7. PMID:28275595. Copyright © 2017 Karger Publishers, Basel, Switzerland.
3.15	Mudhar H.S.
3.16	Poole Perry LJ, Jakobiec FA, Zakka FR, Reichel E, Herwig MC, Perry A, et al. (2013). Reactive retinal astrocytic tumors (so-called vasoproliferative tumors): histopathologic, immunohistochemical, and genetic studies of four cases. Am J Ophthalmol. 155(3):593–608.e1. PMID:23219067. Copyright 2013, with permission from Elsevier.
3.17–3.18	Wilson D.
3.19	Eagle R.C. Jr
3.20–3.21	Wilson D.
3.22	White V.A.
3.23	Dr Jay S. Duker Department of Ophthalmology and New England Eye Center Tufts University School of Medicine Boston MA USA
3.24–3.26	Eagle R.C. Jr
3.27	Grossniklaus H.E.
3.28	Eagle R.C. Jr
3.29	Kivelä T.T.
3.30 A	Dr Carol Shields Ocular Oncology Service Wills Eye Hospital Philadelphia PA USA
3.30 B	Dr Ramon Font Department of Ophthalmology Baylor College of Medicine Houston TX USA
3.30 C	Eagle R.C. Jr
3.31–3.32	Eagle R.C. Jr
4.01	International Agency for Research on Cancer (IARC)
4.02–4.05	Cummings T.
4.06 A	Rodriguez F.
4.06 B	Cummings T.
4.07–4.08	Eberhart C.G.
4.09–4.11	Rodriguez F.
4.12–4.13	Eberhart C.G.
5.01	Dr Thonnie Rose O. See Emory Eye Center Atlanta GA USA Modified, with permission, from Grossniklaus HE, Abbuhl MF, McLean IW (1990). Immunohistologic properties of benign and malignant mixed tumor of the lacrimal gland. Am J Ophthalmol. 110(5):540–9. PMID:1700612
5.02	Grossniklaus H.E.
5.03	Dr Antonio A.V. Cruz Department of Ophthalmology, Otorhinolaryngology and Head and Neck Surgery Ribeirão Preto Medical School University of São Paulo São Paulo BRAZIL
5.04–5.05	Alkatan H.
5.06	Adapted from Alkatan HM, Al-Harkan DH, Al-Mutlaq M, Maktabi A, Elkhamary SM (2014). Epithelial lacrimal gland tumors: a comprehensive clinicopathologic review of 26 lesions with radiologic correlation. Saudi J Ophthalmol. 28(1):49–57. PMID:24526859. With permission from Elsevier.
5.07	Mudhar H.S.
5.08	Alkatan H.
5.09	Grossniklaus H.E.
5.10	White V.A.
5.11	Mudhar H.S.
5.12	Salomao D.R.
5.13	Grossniklaus H.E.
5.14	Thaung C.
5.15–5.16	Iacob C.E.
5.17–5.18	Grossniklaus H.E.
5.19	Iacob C.E.
5.20 A,D,E	Reprinted, with permission, from Wiwatwongwana D, Berean KW, Dolman PJ, Rootman J, White VA (2009). Unusual carcinomas of the lacrimal gland: epithelial-myoepithelial carcinoma and myoepithelial carcinoma. Arch Ophthalmol. 127(8):1054–6. PMID:19667347
5.20 B,C	White V.A.
5.21–5.22	Dr Martin Hyrcza Department of Pathology and Molecular Medicine McMaster University Hamilton ON CANADA
5.23 A,B	Reprinted from Hyrcza MD, Andreasen S, Melchior LC, Tucker T, Heegaard S, White VA (2018). Primary secretory carcinoma of the lacrimal gland: report of a new entity. Am J Ophthalmol. 193:178–83. PMID:29963997, with permission from Elsevier.
5.23 C	White V.A.
5.24	Reprinted from Hyrcza MD, Andreasen S, Melchior LC, Tucker T, Heegaard S, White VA (2018). Primary secretory carcinoma of the lacrimal gland: report of a new entity. Am J Ophthalmol. 193:178–83. PMID:29963997, with permission from Elsevier.

5.25	Dr Tracy Tucker Cancer Genetics and Genomics Laboratory BC Cancer Agency Department of Pathology and Laboratory Medicine, UBC Vancouver BC CANADA Reprinted from Hyrcza MD, Andreasen S, Melchior LC, Tucker T, Heegaard S, White VA (2018). Primary secretory carcinoma of the lacrimal gland: report of a new entity. Am J Ophthalmol. 193:178–83. PMID:29963997, with permission from Elsevier.
5.26–5.27	Reprinted, with permission, from Rosenbaum PS, Mahadevia PS, Goodman LA, Kress Y (1995). Acinic cell carcinoma of the lacrimal gland. Arch Ophthalmol. 113(6):781–5. PMID:7540387
5.28	Grossniklaus H.E.
5.29	Dr Sunny Shen General Cataract and Comprehensive Ophthalmology Department Singapore National Eye Centre SINGAPORE
5.30	Chan A.S.Y.
5.31	Coupland S.E.
5.32	Grossniklaus H.E.
5.33	Coupland S.E.
5.34	Verdijk R.M.

6.01	International Agency for Research on Cancer (IARC)
6.02–6.03	Heegaard S.
6.04	Mudhar H.S.
6.05 A,B	Heegaard S.
6.05 C,D	Mudhar H.S.
6.06–6.10	Heegaard S.
6.11 A,B	Heegaard S.
6.11 C	Rašić D.M.
6.12	Heegaard S.
6.13	Mittal R.
6.14–6.15	Heathcote G.
6.16–6.18	Eberhart C.G.

Sources of tables

1.01	Gichuhi S, Sagoo MS, Weiss HA, Burton MJ (2013). Epidemiology of ocular surface squamous neoplasia in Africa. Trop Med Int Health. 18(12):1424–43. PMID:24237784. https://creativecommons.org/licenses/by/4.0/
1.02	Coupland S.E.
2.01	Roberts F.
5.01	Verdijk R.M.

Sources of figures on front cover

Top left	Grossniklaus H.E. (Fig. 2.45 C)
Top centre	Eagle R.C. Jr (Fig. 2.45 A)
Top right	Eagle R.C. Jr (Fig. 3.04)
Middle left	Eagle R.C. Jr (Fig. 2.50 A)
Middle centre	Eagle R.C. Jr (Fig. 2.50 B)
Middle right	Eagle R.C. Jr (Fig. 3.06 B)
Bottom left	Mudhar H.S. (Fig. 2.51 B)
Bottom centre	Salomao D.R. (Fig. 2.48)
Bottom right	Eagle R.C. Jr (Fig. 3.08)

References

1. Aaberg TM, Benjamin EP, Biscotti CV, Singh AD (2013). Bilateral choroidal tumors consistent with metastatic malignant paraganglioma. Retin Cases Brief Rep. 7(4):301–3. PMID:25383831

2. Abdellatief A, Mason CM, Ytterberg SR, Boorjian SA, Salomão DR, Pulido J (2015). Choroidal involvement in Erdheim-Chester disease. Ophthalmic Surg Lasers Imaging Retina. 46(6):674–6. PMID:26114850

3. Abdolrahimzadeh S, Plateroti AM, Recupero SM, Lambiase A (2016). An update on the ophthalmologic features in the phakomatoses. J Ophthalmol. 2016:3043026. PMID:27493794

4. Abouzeid H, Balmer A, Moulin AP, Mataftsi A, Zografos L, Munier FL (2012). Phenotypic variability of retinocytomas: preregression and postregression growth patterns. Br J Ophthalmol. 96(6):884–9. PMID:22328814

5. Abramson DH, Dunkel IJ, Brodie SE, Kim JW, Gobin YP (2008). A phase I/II study of direct intraarterial (ophthalmic artery) chemotherapy with melphalan for intraocular retinoblastoma initial results. Ophthalmology. 115(8):1398–404, 1404. PMID:18342944

6. Adachi N, Tsuyama Y, Mizota A, Fujimoto N, Suehiro S, Adachi-Usami E (2003). Optic disc metastasis presenting as an initial sign of recurrence of adenoid cystic carcinoma of the larynx. Eye (Lond). 17(2):270–2. PMID:12640429

7. Addison DJ, Font RL (1984). Glioneuroma of iris and ciliary body. Arch Ophthalmol. 102(3):419–21. PMID:6703991

8. Affeldt JC, Minckler DS, Azen SP, Yeh L (1980). Prognosis in uveal melanoma with extrascleral extension. Arch Ophthalmol. 98(11):1975–9. PMID:7436829

9. Afrogheh AH, Jakobiec FA, Hammon R, Grossniklaus HE, Rocco J, Lindeman NI, et al. (2016). Evaluation for high-risk HPV in squamous cell carcinomas and precursor lesions arising in the conjunctiva and lacrimal sac. Am J Surg Pathol. 40(4):519–28. PMID:26735858

10. Ahamed NA, Sait K, Anfnan N, Farwan K, Nizamuddin SH, Baeesa SS (2015). Gestational choriocarcinoma presenting with lacrimal gland metastasis: a first reported case. Case Rep Obstet Gynecol. 2015:879538. PMID:26075121

11. Akda F, Hamezi F, Heule-Dieleman HA, van den Bosch WA, Luyten GP, Tanghe HL, et al. (2010). Orbital metastases of breast cancer. Radiologic features. Ophthalmologe. 107(8):728–32. [German] PMID:20393728

12. Akinsola FB, Mbadugha CA, Onakoya AO, Adefule-Ositelu AO, Aribaba OT, Rotimi-Samuel A (2012). Pattern of conjunctival masses seen at Guinness Eye Centre Luth Idi-Araba. Nig Q J Hosp Med. 22(1):39–43. PMID:23175879

13. Al-Dahmash SA, Shields CL, Kaliki S, Johnson T, Shields JA (2014). Enhanced depth imaging optical coherence tomography of choroidal metastasis in 14 eyes. Retina. 34(8):1588–93. PMID:24743640

14. Al-Ghadeer H, Al-Assiri A, Al-Odhaib S, Alkatan H (2012). Successful removal of a conjunctival myxoma. Middle East Afr J Ophthalmol. 19(3):352–3. PMID:22837636

15. Al-Jamal RT, Cassoux N, Desjardins L, Damato B, Konstantinidis L, Coupland SE, et al. (2016). The Pediatric Choroidal and Ciliary Body Melanoma Study: a survey by the European Ophthalmic Oncology Group. Ophthalmology. 123(4):898–907. PMID:26854035

16. Al-Jamal RT, Mäkitie T, Kivelä T (2003). Nucleolar diameter and microvascular factors as independent predictors of mortality from malignant melanoma of the choroid and ciliary body. Invest Ophthalmol Vis Sci. 44(6):2381–9. PMID:12766034

17. AlAkeely AG, Alkatan HM, Alsuhaibani AH, AlKhalidi H, Safieh LA, Coupland SE, et al. (2017). Benign reactive lymphoid hyperplasia of the conjunctiva in childhood. Br J Ophthalmol. 101(7):933–9. PMID:27899370

18. Alameddine RM, Mansour AM, Kahtani E (2014). Review of choroidal osteomas. Middle East Afr J Ophthalmol. 21(3):244–50. PMID:25100910

19. Albert DM, Dryja TP (1988). Recent studies of the retinoblastoma gene. What it means to the ophthalmologist. Arch Ophthalmol. 106(2):181–2. PMID:3422555

20. Ali MJ, Bothra N, Naik MN (2018). Transitional cell carcinoma of lacrimal sac. Ophthal Plast Reconstr Surg. 34(3):e106. PMID:28582372

21. Ali MJ, Honavar SG, Vemuganti GK (2013). Ciliary body medulloepithelioma in an adult. Surv Ophthalmol. 58(3):266–72. PMID:23218809

22. Alkatan H, Al-Qurashi M (2017). Is routine histopathological examination of dacryocystorhinostomy/dacryocystectomy specimens necessary? A tertiary eye hospital experience. Can J Ophthalmol. 52(1):34–41. PMID:28237146

23. Alkatan HM, Al Qahtani AA, Maktabi AM (2016). Intraocular adenocarcinoma: histopathological report of two cases with different origin. Can J Ophthalmol. 51(2):e67–70. PMID:27085283

24. Alkatan HM, Al-Arfaj KM, Maktabi A (2010). Conjunctival nevi: clinical and histopathologic features in a Saudi population. Ann Saudi Med. 30(4):306–12. PMID:20622349

25. Alkatan HM, Al-Harkan DH, Al-Mutlaq M, Maktabi A, Elkhamary SM (2014). Epithelial lacrimal gland tumors: a comprehensive clinicopathologic review of 26 lesions with radiologic correlation. Saudi J Ophthalmol. 28(1):49–57. PMID:24526859

26. Alkatan HM, Al-Motlak MA, Al-Shedoukhy AA (2010). Metastatic squamous spindle cell carcinoma of the conjunctiva. Saudi J Ophthalmol. 24(4):155–8. PMID:23960894

27. Alkatan HM, Al-Rajhi AA (2016). Corneal xanthogranuloma in association with multiple endocrine neoplasia 1: a clinicopathologic case report and review of the literature. Saudi J Ophthalmol. 30(1):49–52. PMID:26949359

28. Allen CE, Parsons DW (2015). Biological and clinical significance of somatic mutations in Langerhans cell histiocytosis and related histiocytic neoplastic disorders. Hematology (Am Soc Hematol Educ Program). 2015(1):559–64. PMID:26637772

29. Allen RA, Straatsma BR (1961). Ocular involvement in leukemia and allied disorders. Arch Ophthalmol. 66(4):490–508. PMID:13860566

30. Allingham RR, Seo B, Rampersaud E, Bembe M, Challa P, Liu N, et al. (2001). A duplication in chromosome 4q35 is associated with hereditary benign intraepithelial dyskeratosis. Am J Hum Genet. 68(2):491–4. PMID:11170897

31. Almeida A, Kaliki S, Shields CL (2013). Autofluorescence of intraocular tumours. Curr Opin Ophthalmol. 24(3):222–32. PMID:23429597

32. Alves LF, Fernandes BF, Burnier JV, Zoroquiain P, Eskenazi DT, Burnier MN Jr (2011). Incidence of epithelial lesions of the conjunctiva in a review of 12,102 specimens in Canada (Quebec). Arq Bras Oftalmol. 74(1):21–3. PMID:21670902

33. Amin MB, Edge S, Greene F, Byrd DR, Brookland RK, Washington MK, et al., editors (2017). AJCC cancer staging manual. 8th ed. New York: Springer.

34. Amin RM, Hussein FA, Idriss HF, Hanafy NF, Abdallah DM (2013). Pathological, immunohistochemical and microbiologicalal analysis of lacrimal sac biopsies in patients with chronic dacrocystitis. Int J Ophthalmol. 6(6):817–26. PMID:24392331

35. Amoli FA, Heidari AB (2006). Survey of 447 patients with conjunctival neoplastic lesions in Farabi Eye Hospital, Tehran, Iran. Ophthalmic Epidemiol. 13(4):275–9. PMID:16877286

36. Anastassiou G, Heiligenhaus A, Bechrakis N, Bader E, Bornfeld N, Steuhl KP (2002). Prognostic value of clinical and histopathological parameters in conjunctival melanomas: a retrospective study. Br J Ophthalmol. 86(2):163–7. PMID:11815341

37. Anderson BH, Kasher PR, Mayer J, Szynkiewicz M, Jenkinson EM, Bhaskar SS, et al. (2012). Mutations in CTC1, encoding conserved telomere maintenance component 1, cause Coats plus. Nat Genet. 44(3):338–42. PMID:22267198

38. Anderson KK, Lessner AM, Hood I, Mendenhall W, Stringer S, Warren R (1994). Invasive transitional cell carcinoma of the lacrimal sac arising in an inverted papilloma. Arch Ophthalmol. 112(3):306–7. PMID:8129653

39. Andreasen S, Esmaeli B, Holstein SL, Mikkelsen LH, Rasmussen PK, Heegaard S (2017). An update on tumors of the lacrimal gland. Asia Pac J Ophthalmol (Phila). 6(2):159–72. PMID:28399336

40. Andreasen S, Grauslund M, Heegaard S (2017). Lacrimal gland ductal carcinomas: clinical, morphological and genetic characterization and implications for targeted treatment. Acta Ophthalmol. 95(3):299–306. PMID:27808478

41. Andreasen S, Heegaard S, Grauslund M, Homøe P (2016). The interleukin-6/Janus kinase/STAT3 pathway in pleomorphic adenoma and carcinoma ex pleomorphic adenoma of the lacrimal gland. Acta Ophthalmol. 94(8):798–804. PMID:27286739

42. Andreoli MT, Aakalu V, Setabutr P (2015). Epidemiological trends in malignant lacrimal gland tumors. Otolaryngol Head Neck Surg. 152(2):279–83. PMID:25385802

43. Andrew NH, Coupland SE, Pirbhai A, Selva D (2016). Lymphoid hyperplasia of the orbit and ocular adnexa: a clinical pathologic review. Surv Ophthalmol. 61(6):778–90. PMID:27127077

44. Andrew NH, Sladden N, Kearney DJ, Selva D (2015). An analysis of IgG4-related disease (IgG4-RD) among idiopathic orbital inflammations and benign lymphoid hyperplasias using two consensus-based diagnostic criteria for IgG4-RD. Br J Ophthalmol. 99(3):376–81. PMID:25185258

45. Angell LK, Burton TC (1978). Posterior choroidal involvement in Letterer-Siwe disease. J Pediatr Ophthalmol Strabismus. 15(2):79–81. PMID:739337

46. Annels NE, Da Costa CE, Prins FA, Willemze A, Hogendoorn PC, Egeler RM (2003). Aberrant chemokine receptor expression and chemokine production by Langerhans cells underlies the pathogenesis of Langerhans cell histiocytosis. J Exp Med. 197(10):1385–90. PMID:12743170

47. Apple DJ, Craythorn JM, Reidy JJ, Steinmetz RL, Brady SE, Bohart WA (1984). Malignant transformation of an optic nerve melanocytoma. Can J Ophthalmol. 19(7):320–5. PMID:6525581

48. Apushkin MA, Apushkin MA, Shapiro MJ, Mafee MF (2005). Retinoblastoma and simulating lesions: role of imaging. Neuroimaging Clin N Am. 15(1):49–67. PMID:15927860

49. Araujo I, Coupland SE (2017). Primary vitreoretinal lymphoma – a review. Asia Pac J Ophthalmol (Phila). 6(3):283–9. PMID:28558176

50. Arepalli S, Kaliki S, Shields CL (2015). Choroidal metastases: origin, features, and therapy. Indian J Ophthalmol. 63(2):122–7. PMID:25827542

51. Arepalli S, Kaliki S, Shields JA, Shields CL (2012). Growth of congenital hypertrophy of the retinal pigment epithelium over 22 years. J Pediatr Ophthalmol Strabismus. 49 Online:e73–5. PMID:23244302

52. Arepalli S, Shields CL, Kaliki S, Emrich J, Komarnicky L, Shields JA (2013). Diffuse choroidal hemangioma management with plaque radiotherapy in 5 cases. Ophthalmology. 120(11):2358–9. PMID:24182566

53. Argyris PP, Pambuccian SE, Cayci Z, Singh C, Tosios KI, Koutlas IG (2013). Lacrimal gland adenoid cystic carcinoma with high-grade transformation to myoepithelial carcinoma: report of a case and review of literature. Head Neck Pathol. 7(1):85–92. PMID:22829347

54. Aronow ME, Nakagawa JA, Gupta A, Traboulsi EI, Singh AD (2012). Tuberous sclerosis complex: genotype/phenotype correlation of retinal findings. Ophthalmology. 119(9):1917–23. PMID:22608477

55. Arora R, Monga S, Mehta DK, Raina UK, Gogi A, Gupta SD (2006). Malignant fibrous histiocytoma of the conjunctiva. Clin Experiment Ophthalmol. 34(3):275–8. PMID:16671910

56. Ash JE (1950). Epibulbar tumors. Am J Ophthalmol. 33(8):1203–19. PMID:15432557

57. Ashkenazy N, Henry CR, Abbey AM, McKeown CA, Berrocal AM, Murray TG (2014). Successful treatment of juvenile xanthogranuloma using bevacizumab. J AAPOS. 18(3):295–7. PMID:24767830

58. Ashton N, Ward B, Serpell G (1954). Effect of oxygen on developing retinal vessels with particular reference to the problem of retrolental fibroplasia. Br J Ophthalmol. 38(7):397–432. PMID:13172417

59. Asnaghi L, Alkatan H, Mahale A, Othman M, Alwadani S, Al-Hussain H, et al. (2014). Identification of multiple DNA copy number alterations including frequent 8p11.22 amplification in conjunctival squamous cell carcinoma. Invest Ophthalmol Vis Sci. 55(12):8604–13. PMID:25491297

60. Collaborative Ocular Melanoma Study

Group (2001). Assessment of metastatic disease status at death in 435 patients with large choroidal melanoma in the Collaborative Ocular Melanoma Study (COMS): COMS report no. 15. Arch Ophthalmol. 119(5):670–6. PMID:11346394
61. Assheton DC, Guerin EP, Sheridan CM, Bishop PN, Hiscott PS (2007). Neoplastic transformation of ciliary body epithelium is associated with loss of opticin expression. Br J Ophthalmol. 91(2):230–2. PMID:17005546
62. Augsburger JJ, Henson GL, Hershberger VS, Trichopoulos N (2006). Topographical distribution of typical unifocal congenital hypertrophy of retinal pigment epithelium. Graefes Arch Clin Exp Ophthalmol. 244(11):1412–4. PMID:16568286
63. Avdagic E, Farber N, Katabi N, Shinder R (2017). Carcinoma ex pleomorphic adenoma of the lacrimal gland with epithelial-myoepithelial carcinoma histologic type. Ophthal Plast Reconstr Surg. 33(3S Suppl 1):S136–8. PMID:26934566
64. Avedschmidt SE, Stagner AM, Eagle RC Jr, Harocopos GJ, Dou Y, Rao RC (2016). The targetable epigenetic tumor protein EZH2 is enriched in intraocular medulloepithelioma. Invest Ophthalmol Vis Sci. 57(14):6242–6. PMID:27842164
65. Awaji S, Alkatan H, Al-Kharashi S, Al-Rajhi A (2013). Iris melanocytoma in child diagnosed by fine needle aspiration biopsy. Saudi J Ophthalmol. 27(4):277–80. PMID:24371424
66. Aylward GW, Chang TS, Pautler SE, Gass JD (1998). A long-term follow-up of choroidal osteoma. Arch Ophthalmol. 116(10):1337–41. PMID:9790633
67. Diaz-Perez JA, Barajas-Gamboa JS (2012). Complex choristoma of the lacrimal caruncle: a case report of an unusual congenital tumor with clinical and histopathological classification. Int Ophthalmol. 32(1):37–9. PMID:22213061
68. Azari AA, Barney NP (2013). Conjunctivitis: a systematic review of diagnosis and treatment. JAMA. 310(16):1721–9. PMID:24150468
69. Azari AA, Kanavi MR, Saipe N, Lee V, Lucarelli M, Potter HD, et al. (2013). Transitional cell carcinoma of the lacrimal sac presenting with bloody tears. JAMA Ophthalmol. 131(5):689–90. PMID:23471524
70. Babu NA, Rajesh E, Krupaa J, Gnanandar G (2015). Genodermatoses. J Pharm Bioallied Sci. 7(Suppl 1):S203–6. PMID:26015711
71. Badalian-Very G, Vergilio JA, Degar BA, MacConaill LE, Brandner B, Calicchio ML, et al. (2010). Recurrent BRAF mutations in Langerhans cell histiocytosis. Blood. 116(11):1919–23. PMID:20519626
72. Baines PS, Hiscott PS, McLeod D (1982). Posterior non-vascularized proliferative extraretinopathy and peripheral nodular retinal telangiectasis. Trans Ophthalmol Soc U K. 102(Pt 4):487–91. PMID:6964653
73. Bakalian S, Marshall JC, Logan P, Faingold D, Maloney S, Di Cesare S, et al. (2008). Molecular pathways mediating liver metastasis in patients with uveal melanoma. Clin Cancer Res. 14(4):951–6. PMID:18281525
74. Balachandran C, Millar MJ, Murali R, Bulliard C, Malcolm CM, Maloof A (2009). Malignant optic glioma presenting as an acute anterior optic neuropathy. Retin Cases Brief Rep. 3(2):156–60. PMID:25391062
75. Bannister M, Lawson G (2014). Papillary-cystic variant of acinic cell carcinoma in the lacrimal gland. Case Rep Ophthalmol Med. 2014:285485. PMID:24959368
76. Bansal S, Khan AL, Hsuan J (2008). Lacrimal sac mucus-secreting adenocarcinoma. Orbit. 27(3):199–201. PMID:18569829
77. Barak Y, Tong MG, Purkiss TJ, Schaal S (2012). Rosai-Dorfman disease diagnosed because of bilateral choroidal masses. Retin Cases Brief Rep. 6(3):326–9. PMID:25389746
78. Barbaro NM, Rosenblum ML, Maitland CG, Hoyt WF, Davis RL (1982). Malignant optic glioma presenting radiologically as a "cystic" suprasellar mass: case report and review of the literature. Neurosurgery. 11(6):787–9. PMID:6298650
79. Baredes S, Ludwin DB, Troublefield YL, Langer PD, Mirani N (2003). Adenocarcinoma ex-pleomorphic adenoma of the lacrimal sac and nasolacrimal duct: a case report. Laryngoscope. 113(6):940–2. PMID:12782801
80. Barker D, Wright E, Nguyen K, Cannon L, Fain P, Goldgar D, et al. (1987). Gene for von Recklinghausen neurofibromatosis is in the pericentromeric region of chromosome 17. Science. 236(4805):1100–2. PMID:3107130
81. Barker-Griffith AE, McDonald PR, Green WR (1976). Malignant melanoma arising in a choroidal magnacellular nevus (melanocytoma). Can J Ophthalmol. 11(2):140–6. PMID:1078332
82. Barr CC, Rice TA, Michels RG (1980). Angioma-like mass in a patient with retrolental fibroplasia. Am J Ophthalmol. 89(5):647–50. PMID:6155069
83. Barros JN, Almeida SR, Lowen MS, Cunha MC, Gomes JA (2015). Impression cytology in the evaluation of ocular surface tumors: review article. Arq Bras Oftalmol. 78(2):126–32. PMID:25945538
84. Barry JS, Reddy MA (2008). The association of an epibulbar dermoid and Duane syndrome in a patient with a SALL1 mutation (Townes-Brocks syndrome). Ophthalmic Genet. 29(4):177–80. PMID:19005989
85. Bastian BC (2014). The molecular pathology of melanoma: an integrated taxonomy of melanocytic neoplasia. Annu Rev Pathol. 9(1):239–71. PMID:24460190
86. Batra R, Mudhar HS, Sandramouli S (2012). A unique case of IgG4 sclerosing dacryocystitis. Ophthal Plast Reconstr Surg. 28(3):e70–2. PMID:21946772
87. Baysal BE, Maher ER (2015). 15 years of paraganglioma: genetics and mechanism of pheochromocytoma-paraganglioma syndromes characterized by germline SDHB and SDHD mutations. Endocr Relat Cancer. 22(4):T71–82. PMID:26113606
88. Beadling C, Jacobson-Dunlop E, Hodi FS, Le C, Warrick A, Patterson J, et al. (2008). KIT gene mutations and copy number in melanoma subtypes. Clin Cancer Res. 14(21):6821–8. PMID:18980976
89. Bechrakis NE, Lee WR (1991). Dedifferentiation potential of iris melanomas. Fortschr Ophthalmol. 88(6):651–6. PMID:1794785
90. Behbehani RS, Vacarezza N, Sergott RC, Bilyk JR, Hochberg F, Savino PJ (2005). Isolated optic nerve lymphoma diagnosed by optic nerve biopsy. Am J Ophthalmol. 139(6):1128–30. PMID:15953457
91. Bell D, Sniegowski MC, Wani K, Prieto V, Esmaeli B (2016). Mutational landscape of lacrimal gland carcinomas and implications for treatment. Head Neck. 38 Suppl 1:E724–9. PMID:25899808
92. Bell WR, Singh K, Rajan Kd A, Eberhart CG (2015). Expression of p16 and p53 in intraepithelial periocular sebaceous carcinoma. Ocul Oncol Pathol. 2(2):71–5. PMID:27171611
93. Bellmann C, Lumbroso-Le Rouic L, Levy C, Plancher C, Dendale R, Sastre-Garau X, et al. (2010). Uveal melanoma: management and outcome of patients with extraocular spread. Br J Ophthalmol. 94(5):569–74. PMID:19965816
94. Berard M, Sordello S, Ortega N, Carrier JL, Peyri N, Wassef M, et al. (1997). Vascular endothelial growth factor confers a growth advantage in vitro and in vivo to stromal cells cultured from neonatal hemangiomas. Am J Pathol. 150(4):1315–26. PMID:9094988
95. Berg JN, Walter JW, Thisanagayam U, Evans M, Blei F, Waner M, et al. (2001). Evidence for loss of heterozygosity of 5q in sporadic haemangiomas: are somatic mutations involved in haemangioma formation? J Clin Pathol. 54(3):249–52. PMID:11253142
96. Berman EL, Shields CL, Sagoo MS, Eagle RC Jr, Shields JA (2008). Multifocal blue nevus of the conjunctiva. Surv Ophthalmol. 53(1):41–9. PMID:18191656
97. Bernardini FP, Croxatto JO, Nozza P, Rossi A, Capris P (2013). Primary diffuse leptomeningeal gliomatosis in children: a clinical pathologic correlation. Ophthal Plast Reconstr Surg. 29(2):93–7. PMID:23247038
98. Bernardini FP, Orcioni GF, Croxatto JO (2010). Oncocytic carcinoma of the lacrimal gland in a patient with neurofibromatosis. Ophthal Plast Reconstr Surg. 26(6):486–8. PMID:20700068
99. Bernstein-Lipschitz L, Lahav M, Chen V, Gutman I, Gal R, Lipschitz M (1990). Metastatic thyroid carcinoma masquerading as lacrimal gland tumor. Graefes Arch Clin Exp Ophthalmol. 228(2):112–5. PMID:2186969
100. Bertelmann E, Pahl S, Rieck P (2011). Malignant neoplasms of the lacrimal sac: rarity among tear duct diseases. Ophthalmologe. 108(5):440–4. [German] PMID:21125284
101. Bertschinger D, Oberic A, Moulin A, Hamédani M (2010). Malignant transformation of a "benign" lacrimal gland tumor. Klin Monatsbl Augenheilkd. 227(4):321–3. PMID:20408086
102. Betz CS, Leunig A, Janda P, Jund R (2005). Adenocarcinoma in the tear sack after endonasal dacryocystorhinostomy. HNO. 53(3):257–62. [German] PMID:15060716
103. Bhatnagar R, Vine AK (1991). Diffuse infiltrating retinoblastoma. Ophthalmology. 98(11):1657–61. PMID:1800925
104. Bhawan J, Silva C, Taungjaruwinai WM (2013). Inconsistent immunohistochemical expression of lymphatic and blood endothelial cell markers in cutaneous lymphangiomas. J Cutan Pathol. 40(9):801–6. PMID:23782346
105. Bi YW, Chen RJ, Li XP (2007). Clinical and pathological analysis of primary lacrimal sac tumors. Zhonghua Yan Ke Za Zhi. 43(6):499–504. [Chinese] PMID:17897525
106. Bianciotto C, Shields CL, Guzman JM, Romanelli-Gobbi M, Mazzuca D Jr, Green WR, et al. (2011). Assessment of anterior segment tumors with ultrasound biomicroscopy versus anterior segment optical coherence tomography in 200 cases. Ophthalmology. 118(7):1297–302. PMID:21377736
107. Bissig A, Moulin A, Spahn B, Zembowicz A, Schalenbourg A (2012). Conjunctival pigmented epithelioid melanocytoma: a clinicopathological case report. Arch Ophthalmol. 130(11):1478–9. PMID:23143456
108. Biswas J, Bhushan B, Jayakumar N, Chidambaram B (1999). Teratoid malignant medulloepithelioma of the optic nerve: report of a case and review of the literature. Orbit. 18(3):191–6. PMID:12045984
109. Biswas J, Kabra S, Krishnakumar S, Shanmugam MP (2004). Clinical and histopathological characteristics of uveal melanoma in Asian Indians. A study of 103 patients. Indian J Ophthalmol. 52(1):41–4. PMID:15132378
110. Blakeley JO, Bakker A, Barker A, Clapp W, Ferner R, Fisher MJ, et al. (2017). The path forward: 2015 International Children's Tumor Foundation conference on neurofibromatosis type 1, type 2, and schwannomatosis. Am J Med Genet A. 173(6):1714–21. PMID:28436162
111. Blei F, Walter J, Orlow SJ, Marchuk DA (1998). Familial segregation of hemangiomas and vascular malformations as an autosomal dominant trait. Arch Dermatol. 134(6):718–22. PMID:9645641
112. Blicker JA, Rootman J, White VA (1992). Cellular blue nevus of the conjunctiva. Ophthalmology. 99(11):1714–7. PMID:1454347
113. Boehlke CS, Frueh BR, Flint A, Elner VM (2007). Malignant fibrous histiocytoma of the lateral conjunctiva and anterior orbit. Ophthal Plast Reconstr Surg. 23(4):338–40. PMID:17667121
114. Boldrey EE, Schwartz A (1982). Enlargement of congenital hypertrophy of the retinal pigment epithelium. Am J Ophthalmol. 94(1):64–6. PMID:7091284
115. Boley S, Sloan JL, Pemov A, Stewart DR (2009). A quantitative assessment of the burden and distribution of Lisch nodules in adults with neurofibromatosis type 1. Invest Ophthalmol Vis Sci. 50(11):5035–43. PMID:19516012
116. Bolzoni A, Pianta L, Farina D, Nicolai P (2005). Benign myoepithelioma of the lacrimal gland: report of a case. Eur Arch Otorhinolaryngol. 262(3):186–8. PMID:15138773
117. Bonavolontà G, Strianese D, Grassi P, Comune C, Tranfa F, Uccello G, et al. (2013). An analysis of 2,480 space-occupying lesions of the orbit from 1976 to 2011. Ophthal Plast Reconstr Surg. 29(2):79–86. PMID:23470516
118. Bonavolontà G, Tranfa F, Staibano S, Di Matteo G, Orabona P, De Rosa G (1997). Warthin tumor of the lacrimal gland. Am J Ophthalmol. 124(6):857–8. PMID:9402842
119. Bonder D, Fischer MJ, Levine MR (1983). Squamous cell carcinoma of the lacrimal sac. Ophthalmology. 90(9):1133–5. PMID:6646653
120. Boniuk M, Messmer EP, Font RL (1985). Hemangiopericytoma of the meninges of the optic nerve. A clinicopathologic report including electron microscopic observations. Ophthalmology. 92(12):1780–7. PMID:4088633
121. Boniuk M, Zimmerman LE (1962). Epibulbar osteoma (episcleral osseous choristoma). Am J Ophthalmol. 53(2):290–6. PMID:13871021
122. Bonzheim I, Giese S, Deuter C, Süsskind D, Zierhut M, Waizel M, et al. (2015). High frequency of MYD88 mutations in vitreoretinal B-cell lymphoma: a valuable tool to improve diagnostic yield of vitreous aspirates. Blood. 126(1):76–9. PMID:25900979
123. Bor-Shavit E, Hammel N, Nahum Y, Rappaport ZH, Stiebel-Kalish H (2015). Visual disability rates in a ten-year cohort of patients with anterior visual pathway meningiomas. Disabil Rehabil. 37(11):958–62. PMID:25133857
124. Borit A, Richardson EP Jr (1982). The biological and clinical behaviour of pilocytic astrocytomas of the optic pathways. Brain. 105(Pt 1):161–87. PMID:7066671
125. Bosch MM, Wichmann WW, Boltshauser E, Landau K (2006). Optic nerve sheath meningiomas in patients with neurofibromatosis type 2. Arch Ophthalmol. 124(3):379–85. PMID:16534058
126. Boye E, Yu Y, Paranya G, Mulliken JB, Olsen BR, Bischoff J (2001). Clonality and altered behavior of endothelial cells from hemangiomas. J Clin Invest. 107(6):745–52. PMID:11254674
127. Boztug K, Frimpong-Ansah K, Nanduri VR, Lawson J, Russell-Eggitt I, Brock P (2006). Intraocular Langerhans cell histiocytosis in a neonate resulting in bilateral loss of vision. Pediatr Blood Cancer. 47(5):633–5. PMID:16444678
128. Brandwein-Gensler M, Hille J, Wang BY, Urken M, Gordon R, Wang LJ, et al. (2004). Low-grade salivary duct carcinoma: description of 16 cases. Am J Surg Pathol. 28(8):1040–4. PMID:15252310
129. Brannan PA, Kersten RC, Schneider S, Kulwin DR (2005). A case of primary

adenocarcinoma of the lacrimal sac. Orbit. 24(4):291–3. PMID:16354642
130. Brantley MA Jr, Harbour JW (2001). The molecular biology of retinoblastoma. Ocul Immunol Inflamm. 9(1):1–8. PMID:11262663
131. Bredow L, Martin G, Reinhard T, Mittelviefhaus H, Auw-Haedrich C (2009). Recurrent conjunctival papilloma progressing into squamous cell carcinoma with change of HPV-finding during the course. Br J Ophthalmol. 93(11):1437,1451. PMID:19692355
132. Brierly JD, Gospodarowicz MK, Wittekind C, editors (2017). TNM classification of malignant tumours. 8th ed. Oxford: Wiley Blackwell.
133. Broaddus E, Topham A, Singh AD (2009). Incidence of retinoblastoma in the USA: 1975-2004. Br J Ophthalmol. 93(1):21–3. PMID:18621794
134. Bronkhorst IH, Ly LV, Jordanova ES, Vrolijk J, Versluis M, Luyten GP, et al. (2011). Detection of M2-macrophages in uveal melanoma and relation with survival. Invest Ophthalmol Vis Sci. 52(2):643–50. PMID:20811059
135. Bronkhorst IH, Vu TH, Jordanova ES, Luyten GP, Burg SH, Jager MJ (2012). Different subsets of tumor-infiltrating lymphocytes correlate with macrophage influx and monosomy 3 in uveal melanoma. Invest Ophthalmol Vis Sci. 53(9):5370–8. PMID:22743317
136. Broughton WL, Zimmerman LE (1978). A clinicopathologic study of 56 cases of intraocular medulloepitheliomas. Am J Ophthalmol. 85(3):407–18. PMID:655220
137. Brown GC, Shields JA (1985). Tumors of the optic nerve head. Surv Ophthalmol. 29(4):239–64. PMID:3885451
138. Brown HH, Glasgow BJ, Holland GN, Foos RY (1989). Keratinizing corneal intraepithelial neoplasia. Cornea. 8(3):220–4. PMID:2472930
139. Brown NA, Furtado LV, Betz BL, Kiel MJ, Weigelin HC, Lim MS, et al. (2014). High prevalence of somatic MAP2K1 mutations in BRAF V600E-negative Langerhans cell histiocytosis. Blood. 124(10):1655–8. PMID:24982505
140. Brownstein S (1981). Mucoepidermoid carcinoma of the conjunctiva with intraocular invasion. Ophthalmology. 88(12):1226–30. PMID:7322472
141. Brownstein S, Little JM (1983). Ocular neurofibromatosis. Ophthalmology. 90(12):1595–9. PMID:6429597
142. Abu el-Asrar AM, al-Momen AK, Kangave D, Harakati MS (1995). Prognostic importance of retinopathy in acute leukemia. Doc Ophthalmol. 91(3):273–81. PMID:8886591
143. Buckley RJ (1988). Vernal keratoconjunctivitis. Int Ophthalmol Clin. 28(4):303–8. PMID:3053489
144. Buder K, Gesierich A, Gelbrich G, Goebeler M (2013). Systemic treatment of metastatic uveal melanoma: review of literature and future perspectives. Cancer Med. 2(5):674–86. PMID:24403233
145. Buettner H (1975). Congenital hypertrophy of the retinal pigment epithelium. Am J Ophthalmol. 79(2):177–89. PMID:1115190
146. Bui T, Young JW, Frausto RF, Markello TC, Glasgow BJ, Aldave AJ (2016). Hereditary benign intraepithelial dyskeratosis: report of a case and re-examination of the evidence for locus heterogeneity. Ophthalmic Genet. 37(1):76–80. PMID:24555743
147. Bunt AH, Tso MO (1981). Feulgen-positive deposits in retinoblastoma. Incidence, composition, and ultrastructure. Arch Ophthalmol. 99(1):144–50. PMID:7006579
148. Burnier MN, McLean IW, Zimmerman LE, Rosenberg SH (1990). Retinoblastoma. The relationship of proliferating cells to blood vessels. Invest Ophthalmol Vis Sci. 31(10):2037–40. PMID:2211003
149. Burr JM, Mitry E, Rachet B, Coleman MP (2007). Survival from uveal melanoma in England and Wales 1986 to 2001. Ophthalmic Epidemiol. 14(1):3–8. PMID:17365812
150. Burris CK, Rodriguez ME, Raven ML (2015). Melanomalytic glaucoma. Ophthalmology. 122(12):2422. PMID:26592671
151. Bursztyn LL, Hyrcza MD, Allen LH, Berean KW, Wehrli B (2014). Low-grade intraductal carcinoma of the lacrimal gland. Orbit. 33(2):135–8. PMID:24195727
152. Calle CA, Castillo IG, Eagle RC Jr, Daza MT (2006). Oncocytoma of the lacrimal gland: case report and review of the literature. Orbit. 25(3):243–7. PMID:16987774
153. Campbell AA, Jakobiec FA, Rashid A, Dana R, Yoon MK (2016). Bilateral sequential dacryocystitis in a patient with graft-versus-host disease. Ophthal Plast Reconstr Surg. 32(4):e89–92. PMID:25192327
154. Campbell RJ, Min KW, Bolling JP (1997). Skeinoid fibers in mesectodermal leiomyoma of the ciliary body. Ultrastruct Pathol. 21(6):559–67. PMID:9355238
155. Campo E, Swerdlow SH, Harris NL, Pileri S, Stein H, Jaffe ES (2011). The 2008 WHO classification of lymphoid neoplasms and beyond: evolving concepts and practical applications. Blood. 117(19):5019–32. PMID:21300984
156. Cani AK, Soliman M, Hovelson DH, Liu CJ, McDaniel AS, Haller MJ, et al. (2016). Comprehensive genomic profiling of orbital and ocular adnexal lymphomas identifies frequent alterations in MYD88 and chromatin modifiers: new routes to targeted therapies. Mod Pathol. 29(7):685–97. PMID:27102345
157. Canturk S, Qaddoumi I, Khetan V, Ma Z, Furmanchuk A, Antoneli CB, et al. (2010). Survival of retinoblastoma in less-developed countries impact of socioeconomic and health-related indicators. Br J Ophthalmol. 94(11):1432–6. PMID:20733021
158. Cao J, Heijkants RC, Jochemsen AG, Dogrusöz M, de Lange MJ, van der Velden PA, et al. (2016). Targeting of the MAPK and AKT pathways in conjunctival melanoma shows potential synergy. Oncotarget. 8(35):58021–36. PMID:28938534
159. Capó H, Palmer E, Nicholson DH (1993). Congenital cysts of the iris stroma. Am J Ophthalmol. 116(2):228–32. PMID:8352310
160. Caraballo JN, Snyder MR, Johnston PB, O Neill BP, Raja H, Balsanek JG, et al. (2014). Vitreoretinal lymphoma versus uveitis: cytokine profile and correlations. Ocul Immunol Inflamm. 22(1):34–41. PMID:24490677
161. Carbone M, Ferris LK, Baumann F, Napolitano A, Lum CA, Flores EG, et al. (2012). BAP1 cancer syndrome: malignant mesothelioma, uveal and cutaneous melanoma, and MBAITs. J Transl Med. 10:179. PMID:22935333
162. Carney JA (1995). Carney complex: the complex of myxomas, spotty pigmentation, endocrine overactivity, and schwannomas. Semin Dermatol. 14(2):90–8. PMID:7640202
163. Carrau RL, Stillman E, Canaan RE (1994). Mucoepidermoid carcinoma of the conjunctiva. Ophthal Plast Reconstr Surg. 10(3):163–8. PMID:7947443
164. Carreño E, Saornil MA, Garcia-Alvarez C, Lopez-Lara F, De Frutos-Baraja JM, Almaraz A (2012). Prevalence of ocular and oculodermal melanocytosis in Spanish population with uveal melanoma. Eye (Lond). 26(1):159–62. PMID:22020174
165. Carvalho RM, Taleb A, Carvalho GL, Avila M (2010). Conjunctival fibrous histiocytoma simulating atipical pterygium in the Amazon region: case report. Arq Bras Oftalmol. 73(6):534–6. [Portuguese] PMID:21271031
166. Cassiman C, Casteels I, Jacob J, Plasschaert E, Brems H, Dubron K, et al. (2017). Choroidal abnormalities in café-au-lait syndromes: a new differential diagnostic tool? Clin Genet. 91(4):529–35. PMID:27716896
167. Cassoux N, Giron A, Bodaghi B, Tran TH, Baudet S, Davy F, et al. (2007). IL-10 measurement in aqueous humor for screening patients with suspicion of primary intraocular lymphoma. Invest Ophthalmol Vis Sci. 48(7):3253–9. PMID:17591896
168. Cervantes G, Rodríguez AA Jr, Leal AG (2002). Squamous cell carcinoma of the conjunctiva: clinicopathological features in 287 cases. Can J Ophthalmol. 37(1):14–9. PMID:11865953
169. Chacko JG, Lam BL, Adusumilli J, Dubovy SR (2010). Multicentric malignant glioma of adulthood masquerading as optic neuritis. Br J Ophthalmol. 94(6):782–3,812. PMID:18977790
170. Chahud F, Young RH, Remulla JF, Khadem JJ, Dryja TP (2001). Bilateral diffuse uveal melanocytic proliferation associated with extraocular cancers: review of a process particularly associated with gynecologic cancers. Am J Surg Pathol. 25(2):212–8. PMID:11176070
171. Chakraborty R, Hampton OA, Abhyankar H, Zinn DJ, Grimes A, Skull B, et al. (2017). Activating MAPK1 (ERK2) mutation in an aggressive case of disseminated juvenile xanthogranuloma. Oncotarget. 8(28):46065–70. PMID:28512266
172. Chakraborty R, Hampton OA, Shen X, Simko SJ, Shih A, Abhyankar H, et al. (2014). Mutually exclusive recurrent somatic mutations in MAP2K1 and BRAF support a central role for ERK activation in LCH pathogenesis. Blood. 124(19):3007–15. PMID:25202140
173. Chalkia AK, Spandidos DA, Detorakis ET (2013). Viral involvement in the pathogenesis and clinical features of ophthalmic pterygium (review). Int J Mol Med. 32(3):539–43. PMID:23856952
174. Champion R, Daicker BC (1989). Congenital hypertrophy of the pigment epithelium: light microscopic and ultrastructural findings in young children. Retina. 9(1):44–8. PMID:2717803
175. Chan CC, Collins AB, Chew EY (2007). Molecular pathology of eyes with von Hippel-Lindau (VHL) disease: a review. Retina. 27(1):1–7. PMID:17218907
176. Chan CC, Whitcup SM, Solomon D, Nussenblatt RB (1995). Interleukin-10 in the vitreous of patients with primary intraocular lymphoma. Am J Ophthalmol. 120(5):671–3. PMID:7485372
177. Chan WM, Liu DT, Lam LY, Choi PC, Chan CK, Lam DS, et al. (2004). Primary epithelial-myoepithelial carcinoma of the lacrimal gland. Arch Ophthalmol. 122(11):1714–7. PMID:15534138
178. Chang MW, Frieden IJ, Good W (1996). The risk intraocular juvenile xanthogranuloma: survey of current practices and assessment of risk. J Am Acad Dermatol. 34(3):445–9. PMID:8609257
179. Chang SH, Worley LA, Onken MD, Harbour JW (2008). Prognostic biomarkers in uveal melanoma: evidence for a stem cell-like phenotype associated with metastasis. Melanoma Res. 18(3):191–200. PMID:18477893
180. Chang TC, Estes R (2014). Beta blocker treatment of infantile conjunctival hemangiomas–observations from 2 cases. J AAPOS. 18(1):80–2. PMID:24568991
181. Chang TS, Byrne SF, Gass JD, Hughes JR, Johnson RN, Murray TG (1996). Echographic findings in benign reactive lymphoid hyperplasia of the choroid. Arch Ophthalmol. 114(6):669–75. PMID:8639077
182. Chang Y, Moore P (2014). Twenty years of KSHV. Viruses. 6(11):4258–64. PMID:25386844
183. Chang Y, Wei WB, Shi JT, Xian JF, Yang WL, Xu XL, et al. (2016). Clinical and histopathological features of adenomas of the ciliary pigment epithelium. Acta Ophthalmol. 94(7):e637–43. PMID:27130243
184. Chanudet E, Ye H, Ferry J, Bacon CM, Adam P, Müller-Hermelink HK, et al. (2009). A20 deletion is associated with copy number gain at the TNFA/B/C locus and occurs preferentially in translocation-negative MALT lymphoma of the ocular adnexa and salivary glands. J Pathol. 217(3):420–30. PMID:19006194
185. Chanudet E, Zhou Y, Bacon CM, Wotherspoon AC, Müller-Hermelink HK, Adam P, et al. (2006). Chlamydia psittaci is variably associated with ocular adnexal MALT lymphoma in different geographical regions. J Pathol. 209(3):344–51. PMID:16583361
185A. Chao AN, Shields CL, Krema H, Shields JA (2001). Outcome of patients with periocular sebaceous gland carcinoma with and without conjunctival intraepithelial invasion. Ophthalmology. 108(10):1877–83. PMID:11581065
186. Chaput F, Amer R, Baglivo E, Touitou V, Kozyreff A, Bron D, et al. (2017). Intraocular T-cell lymphoma: clinical presentation, diagnosis, treatment, and outcome. Ocul Immunol Inflamm. 25(5):639–48. PMID:27002464
187. Char DH, Miller T, Kroll S (1997). Orbital metastases: diagnosis and course. Br J Ophthalmol. 81(5):386–90. PMID:9227204
188. Char DH, Stone RD, Crawford JB, Wallyn R, Irvine AR, Hilton GF, et al. (1980). Diffuse melanoma of the choroid. Br J Ophthalmol. 64(3):178–80. PMID:6966937
189. Charles NC, Fox DM, Avendaño JA, Marroquín LS, Appleman W (1997). Conjunctival neurilemoma. Report of 3 cases. Arch Ophthalmol. 115(4):547–9. PMID:9109769
190. Chavez M, Mafee MF, Castillo B, Kaufman LM, Johnstone H, Edward DP (2004). Medulloepithelioma of the optic nerve. J Pediatr Ophthalmol Strabismus. 41(1):48–52. PMID:14974835
191. Chawla B, Kashyap S, Sen S, Bajaj MS, Pushker N, Gupta K, et al. (2013). Clinicopathologic review of epithelial tumors of the lacrimal gland. Ophthal Plast Reconstr Surg. 29(6):440–5. PMID:24145905
192. Chen H, Li J, Wang L, Cong N, Shi C, Song J, et al. (2014). Hepatocellular carcinoma metastasis to the lacrimal gland: a case report. Oncol Lett. 8(2):911–3. PMID:25013516
193. Chen JJ, Costello F, Kardon RH (2015). Sex disparities in neuro-ophthalmologic disorders. Curr Eye Res. 40(2):247–65. PMID:24911098
194. Chen TY, Keeney MG, Chintakuntlawar AV, Knutson DL, Kloft-Nelson S, Greipp PT, et al. (2017). Adenoid cystic carcinoma of the lacrimal gland is frequently characterized by MYB rearrangement. Eye (Lond). 31(5):720–5. PMID:28085142
195. Chen X, Maniotis AJ, Majumdar D, Pe'er J, Folberg R (2002). Uveal melanoma cell staining for CD34 and assessment of tumor vascularity. Invest Ophthalmol Vis Sci. 43(8):2533–9. PMID:12147581
196. Chen X, Wu Q, Tan L, Porter D, Jager MJ, Emery C, et al. (2014). Combined PKC and MEK inhibition in uveal melanoma with GNAQ and GNA11 mutations. Oncogene. 33(39):4724–34. PMID:24141786
197. Chew EY (2005). Ocular manifestations of von Hippel-Lindau disease: clinical and genetic investigations. Trans Am Ophthalmol Soc. 103:495–511. PMID:17057815
198. Chhablani PP, Ambiya V, Nair AG, Bondalapati S, Chhablani J (2018). Retinal findings on OCT in systemic conditions. Semin Ophthalmol. 33(4):525–46. PMID:28640657
199. Chi MJ, Baek SH (2006). Clinical analysis

of benign eyelid and conjunctival tumors. Ophthalmologica. 220(1):43–51. PMID:16374048
200. Chien JL, Sioufi K, Surakiatchanukul T, Shields JA, Shields CL (2017). Choroidal nevus: a review of prevalence, features, genetics, risks, and outcomes. Curr Opin Ophthalmol. 28(3):228–37. PMID:28141766
201. Chilton J, Caughron MR, Kepes JJ (1990). Ganglioglioma of the optic chiasm: case report and review of the literature. Neurosurgery. 26(6):1042–5. PMID:2194139
202. Chmielecki J, Crago AM, Rosenberg M, O'Connor R, Walker SR, Ambrogio L, et al. (2013). Whole-exome sequencing identifies a recurrent NAB2-STAT6 fusion in solitary fibrous tumors. Nat Genet. 45(2):131–2. PMID:23313954
203. Cho HK, Park SH, Shin SY (2011). Isolated optic nerve metastasis of breast cancer initially mimicking retrobulbar optic neuritis. Eur J Ophthalmol. 21(4):513–5. PMID:21140366
204. Choi EK, Chévez-Barrios P (2014). Inflamed conjunctival nevi: histopathological criteria. Arch Pathol Lab Med. 138(9):1242–6. PMID:25171709
205. Choi M, Koo JS, Yoon JS (2015). Recurred adenoid cystic carcinoma of lacrimal gland with aggressive local invasion to the maxillary bone marrow without increased uptake in PET-CT. Korean J Ophthalmol. 29(1):68–70. PMID:25646064
206. Chong EM, Coffee RE, Chintagumpala M, Hurwitz RL, Hurwitz MY, Chévez-Barrios P (2006). Extensively necrotic retinoblastoma is associated with high-risk prognostic factors. Arch Pathol Lab Med. 130(11):1669–72. PMID:17076529
207. Chowers I, Folberg R, Livni N, Pe'er J (2002). p53 immunoreactivity, Ki-67 expression, and microcirculation patterns in melanoma of the iris, ciliary body, and choroid. Curr Eye Res. 24(2):105–8. PMID:12187481
208. Christmas NJ, Mead MD, Richardson EP, Albert DM (1991). Secondary optic nerve tumors. Surv Ophthalmol. 36(3):196–206. PMID:1776123
209. Chung A, Mudhar HS (2014). Conjunctival metastasis from pleural mesothelioma. Ocul Oncol Pathol. 1(1):19–23. PMID:27175358
210. Coban-Karatas M, Bal N, Altan-Yaycioglu R, Terzi A (2016). Spindle cell carcinoma of the conjunctiva: a rare entity. Indian J Ophthalmol. 64(5):402–4. PMID:27380985
211. Cockerham GC, Hidayat AA, Bijwaard KE, Sheng ZM (2000). Re-evaluation of "reactive lymphoid hyperplasia of the uvea": an immunohistochemical and molecular analysis of 10 cases. Ophthalmology. 107(1):151–8. PMID:10647734
212. Cohen BH, Green WR, Iliff NT, Taxy JB, Schwab LT, de la Cruz Z (1980). Spindle cell carcinoma of the conjunctiva. Arch Ophthalmol. 98(10):1809–13. PMID:7425908
213. Cohen VM, Shields CL, Furuta M, Shields JA (2008). Vitreous seeding from retinal astrocytoma in three cases. Retina. 28(6):884–8. PMID:18536607
214. Cohen VM, Tsimpida M, Hungerford JL, Jan H, Cerio R, Moir G (2013). Prospective study of sentinel lymph node biopsy for conjunctival melanoma. Br J Ophthalmol. 97(12):1525–9. PMID:24064944
215. Colarossi C, Milazzo M, Paglierani M, Massi D, Memeo L, Canzonieri V (2013). A juvenile case of conjunctival atypical nevus. Diagn Pathol. 8:64. PMID:23607499
216. Collins VP, Jones DT, Giannini C (2015). Pilocytic astrocytoma: pathology, molecular mechanisms and markers. Acta Neuropathol. 129(6):775–88. PMID:25792358
217. Colman SD, Williams CA, Wallace MR (1995). Benign neurofibromas in type 1 neurofibromatosis (NF1) show somatic deletions of the NF1 gene. Nat Genet. 11(1):90–2. PMID:7550323
218. Conway VH, Brownstein S, Chisholm IA (1985). Lacrimal gland choristoma of the ciliary body. Ophthalmology. 92(3):449–53. PMID:3991133
219. Cook N, Mushtaq F, Leitner C, Ilchyshyn A, Smith GT, Cree IA (2016). Chronic tarsal conjunctivitis. BMC Ophthalmol 16:130. PMID:27473439
220. Cooling RJ, Wright JE (1979). Arachnoid hyperplasia in optic nerve glioma: confusion with orbital meningioma. Br J Ophthalmol. 63(9):596–9. PMID:486377
221. Copson B, McKelvie PA, Khong JJ (2017). Massive retinal gliosis with episcleral extension. Clin Experiment Ophthalmol. 45(9):923–4. PMID:28516476
222. Corrêa ZM, Augsburger JJ (2016). Independent prognostic significance of gene expression profile class and largest basal diameter of posterior uveal melanomas. Am J Ophthalmol. 162:20–7.e1. PMID:26596399
223. Costa S, Byrne M, Pissaloux D, Haddad V, Paindavoine S, Thomas L, et al. (2016). Melanomas associated with blue nevi or mimicking cellular blue nevi: clinical, pathologic, and molecular study of 11 cases displaying a high frequency of GNA11 mutations, BAP1 expression loss, and a predilection for the scalp. Am J Surg Pathol. 40(3):368–77. PMID:26645730
224. Coupland S, Heegaard S (2014). Can conjunctival lymphoma be a clinical diagnosis? Br J Ophthalmol. 98(5):574–5. PMID:24307715
225. Coupland SE, Anastassiou G, Bornfeld N, Hummel M, Stein H (2005). Primary intraocular lymphoma of T-cell type: report of a case and review of the literature. Graefes Arch Clin Exp Ophthalmol. 243(3):189–97. PMID:15806372
225A. Coupland SE, Campbell I, Damato B (2008). Routes of extraocular extension of uveal melanoma: risk factors and influence on survival probability. Ophthalmology. 115(10):1778–85. PMID:1855472
226. Coupland SE, Damato B (2008). Understanding intraocular lymphomas. Clin Experiment Ophthalmol. 36(6):564–78. PMID:18954321
227. Coupland SE, Foss HD, Assaf C, Auw-Haedrich C, Anastassiou G, Anagnostopoulos I, et al. (1999). T-cell and T/natural killer-cell lymphomas involving ocular and ocular adnexal tissues: a clinicopathologic, immunohistochemical, and molecular study of seven cases. Ophthalmology. 106(11):2109–20. PMID:10571346
228. Coupland SE, Foss HD, Bechrakis NE, Hummel M, Stein H (2001). Secondary ocular involvement in systemic "memory" B-cell lymphocytic leukemia. Ophthalmology. 108(7):1289–95. PMID:11425689
229. Coupland SE, Heimann H, Kellner U, Bornfeld N, Foerster MH, Lee WR (1998). Keratoacanthoma of the bulbar conjunctiva. Br J Ophthalmol. 82(5):586. PMID:9713071
230. Coupland SE, Hummel M, Müller HH, Stein H (2005). Molecular analysis of immunoglobulin genes in primary intraocular lymphoma. Invest Ophthalmol Vis Sci. 46(10):3507–14. PMID:16186327
231. Coupland SE, Krause L, Delecluse HJ, Anagnostopoulos I, Foss HD, Hummel M, et al. (1998). Lymphoproliferative lesions of the ocular adnexa. Analysis of 112 cases. Ophthalmology. 105(8):1430–41. PMID:9709754
232. Coupland SE, Loddenkemper C, Smith JR, Braziel RM, Charlotte F, Anagnostopoulos I, et al. (2005). Expression of immunoglobulin transcription factors in primary intraocular lymphoma and primary central nervous system lymphoma. Invest Ophthalmol Vis Sci. 46(11):3957–64. PMID:16249468
233. Coupland SE, White VA, Rootman J, Damato B, Finger PT (2009). A TNM-based clinical staging system of ocular adnexal lymphomas. Arch Pathol Lab Med. 133(8):1262–7. PMID:19653722
234. Crawford JB, Howes EL Jr, Char DH (1999). Combined nevi of the conjunctiva. Trans Am Ophthalmol Soc. 97:170–85. PMID:10703123
235. Cree IA, Foss AJ, Luthert PJ, McCulloch P (1996). Undefined high-power fields. Lancet. 347(8996):273–4. PMID:8551926
236. Crosby MB, Crosby CV, Wojno TH, Grossniklaus HE (2009). Conjunctival lichen planus in a patient with herpes simplex virus keratitis. Cornea. 28(8):936–7. PMID:19654517
237. Croxatto JO, Font RL (1982). Hemangiopericytoma of the orbit: a clinicopathologic study of 30 cases. Hum Pathol. 13(3):210–8. PMID:7076208
238. Cummings TJ, Dodd LG, Eedes CR, Klintworth GK (2008). Hereditary benign intraepithelial dyskeratosis: an evaluation of diagnostic cytology. Arch Pathol Lab Med. 132(8):1325–8. PMID:18684035
239. Curado MP, Edwards B, Shin HR, Storm H, Ferlay J, Heanue M, et al., editors (2007). Cancer incidence in five continents, Vol. IX. Lyon: International Agency for Research on Cancer. IARC Scientific Publication No. 160. Available from: http://publications.iarc.fr/315.
240. Cursiefen C, Schlötzer-Schrehardt U, Breiteneder-Geleff S, Holbach LM (2001). Orbital lymphangioma with positive immunohistochemistry of lymphatic endothelial markers (vascular endothelial growth factor receptor 3 and podoplanin). Graefes Arch Clin Exp Ophthalmol. 239(8):628–32. PMID:11585321
241. Cursiefen C, Schlötzer-Schrehardt U, Küchle M, Sorokin L, Breiteneder-Geleff S, Alitalo K, et al. (2002). Lymphatic vessels in vascularized human corneas: immunohistochemical investigation using LYVE-1 and podoplanin. Invest Ophthalmol Vis Sci. 43(7):2127–35. PMID:12091407
242. Damasceno RW, Holbach LM (2012). Primary ductal adenocarcinoma of the lacrimal gland: case report. Arq Bras Oftalmol. 75(1):64–6. PMID:22552422
243. Damato B, Coupland SE (2008). Conjunctival melanoma and melanosis: a reappraisal of terminology, classification and staging. Clin Experiment Ophthalmol. 36(8):786–95. PMID:19128387
244. Damato B, Coupland SE (2009). An audit of conjunctival melanoma treatment in Liverpool. Eye (Lond). 23(4):801–9. PMID:18535601
245. Damato B, Coupland SE (2009). Management of conjunctival melanoma. Expert Rev Anticancer Ther. 9(9):1227–39. PMID:19761427
246. Damato BE, Coupland SE (2012). Differences in uveal melanomas between men and women from the British Isles. Eye (Lond). 26(2):292–9. PMID:22079972
247. Daniel L, Rao S, Muthusamy R, Yerramsetti D (2014). Mucoepidermoid carcinoma ex pleomorphic adenoma of the lacrimal gland: a rare presentation. Indian J Ophthalmol. 62(6):743–6. PMID:25005213
248. Dark AJ, Streeten BW (1980). Preinvasive carcinoma of the cornea and conjunctiva. Br J Ophthalmol. 64(7):506–14. PMID:7426564
249. Dasgupta T, Wilson LD, Yu JB (2009). A retrospective review of 1349 cases of sebaceous carcinoma. Cancer. 115(1):158–65. PMID:18988294
250. Davis JL, Viciana AL, Ruiz P (1997). Diagnosis of intraocular lymphoma by flow cytometry. Am J Ophthalmol. 124(3):362–72. PMID:9439362
251. Dayan MR, Elston JS, McDonald B (2000). Bilateral lymphomatous optic neuropathy diagnosed on optic nerve biopsy. Arch Ophthalmol. 118(10):1455–7. PMID:11030839
252. de Alba MA, Villegas VM, Gold AS, Wildner A, Ehlies FJ, Latiff A, et al. (2015). Clinical findings and genetic expression profiling of three pigmented lesions of the optic nerve. Case Rep Ophthalmol Med. 2015:590659. PMID:25984377
253. de Brito BS, Gaspar NG, Egal ES, Sanchez-Romero C, Martins AS, Tincani AJ, et al. (2016). PLAG1 expression is maintained in recurrent pleomorphic adenoma. Virchows Arch. 469(4):477–81. PMID:27381214
254. de Brito BS, Giovanelli N, Egal ES, Sánchez-Romero C, Nascimento JS, Martins AS, et al. (2016). Loss of expression of Plag1 in malignant transformation from pleomorphic adenoma to carcinoma ex pleomorphic adenoma. Hum Pathol. 57:152–9. PMID:27473265
255. de Jong MC, Kors WA, de Graaf P, Castelijns JA, Kivelä T, Moll AC (2014). Trilateral retinoblastoma: a systematic review and meta-analysis. Lancet Oncol. 15(10):1157–67. PMID:25126964
256. de Keizer RJ, de Wolff-Rouendaal D, Nooy MA (2008). Angiosarcoma of the eyelid and periorbital region. Experience in Leiden with iridium192 brachytherapy and low-dose doxorubicin chemotherapy. Orbit. 27(1):5–12. PMID:18307140
257. De Laey JJ, De Gersem R (1989). Clinical aspects of leukemic infiltration of the choroid and the optic nerve. J Fr Ophtalmol. 12(11):819–25. [French] PMID:2700993
258. De Silva DJ, Tumuluri K, Joshi N (2005). Conjunctival squamous cell carcinoma: atypical presentation of HIV. Clin Experiment Ophthalmol. 33(4):419–20. PMID:16033363
259. de Camargo B, de Oliveira Ferreira JM, de Souza Reis R, Ferman S, de Oliveira Santos M, Pombo-de-Oliveira MS (2011). Socioeconomic status and the incidence of non-central nervous system childhood embryonic tumours in Brazil. BMC Cancer. 11:160. PMID:21545722
260. De Rosa G, Zeppa P, Tranfa F, Bonavolontà G (1986). Acinic cell carcinoma arising in a lacrimal gland. First case report. Cancer. 57(10):1988–91. PMID:3955504
261. De Salvo G, Krebs I, Binder S (2010). High-definition optical coherence tomography in a case of congenital hypertrophy of the retinal pigment epithelium. Ophthalmic Surg Lasers Imaging. 41 Suppl:S93–5. PMID:21117611
262. DeBarge LR, Chan CC, Greenberg SC, McLean IW, Yannuzzi LA, Nussenblatt RB (1994). Chorioretinal, iris, and ciliary body infiltration by juvenile xanthogranuloma masquerading as uveitis. Surv Ophthalmol. 39(1):65–71. PMID:7974193
263. Decatur CL, Ong E, Garg N, Anbunathan H, Bowcock AM, Field MG, et al. (2016). Driver mutations in uveal melanoma: associations with gene expression profile and patient outcomes. JAMA Ophthalmol. 134(7):728–33. PMID:27123562
264. Dei Tos AP, Seregard S, Calonje E, Chan JK, Fletcher CD (1995). Giant cell angiofibroma. A distinctive orbital tumor in adults. Am J Surg Pathol. 19(11):1286–93. PMID:7573691
265. Deliganis AV, Geyer JR, Berger MS (1996). Prognostic significance of type 1 neurofibromatosis (von Recklinghausen Disease) in childhood optic glioma. Neurosurgery. 38(6):1114–9. PMID:8727140
266. Demicco EG, Harms PW, Patel RM, Smith SC, Ingram D, Torres K, et al. (2015). Extensive survey of STAT6 expression in a large series of mesenchymal tumors. Am J Clin Pathol. 143(5):672–82. PMID:25873501
267. Demirci H, Christanson MD (2013). Eyelid angiosarcoma: a case report and review of

the literature. Middle East Afr J Ophthalmol. 20(3):259–62. PMID:24014993
268. Demirci H, Mashayekhi A, Shields CL, Eagle RC Jr, Shields JA (2005). Iris melanocytoma: clinical features and natural course in 47 cases. Am J Ophthalmol. 139(3):468–75. PMID:15767055
269. Demirci H, Shields CL, Chao AN, Shields JA (2003). Uveal metastasis from breast cancer in 264 patients. Am J Ophthalmol. 136(2):264–71. PMID:12888048
270. Demirci H, Shields CL, Eagle RC Jr, Shields JA (2006). Report of a conjunctival myxoma case and review of the literature. Arch Ophthalmol. 124(5):735–8. PMID:16682598
271. Demirci H, Shields CL, Shields JA (2003). Bilateral optic disk melanocytoma in a 10-month-old infant. Am J Ophthalmol. 136(1):190–2. PMID:12834694
272. Demirci H, Shields CL, Shields JA, Eagle RC Jr (2000). Malignant melanoma arising from unusual conjunctival blue nevus. Arch Ophthalmol. 118(11):1581–4. PMID:11074819
273. Demirci H, Shields CL, Shields JA, Eagle RC Jr, Honavar S (2001). Ring melanoma of the anterior chamber angle: a report of fourteen cases. Am J Ophthalmol. 132(3):336–42. PMID:11530045
274. Denby P, Harvey L, English MG (1986). Solitary metastasis from an occult renal cell carcinoma presenting as a primary lacrimal gland tumour. Orbit. 5:21–4.
275. DeParis SW, Bloomer M, Han Y, Vagefi MR, Shieh JTC, Solomon DA, et al. (2017). Uveal ganglioneuroma due to germline PTEN mutation (Cowden syndrome) presenting as unilateral infantile glaucoma. Ocul Oncol Pathol. 3(2):122–8. PMID:28868283
276. Dharmasena A, Lee PW, Irion LC, Bonshek R, Abdullah M, Nolan D (2016). Non-keratinising undifferentiated nasopharyngeal-type carcinoma of the lacrimal sac. Int J Ophthalmol. 9(8):1238–42. PMID:27588283
277. Dhupper M, Biswas J, Gopal L, Kumar SK, Khetan V (2012). Clinicopathological correlation of choroidal melanoma in Indian population: a study of 113 cases. Oman J Ophthalmol. 5(1):42–5. PMID:22557876
278. Di Cesare S, Marshall JC, Fernandes BF, Logan P, Antecka E, Filho VB, et al. (2007). In vitro characterization and inhibition of the CXCR4/CXCL12 chemokine axis in human uveal melanoma cell lines. Cancer Cell Int. 7:17. PMID:18001467
279. Di Cesare S, Marshall JC, Logan P, Antecka E, Faingold D, Maloney SC, et al. (2007). Expression and migratory analysis of 5 human uveal melanoma cell lines for CXCL12, CXCL8, CXCL1, and HGF. J Carcinog. 6:2. PMID:17261188
280. Di Girolamo N (2012). Association of human papilloma virus with pterygia and ocular-surface squamous neoplasia. Eye (Lond). 26(2):202–11. PMID:22134594
281. Diltoer E, Ten Tusscher MP (2015). Breast cancer metastasis presenting as conjunctival chemosis. Case Rep Ophthalmol. 6(3):439–42. PMID:26955345
282. Dimaras H, Khetan V, Halliday W, Héon E, Chan HS, Gallie BL (2009). Retinoma underlying retinoblastoma revealed after tumor response to 1 cycle of chemotherapy. Arch Ophthalmol. 127(8):1066–8. PMID:19667353
283. Dimaras H, Khetan V, Halliday W, Orlic M, Prigoda NL, Piovesan B, et al. (2008). Loss of RB1 induces non-proliferative retinoma: increasing genomic instability correlates with progression to retinoblastoma. Hum Mol Genet. 17(10):1363–72. PMID:18211953
284. Dingemans KP, van den Bergh Weerman MA (1990). Rapid contrasting of extracellular elements in thin sections. Ultrastruct Pathol. 14(6):519–27. PMID:1704157
285. Dithmar S, Völcker HE, Grossniklaus HE (1999). Multifocal intraocular malignant melanoma: report of two cases and review of the literature. Ophthalmology. 106(7):1345–8. PMID:10406619
286. Dithmar SA, Rusciano DA, Armstrong CA, Lynn MJ, Grossniklaus HE (1999). Depletion of NK cell activity results in growth of hepatic micrometastases in a murine ocular melanoma model. Curr Eye Res. 19(5):426–31. PMID:10520219
287. Divine RD, Anderson RL, Ossoinig KC (1982). Metastatic carcinoid unresponsive to radiation therapy presenting as a lacrimal fossa mass. Ophthalmology. 89(5):516–20. PMID:7099572
288. Dobyns WB, Michels VV, Groover RV, Mokri B, Trautmann JC, Forbes GS, et al. (1987). Familial cavernous malformations of the central nervous system and retina. Ann Neurol. 21(6):578–83. PMID:3606045
289. Dogrusöz M, Bagger M, van Duinen SG, Kroes WG, Ruivenkamp CA, Böhringer S, et al. (2017). The prognostic value of AJCC staging in uveal melanoma is enhanced by adding chromosome 3 and 8q status. Invest Ophthalmol Vis Sci. 58(2):833–42. PMID:28159971
290. Dolin PJ, Foss AJ, Hungerford JL (1994). Uveal melanoma: is solar ultraviolet radiation a risk factor? Ophthalmic Epidemiol. 1(1):27–30. PMID:8790610
291. Domingo RE, Manganip LE, Castro RM (2015). Tumors of the eye and ocular adnexa at the Philippine Eye Research Institute: a 10-year review. Clin Ophthalmol. 9:1239–47. PMID:26185414
292. Doro D, Parrozzani R, Midena E (2012). Ultrasound biomicroscopy examination of anterior uveal tumors: information on location and size only? Acta Clin Croat. 51 Suppl 1:37–44. PMID:23431723
293. Dorsey CS, Montgomery H (1954). Blue nevus and its distinction from Mongolian spot and the nevus of Ota. J Invest Dermatol. 22(3):225–36. PMID:13130904
294. Dotto JE, Glusac EJ (2006). p63 is a useful marker for cutaneous spindle cell squamous cell carcinoma. J Cutan Pathol. 33(6):413–7. PMID:16776716
295. Doycheva D, Zierhut M, Süsskind D, Bartz-Schmidt KU, Deuter C (2015). Diagnostics and treatment of choroidal lymphoma. Ophthalmologe. 112(3):217–22. [German] PMID:25693876
296. Doyle LA, Vivero M, Fletcher CD, Mertens F, Hornick JL (2014). Nuclear expression of STAT6 distinguishes solitary fibrous tumor from histologic mimics. Mod Pathol. 27(3):390–5. PMID:24030747
297. Dratviman-Storobinsky O, Cohen Y, Frenkel S, Pe'er J, Goldenberg-Cohen N (2010). Lack of oncogenic GNAQ mutations in melanocytic lesions of the conjunctiva as compared to uveal melanoma. Invest Ophthalmol Vis Sci. 51(12):6180–2. PMID:20631239
298. Dryja TP, Cavenee W, White R, Rapaport JM, Petersen R, Albert DM, et al. (1984). Homozygosity of chromosome 13 in retinoblastoma. N Engl J Med. 310(9):550–3. PMID:6694706
299. Dryja TP, Zakov ZN, Albert DM (1980). Adenocarcinoma arising from the epithelium of the iris and ciliary body. Int Ophthalmol Clin. 20(2):177–90. PMID:6995386
300. Duncan JL, Golabi M, Fredrick DR, Hoyt CS, Hwang DG, Kramer SG, et al. (1998). Complex limbal choristomas in linear nevus sebaceous syndrome. Ophthalmology. 105(8):1459–65. PMID:9709758
301. Duprez R, Lacoste V, Brière J, Couppié P, Frances C, Sainte-Marie D, et al. (2007). Evidence for a multiclonal origin of multicentric advanced lesions of Kaposi sarcoma. J Natl Cancer Inst. 99(14):1086–94. PMID:17623796
302. Durieux E, Descotes F, Nguyen AM, Grange JD, Devouassoux-Shisheboran M (2015). Somatic DICER1 gene mutation in sporadic intraocular medulloepithelioma without pleuropulmonary blastoma syndrome. Hum Pathol. 46(5):783–7. PMID:25791583
303. Dutton JJ (1991). Optic nerve gliomas and meningiomas. Neurol Clin. 9(1):163–77. PMID:2011108
304. Eagle RC Jr (2009). High-risk features and tumor differentiation in retinoblastoma: a retrospective histopathologic study. Arch Pathol Lab Med. 133(8):1203–9. PMID:19653710
305. Eagle RC Jr, Font RL, Swerczek TW (1978). Malignant medulloepithelioma of the optic nerve in a horse. Vet Pathol. 15(4):488–94. PMID:695223
306. Eagle RC Jr, Shields JA, Donoso L, Milner RS (1989). Malignant transformation of spontaneously regressed retinoblastoma, retinoma/retinocytoma variant. Ophthalmology. 96(9):1389–95. PMID:2780006
307. Easton DF, Ponder MA, Huson SM, Ponder BA (1993). An analysis of variation in expression of neurofibromatosis (NF) type 1 (NF1): evidence for modifying genes. Am J Hum Genet. 53(2):305–13. PMID:8328449
308. Edelstein C, Shields CL, Shields JA, Eagle RC Jr (1998). Presumed adenocarcinoma of the retinal pigment epithelium in a blind eye with a staphyloma. Arch Ophthalmol. 116(4):525–8. PMID:9565054
309. Edward DP, Alkatan H, Rafiq Q, Eberhart C, Al Mesfer S, Ghazi N, et al. (2015). MicroRNA profiling in intraocular medulloepitheliomas. PLoS One. 10(3):e0121706. PMID:25807141
310. Egan KM, Seddon JM, Glynn RJ, Gragoudas ES, Albert DM (1988). Epidemiologic aspects of uveal melanoma. Surv Ophthalmol. 32(4):239–51. PMID:3279559
311. Egbert PR, Chan CC, Winter FC (1976). Flat preparations of the retinal vessels in Coats' disease. J Pediatr Ophthalmol. 13(6):336–9. PMID:798026
312. Eggers H, Jakobiec FA, Jones IS (1976). Tumors of the optic nerve. Doc Ophthalmol. 41(1):43–128. PMID:773617
313. El Demellawy D, McGowan-Jordan J, de Nanassy J, Chernetsova E, Nasr A (2017). Update on molecular findings in rhabdomyosarcoma. Pathology. 49(3):238–46. PMID:28256213
314. El-Naggar AK, Chan JKC, Grandis JR, Takata T, Slootweg PJ, editors (2017). WHO classification of head and neck tumours. 4th ed. Lyon: International Agency for Research on Cancer. Available from: http://publications.iarc.fr/548.
315. El-Sawy T, Frank SJ, Hanna E, Sniegowski M, Lai SY, Nasser QJ, et al. (2013). Multidisciplinary management of lacrimal sac/nasolacrimal duct carcinomas. Ophthal Plast Reconstr Surg. 29(6):454–7. PMID:24195987
316. Eldaly H, Eldaly Z (2015). Melanocytoma of the optic nerve head, thirty-month follow-up. Semin Ophthalmol. 30(5–6):464–9. PMID:24506313
317. Eldesouky MA, Elbakary MA, Sabik S, Shareef MM (2014). Lacrimal fossa lesions: a review of 146 cases in Egypt. Clin Ophthalmol. 8:1603–9. PMID:25210428
318. Eletr ZM, Wilkinson KD (2011). An emerging model for BAP1's role in regulating cell cycle progression. Cell Biochem Biophys. 60(1–2):3–11. PMID:21484256
319. Eller AW, Bernardino VB Jr (1983). Blue nevi of the conjunctiva. Ophthalmology. 90(12):1469–71. PMID:6677846
320. Ellis FJ, Eagle RC Jr, Shields JA, Shields CL, Fessler JN, Takemoto LJ (1993). Phakomatous choristoma (Zimmerman's tumor). Immunohistochemical confirmation of lens-specific proteins. Ophthalmology. 100(6):955–60. PMID:7685513
321. Ellis GS Jr, Pakalnis VA, Worley G, Green JA, Frothingham TE, Sturner RA, et al. (1986). Toxocara canis infestation. Clinical and epidemiological associations with seropositivity in kindergarten children. Ophthalmology. 93(8):1032–7. PMID:3763150
322. Elsas FJ, Green WR (1975). Epibulbar tumors in childhood. Am J Ophthalmol. 79(6):1001–7. PMID:166560
322A. Emile JF, Abla O, Fraitag S, Horne A, Haroche J, Donadieu J, et al. (2016). Revised classification of histiocytoses and neoplasms of the macrophage-dendritic cell lineages. Blood. 127(22):2672–81. PMID:26966089
322B. Emile JF, Charlotte F, Amoura Z, Haroche J (2013). BRAF mutations in Erdheim-Chester disease. J Clin Oncol. 31(3):398. PMID:23248255
323. Emmanuel B, Ruder E, Lin SW, Abnet C, Hollenbeck A, Mbulaiteye S (2012). Incidence of squamous-cell carcinoma of the conjunctiva and other eye cancers in the NIH-AARP Diet and Health Study. Ecancermedicalscience. 6:254. PMID:22654961
324. Enescu AS, Mărgăritescu CL, Crăiţoiu MM, Enescu A, Crăiţoiu Ş (2013). The involvement of growth differentiation factor 5 (GDF5) and aggrecan in the epithelial-mesenchymal transition of salivary gland pleomorphic adenoma. Rom J Morphol Embryol. 54(4):969–76. PMID:24398992
325. Erickson BP, Modi YS, Ko MJ, Hussain RM, Gomez-Fernandez C, Johnson TE (2014). Transitional cell-type papillary carcinoma of the lacrimal sac manifesting as a medial canthal skin lesion. Orbit. 33(5):378–81. PMID:24911210
326. Erşahin Y, Yünten N (1999). Bilateral optic nerve glioma. Pediatr Neurosurg. 31(3):168. PMID:10708361
327. Eskelin S, Kivelä T (2002). Mode of presentation and time to treatment of uveal melanoma in Finland. Br J Ophthalmol. 86(3):333–8. PMID:11864894
328. Eskelin S, Tommila P, Palosaari T, Kivelä T (2008). Photodynamic therapy with verteporfin to induce regression of aggressive retinal astrocytomas. Acta Ophthalmol. 86(7):794–9. PMID:18759802
329. Esmaeli B, Roberts D, Ross M, Fellman M, Cruz H, Kim SK, et al. (2012). Histologic features of conjunctival melanoma predictive of metastasis and death (an American Ophthalmological thesis). Trans Am Ophthalmol Soc. 110:64–73. PMID:23818735
330. Esmaili DD, Mukai S, Jakobiec FA, Kim IK, Gragoudas ES (2009). Ocular melanocytoma. Int Ophthalmol Clin. 49(1):165–75. PMID:19125075
331. Esteban F, González-Pérez JM, Benaixa JP, Redondo M, Nevado M, López-Garrido J, et al. (2007). Malignant melanomas of the nasolacrimal duct. J Laryngol Otol. 121(3):285–8. PMID:17123453
332. Evans DG, Baser ME, McGaughran J, Sharif S, Howard E, Moran A (2002). Malignant peripheral nerve sheath tumours in neurofibromatosis 1. J Med Genet. 39(5):311–4. PMID:12011145
333. Eweiss AZ, Lund VJ, Jay A, Rose G (2013). Transitional cell tumours of the lacrimal drainage apparatus. Rhinology. 51(4):349–54. PMID:24260768
334. Ewens KG, Bhatti TR, Moran KA, Richards-Yutz J, Shields CL, Eagle RC, et al. (2017). Phosphorylation of pRb: mechanism for RB pathway inactivation in MYCN-amplified retinoblastoma. Cancer Med. 6(3):619–30.

PMID:28211617
335. Faber DL, Galili R, Nitzan O, Sharoni E (2015). Systemic generalized lymphangiomatosis: a diagnostic challenge. Isr Med Assoc J. 17(12):785–6. PMID:26897985
336. Fajardo-Gutiérrez A, Juárez-Ocaña S, González-Miranda G, Palma-Padilla V, Carreón-Cruz R, Ortega-Alvárez MC, et al. (2007). Incidence of cancer in children residing in ten jurisdictions of the Mexican Republic: importance of the cancer registry (a population-based study). BMC Cancer. 7:68. PMID:17445267
337. Fan JT, Robertson DM, Campbell RJ (1995). Clinicopathologic correlation of a case of adenocarcinoma of the retinal pigment epithelium. Am J Ophthalmol. 119(2):243–5. PMID:7832240
338. Farah SE, Konrad H, Huang DT, Geist CE (1999). Ectopic orbital meningioma: a case report and review. Ophthal Plast Reconstr Surg. 15(6):463–6. PMID:10588262
339. Faris B, Tolentino FI, Freeman HM, Brockhurst RJ, Schepens CL (1971). Retrolental fibroplasia in the cicatricial stage. Fundus and vitreous findings. Arch Ophthalmol. 85(6):661–8. PMID:5109298
340. Farmer JP, Lamba M, Lamba WR, Jordan DR, Gilberg S, Sengar DP, et al. (2005). Lymphoproliferative lesions of the lacrimal gland: clinicopathological, immunohistochemical and molecular genetic analysis. Can J Ophthalmol. 40(2):151–60. PMID:16049528
341. Fatima A, Matalia HP, Vemuganti GK, Honavar SG, Sangwan VS (2006). Pseudoepitheliomatous hyperplasia mimicking ocular surface squamous neoplasia following cultivated limbal epithelium transplantation. Clin Experiment Ophthalmol. 34(9):889–91. PMID:17181623
342. Felder KS, Brockhurst RJ (1982). Neovascular fundus abnormalities in peripheral uveitis. Arch Ophthalmol. 100(5):750–4. PMID:6177305
343. Feng L, Cai D, Muhetaer A, Yang YL, Ren F, Yishake M, et al. (2017). Spindle cell carcinoma: the general demographics, basic clinico-pathologic characteristics, treatment, outcome and prognostic factors. Oncotarget. 8(26):43228–36. PMID:28591732
344. Feng X, Degese MS, Iglesias-Bartolome R, Vaque JP, Molinolo AA, Rodrigues M, et al. (2014). Hippo-independent activation of YAP by the GNAQ uveal melanoma oncogene through a trio-regulated rho GTPase signaling circuitry. Cancer Cell. 25(6):831–45. PMID:24882515
345. Fernandes BF, Odashiro AN, Saraiva VS, Logan P, Antecka E, Burnier MN Jr. (2007). Immunohistochemical expression of melan-A and tyrosinase in uveal melanoma. J Carcinog. 6:6. PMID:17445277
346. Fernández-Vega Cueto L, Tresserra F, de la Paz MF (2014). De novo growth of a capillary hemangioma of the conjunctiva. Arch Soc Esp Oftalmol. 89(3):127–9. [Spanish] PMID:24269394
347. Ferry AP (1981). Granular cell tumor (myoblastoma) of the palpebral conjunctiva causing pseudoepitheliomatous hyperplasia of the conjunctival epithelium. Am J Ophthalmol. 91(2):234–8. PMID:6258438
348. Ferry AP, Font RL (1974). Carcinoma metastatic to the eye and orbit. I. A clinicopathologic study of 227 cases. Arch Ophthalmol. 92(4):276–86. PMID:4412321
349. Ferry AP, Hein HF (1970). Epibulbar osseous choristoma within an epibulbar dermoid. Am J Ophthalmol. 70(5):764–6. PMID:5477166
350. Ferry JA, Fung CY, Zukerberg L, Lucarelli MJ, Hasserjian RP, Preffer FI, et al. (2007). Lymphoma of the ocular adnexa: a study of 353 cases. Am J Surg Pathol. 31(2):170–84. PMID:17255761
351. Field MG, Decatur CL, Kurtenbach S, Gezgin G, van der Velden PA, Jager MJ, et al. (2016). PRAME as an independent biomarker for metastasis in uveal melanoma. Clin Cancer Res. 22(5):1234–42. PMID:26933176
352. Fine SW, McClain SA, Li M (2004). Immunohistochemical staining for calretinin is useful for differentiating schwannomas from neurofibromas. Am J Clin Pathol. 122(4):552–9. PMID:15487453
353. Fishman ML, Tomaszewski MM, Kuabara T (1976). Malignant melanoma of the skin metastatic to the eye. Frequency in autopsy series. Arch Ophthalmol. 94(8):1309–11. PMID:949273
354. Fisson S, Ouakrim H, Touitou V, Baudet S, Ben Abdelwahed R, Donnou S, et al. (2013). Cytokine profile in human eyes: contribution of a new cytokine combination for differential diagnosis between intraocular lymphoma or uveitis. PLoS One. 8(2):e52385. PMID:23405064
355. Flanagan JC, Stokes DP (1978). Lacrimal sac tumors. Ophthalmology. 85(12):1282–7. PMID:745835
356. Fleming MD, Pinkus JL, Fournier MV, Alexander SW, Tam C, Loda M, et al. (2003). Coincident expression of the chemokine receptors CCR6 and CCR7 by pathologic Langerhans cells in Langerhans cell histiocytosis. Blood. 101(7):2473–5. PMID:12642342
357. Fletcher CDM, Bridge JA, Hogendoorn PCW, Mertens F, editors (2013). WHO classification of tumours of soft tissue and bone. 4th ed. Lyon: International Agency for Research on Cancer. Available from: http://publications.iarc.fr/15.
358. Folberg R, Hendrix MJ, Maniotis AJ (2000). Vasculogenic mimicry and tumor angiogenesis. Am J Pathol. 156(2):361–81. PMID:10666364
359. Folberg R, Jakobiec FA, Bernardino VB, Iwamoto T (1989). Benign conjunctival melanocytic lesions. Clinicopathologic features. Ophthalmology. 96(4):436–61. PMID:2657539
360. Folberg R, McLean IW, Zimmerman LE (1985). Primary acquired melanosis of the conjunctiva. Hum Pathol. 16(2):129–35. PMID:3972395
361. Folberg R, Rummelt V, Parys-Van Ginderdeuren R, Hwang T, Woolson RF, Pe'er J, et al. (1993). The prognostic value of tumor blood vessel morphology in primary uveal melanoma. Ophthalmology. 100(9):1389–98. PMID:8371929
362. Font RL, Chaqués-Alepuz V (2011). Giant optic disk melanocytoma complicated with massive intraocular seeding. Arch Soc Esp Oftalmol. 86(5):158–61. [Spanish] PMID:21624657
363. Font RL, Del Valle M, Avedaño J, Longo M, Boniuk M (2008). Primary adenoid cystic carcinoma of the conjunctiva arising from the accessory lacrimal glands: a clinicopathologic study of three cases. Cornea. 27(4):494–7. PMID:18434856
364. Font RL, Ferry AP (1976). Carcinoma metastatic to the eye and orbit III. A clinicopathologic study of 28 cases metastatic to the orbit. Cancer. 38(3):1326–35. PMID:953971
365. Font RL, Moura RA, Shetlar DJ, Martinez JA, McPherson AR (1989). Combined hamartoma of sensory retina and retinal pigment epithelium. Retina. 9(4):302–11. PMID:2697919
366. Font RL, Smith SL, Bryan RG (1998). Malignant epithelial tumors of the lacrimal gland: a clinicopathologic study of 21 cases. Arch Ophthalmol. 116(5):613–6. PMID:9596497
367. Font RL, Yanoff M, Zimmerman LE (1969). Intraocular adipose tissue and persistent hyperplastic primary vitreous. Arch Ophthalmol. 82(1):43–50. PMID:5791501
368. Font RL, Croxatto JO, Rao NA (2006). Tumors of the orbit. In: AFIP atlas of tumor pathology: tumors of the eye and ocular adnexa. Series 4, Fascicle 5. Washington, DC: American Registry of Pathology; pp. 265–319.
369. Foss AJ, Alexander RA, Hungerford JL, Harris AL, Cree IA, Lightman S (1997). Reassessment of the PAS patterns in uveal melanoma. Br J Ophthalmol. 81(3):240–8. PMID:9135390
370. Foss AJ, Alexander RA, Jefferies LW, Hungerford JL, Harris AL, Lightman S (1996). Microvessel count predicts survival in uveal melanoma. Cancer Res. 56(13):2900–3. PMID:8674036
371. Foss AJ, Pecorella I, Alexander RA, Hungerford JL, Garner A (1994). Are most intraocular "leiomyomas" really melanocytic lesions? Ophthalmology. 101(5):919–24. PMID:8190481
372. Francis JH, Wiesner T, Milman T, Won HH, Lin A, Lee V, et al. (2016). Investigation of somatic GNAQ, GNA11, BAP1 and SF3B1 mutations in ophthalmic melanocytomas. Ocul Oncol Pathol. 2(3):171–7. PMID:27239460
373. Frank RN, Ryan SJ Jr (1972). Peripheral retinal neovascularization with chronic myelogenous leukemia. Arch Ophthalmol. 87(5):585–9. PMID:4503298
374. Frayer WC (1966). Reactivity of the retinal pigment epithelium: an experimental and histopathologic study. Trans Am Ophthalmol Soc. 64:586–643. PMID:5965122
375. Fredrick DR, Char DH, Ljung BM, Brinton DA (1989). Solitary intraocular lymphoma as an initial presentation of widespread disease. Arch Ophthalmol. 107(3):395–7. PMID:2647068
376. Freedman SF, Elner VM, Donev I, Gunta R, Albert DM (1988). Intraocular neurilemmoma arising from the posterior ciliary nerve in neurofibromatosis. Pathologic findings. Ophthalmology. 95(11):1559–64. PMID:3145478
377. Freeman RG, Cloud TM, Knox JM (1961). Keratocanthoma of the conjunctiva. A case report. Arch Ophthalmol. 65(6):817–9. PMID:13701646
378. Freiberg FJ, Kunstmann E, König T, Matlach J, Kampik D (2016). Conjunctival lymphangioma in a 4-year-old girl revealed tuberous sclerosis complex. GMS Ophthalmol Cases. 6:Doc09. PMID:27703871
379. Fried I, Tabori U, Tihan T, Reginald A, Bouffet E (2013). Optic pathway gliomas: a review. CNS Oncol. 2(2):143–59. PMID:25057976
380. Friedman JM (1999). Epidemiology of neurofibromatosis type 1. Am J Med Genet. 89(1):1–6. PMID:10469430
381. Fritz A, Percy C, Jack A, Shanmugaratnam K, Sobin L, Parkin DM, et al., editors (2013). International classification of diseases for oncology (ICD-O). 3rd ed. 1st revision. Geneva: World Health Organization.
382. Fritz D, van de Beek D, Brouwer MC (2016). Clinical features, treatment and outcome in neurosarcoidosis: systematic review and meta-analysis. BMC Neurol. 16(1):220. PMID:27846819
383. Fuchs U, Kivelä T, Tarkkanen A (1991). Cytoskeleton in normal and reactive human retinal pigment epithelial cells. Invest Ophthalmol Vis Sci. 32(13):3178–86. PMID:1748549
384. Fukuda R, Tanabe T, Sawamura H, Kawata M, Tsuji H, Kaburaki T (2011). Case of metastatic pulmonary carcinoma in optic disc diagnosed from results of biopsy performed during vitrectomy surgery. Graefes Arch Clin Exp Ophthalmol. 249(12):1883–7. PMID:21845391
385. Fung AT, Pellegrini M, Shields CL (2014). Congenital hypertrophy of the retinal pigment epithelium: enhanced-depth imaging optical coherence tomography in 18 cases. Ophthalmology. 121(1):251–6. PMID:24126031
386. Gahankari MD, Jehangir R, Bhatti SS (1992). Melanocytoma of the optic disc. J Postgrad Med. 38(3):135–6. PMID:1303415
387. Galinos SO, Smith TR, Brockhurst RJ (1979). Angioma-like lesion in hemoglobin sickle cell disease. Ann Ophthalmol. 11(10):1549–52. PMID:555848
388. Gallagher RP, Elwood JM, Rootman J, Spinelli JJ, Hill GB, Threlfall WJ, et al. (1985). Risk factors for ocular melanoma: Western Canada Melanoma Study. J Natl Cancer Inst. 74(4):775–8. PMID:3857374
389. Gallego Melcón S, Sánchez de Toledo Codina J (2007). Molecular biology of rhabdomyosarcoma. Clin Transl Oncol. 9(7):415–9. PMID:17652054
390. Galletti JG, Guzmán M, Giordano MN (2017). Mucosal immune tolerance at the ocular surface in health and disease. Immunology. 150(4):397–407. PMID:28108991
391. Gao Y, Moonis G, Cunnane ME, Eisenberg RL (2013). Lacrimal gland masses. AJR Am J Roentgenol. 201(3):W371–81. PMID:23971467
391A. Garrett M. Ocular metastasis from seminoma (1959). Br J Ophthalmol. 43:759–61. PMID:13826650
392. Gass JD (1971). Cavernous hemangioma of the retina. A neuro-oculo-cutaneous syndrome. Am J Ophthalmol. 71(4):799–814. PMID:5553009
393. Gass JD, Gieser RG, Wilkinson CP, Beahm DE, Pautler SE (1990). Bilateral diffuse uveal melanocytic proliferation in patients with occult carcinoma. Arch Ophthalmol. 108(4):527–33. PMID:2322154
394. Gass JD, Guerry RK, Jack RL, Harris G (2003). Choroidal osteoma. 1978. Retina. 23(6 Suppl):428–35. PMID:15035392
395. Gayre GS, Proia AD, Dutton JJ (2002). Epibulbar osseous choristoma: case report and review of the literature. Ophthalmic Surg Lasers. 33(5):410–5. PMID:12358295
396. Geneva II, Eagle RC, Barker-Griffith A, Stefanyszyn M, Weisenthal R (2013). Squamous metaplasia of the conjunctiva: a previously unrecognized adverse effect of risedronate sodium. JAMA Ophthalmol. 131(2):249–51. PMID:23411897
397. George RS, Lewis DR, Archibald CW, Heathcote G (2018). Bilateral HPV positive squamous cell carcinoma in situ of conjunctiva. Ophthalmic Plast Reconstr Surg. 34(1):e1–3. PMID:28622197
398. Gerner N, Nørregaard JC, Jensen OA, Prause JU (1996). Conjunctival naevi in Denmark 1960-1980. A 21-year follow-up study. Acta Ophthalmol Scand. 74(4):334–7. PMID:8883545
399. Gezgin G, Dogrusöz M, van Essen TH, Kroes WGM, Luyten GPM, van der Velden PA, et al. (2017). Genetic evolution of uveal melanoma guides the development of an inflammatory microenvironment. Cancer Immunol Immunother. 66(7):903–12. PMID:28391358
400. Ghosh K, Mitra S, Hiwase D (2000). Choroidal infiltrates simulating fundal changes of acute leukemia during hematological recovery following high-dose chemotherapy in acute myelomonocytic leukemia in remission. Am J Hematol. 63(1):42–5. PMID:10602168
401. Giaconi JA, Karp CL (2003). Current treatment options for conjunctival and corneal intraepithelial neoplasia. Ocul Surf. 1(2):66–73. PMID:17075634
402. Gichuhi S, Irlam JJ (2013). Interventions for squamous cell carcinoma of the conjunctiva in HIV-infected individuals. Cochrane Database Syst Rev. (2):CD005643. PMID:23450564
403. Gichuhi S, Ohnuma S, Sagoo MS, Burton MJ (2014). Pathophysiology of ocular surface squamous neoplasia. Exp Eye Res. 129:172–82. PMID:25447808
404. Gichuhi S, Sagoo MS, Weiss HA, Burton MJ (2013). Epidemiology of ocular surface

squamous neoplasia in Africa. Trop Med Int Health. 18(12):1424–43. PMID:24237784
405. Ginderdeuren RV, Missotten GS, van den Oord J (2013). Choroidal paraganglioma with metastases to the fellow eye. Case Rep Ophthalmol. 4(1):17–22. PMID:23525329
406. Godfrey KJ, Kinori M, Lin JH, Snyder VS, Granet DB Heichel CW, et al. (2016). Large benign de novo conjunctival hemangioma in an 11-year-old boy: case report and literature review. J AAPOS. 20(5):462–4. PMID:27647119
407. Gogos K, Tyradellis C, Spaulding AG, Kranias G (2004). Iris cyst simulating melanoma. J AAPOS. 8(5):502–3. PMID:15492747
408. Goldberg RA, Rootman J, Cline RA (1990). Tumors metastatic to the orbit: a changing picture Surv Ophthalmol. 35(1):1–24. PMID:2204127
409. Goldberg RE, Pheasant TR, Shields JA (1979). Cavernous hemangioma of the retina. A four-generation pedigree with neurocutaneous manifestations and an example of bilateral retinal involvement. Arch Ophthalmol. 97(12):2321–4. PMID:229814
410. Goldenberg-Cohen N, Cohen Y, Rosenbaum E, Herscovici Z, Chowers I, Weinberger D, et al. (2005). T1799A BRAF mutations in conjunctival melanocytic lesions. Invest Ophthalmol Vis Sci. 46(9):3027–30. PMID:16123397
411. Gonçalves AC, de Lima PP, Monteiro ML (2016). Epithelial-myoepithelial carcinoma of the lacrimal gland 14 years after en bloc resection of a pleomorphic lacrimal gland adenoma. Ophthal Plast Reconstr Surg. 32(2):e42–4. PMID:25025382
412. Gonder JR, Ezell PC, Shields JA, Augsburger JJ (1982). Ocular melanocytosis. A study to determine the prevalence rate of ocular melanocytosis. Ophthalmology. 89(8):950–2. PMID:7133640
413. Gorham JP, Szalai E, Wells JR, Grossniklaus HE (2017). Retinoinvasive uveal melanoma: report of 2 cases and review of the literature. Ocul Oncol Pathol. 3(4):292–5. PMID:29344483
414. Goto H, Takahira M, Azumi A (2015). Diagnostic criteria for IgG4-related ophthalmic disease. Jpn J Ophthalmol. 59(1):1–7. PMID:25392273
415. Gottlieb F, Fammartino JJ, Stratford TP, Brockhurst RJ (1984). Retinal angiomatous mass. A complication of retinal detachment surgery. Retina. 4(3):152–7. PMID:6494632
416. Gravanis MB (1989). Allograft heart accelerated atherosclerosis: evidence for cell-mediated immunity in pathogenesis. Mod Pathol. 2(5):495–505. PMID:2813347
417. Green WR, Iliff WJ, Trotter RR (1974). Malignant teratoid medulloepithelioma of the optic nerve. Arch Ophthalmol. 91(6):451–4. PMID:4827430
418. Greene DP, Shield DR, Shields CL, Shields JA, Servat JJ, Lin CJ, et al. (2014). Cutaneous melanoma metastatic to the orbit: review of 15 cases. Ophthalmic Plast Reconstr Surg. 30(3):233–7. PMID:24811686
420. Greenstein MB, Myers CE, Meuer SM, Klein BE, Cotch MF, Wong TY, et al. (2011). Prevalence and characteristics of choroidal nevi: the multi-ethnic study of atherosclerosis. Ophthalmology. 118(12):2468–73. PMID:21820181
421. Griewank KG, Murali R, Schilling B, Scholz S, Sucker A, Song M, et al. (2013). TERT promoter mutations in ocular melanoma distinguish between conjunctival and uveal tumours. Br J Cancer. 109(2):497–501. PMID:23799844
422. Griewank KG, Westekemper H, Murali R, Mach M, Schilling B, Wiesner T, et al. (2013). Conjunctival melanomas harbor BRAF and NRAS mutations and copy number changes similar to cutaneous and mucosal melanomas. Clin Cancer Res. 19(12):3143–52. PMID:23633454
423. Grimm SA, Pulido JS, Jahnke K, Schiff D, Hall AJ, Shenkier TN, et al. (2007). Primary intraocular lymphoma: an International Primary Central Nervous System Lymphoma Collaborative Group report. Ann Oncol. 18(11):1851–5. PMID:17804469
424. Grob SR, Jakobiec FA, Rashid A, MacIntosh P, Kelly H, Fay A (2016). Pediatric optic nerve meningioma: diagnostic and therapeutic challenges. Ophthal Plast Reconstr Surg. 32(6):e160–4. PMID:25585303
425. Grob SR, Jakobiec FA, Stagner AM, Colby KA (2015). Diffuse epibulbar complex lacrimal-cartilaginous choristoma: diagnostic clues and management. Cornea. 34(10):1321–3. PMID:26147834
426. Grossniklaus HE (2013). Progression of ocular melanoma metastasis to the liver: the 2012 Zimmerman Lecture. JAMA Ophthalmol. 131(4):462–9. PMID:23392528
427. Grossniklaus HE, Albert DM, Green WR, Conway BP, Hovland KR (1997). Clear cell differentiation in choroidal melanoma. COMS report no. 8. Arch Ophthalmol. 115(7):894–8. PMID:9230830
428. Grossniklaus HE, Green WR, Luckenbach M, Chan CC (1987). Conjunctival lesions in adults. A clinical and histopathologic review. Cornea. 6(2):78–116. PMID:3301209
429. Grossniklaus HE, Martin DF, Avery R, Shields JA, Shields CL, Kuo IC, et al. (1998). Uveal lymphoid infiltration. Report of four cases and clinicopathologic review. Ophthalmology. 105(7):1265–73. PMID:9663232
430. Grossniklaus HE, Martin DF, Solomon AR (1990). Invasive conjunctival tumor with keratoacanthoma features. Am J Ophthalmol. 109(6):736–8. PMID:2346208
431. Grossniklaus HE, Wojno TH, Wilson MW, Someren AO (1997). Myoepithelioma of the lacrimal gland. Arch Ophthalmol. 115(12):1588–90. PMID:9400797
432. Grossniklaus HE, Zhang Q, You S, McCarthy C, Heegaard S, Coupland SE (2016). Metastatic ocular melanoma to the liver exhibits infiltrative and nodular growth patterns. Hum Pathol. 57:165–75. PMID:27476775
433. Grossniklaus HE, Zimmerman LE, Kachmer ML (1990). Pleomorphic adenocarcinoma of the ciliary body. Immunohistochemical and electron microscopic features. Ophthalmology. 97(6):763–8. PMID:2197590
434. Grulich AE, van Leeuwen MT, Falster MO, Vajdic CM (2007). Incidence of cancers in people with HIV/AIDS compared with immunosuppressed transplant recipients: a meta-analysis. Lancet. 370(9581):59–67. PMID:17617273
435. Guerriero S, Sborgia A, Giancipoli G, Fiore MG, Ross R, Piscitelli D (2011). A rare case of primitive epithelioid leiomyosarcoma of the conjunctiva. Orbit. 30(3):169–71. PMID:21574810
436. Guijarro-Oria FJ, Mencía-Gutiérrez E, Gutiérrez-Díaz E, López-Tizón E (2013). Orbital giant conjunctival epithelial primary cyst. Arch Soc Esp Oftalmol. 88(4):157–9. PMID:23597646
437. Gulati R, Alkhatib Y, Donthireddy V, Felicella MM, Menon MP, Inamdar KV (2015). Isolated ocular manifestation of relapsed chronic myelogenous leukemia presenting as myeloid blast crisis in a patient on imatinib therapy: a case report and review of the literature. Case Rep Pathol. 2015:380451. PMID:26819793
438. Gündüz K, Eagle RC Jr, Shields CL, Shields JA, Augsburger JJ (1999). Invasive giant cell astrocytoma of the retina in a patient with tuberous sclerosis. Ophthalmology. 106(3):639–42. PMID:10080228
439. Gündüz K, Shields CL, Shields JA, Mercado G, Eagle RC Jr (1998). Intraocular neoplastic cyst from mucoepidermoid carcinoma of the conjunctiva. Arch Ophthalmol. 116(11):1521–3. PMID:9823358
440. Gündüz K, Shields JA, Shields CL, Eagle RC Jr, Diniz W, Mercado G, et al. (1999). Transscleral choroidal biopsy in the diagnosis of choroidal lymphoma. Surv Ophthalmol. 43(6):551–5. PMID:10416797
441. Guo P, Yan F, Tian C, Zhao P, Wang Z, Xian J (2014). Imaging and histopathological findings of lacrimal sac lymphoma. Chin Med J (Engl). 127(1):120–4. PMID:24384436
442. Gupta MP, Lane AM, DeAngelis MM, Mayne K, Crabtree M, Gragoudas ES, et al. (2015). Clinical characteristics of uveal melanoma in patients with germline BAP1 mutations. JAMA Ophthalmol. 133(8):881–7. PMID:25974357
443. Gupta N, Kaur J, Rajwanshi A, Nijhawan R, Srinivasan R, Dey P, et al. (2012). Spectrum of orbital and ocular adnexal lesions: an analysis of 389 cases diagnosed by fine needle aspiration cytology. Diagn Cytopathol. 40(7):582–5. PMID:21309008
444. Gupta R, Singh S, Hedau S, Nigam S, Das BC, Singh I, et al. (2007). Spindle cell carcinoma of head and neck: an immunohistochemical and molecular approach to its pathogenesis. J Clin Pathol. 60(5):472–5. PMID:16731596
445. Gupta S, Gupta S, Urs AB, Singh K (2017). Leukoplakia of buccal mucosa with transformation into spindle cell carcinoma: a rare case report. J Oral Maxillofac Pathol. 21(1):119–23. PMID:28479698
446. Gutmann DH, Donahoe J, Brown T, James CD, Perry A (2000). Loss of neurofibromatosis 1 (NF1) gene expression in NF1-associated pilocytic astrocytomas. Neuropathol Appl Neurobiol. 26(4):361–7. PMID:10931370
447. Guyer DR, Schachat AP, Vitale S, Markowitz JA, Braine H, Burke PJ, et al. (1989). Leukemic retinopathy. Relationship between fundus lesions and hematologic parameters at diagnosis. Ophthalmology. 96(6):860–4. PMID:2740081
448. Hadden PW, Damato BE, McKay IC (2003). Bilateral uveal melanoma: a series of four cases. Eye (Lond). 17(5):613–6. PMID:12855969
449. Haisley-Royster CA, Allingham RR, Klintworth GK, Prose NS (2001). Hereditary benign intraepithelial dyskeratosis: report of two cases with prominent oral lesions. J Am Acad Dermatol. 45(4):634–6. PMID:11568764
450. Hale PN, Allen RA, Straatsma BR (1965). Benign melanomas (nevi) of the choroid and ciliary body. Arch Ophthalmol. 74(4):532–8. PMID:5838370
451. Hamam R, Bhat P, Foster CS (2009). Conjunctival/corneal intraepithelial neoplasia. Int Ophthalmol Clin. 49(1):63–70. PMID:19125065
452. Hanafi H, Verdijk RM, Paridaens D (2016). Malignant pleural mesothelioma with lacrimal gland metastasis. Acta Ophthalmol. 94(8):836–8. PMID:27422678
453. Handorf CR, Kulkarni A, Grenert JP, Weiss LM, Rogers WM, Kim OS, et al. (2013). A multicenter study directly comparing the diagnostic accuracy of gene expression profiling and immunohistochemistry for primary site identification in metastatic tumors. Am J Surg Pathol. 37(7):1067–75. PMID:23648464
454. Harbour JW, Brantley MA Jr, Hollingsworth H, Gordon M (2004). Association between posterior uveal melanoma and iris freckles, iris naevi, and choroidal naevi. Br J Ophthalmol. 88(1):36–8. PMID:14693769
455. Harbour JW, Onken MD, Roberson ED, Duan S, Cao L, Worley LA, et al. (2010). Frequent mutation of BAP1 in metastasizing uveal melanomas. Science. 330(6009):1410–3. PMID:21051595
456. Harbour JW, Roberson ED, Anbunathan H, Onken MD, Worley LA, Bowcock AM (2013). Recurrent mutations at codon 625 of the splicing factor SF3B1 in uveal melanoma. Nat Genet. 45(2):133–5. PMID:23313955
457. Harold Lee HB, Garrity JA, Cameron JD, Strianese D, Bonavolontà G, Patrinely JR (2008). Primary optic nerve sheath meningioma in children. Surv Ophthalmol. 53(6):543–58. PMID:19026318
458. Harooni H, Schoenfield LR, Singh AD (2011). Current appraisal of conjunctival melanocytic tumors: classification and treatment. Future Oncol. 7(3):435–46. PMID:21417906
459. Harris DC, Clark CV, Bartholomew RS (1989). Carcinoid tumour in the lacrimal gland. Doc Ophthalmol. 73(1):43–51. PMID:2630240
460. Harris JL, Gumucio CC, Ohanion MB (1968). Adenocarcinoma of the ciliary epithelium. Arch Ophthalmol. 80(2):217–9. PMID:5661889
461. Harvey P, Lee JA, Talbot JF, Goepel JR (1994). Isolated xanthogranuloma of the limbus in an adult. Br J Ophthalmol. 78(8):657–9. PMID:7918298
462. Hasche H, Eck M, Lieb W (2003). Immunochemical demonstration of human herpes virus 8 in conjunctival Kaposi's sarcoma. Ophthalmologe. 100(2):142–4. [German] PMID:12589459
463. Hashemi H, Mohebbi M, Mehravaran S, Mazloumi M, Jahanbani-Ardakani H, Abtahi SH (2017). Hyperimmunoglobulin E syndrome: genetics, immunopathogenesis, clinical findings, and treatment modalities. J Res Med Sci. 22:53. PMID:28567072
464. Hashimoto K, Sasajima Y, Ando M, Yonemori K, Hirakawa A, Furuta K, et al. (2012). Immunohistochemical profile for unknown primary adenocarcinoma. PLoS One. 7(1):e31181. PMID:22299055
465. Hau SC, Papastefanou V, Shah S, Sagoo MS, Restori M, Cohen V (2015). Evaluation of iris and iridociliary body lesions with anterior segment optical coherence tomography versus ultrasound B-scan. Br J Ophthalmol. 99(1):81–6. PMID:25091953
466. Hayward DM, Yoo D, Lee JM, Wild E, Prabhu VC (2014). Myoepithelioma of the orbital apex and middle cranial fossa: case report and review of the literature. Neuroophthalmology. 38(1):14–20. PMID:27928268
467. Heathcote JG (2012). Transitional neoplasms of the naso-lacrimal system: a review of the histopathology and histogenesis. Saudi J Ophthalmol. 26(2):125–31. PMID:23960982
468. Heathcote JG, Schoales BA, Willis NR (1991). Incontinentia pigmenti (Bloch-Sulzberger syndrome): a case report and review of the ocular pathological features. Can J Ophthalmol. 26(4):229–37. PMID:1889027
469. Heddi A, Faure-Vigny H, Wallace DC, Stepien G (1996). Coordinate expression of nuclear and mitochondrial genes involved in energy production in carcinoma and oncocytoma. Biochim Biophys Acta. 1316(3):203–9. PMID:8781539
470. Salomão D, Tóth J, Kennedy S (2015). Eyelid pathology. In: Heegaard S, Grossniklaus H, editors. Eye pathology: an illustrated guide. Berlin: Springer-Verlag; pp. 443–546.
472. Heegaard S, Larsen JN, Fledelius HC, Prause JU (2001). Neoplasia versus hyperplasia of the retinal pigment epithelium. A comparison of two cases. Acta Ophthalmol Scand. 79(6):626–33. PMID:11782230
473. Heindl LM, Jünemann AG, Kruse FE, Holbach LM (2010). Tumors of the lacrimal drainage system. Orbit. 29(5):298–306. PMID:20958177
474. Heindl LM, Naumann GO, Kruse FE,

Holbach LM (2008). Aggressive metastasising adenocarcinoma of the retinal pigment epithelium with trisomy 21. Br J Ophthalmol. 92(3):389–91. PMID:18303161
475. Hellquist H, Skalova A, Azadeh B (2016). Salivary gland hybrid tumour revisited: could they represent high-grade transformation in a low-grade neoplasm? Virchows Arch. 469(6):643–50. PMID:27605055
475A. Henriquez F, Janssen C, Kemp EG, Roberts F (2007). The T1799A BRAF mutation is present in iris melanoma. Invest Ophthalmol Vis Sci. 48(11):4897–900. PMID:17962436
476. Hendrix MJ, Seftor EA, Seftor RE, Kirschmann DA, Gardner LM, Boldt HC, et al. (1998). Regulation of uveal melanoma interconverted phenotype by hepatocyte growth factor/scatter factor (HGF/SF). Am J Pathol. 152(4):855–63. PMID:9546344
477. Hennessy MP, Collins F, Coroneo MT (1993). The distinction between multiple retinal pigment epithelial hamartomata (MRPEH) in familial adenomatous polyposis (FAP) and congenital hypertrophy of the retinal pigment epithelium (CHRPE). Aust N Z J Ophthalmol. 21(4):275–6. PMID:8148147
478. Hered RW, Hiles DA (1987). Epibulbar osseous choristoma and ectopic lacrimal gland underlying a dermolipoma. J Pediatr Ophthalmol Strabismus. 24(5):255–8. PMID:3681614
479. Héritier S, Hélias-Rodzewicz Z, Chakraborty R, Sengal AG, Bellanné-Chantelot C, Thomas C, et al. (2017). New somatic BRAF splicing mutation in Langerhans cell histiocytosis. Mol Cancer. 16(1):115. PMID:28679432
480. Herschorn BJ, Jakobiec FA, Hornblass A, Iwamoto T, Harrison WG (1983). Mucoepidermoid carcinoma of the palpebral mucocutaneous junction. A clinical, light microscopic and electron microscopic study of an unusual tubular variant. Ophthalmology. 90(12):1437–46. PMID:6677843
481. Herwig MC, Fassunke J, Merkelbach-Bruse S, Holz FG, Fischer HP, Loeffler KU (2012). Reactive lymphoid hyperplasia of the ocular surface: clinicopathologic features and search for infectious agents. Acta Ophthalmol. 90(4):e331–2. PMID:22067517
482. Herwig MC, Fischer HP, Holz FG, Loeffler KU (2010). Conjunctival myxoma: two cases. Histopathological examination and clinical course. Ophthalmologe. 107(9):843–7. [German] PMID:20376460
483. Herwig MC, Wells JR, Grossniklaus HE (2012). Conjunctival stromal tumor: report of 4 cases. Ophthalmology. 119(4):682–7. PMID:22200094
484. Hine JE, Kingham JD (1979). Myelogenous leukemia and bilateral exudative retinal detachment. Ann Ophthalmol. 11(12):1867–72. PMID:299244
485. Ho CY, Mosier S, Safneck J, Salomao DR, Miller NR, Eberhart CG, et al. (2015). Genetic profiling by single-nucleotide polymorphism-based array analysis defines three distinct subtypes of orbital meningioma. Brain Pathol. 25(2):193–201. PMID:24773246
486. Hodgson N, Whipple K, Lin JH, Brumund KT, Kikkawa DO, Korn BS (2013). Bilateral squamous cell carcinoma of the lacrimal sac. Ophthal Plast Reconstr Surg. 29(6):e149–51. PMID:24217491
487. Hoepner J, Yanoff M (1972). Ocular anomalies in trisomy 13-15: an analysis of 13 eyes with two new findings. Am J Ophthalmol. 74(4):729–37. PMID:4627577
488. Holz FG, Boehmer HV, Mechtersheimer G, Ott G, Völcker HE (1999). Uveal non-Hodgkin's lymphoma with epibulbar extension simulating choroidal effusion syndrome. Retina. 19(4):343–6. PMID:10458303
489. Honavar SG, Manjandavida FP (2015). Tumors of the ocular surface: a review. Indian J Ophthalmol. 63(3):187–203. PMID:25971163
490. Honavar SG, Shields CL, Maus M, Shields JA, Demirci H, Eagle RC Jr (2001). Primary intraepithelial sebaceous gland carcinoma of the palpebral conjunctiva. Arch Ophthalmol. 119(5):764–7. PMID:11346408
491. Hoover DL, Smith LE, Turner SJ, Gelber RD, Sallan SE (1988). Ophthalmic evaluation of survivors of acute lymphoblastic leukemia. Ophthalmology. 95(2):151–5. PMID:3173990
492. Hornblass A, Jakobiec FA, Bosniak S, Flanagan J (1980). The diagnosis and management of epithelial tumors of the lacrimal sac. Ophthalmology. 87(6):476–90. PMID:7413136
493. Horvath A, Bertherat J, Groussin L, Guillaud-Bataille M, Tsang K, Cazabat L, et al. (2010). Mutations and polymorphisms in the gene encoding regulatory subunit type 1-alpha of protein kinase A (PRKAR1A): an update. Hum Mutat. 31(4):369–79. PMID:20358582
494. House RJ, Mashayekhi A, Shields JA, Shields CL (2016). Total regression of acquired retinal astrocytoma using photodynamic therapy. Retin Cases Brief Rep. 10(1):41–3. PMID:26164044
495. Hsieh CY, Liao YP, Wu CC, Yuan SP, Ho JH, Roan R, et al. (2016). Nasal dissemination of a single-clone IgH-rearranged conjunctival MALT lymphoma through the nasolacrimal duct: a case report. Oncol Lett. 12(2):1007–10. PMID:27446385
496. Hu DN, McCormick SA, Yu GP (2008). Latitude and uveal melanoma. Ophthalmology. 115(4):757–9. PMID:18387420
497. Hu DN, Yu G, McCormick SA, Finger PT (2008). Population-based incidence of conjunctival melanoma in various races and ethnic groups and comparison with other melanomas. Am J Ophthalmol. 145(3):418–23. PMID:18191091
498. Hu DN, Yu GP, McCormick SA, Schneider S, Finger PT (2005). Population-based incidence of uveal melanoma in various races and ethnic groups. Am J Ophthalmol. 140(4):612–7. PMID:16226513
499. Hubbard KB, Hepler JR (2006). Cell signalling diversity of the Gqalpha family of heterotrimeric G proteins. Cell Signal. 18(2):135–50. PMID:16182515
500. Hudson LE, Mendoza PR, Yan J, Grossniklaus HE (2017). Reactive retinal astrocytic tumor (focal nodular gliosis): a case report. Ocul Oncol Pathol. 3(1):1–7. PMID:28275595
501. Hufnagel TJ, Sears ML, Shapiro M, Kim JH (1988). Ciliary body neurilemoma recurring after 15 years. Graefes Arch Clin Exp Ophthalmol. 226(5):443–6. PMID:3192095
502. IARC Working Group on the Evaluation of Carcinogenic Risks to Humans (2007). Human papillomaviruses. IARC Monogr Eval Carcinog Risks Hum. 90:1–636. PMID:18354839
503. Huson S, Jones D, Beck L (1987). Ophthalmic manifestations of neurofibromatosis. Br J Ophthalmol. 71(3):235–8. PMID:3103673
504. Hussain RM, Matthews JL, Dubovy SR, Thompson JM, Wang G (2014). UV-independent p53 mutations in sebaceous carcinoma of the eyelid. Ophthal Plast Reconstr Surg. 30(5):392–5. PMID:24777261
505. Inayama Y, Hanashi M, Yazawa T, Mitsui H, Kimura A, Ito D (2005). Massive gliosis of the retina: report of a case investigated by immunohistochemistry and clonality assays. Hum Pathol. 36(6):702–5. PMID:16021579
506. Inoue R, Saishin Y, Shima C, Yoshikawa H, Ohguro N, Tano Y (2009). A case of iris melanocytoma transformed to malignant melanoma. Jpn J Ophthalmol. 53(3):271–3. PMID:19484449
507. AJCC Ophthalmic Oncology Task Force (2015). International validation of the American Joint Committee on Cancer's 7th edition classification of uveal melanoma. JAMA Ophthalmol. 133(4):376–83. PMID:25555246
508. Iordanous Y, Belrose JC, Cadieux DC, Chakrabarti S, Farmer JP, Allen LH (2015). p63 positive mucoepidermoid tumor of the lacrimal sac with associated papilloma. Orbit. 34(4):220–2. PMID:26121166
509. Isaacs TW, Vermeulen TL, Spagnolo D, Amanuel B (2015). Choroidal involvement in Rosai-Dorfman syndrome may be depicted and followed using enhanced depth imaging optical coherence tomography (EDI-OCT). Graefes Arch Clin Exp Ophthalmol. 253(10):1821–2. PMID:25825230
510. Isaacson PG, Du MQ (2004). MALT lymphoma: from morphology to molecules. Nat Rev Cancer. 4(8):644–53. PMID:15286744
511. Ishida M, Iwai M, Yoshida K, Kagotani A, Kohzaki H, Arikata M, et al. (2013). Primary ductal adenocarcinoma of the lacrimal sac: the first reported case. Int J Clin Exp Pathol. 6(9):1929–34. PMID:24040460
512. Ishijima K, Kase S, Noda M, Ishida S (2011). Intraocular neovascularization associated with choroidal ganglioneuroma in neurofibromatosis type 1. Eur J Ophthalmol. 21(6):837–40. PMID:21574161
513. Islam S, Thomas A, Eisenberg RL, Hoffman GR (2012). Surgical management of transitional cell carcinoma of the lacrimal sac: is it time for a new treatment algorithm? J Plast Reconstr Aesthet Surg. 65(2):e33–6. PMID:21986110
514. Aït-Khaled N, Pearce N, Anderson HR, Ellwood P, Montefort S, Shah J, et al. (2009). Global map of the prevalence of symptoms of rhinoconjunctivitis in children: the International Study of Asthma and Allergies in Childhood (ISAAC) Phase Three. Allergy. 64(1):123–48. PMID:19132975
515. Iwamoto T, Jakobiec FA, Darrell RW (1981). Fibrous histiocytoma of the corneoscleral limbus: the ultrastructure of a distinctive inclusion. Ophthalmology. 88(12):1260–8. PMID:6275324
516. Jabs DA, Hirst LW, Green WR, Tutschka PJ, Santos GW, Beschorner WE (1983). The eye in bone marrow transplantation. II. Histopathology. Arch Ophthalmol. 101(4):585–90. PMID:6340649
517. Jacobs M, Benger R (1989). Metastatic breast carcinoma of the orbit. Aust N Z J Ophthalmol. 17(4):357–61. PMID:2560382
518. Jacoby LB, MacCollin M, Louis DN, Mohney T, Rubio MP, Pulaski K, et al. (1994). Exon scanning for mutation of the NF2 gene in schwannomas. Hum Mol Genet. 3(3):413–9. PMID:8012353
519. Jaffe MS, Shields JA, Canny CL, Eagle RC Jr, Fry RL (1977). Retinoblastoma simulating Coats' disease: a clinicopathologic report. Ann Ophthalmol. 9(7):863–8. PMID:900721
520. Jahnke K, Korfel A, Komm J, Bechrakis NE, Stein H, Thiel E, et al. (2006). Intraocular lymphoma 2000-2005: results of a retrospective multicentre trial. Graefes Arch Clin Exp Ophthalmol. 244(6):663–9. PMID:16228920
521. Jain D, Ebrahimi KB, Miller NR, Eberhart CG (2010). Intraorbital meningiomas: a pathologic review using current World Health Organization criteria. Arch Pathol Lab Med. 134(5):766–70. PMID:20441509
522. Jakobiec FA (2016). Conjunctival primary acquired melanosis: is it time for a new terminology? Am J Ophthalmol. 162:3–19.e1. PMID:26556007
523. Jakobiec FA, Bhat P, Colby KA (2010). Immunohistochemical studies of conjunctival nevi and melanomas. Arch Ophthalmol. 128(2):174–83. PMID:20142539
524. Jakobiec FA, Brodie SE, Haik B, Iwamoto T (1983). Giant cell astrocytoma of the retina. A tumor of possible Mueller cell origin. Ophthalmology. 90(12):1565–76. PMID:6677857
525. Jakobiec FA, Colby K, Bajart AM, Saragas SJ, Moulin A (2009). Immunohistochemical studies of atypical conjunctival melanocytic nevi. Arch Ophthalmol. 127(8):970–80. PMID:19667333
526. Jakobiec FA, Folberg R, Iwamoto T (1989). Clinicopathologic characteristics of premalignant and malignant melanocytic lesions of the conjunctiva. Ophthalmology. 96(2):147–66. PMID:2649838
527. Jakobiec FA, Font RL, Tso MO, Zimmerman LE (1977). Mesectodermal leiomyoma of the ciliary body: a tumor of presumed neural crest origin. Cancer. 39(5):2102–13. PMID:870167
528. Jakobiec FA, Kool M, Stagner AM, Pfister SM, Eagle RC, Proia AD, et al. (2015). Intraocular medulloepitheliomas and embryonal tumors with multilayered rosettes of the brain: comparative roles of LIN28A and C19MC. Am J Ophthalmol. 159(6):1065–74.e1. PMID:25748578
529. Jakobiec FA, Rai R, Yoon MK (2014). Fibrous histiocytoma of the tarsus: clinical and immunohistochemical observations with a differential diagnosis. Cornea. 33(5):536–9. PMID:24608257
530. Jakobiec FA, Rashid A, Lewis K (2015). Massive retinal gliosis in neurofibromatosis type 1. JAMA Ophthalmol. 133(1):100–2. PMID:25317586
531. Jakobiec FA, Rose MF, Trief D, Stagner AM, Kim I, Gragoudas ES (2015). Immunohistochemical investigations of adult intraocular medulloepitheliomas. Clin Experiment Ophthalmol. 43(4):379–85. PMID:25251824
532. Jakobiec FA, Silbert G (1981). Are most iris 'melanomas' really nevi? A clinicopathologic study of 189 lesions. Arch Ophthalmol. 99(12):2117–32. PMID:7305709
533. Jakobiec FA, Stacy RC, Thakker MM (2011). Blue nevus of the tarsus as the predominant component of a combined nevus of the eyelid. Ophthal Plast Reconstr Surg. 27(4):e94–6. PMID:20940655
534. Jakobiec FA, Stagner AM, Eagle RC Jr, Lally SE, Krane JF (2017). Unusual pleomorphic adenoma of the lacrimal gland: immunohistochemical demonstration of PLAG1 and HMGA2 oncoproteins. Surv Ophthalmol. 62(2):219–26. PMID:27567603
535. Jakobiec FA, Stagner AM, Lefebvre DR (2017). Uniformly sclerotic diffuse large b-cell lymphoma of the orbit. Ophthal Plast Reconstr Surg. 33(3S Suppl 1):S127–9. PMID:26561954
536. Jakobiec FA, Stagner AM, Rubin PAD (2017). Lymphoepithelial carcinoma of the nasolacrimal duct: clinical, radiologic, and immunopathologic features. Ophthal Plast Reconstr Surg. 33(3S Suppl 1):S18–21. PMID:25902392
537. Jakobiec FA, Stagner AM, Sutula FC, Freitag SK, Yoon MK (2016). Pigmentation of the lacrimal sac epithelium. Ophthal Plast Reconstr Surg. 32(6):415–23. PMID:26348325
538. Jakobiec FA, Thanos A, Stagner AM, Grossniklaus HE, Proia AD (2016). So-called massive retinal gliosis: a critical review and reappraisal. Surv Ophthalmol. 61(3):339–56. PMID:26703887
539. Jakobiec FA, Trief D, Rashid A, Rose MF, Minckler D, Vanderveen D, et al. (2014). New insights into the development of infantile intraocular medulloepithelioma. Am J Ophthalmol. 158(6):1275–96.e1. PMID:25174896
540. Jakobiec FA, Werdich XQ, Chodosh J, Freitag SK (2014). An analysis of conjunctival and periocular venous malformations: clinicopathologic and immunohistochemical features with a comparison of racemose and

cirsoid lesions. Surv Ophthalmol. 59(2):236–44. PMID:24355066
541. Jakobiec FA, Zimmerman LE, Spencer WH, Slakter JS, Krebs W (1987). Metastatic colloid carcinoma versus primary carcinoma of the ciliary epithelium. Ophthalmology. 94(11):1469–80. PMID:2825094
542. Jakobiec FA, Zuckerman BD, Berlin AJ, Odell P, MacRae DW, Tuthill RJ (1985). Unusual melanocytic nevi of the conjunctiva. Am J Ophthalmol. 100(1):100–13. PMID:4014368
543. Jampol LM, Goldberg MF, Busse B (1975). Peripheral retinal microaneurysms in chronic leukemia. Am J Ophthalmol. 80(2):242–8. PMID:1057377
544. Janakiram TN, Sagar S, Sharma SB, Subramaniam V (2016). Primary mucoepidermoid carcinoma of the lacrimal sac - a case report and literature review. Klin Onkol. 29(4):291–4. PMID:27534787
545. Jang J, Kie JH, Lee SY, Kim SJ, Lew H, Hong SW, et al. (2001). Acinic cell carcinoma of the lacrimal gland with intracranial extension: a case report. Ophthal Plast Reconstr Surg. 17(6):454–7. PMID:11766029
546. Jang JH, Chang SD, Choe MS (2009). A case of recurrent Schneiderian papilloma of the lacrimal sac invading the nasal cavity. Korean J Ophthalmol. 23(2):100–3. PMID:19568358
547. Jans SR, Schomerus E, Bygum A (2015). Neurofibromatosis type 1 diagnosed in a child based on multiple juvenile xanthogranulomas and juvenile myelomonocytic leukemia. Pediatr Dermatol. 32(1):e29–32. PMID:25516272
548. Jansen JC, Van Calster J, Pulido JS, Miles SL, Vile RG, Van Bergen T, et al. (2015). Early diagnosis and successful treatment of paraneoplastic melanocytic proliferation. Br J Ophthalmol. 99(7):943–8. PMID:25908835
549. Janssens K, Mertens M, Lauwers N, de Keizer RJ, Mathysen DG, De Groot V (2016). To study and determine the role of anterior segment optical coherence tomography and ultrasound biomicroscopy in corneal and conjunctival tumors. J Ophthalmol. 2016:1048760. PMID:28050274
550. Jastrzebski A, Brownstein S, Jordan DR, Gilberg SM (2012). Histochemical analysis and immunohistochemical profile of mucoepidermoid carcinoma of the conjunctiva. Saudi J Ophthalmol. 26(2):205–10. PMID:23960993
551. Jastrzebski A, Brownstein S, Manusow J, Rubab S (2011). Isolated conjunctival lymphangioma. Can J Ophthalmol. 46(4):369–70. PMID:21816261
552. Javitt NB (1992). Polyethylene glycol 900: useful marker rather than notable exception. Gastroenterology. 102(6):2190–2. PMID:1587453
553. Jaworski A, Wolffsohn JS, Napper GA (2000). Detection, aetiology and management of conjunctival intraepithelial neoplasia. Ophthalmic Physiol Opt. 20(5):371–80. PMID:11045245
554. Jett K, Friedman JM (2010). Clinical and genetic aspects of neurofibromatosis 1. Genet Med. 12(1):1–11. PMID:20027112
555. Jittapiromsak N, Hou P, Williams MD, Chi TL (2017). Orbital oncocytoma: evaluation with dynamic contrast-enhanced magnetic resonance imaging using a time-signal intensity curve and positive enhancement integral images. Clin Imaging. 42:161–4. PMID:28033355
556. Joag MG, Gupta A, Galor A, Dubovy SR, Bermudez-Magner JA, Wang J, et al. (2015). Conjunctival intraepithelial neoplasia with mucoepidermoid differentiation: a case report of a subtle lesion. Ocul Oncol Pathol. 1(4):278–82. PMID:27171853
557. Jonas JB, You QS, Xu L, Wang YX (2008). Choroidal nevi in adult Chinese. Ophthalmology. 115(6):1102–1102.e1. PMID:18519073
558. Juarez CP, Tso MO (1980). An ultrastructural study of melanocytomas (magnocellular nevi) of the optic disk and uvea. Am J Ophthalmol. 90(1):48–62. PMID:7395958
559. Jünemann A, Holbach LM (1998). Epithelial giant inclusion cyst 50 years after enucleation without orbital implant. Klin Monbl Augenheilkd. 212(2):127–8. [German] PMID:9577816
560. Jung JH, Shin DH, Cho KS, Choi HY (2013). Nasolacrimal duct obstruction caused by oncocytic carcinoma. Korean J Ophthalmol. 27(2):126–9. PMID:23543280
561. Jung JJ, Chen MH, Rofagha S, Lee SS (2017). Graft-versus-host disease panuveitis and bilateral serous detachments: multimodal imaging analysis. Retin Cases Brief Rep. 11 Suppl 1:S54–61. PMID:27571426
562. Kaeser PF, Uffer S, Zografos L, Hamédani M (2006). Tumors of the caruncle: a clinicopathologic correlation. Am J Ophthalmol. 142(3):448–55. PMID:16935590
563. Kaikov Y (1996). Optic nerve head infiltration in acute leukemia in children: an indication for emergency optic nerve radiation therapy. Med Pediatr Oncol. 26(2):101–4. PMID:8531846
564. Kaiserman I, Amer R, Pe'er J (2004). Liver function tests in metastatic uveal melanoma. Am J Ophthalmol. 137(2):236–43. PMID:14962411
565. Kaliki S, Arepalli S, Shields CL, Klein K, Sun H, Hysenj E, et al. (2013). Conjunctival papilloma: features and outcomes based on age at initial examination. JAMA Ophthalmol. 131(5):585–93. PMID:23538642
566. Kaliki S, Eagle RC, Grossniklaus HE, Campbell RJ, Shields CL, Shields JA (2013). Inadvertent implantation of aqueous tube shunts in glaucomatous eyes with unrecognized intraocular neoplasms: report of 5 cases. JAMA Ophthalmol. 131(7):925–8. PMID:23699787
567. Kaliki S, Shields CL, Eagle RC Jr, Vemuganti GK, Almeida A, Manjandavida FP, et al. (2013). Ciliary body medulloepithelioma: analysis of 41 cases. Ophthalmology. 120(12):2552–9. PMID:23796765
568. Kaliki S, Shields CL, Shah SU, Eagle RC Jr, Shields JA, Leahey A (2011). Postenucleation adjuvant chemotherapy with vincristine, etoposide, and carboplatin for the treatment of high-risk retinoblastoma. Arch Ophthalmol. 129(11):1422–7. PMID:22084213
569. Kaliki S, Shields CL, Shields JA (2015). Uveal melanoma: estimating prognosis. Indian J Ophthalmol. 63(2):93–102. PMID:25827538
570. Kalina PH, Bartley GB, Campbell RJ, Buettner H (1991). Isolated neurofibromas of the conjunctiva. Am J Ophthalmol. 111(6):694–8. PMID:2039037
571. Kalirai H, Dodson A, Faqir S, Damato BE, Coupland SE (2014). Lack of BAP1 protein expression in uveal melanoma is associated with increased metastatic risk and has utility in routine prognostic testing. Br J Cancer. 111(7):1373–80. PMID:25058347
572. Kamada Y, Sakata A, Nakadomari S, Takehana M (1998). Phakomatous choristoma of the eyelid: immunohistochemical observation. Jpn J Ophthalmol. 42(1):41–5. PMID:9507364
573. Kanavi MR, Hosseini SB, Aliakbar-Navahi R, Aghaei H (2017). Impression cytology in a series of clinically diagnosed ocular surface melanocytic lesions. J Ophthalmic Vis Res. 12(1):17–22. PMID:28299002
574. Kaneko A (1993). Malignant ophthalmic tumors. Nihon Rinsho. 51 Suppl:1013–20. [Japanese] PMID:8459526
575. Kanoff JM, Colby K, Jakobiec FA (2010). Incipient corneoscleral xanthogranuloma with S-100 positivity in a teenager. Cornea. 29(6):688–90. PMID:20458239
576. Kantelip B, Boccard R, Nores JM, Bacin F (1989). A case of conjunctival Spitz nevus: review of literature and comparison with cutaneous locations. Ann Ophthalmol. 21(5):176–9. PMID:2662866
577. Kantelip B, Nores JM, Boccard R, Souedan M, Bacin F (1988). A case of fibrous histiocytoma of the conjunctiva. Presse Med. 17(17):859–61. [French] PMID:2838836
578. Kapatai G, Brundler MA, Jenkinson H, Kearns P, Parulekar M, Peet AC, et al. (2013). Gene expression profiling identifies different sub-types of retinoblastoma. Br J Cancer. 109(2):512–25. PMID:23756868
579. Karacorlu M, Hocaoglu M, Sayman Muslubas I, Ersoz MG, Arf S (2018). Therapeutic outcomes after endoresection of complex retinal capillary hemangioblastoma. Retina. 38(3):569–77. PMID:28196061
580. Karcioglu ZA, Mullaney PB (1997). Diagnosis and management of iris juvenile xanthogranuloma. J Pediatr Ophthalmol Strabismus. 34(1):44–51. PMID:9027680
581. Karesh JW, Goldman EJ, Reck K, Kelman SE, Lee EJ, Schiffer CA (1989). A prospective ophthalmic evaluation of patients with acute myeloid leukemia: correlation of ocular and hematologic findings. J Clin Oncol. 7(10):1528–32. PMID:2778482
582. Karim R, Ghabrial R, Lin B (2009). Transitional cell carcinoma of the nasolacrimal sac. Clin Ophthalmol. 3:587–91. PMID:19898663
583. Karlsson M, Boeryd B, Carstensen J, Frånlund B, Gustafsson B, Kågedal B, et al. (1996). Correlations of Ki-67 and PCNA to DNA ploidy, S-phase fraction and survival in uveal melanoma. Eur J Cancer. 32A(2):357–62. PMID:8664054
584. Karp CL, Moore JK, Rosa RH Jr (2001). Treatment of conjunctival and corneal intraepithelial neoplasia with topical interferon alpha-2b. Ophthalmology. 108(6):1093–8. PMID:11382635
585. Karp LA, Zimmerman LE, Borit A, Spencer W (1974). Primary intraorbital meningiomas. Arch Ophthalmol. 91(1):24–8. PMID:4202807
586. Kass LG, Hornblass A (1989). Sebaceous carcinoma of the ocular adnexa. Surv Ophthalmol. 33(6):477–90. PMID:2658172
587. Katayama K, Asano K, Ohkuma H, Terui K, Sasaki S, Sato T, et al. (2014). Case of pediatric optic pathway oligodendroglioma presenting widespread invasion and dissemination in the cerebrospinal fluid. Brain Tumor Pathol. 31(3):208–14. PMID:23996461
588. Kathil P, Milman T, Finger PT (2011). Characteristics of anterior uveal melanocytomas in 17 cases. Ophthalmology. 118(9):1874–80. PMID:21561663
589. Katircioglu YA, Altiparmak UE, Akmansu H, Ustün H, Zorlu F, Duman S (2003). Squamous cell carcinoma of the lacrimal sac. Orbit. 22(3):151–3. PMID:12868021
590. Kattah JC, Suski ET, Killen JY, Smith FP, Limaye SR (1980). Optic neuritis and systemic lymphoma. Am J Ophthalmol. 89(3):431–6. PMID:6966134
591. Katz SE, Rootman J, Dolman PJ, White VA, Berean KW (1996). Primary ductal adenocarcinoma of the lacrimal gland. Ophthalmology. 103(1):157–62. PMID:8628547
592. Kausar A, Zafar SN, Altaf S, Khan A (2015). Ophthalmic manifestations of linear nevus sebaceous/organoid nevus syndrome. J Coll Physicians Surg Pak. 25(3):220–2. PMID:25772967
593. Keijser S, Missotten GS, De Wolff-Rouendaal D, Verbeke SL, Van Luijk CM, Veselic-Charvat M, et al. (2007). Impression cytology of melanocytic conjunctival tumours using the Biopore membrane. Eur J Ophthalmol. 17(4):501–6. PMID:17671922
594. Kelishadi M, Kelishadi M, Moradi A, Javid N, Bazouri M, Tabarraei A (2015). Human adenoviruses role in ophthalmic pterygium formation. Jundishapur J Microbiol. 8(4):e16871. PMID:26034543
595. Kenawy N, Lake SL, Coupland SE, Damato BE (2013). Conjunctival melanoma and melanocytic intra-epithelial neoplasia. Eye (Lond). 27(2):142–52. PMID:23222568
596. Khafaga Y, Hassounah M, Kandil A, Kanaan I, Allam A, El Husseiny G, et al. (2003). Optic gliomas: a retrospective analysis of 50 cases. Int J Radiat Oncol Biol Phys. 56(3):807–12. PMID:12788189
597. Khalil MK (1983). Balloon cell malignant melanoma of the choroid: ultrastructural studies. Br J Ophthalmol. 67(9):579–84. PMID:6882713
598. Khan AA, Sarwar S, Sadiq MA, Ahmad I, Tariq N, Sibghat-Ul-Noor (2017). Analysis of orbital malignancies presenting in a tertiary care hospital in Pakistan. Pak J Med Sci. 33(1):70–4. PMID:28367175
599. Khong JJ, Hardy TG, McNab AA (2013). Prevalence of oculo-auriculo-vertebral spectrum in dermolipoma. Ophthalmology. 120(8):1529–32. PMID:23683920
600. Kiire CA, Dhillon B (2006). The aetiology and associations of conjunctival intraepithelial neoplasia. Br J Ophthalmol. 90(1):109–13. PMID:16361679
601. Kilcline C, Frieden IJ (2008). Infantile hemangiomas: how common are they? A systematic review of the medical literature. Pediatr Dermatol. 25(2):168–73. PMID:18429772
602. Kim HJ, McCormick SA, Nath S, Moskowitz B, Milman T (2010). Melanocytic nevi of the tarsal conjunctiva: clinicopathologic case series with review of literature. Ophthal Plast Reconstr Surg. 26(6):438–42. PMID:20683369
603. Kim HJ, Shields CL, Eagle RC Jr, Shields JA (2006). Fibrous histiocytoma of the conjunctiva. Am J Ophthalmol. 142(6):1036–43. PMID:17157587
604. Kim IT, Lee SM (2000). Choroidal Langerhans' cell histiocytosis. Acta Ophthalmol Scand. 78(1):97–100. PMID:10726800
605. Kim JE, Kim BJ, Kang H (2014). A recurrent angiosarcoma isolated to the eyelid without the recurrence on the primary lesion of the forehead. Ann Dermatol. 26(2):231–5. PMID:24882979
606. Kim JL, Mendoza PR, Rashid A, Hayek B, Grossniklaus HE (2015). Optic nerve lymphoma: report of two cases and review of the literature. Surv Ophthalmol. 60(2):153–65. PMID:25595061
607. Kim MM, Dabaja BS, Medeiros J, Kim S, Allen P, Chevez-Barrios P, et al. (2016). Survival outcomes of primary intraocular lymphoma: a single-institution experience. Am J Clin Oncol. 39(2):109–13. PMID:24390272
608. Kim MS, Kim SA, Sa HS (2014). Old-age-onset subconjunctival juvenile xanthogranuloma without limbal involvement. BMC Ophthalmol. 14:24. PMID:24602225
609. Kim YD, Goldberg RA (1994). Orbital fat prolapse and dermolipoma: two distinct entities. Korean J Ophthalmol. 8(1):42–3. PMID:7933633
610. Kincaid MC, Green WR (1983). Ocular and orbital involvement in leukemia. Surv Ophthalmol. 27(4):211–32. PMID:6342189
611. Kincaid MC, Meis JM, Lee MW (1989). Adenoid cystic carcinoma of the lacrimal sac. Ophthalmology. 96(11):1655–8. PMID:2559385
612. Kiratli H, Shields CL, Shields JA, DePotter P (1996). Metastatic tumours to the conjunctiva: report of 10 cases. Br J Ophthalmol. 80(1):5–8. PMID:8664233
613. Kiratli H, Uzun S, Tarlan B, Ateş D, Baydar DE, Söylemezoğlu F (2015). Renal carcinoid

tumor metastatic to the uvea, medial rectus muscle, and the contralateral lacrimal gland. Ophthal Plast Reconstr Surg. 31(4):e91–3. PMID:24777267

614. Kirkegaard MM, Coupland SE, Prause JU, Heegaard S (2015). Malignant lymphoma of the conjunctiva. Surv Ophthalmol. 60(5):444–58. PMID:26003619

615. Kirmani MH, Thomas EL, Rao NA, Laborde RP (1987). Intraocular reticulum cell sarcoma: diagnosis by choroidal biopsy. Br J Ophthalmol. 71(10):748–52. PMID:3314978

616. Kitamura Y, Akiyama T, Hirose S, Yoshida K (2012). Optic nerve sheath solitary fibrous tumor. Acta Neurochir (Wien). 154(4):633–5. PMID:22215145

617. Kitamura Y, Akiyama T, Sasaki H, Hayashi Y, Yoshida K (2013). Optic nerve seeding of atypical meningiomas presenting with subacute visual loss: 2 case reports with genetic characterization. J Neurosurg. 119(2):494–8. PMID:23432529

618. Kivelä T (2014). Incidence, prevalence and epidemiology of ocular melanoma. In: Murray TG, Boldt HC, editors. Ocular melanoma: advances in diagnostic and therapeutic strategies. London: Future Medicine; pp. 20–38.

619. Kivelä T, Simpson ER, Grossniklaus HE, Jager MJ, Singh AD, Caminal JM, et al. (2017). Uveal melanoma. In: Amin MB, Edge S, Greene F, Byrd DR, Brookland RK, Washington MK, et al., editors. AJCC cancer staging manual. 8th ed. New York: Springer; pp. 805–17.

620. Kivelä T (2009). The epidemiological challenge of the most frequent eye cancer: retinoblastoma, an issue of birth and death. Br J Ophthalmol. 93(9):1129–31. PMID:19704035

621. Kivelä T, Eskelin S (2006). Transformation of nevus to melanoma. Ophthalmology. 113(5):887–8.e1. PMID:16650691

622. Kivelä T, Kauniskangas L, Miettinen P, Tarkkanen A (1989). Glioneuroma associated with colobomatous dysplasia of the anterior uvea and retina. A case simulating medulloepithelioma. Ophthalmology. 96(12):1799–808. PMID:2622623

623. Kivelä T, Summanen P (1997). Retinoinvasive malignant melanoma of the uvea. Br J Ophthalmol. 81(8):691–7. PMID:9349160

624. Kivelä T, Tarkkanen A, Virtanen I (1989). Synaptophysin in the human retina and retinoblastoma. An immunohistochemical and western blotting study. Invest Ophthalmol Vis Sci. 30(2):212–9. PMID:2464554

625. Kivelä TT, Piperno-Neumann S, Desjardins L, Schmittel A, Bechrakis N, Midena E, et al. (2016). Validation of a prognostic staging for metastatic uveal melanoma: a collaborative study of the European Ophthalmic Oncology Group. Am J Ophthalmol. 168:217–26. PMID:27296487

626. Klein A, Barak A, Habot-Wilner Z, Goldenberg D, Neudorfer M (2011). The appearance of congenital hypertrophy of retinal pigment epithelium by high-resolution optical coherence tomography. Retina. 31(8):1740–1. PMID:21817965

627. Klein KA, Lally DR, Taney LS, Laver NV, Duker JS (2015). Retinal pigment epithelial adenocarcinoma presenting as an amelanotic mass. Ophthalmic Surg Lasers Imaging Retina. 46(3):369–72. PMID:26180844

628. Kline LB, Garcia JH, Harsh GR 3rd (1984). Lymphomatous optic neuropathy. Arch Ophthalmol. 102(11):1655–7. PMID:6497749

629. Klingele TG, Hogan MJ (1975). Ocular reticulum cell sarcoma. Am J Ophthalmol. 79(1):39–47. PMID:1089097

630. Klufas MA, McCannel CA, McCannel TA (2016). Simultaneous retinal and choroidal metastases in lung adenocarcinoma. JAMA Ophthalmol. 134(5):e155368. PMID:27258608

631. Klüppel M, Müller W, Sundmacher R (1999). Lacrimal gland choristoma of the iris. Arch Ophthalmol. 117(1):110–1. PMID:9930171

632. Knackstedt T, Samie FH (2017). Sebaceous carcinoma: a review of the scientific literature. Curr Treat Options Oncol. 18(8):47. PMID:28681210

633. Knapp AN, Samara WA, Shields CL, Shields JA, Eagle RC Jr (2016). Conjunctival fibrous histiocytoma in an 8-year-old boy. J AAPOS. 20(4):368–70. PMID:27282913

634. Knežević M, Stojković M, Jovanović M, Stanković Z, Rašić DM (2012). A 7-year prospective study of routine histopathological evaluation of the lacrimal sac wall incisional biopsy specimens obtained during external dacryocystorhinostomy in adults and a review of the literature. Med Oncol. 29(1):396–400. PMID:21264538

635. Kniggendorf VF, Neto ET, Maia EM, Grando JPS, Bardal AMC, Beato PMM, et al. (2016). Bilateral diffuse uveal melanocytic proliferation associated with renal cancer: the importance of indocyanine green angiography and early diagnosis. Retin Cases Brief Rep. 12(3):166–71. PMID:27861254

636. Kobrin EG, Shields CL, Danzig CJ, Ehya H, King RA, Shields JA (2007). Intraocular lacrimal gland choristoma diagnosed by fine-needle aspiration biopsy. Cornea. 26(6):753–5. PMID:17592332

637. Koch KR, Ortmann M, Heindl LM (2015). Extraocular extension of a benign ciliary body nevus. JAMA Ophthalmol. 133(12):e153137. PMID:26659447

638. Kodjikian L, Gain P, Donate D, Gambrelle J, Rouberol F, de la Fouchardiere A, et al. (2004). Cataract formation with a primary iris stromal cyst. J Pediatr Ophthalmol Strabismus. 41(4):232–5. PMID:15305534

639. Kohn R, Nofsinger K, Freedman SI (1981). Rapid recurrence of papillary squamous cell carcinoma of the canaliculus. Am J Ophthalmol. 92(3):363–7. PMID:7294095

640. Koletsa T, Karayannopoulou G, Dereklis D, Vasileiadis I, Papadimitriou CS, Hytiroglou P (2009). Mesectodermal leiomyoma of the ciliary body: report of a case and review of the literature. Pathol Res Pract. 205(2):125–30. PMID:18930601

641. Konstantinidis L, Damato B (2017). Intraocular metastases–a review. Asia Pac J Ophthalmol (Phila). 6(2):208–14. PMID:28399345

642. Konstantinidis L, Rospond-Kubiak I, Zeolite I, Heimann H, Groenewald C, Coupland SE, et al. (2014). Management of patients with uveal metastases at the Liverpool Ocular Oncology Centre. Br J Ophthalmol. 98(1):92–8. PMID:24169654

643. Kontos G, Borooah S, Khan A, Fleck BW, Coupland SE (2016). The epidemiology, clinical characteristics, histopathology and management of juvenile- and adult-onset corneoscleral limbus xanthogranuloma. Graefes Arch Clin Exp Ophthalmol. 254(3):413–20. PMID:26794218

644. Kontos GT, Coupland SE, Quah SA (2014). A case of a limbal adult onset xanthogranuloma. Acta Ophthalmol. 92(8):e692–3. PMID:24930575

645. Kooi IE, Mol BM, Moll AC, van der Valk P, de Jong MC, de Graaf P, et al. (2015). Loss of photoreceptorness and gain of genomic alterations in retinoblastoma reveal tumor progression. EBioMedicine. 2(7):660–70. PMID:26288838

646. Koopmans AE, Ober K, Dubbink HJ, Paridaens D, Naus NC, Belunek S, et al. (2014). Prevalence and implications of TERT promoter mutation in uveal and conjunctival melanoma and in benign and premalignant conjunctival melanocytic lesions. Invest Ophthalmol Vis Sci. 55(9):6024–30. PMID:25159205

647. Koopmans AE, Verdijk RM, Brouwer RW, van den Bosch TP, van den Berg MM, Vaarwater J, et al. (2014). Clinical significance of immunohistochemistry for detection of BAP1 mutations in uveal melanoma. Mod Pathol. 27(10):1321–30. PMID:24633195

648. Korshunov A, Jakobiec FA, Eberhart CG, Hovestadt V, Capper D, Jones DT, et al. (2015). Comparative integrated molecular analysis of intraocular medulloepitheliomas and central nervous system embryonal tumors with multilayered rosettes confirms that they are distinct nosologic entities. Neuropathology. 35(6):538–44. PMID:26183384

649. Koturović Z, Knežević M, Rašić DM (2017). Clinical significance of routine lacrimal sac biopsy during dacryocystorhinostomy: a comprehensive review of literature. Bosn J Basic Med Sci. 17(1):1–8. PMID:27754826

650. Kraemer KH, Lee MM, Scotto J (1987). Xeroderma pigmentosum. Cutaneous, ocular, and neurologic abnormalities in 830 published cases. Arch Dermatol. 123(2):241–50. PMID:3545087

651. Kramer GD, Arepalli S, Shields CL, Shields JA (2014). Ciliary body medulloepithelioma association with pleuropulmonary blastoma in a familial tumor predisposition syndrome. J Pediatr Ophthalmol Strabismus. 51 Online:e48–50. PMID:25032694

652. Kraus MD, Haley JC, Ruiz R, Essary L, Moran CA, Fletcher CD (2001). "Juvenile" xanthogranuloma: an immunophenotypic study with a reappraisal of histogenesis. Am J Dermatopathol. 23(2):104–11. PMID:11285404

653. Krema H, Simpson ER, Pavlin CJ, Payne D, Vasquez LM, McGowan H (2009). Management of ciliary body melanoma with iodine-125 plaque brachytherapy. Can J Ophthalmol. 44(4):395–400. PMID:19606159

654. Krishna M (2010). Diagnosis of metastatic neoplasms: an immunohistochemical approach. Arch Pathol Lab Med. 134(2):207–15. PMID:20121608

655. Krishna Y, Coupland SE (2017). Lacrimal sac tumors–a review. Asia Pac J Ophthalmol (Phila). 6(2):173–8. PMID:28399337

656. Krishna Y, Irion LD, Karim S, Dharmsena A, McCormick A, Coupland SE (2017). Chronic lymphocytic leukaemia/small-cell lymphocytic lymphoma of the lacrimal sac: a case series. Ocul Oncol Pathol. 3(3):224–8. PMID:29071273

657. Krishna Y, Kalirai H, Thornton S, Damato BE, Heimann H, Coupland SE (2016). Genetic findings in treatment-naïve and proton-beam-radiated iris melanomas. Br J Ophthalmol. 100(7):1012–6. PMID:27098748

658. Krohn J, Frøystein T, Dahl O (2009). Topography of solitary congenital hypertrophy of the retinal pigment epithelium in the ocular fundus. Acta Ophthalmol. 87(8):921–2. PMID:19604161

659. Krohn J, Kjersem B (2011). Stereo fundus photography in the diagnosis of optic disc melanocytoma. Acta Ophthalmol. 89(6):e533–4. PMID:21106045

660. Kubota T, Moritani S (2007). High incidence of autoimmune disease in Japanese patients with ocular adnexal reactive lymphoid hyperplasia. Am J Ophthalmol. 144(1):148–9. PMID:17601445

661. Kubota T, Moritani S, Ichihara S (2013). Clinicopathologic and immunohistochemical features of primary ductal adenocarcinoma of lacrimal gland: five new cases and review of literature. Graefes Arch Clin Exp Ophthalmol. 251(8):2071–6. PMID:23613093

662. Küchle M, Holbach L, Schlötzer-Schrehardt U, Naumann GO (1994). Schwannoma of the ciliary body treated by block excision. Br J Ophthalmol. 78(5):397–400. PMID:8025076

663. Kujala E, Damato B, Coupland SE, Desjardins L, Bechrakis NE, Grange JD, et al. (2013). Staging of ciliary body and choroidal melanomas based on anatomic extent. J Clin Oncol. 31(22):2825–31. PMID:23816968

664. Kujala E, Mäkitie T, Kivelä T (2003). Very long-term prognosis of patients with malignant uveal melanoma. Invest Ophthalmol Vis Sci. 44(11):4651–9. PMID:14578381

665. Kumar A, Kumar Dorairaj S, Prabhakaran VC, Prakash DR, Chakraborty S (2007). Identification of genes associated with tumorigenesis of meibomian cell carcinoma by microarray analysis. Genomics. 90(5):559–66. PMID:17889501

666. Kuo PK, Puliafito CA, Wang KM, Liu HS, Wu BF (1982). Uveal melanoma in China. Int Ophthalmol Clin. 22(3):57–71. PMID:7107133

667. Kupersmith MJ, Martin V, Heller G, Shah A, Mitnick HJ (2004). Idiopathic hypertrophic pachymeningitis. Neurology. 62(5):686–94. PMID:15007115

668. Kurisu Y, Shibayama Y, Tsuji M, Kurokawa A, Akutagawa H, Egashira Y, et al. (2005). A case of primary ductal adenocarcinoma of the lacrimal gland: histopathological and immunohistochemical study. Pathol Res Pract. 201(1):49–53. PMID:15807311

669. Kurli M, Finger PT (2005). Melanocytic conjunctival tumors. Ophthalmol Clin North Am. 18(1):15–24,vii. PMID:15763188

670. Kurli M, Finger PT, Manor T, McCormick SA, Grossniklaus HE (2005). Finding malignant change in a necrotic choroidal melanocytoma: a clinical challenge. Br J Ophthalmol. 89(7):921–2. PMID:15965181

671. Kurosawa A, Kurosawa H (1982). Ovoid bodies in choroidal neurofibromatosis. Arch Ophthalmol. 100(12):1939–41. PMID:6816197

672. Kusunose M, Sakino Y, Noda Y, Daa T, Kubota T (2017). A case of iris melanocytoma demonstrating diffuse melanocytic proliferation with uncontrolled intraocular pressure. Case Rep Ophthalmol. 8(1):190–4. PMID:28512420

673. Kwiek B, Schwartz RA (2016). Keratoacanthoma (KA): an update and review. J Am Acad Dermatol. 74(6):1220–33. PMID:26853179

674. Lach B, Al Shail E, Patay Z (2003). Spontaneous anaplasia in pilocytic astrocytoma of cerebellum. Br J Neurosurg. 17(3):250–2. PMID:14565523

675. Lahav M, Albert DM, Wyand S (1973). Clinical and histopathologic classification of retinal dysplasia. Am J Ophthalmol. 75(4):648–67. PMID:4696669

676. Laird PW, Grossniklaus HE, Hubbard GB (2013). Ciliary body medulloepithelioma associated with pleuropulmonary blastoma. Br J Ophthalmol. 97(8):1079,1086–7. PMID:23613510

677. Lake SL, Jmor F, Dopierala J, Taktak AF, Coupland SE, Damato BE (2011). Multiplex ligation-dependent probe amplification of conjunctival melanoma reveals common BRAF V600E gene mutation and gene copy number changes. Invest Ophthalmol Vis Sci. 52(8):5598–604. PMID:21693616

678. Lally DR, Eagle RC, Wasserman BN (2013). Occult intraorbital conjunctival inclusion cyst discovered almost 70 years after strabismus surgery. J Pediatr Ophthalmol Strabismus. 50 Online:e15–7. PMID:23557018

679. Lambade PN, Lambade D, Saha TK, Bande CR, Ramakrishana A (2015). Malignant fibrous histiocytoma: an uncommon sarcoma with pathological fracture of mandible. J Maxillofac Oral Surg. 14(Suppl 1):283–7. PMID:25838711

680. Lang FF, Miller DC, Pisharody S, Koslow M, Newcomb EW (1994). High frequency of p53 protein accumulation without p53 gene mutation in human juvenile pilocytic, low grade and

anaplastic astrocytomas. Oncogene. 9(3):949–54. PMID:8108140
681. Lang TU, Williams JM, Laver NV (2010). Corneal myxoma. Ophthalmic Surg Lasers Imaging. 9:1–2. PMID:20337333
682. Larsen AC (2016). Conjunctival malignant melanoma in Denmark: epidemiology, treatment and prognosis with special emphasis on tumorigenesis and genetic profile. Acta Ophthalmol. 94 Thesis 1:1–27. PMID:27192168
683. Larsen AC, Dahl C, Dahmcke CM, Lade-Keller J, Siersma VD, Toft PB, et al. (2016). BRAF mutations in conjunctival melanoma: investigation of incidence, clinicopathological features, prognosis and paired premalignant lesions. Acta Ophthalmol. 94(5):463–70. PMID:27009410
684. Larsen AC, Dahmcke CM, Dahl C, Siersma VD, Toft PB, Coupland SE, et al. (2015). A retrospective review of conjunctival melanoma presentation, treatment, and outcome and an investigation of features associated with BRAF mutations. JAMA Ophthalmol. 133(11):1295–303. PMID:26425792
685. Lattier JM, Yang H, Crawford S, Grossniklaus HE (2013). Host pigment epithelium-derived factor (PEDF) prevents progression of liver metastasis in a mouse model of uveal melanoma. Clin Exp Metastasis. 30(8):969–76. PMID:23793989
686. Lau LL, Lung CK, Ahmad SS (2015). A benign presentation of primary ductal adenocarcinoma of lacrimal gland: a rare malignancy. Indian J Ophthalmol. 63(11):856–8. PMID:26669339
687. Laver NM, Hidayat AA, Croxatto JO (1999). Pleomorphic adenocarcinomas of the ciliary epithelium. Immunohistochemical and ultrastructural features of 12 cases. Ophthalmology. 106(1):103–10. PMID:9917789
688. Lee AG, Tang RA, Roberts D, Schiffman JS, Osborne A (2001). Primary central nervous system lymphoma involving the optic chiasm in AIDS. J Neuroophthalmol. 21(2):95–8. PMID:11450910
689. Lee CS, Bae JH, Jeon IH, Byeon SH, Koh HJ, Lee SC (2010). Melanocytoma of the optic disk in the Korean population. Retina. 30(10):1714–20. PMID:20829742
690. Lee GA, Hirst LW (1992). Incidence of ocular surface epithelial dysplasia in metropolitan Brisbane. A 10-year survey. Arch Ophthalmol. 110(4):525–7. PMID:1562262
691. Lee GA, Hirst LW (1995). Ocular surface squamous neoplasia. Surv Ophthalmol. 39(6):429–50. PMID:7660300
692. Lee HB, Pulido JS, Buettner H, Salomão D, Zent CS, Link TP (2006). Intravascular B-cell lymphoma (angiotropic lymphoma) with choroidal involvement. Arch Ophthalmol. 124(9):1357–9. PMID:16966639
693. Lee LC, Howes EL, Bhisitkul RB (2002). Systemic non-Hodgkin's lymphoma with optic nerve infiltration in a patient with AIDS. Retina. 22(1):75–9. PMID:11884882
694. Lee SW, Park SH, Kim IH, Chung H, Kim TY, Heo DS (2007). Nonsurgical treatment of an incompletely excised primary adenocarcinoma of nonpigmented ciliary epithelium. Tumori. 93(5):514–7. PMID:18038890
695. Lee V, Cree IA, Hungerford JL (1999). Ring melanoma–a rare cause of refractory glaucoma. Br J Ophthalmol. 83(2):194–8. PMID:10396198
696. Lee YJ, Oh YH (2009). Primary ductal adenocarcinoma of the lacrimal gland. Jpn J Ophthalmol. 53(3):268–70. PMID:19484447
697. Lehman LJ, Hohberger GG, Buettner H, Campbell RJ (1997). Necrotic melanocytoma of the choroid in a 2-year-old child. J Pediatr Ophthalmol Strabismus. 34(1):40–3. PMID:9027679
698. Leidenix M, Mamalis N, Goodart R, Harrie R, Kjeldsberg C (1994). Malignant transformation of a necrotic melanocytoma of the choroid in an amblyopic eye. Ann Ophthalmol. 26(2):42–6. PMID:8010703
699. Leonardi A, Castegnaro A, Valerio AL, Lazzarini D (2015). Epidemiology of allergic conjunctivitis: clinical appearance and treatment patterns in a population-based study. Curr Opin Allergy Clin Immunol. 15(5):482–8. PMID:26258920
700. Leonardi A, Piliego F, Castegnaro A, Lazzarini D, La Gloria Valerio A, Mattana P, et al. (2015). Allergic conjunctivitis: a cross-sectional study. Clin Exp Allergy. 45(6):1118–25. PMID:25809830
701. Leonardy NJ, Rupani M, Dent G, Klintworth GK (1990). Analysis of 135 autopsy eyes for ocular involvement in leukemia. Am J Ophthalmol. 109(4):436–44. PMID:2330946
702. Levasseur SD, Wittenberg LA, White VA (2013). Vitreoretinal lymphoma: a 20-year review of incidence, clinical and cytologic features, treatment, and outcomes. JAMA Ophthalmol. 131(1):50–5. PMID:23307208
703. Levi-Schaffer F, Micera A, Zamir E, Mechoulam H, Puxeddu I, Piliponsky AM, et al. (2002). Nerve growth factor and eosinophils in inflamed juvenile conjunctival nevus. Invest Ophthalmol Vis Sci. 43(6):1850–6. PMID:12036989
704. Lewis RA, Cohen MH, Wise GN (1975). Cavernous haemangioma of the retina and optic disc. A report of three cases and a review of the literature. Br J Ophthalmol. 59(8):422–34. PMID:1106760
705. Li J, Perry A, James CD, Gutmann DH (2001). Cancer-related gene expression profiles in NF1-associated pilocytic astrocytomas. Neurology. 56(7):885–90. PMID:11294925
706. Li W, Gragoudas ES, Egan KM (2000). Metastatic melanoma death rates by anatomic site after proton beam irradiation for uveal melanoma. Arch Ophthalmol. 118(8):1066–70. PMID:10922199
707. Li X, Huang Y, Bi C, Yuan J, He H, Zhang H, et al. (2017). Primary central nervous system diffuse large B-cell lymphoma shows an activated B-cell-like phenotype with co-expression of C-MYC, BCL-2, and BCL-6. Pathol Res Pract. 213(6):659–65. PMID:28552541
708. Lieb WE, Shields JA, Eagle RC Jr, Kwa D, Shields CL (1990). Cystic adenoma of the pigmented ciliary epithelium. Clinical, pathologic, and immunohistopathologic findings. Ophthalmology. 97(11):1489–93. PMID:1701528
709. Lim LL, Suhler EB, Rosenbaum JT, Wilson DJ (2005). The role of choroidal and retinal biopsies in the diagnosis and management of atypical presentations of uveitis. Trans Am Ophthalmol Soc. 103:84–92. PMID:17057791
710. Lin HC, Chu PH, Jung SM, Yang ML, Ma DH (2012). MUC5AC in juvenile conjunctival nevus. Jpn J Ophthalmol. 56(2):107–12. PMID:22139382
711. Lin TC, Lin PY, Wang LC, Chen SJ, Chang YM, Lee SM (2014). Intraocular involvement of T-cell lymphoma presenting as inflammatory glaucoma, neurotrophic keratopathy, and choroidal detachment. J Chin Med Assoc. 77(7):385–8. PMID:24909374
712. Lincoff NS, Chung C, Balos L, Corbo JC, Sharma A (2012). Combing the globe for terrorism. J Neuroophthalmol. 32(1):82–5. PMID:22330854
713. Lindegaard J, Heegaard S, Toft PB, Nysom K, Prause JU (2010). Malignant transformation of a medulloepithelioma of the optic nerve. Orbit. 29(3):161–4. PMID:20497085
714. Lindegaard J, Isager P, Prause JU, Heegaard S (2006). Optic nerve invasion of uveal melanoma: clinical characteristics and metastatic pattern. Invest Ophthalmol Vis Sci. 47(8):3268–75. PMID:16877391
715. Lindegaard J, Isager P, Prause JU, Heegaard S (2007). Optic nerve invasion of uveal melanoma. APMIS. 115(1):1–16. PMID:17223846
716. Listernick R, Charrow J, Greenwald M, Mets M (1994). Natural history of optic pathway tumors in children with neurofibromatosis type 1: a longitudinal study. J Pediatr. 125(1):63–6. PMID:8021787
717. Listernick R, Charrow J, Gutmann DH (1999). Intracranial gliomas in neurofibromatosis type 1. Am J Med Genet. 89(1):38–44. PMID:10469435
718. Listernick R, Darling C, Greenwald M, Strauss L, Charrow J (1995). Optic pathway tumors in children: the effect of neurofibromatosis type 1 on clinical manifestations and natural history. J Pediatr. 127(5):718–22. PMID:7472822
719. Listernick R, Louis DN, Packer RJ, Gutmann DH (1997). Optic pathway gliomas in children with neurofibromatosis 1: consensus statement from the NF1 Optic Pathway Glioma Task Force. Ann Neurol. 41(2):143–9. PMID:9029062
720. Liu L, Wu J, Geng J, Yuan Z, Huang D (2013). Geographical prevalence and risk factors for pterygium: a systematic review and meta-analysis. BMJ Open. 3(11):e003787. PMID:24253031
721. Liu TYA, Ediriwickrema LS, Vizcaino MA, Wenick A, Miller NR (2017). Optic nerve infiltration and vitreous seeding by a cerebral glioblastoma. JAMA Ophthalmol. 135(4):400–1. PMID:28208187
722. Liu Y, Su M, Yang Y, Zhao B, Qin L, Han Z (2017). Prognostic factors associated with decreased survival in patients with acinic cell carcinoma of the parotid gland. J Oral Maxillofac Surg. 75(2):416–22. PMID:27474461
723. Liy-Wong C, Mohammed J, Carleton A, Pope E, Parkin P, Lara-Corrales I (2017). The relationship between neurofibromatosis type 1, juvenile xanthogranuloma, and malignancy: a retrospective case-control study. J Am Acad Dermatol. 76(6):1084–7. PMID:28189268
724. Lloyd WC 3rd, Eagle RC Jr, Shields JA, Kwa DM, Arbizo VV (1990). Congenital hypertrophy of the retinal pigment epithelium. Electron microscopic and morphometric observations. Ophthalmology. 97(8):1052–60. PMID:2402417
725. Loeffler KU, Kivelä T, Borgmann H, Witschel H (1996). Malignant tumor of the retinal pigment epithelium with extraocular extension in a phthisical eye. Graefes Arch Clin Exp Ophthalmol. 234 Suppl 1:S70–5. PMID:8871153
726. Loeffler KU, McMenamin PG (1987). An ultrastructural study of DNA precipitation in the anterior segment of eyes with retinoblastoma. Ophthalmology. 94(9):1160–8. PMID:3684233
727. Lois N, Shields CL, Shields JA, Eagle RC Jr, De Potter P (1998). Cavitary melanoma of the ciliary body. A study of eight cases. Ophthalmology. 105(6):1091–8. PMID:9627662
728. Lois N, Shields CL, Shields JA, Mercado G (1998). Primary cysts of the iris pigment epithelium. Clinical features and natural course in 234 patients. Ophthalmology. 105(10):1879–85. PMID:9787358
729. Lois N, Shields CL, Shields JA, Mercado G, De Potter P (1998). Primary iris stromal cysts. A report of 17 cases. Ophthalmology. 105(7):1317–22. PMID:9663240
730. LoRusso FJ, Boniuk M, Font RL (2000). Melanocytoma (magnocellular nevus) of the ciliary body: report of 10 cases and review of the literature. Ophthalmology. 107(4):795–800. PMID:10768345
731. Loukianou E, Kisma N, Pal B (2011). Evolution of an astrocytic hamartoma of the optic nerve head in a patient with retinitis pigmentosa - photographic documentation over 2 years of follow-up. Case Rep Ophthalmol. 2(1):45–9. PMID:21347192
732. Low JR, Bian Ng S, Sundar G (2011). Undifferentiated carcinoma of the lacrimal sac: case report and review of literature. Orbit. 30(6):293–6. PMID:21957907
733. Lu WY, Goldman M, Young B, Davis DG (1993). Optic nerve ganglioglioma. Case report. J Neurosurg. 78(6):979–82. PMID:8487083
734. Lubahn JG, Lee RK, Karp CL (2014). Resolution of conjunctival sessile hemangioma with topical timolol. Cornea. 33(1):99–100. PMID:24270678
735. Luthra CL, Doxanas MT, Green WR (1978). Lesions of the caruncle: a clinicohistopathologic study. Surv Ophthalmol. 23(3):183–95. PMID:216128
736. Lynch TM, Gutmann DH (2002). Neurofibromatosis 1. Neurol Clin. 20(3):841–65. PMID:12432832
737. MacCumber MW, Hoffman PN, Wand GS, Epstein JI, Beschorner WE, Green WR (1990). Ophthalmic involvement in aggressive histiocytosis X. Ophthalmology. 97(1):22–7. PMID:2179796
738. Madreperla SA, Green WR, Daniel R, Shah KV (1993). Human papillomavirus in primary epithelial tumors of the lacrimal sac. Ophthalmology. 100(4):569–73. PMID:8386822
739. Maegawa J, Yasumura K, Iwai T, Hata M, Inayama Y, Kobayashi S (2014). Malignant melanoma of the lacrimal sac: a case report. Int J Dermatol. 53(2):243–5. PMID:24261959
740. Mäkitie T, Summanen P, Tarkkanen A, Kivelä T (1999). Microvascular density in predicting survival of patients with choroidal and ciliary body melanoma. Invest Ophthalmol Vis Sci. 40(11):2471–80. PMID:10509639
741. Mäkitie T, Summanen P, Tarkkanen A, Kivelä T (1999). Microvascular loops and networks as prognostic indicators in choroidal and ciliary body melanomas. J Natl Cancer Inst. 91(4):359–67. PMID:10050870
742. Mäkitie T, Summanen P, Tarkkanen A, Kivelä T (2001). Tumor-infiltrating macrophages (CD68(+) cells) and prognosis in malignant uveal melanoma. Invest Ophthalmol Vis Sci. 42(7):1414–21. PMID:11381040
743. Mallen-St Clair J, Arshi A, Tajudeen B, Abemayor E, St John M (2014). Epidemiology and treatment of lacrimal gland tumors: a population-based cohort analysis. JAMA Otolaryngol Head Neck Surg. 140(12):1110–6. PMID:25393577
744. Maly A, Epstein D, Meir K, Pe'er J (2008). Histological criteria for grading of atypia in melanocytic conjunctival lesions. Pathology. 40(7):676–81. PMID:18985522
745. Mamaï O, Boussofara L, Denguezli M, Escande-Beillard N, Kraiem W, Merriman B, et al. (2015). Multiple self-healing palmoplantar carcinoma: a familial predisposition to skin cancer with primary palmoplantar and conjunctival lesions. J Invest Dermatol. 135(1):304–8. PMID:25050600
746. Mandelcorn E, McGuire K, Dixon W, Mandelcorn M (2009). Ocular paraneoplastic syndrome: a case of bilateral diffuse uveal melanocytic proliferation. Retina. 29(9):1375–6. PMID:19934829
747. Manjandavida FP, Arepalli S, Tarlan B, Shields CL (2014). Optical coherence tomography characteristics of epi-iridic membrane in a child with recurrent hyphema and presumed juvenile xanthogranuloma. J AAPOS. 18(1):93–5. PMID:24568997
748. Manjandavida FP, Honavar SG, Gowrishankar S, Mulay K, Reddy VA, Vemuganti GK

(2013). Optic nerve meningeal hemangiopericytoma: a clinicopathologic case report. Surv Ophthalmol. 58(4):341–7. PMID:23294915
749. Mansour AM, Barber JC, Reinecke RD, Wang FM (1989). Ocular choristomas. Surv Ophthalmol. 33(5):339–58. PMID:2655139
750. Manz HJ, Rosen DA, Macklin RD, Willis WE (1973). Neuroectodermal tumor of anterior lip of the optic cup. Glioneuroma transitional to teratoid medullo-epithelioma. Arch Ophthalmol. 89(5):382–6. PMID:4697214
751. Marchuk DA (2001). Pathogenesis of hemangioma. J Clin Invest. 107(6):665–6. PMID:11254664
752. Margo C, Hidayat A, Kopelman J, Zimmerman LE (1983). Retinocytoma. A benign variant of retinoblastoma. Arch Ophthalmol. 101(10):1519–31. PMID:6626001
753. Margo CE, Bombardier T (1985). The diagnostic value of fungal autofluorescence. Surv Ophthalmol. 29(5):374–6. PMID:3992475
754. Margo CE, Brooks HL Jr (1991). Adenocarcinoma of the ciliary epithelium in a 12-year-old black child. J Pediatr Ophthalmol Strabismus. 28(4):232–5. PMID:1919972
755. Margo CE, Groden LR (1989). Intraepithelial neoplasia of the conjunctiva with mucoepidermoid differentiation. Am J Ophthalmol. 108(5):600–1. PMID:2817062
756. Margo CE, Grossniklaus HE (1995). Intraepithelial sebaceous neoplasia without underlying invasive carcinoma. Surv Ophthalmol. 39(4):293–301. PMID:7725228
757. Margo CE, Grossniklaus HE (2001). Pseudoadenomatous hyperplasia of the conjunctiva. Ophthalmology. 108(1):135–8. PMID:11150278
758. Margo CE, Lessner A, Stern GA (1992). Intraepithelial sebaceous carcinoma of the conjunctiva and skin of the eyelid. Ophthalmology. 99(2):227–31. PMID:1553212
759. Margo CE, Lowery RL, Kerschmann RL (1997). Lack of p53 protein immunoreactivity in bilateral diffuse uveal melanocytic proliferation. Retina. 17(5):434–6. PMID:9355192
760. Margo CE, Mulla Z, Billiris K (1998). Incidence of surgically treated uveal melanoma by race and ethnicity. Ophthalmology. 105(6):1087–90. PMID:9627661
761. Martin M, Maßhöfer L, Temming P, Rahmann S, Metz C, Bornfeld N, et al. (2013). Exome sequencing identifies recurrent somatic mutations in EIF1AX and SF3B1 in uveal melanoma with disomy 3. Nat Genet. 45(8):933–6. PMID:23793026
762. Marunaka H, Orita Y, Tachibana T, Miki K, Makino T, Yoshino T, et al. (2018). Diffuse large B-cell lymphoma of the lacrimal sac arising from a patient with IgG4-related disease. Mod Rheumatol. 28(3):559–63. PMID:26708772
763. Mashayekhi A, Kaliki S, Walker B, Park C, Sinha N, Kremer FZ, et al. (2013). Metastasis from uveal melanoma associated with congenital ocular melanocytosis: a matched study. Ophthalmology. 120(7):1465–8. PMID:23522968
764. Mashayekhi A, Shields CL (2003). Circumscribed choroidal hemangioma. Curr Opin Ophthalmol. 14(3):142–9. PMID:12777933
765. Mashayekhi A, Shukla SY, Shields JA, Shields CL (2014). Choroidal lymphoma: clinical features and association with systemic lymphoma. Ophthalmology. 121(1):342–51. PMID:23978622
766. Mashayekhi A, Siu S, Shields CL, Shields JA (2011). Slow enlargement of choroidal nevi: a long-term follow-up study. Ophthalmology. 118(2):382–8. PMID:20801518
767. Mastorakos P, Hays MA, Caruso JP, Chen CJ, Ding D, Taylor DG, et al. (2018). Transtentorial dissemination of optic nerve glioblastoma: case report. J Neurosurg. 128(2):406–13. PMID:28298017
768. Mastropasqua R, Thaung C, Pavesio C, Lightman S, Westcott M, Okhravi N, et al. (2015). The role of chorioretinal biopsy in the diagnosis of intraocular lymphoma. Am J Ophthalmol. 160(6):1127–32.e1. PMID:26344582
769. Matatall KA, Agapova OA, Onken MD, Worley LA, Bowcock AM, Harbour JW (2013). BAP1 deficiency causes loss of melanocytic cell identity in uveal melanoma. BMC Cancer. 13:371. PMID:23915344
770. Mathai A, Lall A, Jain R, Pathengay A (2006). Systemic non-Hodgkin's lymphoma masquerading as Vogt-Koyanagi-Harada disease in an HIV-positive patient. Clin Experiment Ophthalmol. 34(3):280–2. PMID:16671912
771. Matilainen S, Isohanni P, Euro L, Lönnqvist T, Pihko H, Kivelä T, et al. (2017). Mitochondrial encephalomyopathy and retinoblastoma explained by compound heterozygosity of SUCLA2 point mutation and 13q14 deletion. Eur J Hum Genet. 25(3):0–393. PMID:28179631
772. Matsuyama A, Hisaoka M, Nagao Y, Hashimoto H (2011). Aberrant PLAG1 expression in pleomorphic adenomas of the salivary gland: a molecular genetic and immunohistochemical study. Virchows Arch. 458(5):583–92. PMID:21394649
773. Matsuyama J, Ichikawa M, Oikawa T, Sato T, Kishida Y, Oda K, et al. (2014). Primary CNS lymphoma arising in the region of the optic nerve presenting as loss of vision: 2 case reports, including a patient with a massive intracerebral hemorrhage. Brain Tumor Pathol. 31(3):222–8. PMID:23999767
774. Mavrikakis I, Heran MK, Rootman J (2006). MR findings in a patient with isolated intrinsic optic nerve lymphoma. Ophthal Plast Reconstr Surg. 22(6):482–4. PMID:17117111
775. Mayer RR, Frankfort BJ, Strickland BA, Debnam JM, McCutcheon IE, Groves MD, et al. (2017). Leptomeningeal metastases presenting exclusively with ocular disturbance in 34 patients: a tertiary care cancer hospital experience. J Clin Neurosci. 39:151–4. PMID:28215459
776. McDonnell JM, McDonnell PJ, Mounts P, Wu TC, Green WR (1986). Demonstration of papillomavirus capsid antigen in human conjunctival neoplasia. Arch Ophthalmol. 104(12):1801–5. PMID:3024607
777. McKelvie PA, Daniell M, McNab A, Loughnan M, Santamaria JD (2002). Squamous cell carcinoma of the conjunctiva: a series of 26 cases. Br J Ophthalmol. 86(2):168–73. PMID:11815342
778. McLaughlin ME, Pepin SM, Maccollin M, Choopong P, Lessell S (2007). Ocular pathologic findings of neurofibromatosis type 2. Arch Ophthalmol. 125(3):389–94. PMID:17353411
779. McLean IW, Foster WD, Zimmerman LE, Gamel JW (1983). Modifications of Callender's classification of uveal melanoma at the Armed Forces Institute of Pathology. Am J Ophthalmol. 96(4):502–9. PMID:6624832
780. McLean IW, Keefe KS, Burnier MN (1997). Uveal melanoma. Comparison of the prognostic value of fibrovascular loops, mean of the ten largest nucleoli, cell type, and tumor size. Ophthalmology. 104(5):777–80. PMID:9160022
781. McLean IW, Saraiva VS, Burnier MN Jr (2004). Pathological and prognostic features of uveal melanomas. Can J Ophthalmol. 39(4):343–50. PMID:15327098
782. McMahon RT, Font RL, McLean IW (1976). Phakomatous choristoma of eyelid: electron microscopical confirmation of lenticular derivation. Arch Ophthalmol. 94(10):1778–81. PMID:973823
783. Mehta M, Rasheed RA, Duker J, Reichel E, Feinberg E, Husain D, et al. (2015). Vitreous evaluation: a diagnostic challenge. Ophthalmology. 122(3):531–7. PMID:25439597
784. Meisels HI, Goldberg MF (1979). Vascular anastomoses between the iris and persistent hyperplastic primary vitreous. Am J Ophthalmol. 88(2):179–85. PMID:112868
785. Mello PC, Brasil OF, Vidoris A, Morales MC, Belfort RN (2016). Iris metastases from systemic cancer: a report of three cases. Arq Bras Oftalmol. 79(6):407–10. PMID:28076572
786. Memoli VA, Brown EF, Gould VE (1984). Glial fibrillary acidic protein (GFAP) immunoreactivity in peripheral nerve sheath tumors. Ultrastruct Pathol. 7(4):269–75. PMID:6543600
787. Mendoza PR, Grossniklaus HE (2015). The biology of retinoblastoma. Prog Mol Biol Transl Sci. 134:503–16. PMID:26310174
788. Mendoza PR, Jakobiec FA, Krane JF (2013). Immunohistochemical features of lacrimal gland epithelial tumors. Am J Ophthalmol. 156(6):1147–58.e1. PMID:23972314
789. Mendoza PR, Specht CS, Hubbard GB, Wells JR, Lynn MJ, Zhang Q, et al. (2015). Histopathologic grading of anaplasia in retinoblastoma. Am J Ophthalmol. 159(4):764–76. PMID:25528954
790. Merten DF, Gooding CA, Newton TH (1974). The radiographic features of meningiomas in childhood and adolescence. Pediatr Radiol. 2(2):89–96. PMID:15822329
791. Messmer E, Font RL, Laqua H, Höpping W, Naumann GO (1984). Cavernous hemangioma of the retina. Immunohistochemical and ultrastructural observations. Arch Ophthalmol. 102(3):413–8. PMID:6538410
792. Metwalley KA, Farghaly HS, Abd El-Hafeez HA (2013). Evaluation of left ventricular mass and function, lipid profile, and insulin resistance in Egyptian children with growth hormone deficiency: a single-center prospective case-control study. Indian J Endocrinol Metab. 17(5):876–82. PMID:24083170
793. Metz DP, Hingorani M, Calder VL, Buckley RJ, Lightman SL (1997). T-cell cytokines in chronic allergic eye disease. J Allergy Clin Immunol. 100(6 Pt 1):817–24. PMID:9438492
794. Meyer CH, Becker R, Schmidt JC, Kroll P (2002). When is congenital hypertrophy of the retinal pigment epithelium (CHRPE) associated with the Gardner's syndrome? An overview with clinical examples. Klin Monatsbl Augenheilkd. 219(9):644–8. [German] PMID:12410463
795. Meyerle CB, Dahr SS, Wetjen NM, Jirawuthiworavong GV, Butman JA, Lonser RR, et al. (2008). Clinical course of retrobulbar hemangioblastomas in von Hippel-Lindau disease. Ophthalmology. 115(8):1382–9. PMID:18395800
796. Michels RG, Knox DL, Erozan YS, Green WR (1975). Intraocular reticulum cell sarcoma. Diagnosis by pars plana vitrectomy. Arch Ophthalmol. 93(12):1331–5. PMID:1106372
797. Micieli JA, Margolin EA (2016). Optic disc metastasis as the presenting sign of lung adenocarcinoma. J Neuroophthalmol. 36(4):399–401. PMID:27468119
798. Mikhail M, Michel RP, Chankowsky J, Arthurs B (2017). Epiphora as first presenting sign of primary extranodal NK/T-cell lymphoma of the lacrimal sac. Orbit. 36(1):19–21. PMID:28146362
799. Mikropoulos D, Mavrikakis I, Ziakas NG, Konstas AG, Boboridis KG (2011). Kaposi's sarcoma of the bulbar conjunctiva in an immunocompetent patient. Case Rep Ophthalmol. 2(2):193–7. PMID:21734889
800. Miles SL, Niles RM, Pittock S, Vile R, Davies J, Winters JL, et al. (2012). A factor found in the IgG fraction of serum of patients with paraneoplastic bilateral diffuse uveal melanocytic proliferation causes proliferation of cultured human melanocytes. Retina. 32(9):1959–66. PMID:22791177
801. Millar MJ, Tumuluri K, Murali R, Ng T, Beaumont P, Maloof A (2008). Bilateral primary optic nerve lymphoma. Ophthal Plast Reconstr Surg. 24(1):71–3. PMID:18209656
802. Miller CV, Wolf A, Klingenstein A, Decker C, Garip A, Kampik A, et al. (2014). Clinical outcome of advanced squamous cell carcinoma of the conjunctiva. Eye (Lond). 28(8):962–7. PMID:24858526
803. Miller NR (2004). Primary tumours of the optic nerve and its sheath. Eye (Lond). 18(11):1026–37. PMID:15534587
804. Milman T, Petousis V, McCormick SA, Finger PT (2011). Anterior segment tumor aspiration cutter-assisted biopsy: experience with pathology. Am J Ophthalmol. 152(5):776–83.e1. PMID:21794848
805. Milman T, Schear MJ, Eagle RC Jr (2014). Diagnostic utility of adipophilin immunostain in periocular carcinomas. Ophthalmology. 121(4):964–71. PMID:24290802
806. Milman T, Shields JA, Husson M, Marr BP, Shields CL, Eagle RC Jr (2005). Primary ductal adenocarcinoma of the lacrimal gland. Ophthalmology. 112(11):2048–51. PMID:16271319
807. Mimura T, Nakashizuka T, Kami J, Kohmura M, Sato S, Dou K, et al. (2012). Bilateral choroidal detachment after cord blood stem cell transplantation in an adult patient with acute myeloid leukemia. Int Ophthalmol. 32(4):379–81. PMID:22350079
808. Min KW, Park HK, Kim WY, Kim WS, Lim SD, Han HS, et al. (2014). Primary ductal adenocarcinoma of the lacrimal gland, associated with abundant intracytoplasmic lumens containing some eosinophilic hyaline globules: cytological, histological and ultrastructural findings. Ultrastruct Pathol. 38(5):363–6. PMID:24932904
809. Minnetti M, Grossman A (2016). Somatic and germline mutations in NETs: implications for their diagnosis and management. Best Pract Res Clin Endocrinol Metab. 30(1):115–27. PMID:26971848
810. Mishra DK, Veena U, Kaliki S, Kethiri AR, Sangwan VS, Ali MH, et al. (2016). Differential expression of stem cell markers in ocular surface squamous neoplasia. PLoS One. 11(9):e0161800. PMID:27584160
811. Missotten GS, Gambrelle J, de Wolff-Rouendaal D, de Keizer RJ (2010). Epistaxis or epiphora as a sign for extension of a conjunctival melanoma. A series of six patients with nasolacrimal recurrence. Br J Ophthalmol. 94(10):1328–31. PMID:20584717
812. Missotten GS, Keijser S, De Keizer RJ, De Wolff-Rouendaal D (2005). Conjunctival melanoma in the Netherlands: a nationwide study. Invest Ophthalmol Vis Sci. 46(1):75–82. PMID:15623757
813. Mito H, Takahashi Y, Nakano T, Asamoto K, Ikeda H, Kakizaki H (2014). Consecutive microscopic anatomical characteristics of the lacrimal sac and nasolacrimal duct: cases with or without inflammation. Invest Ophthalmol Vis Sci. 55(8):5233–7. PMID:25082889
814. Mittal R, Araujo I, Czanner G, Coupland SE (2016). Perforin expression in eyelid sebaceous carcinomas: a useful and specific immunomarker for the differential diagnosis of eyelid carcinomas. Acta Ophthalmol. 94(5):e325–30. PMID:26843360
815. Mittal R, Cherepanoff S, Thornton S, Kalirai H, Damato B, Coupland SE (2015). Bilateral diffuse uveal melanocytic proliferation: molecular genetic analysis of a case and review of the literature. Ocul Oncol Pathol. 2(2):94–9. PMID:27171825
816. Mitter D, Ullmann R, Muradyan A, Klein-Hitpass L, Kanber D, Ounap K, et al. (2011). Genotype-phenotype correlations in patients with retinoblastoma and interstitial 13q deletions. Eur J Hum Genet. 19(9):947–58.

PMID:21505449
817. Makar J, Kocjan BJ, Hošnjak L, Pižem J, Beltram M, Gale N, et al. (2015). Morphological characteristics of conjunctival squamous papillomas in relation to human papillomavirus infection. Br J Ophthalmol. 99(3):431–6. PMID:25527693
818. Moloney TP, Trinh T, Farrah JJ (2014). A case of conjunctival mucoepidermoid carcinoma in Australia. Clin Ophthalmol. 8:11–4. PMID:24363552
819. Montalban A, Liétin B, Louvrier C, Russier M, Kemeny JL, Mom T, et al. (2010). Malignant lacrimal sac tumors. Eur Ann Otorhinolaryngol Head Neck Dis. 127(5):165–72. PMID:21036121
820. Montes TL, Agra MV, Alonso MSM, Lorenzo AO (2017). Conjunctival leiomyosarcoma: a case report and review of literature. Indian J Ophthalmol. 65(5):406–8. PMID:28573999
821. Mooy CM, Luyten GP, de Jong PT, Luider TM, Stijnen T, van de Ham F, et al. (1995). Immunohistochemical and prognostic analysis of apoptosis and proliferation in uveal melanoma. Am J Pathol. 147(4):1097–104. PMID:7573354
822. Moran S, Martínez-Cardús A, Sayols S, Musulén E, Balañá C, Estival-Gonzalez A, et al. (2016). Epigenetic profiling to classify cancer of unknown primary: a multicentre, retrospective analysis. Lancet Oncol. 17(10):1386–95. PMID:27575023
823. Mori T, Sukeda A, Sekine S, Shibata S, Ryo E, Okano H et al. (2017). SOX10 expression as well as BRAF and GNAQ/11 mutations distinguish pigmented ciliary epithelium neoplasms from uveal melanomas. Invest Ophthalmol Vis Sci. 58(12):5445–51. PMID:29059311
824. Mortuza S, Esmaeli B, Bell D (2014). Primary intraocular ancient schwannoma: a case report and review of the literature. Head Neck. 36(4):E36–8. PMID:23729377
825. Moulin AP, Bucher M, Pournaras JA, Nguyen C, Ambresin A (2010). Fluorescein and indocyanine green angiography findings in B cell lymphoblastic leukemia mimicking acute central serous chorioretinopathy. Klin Monatsbl Augenheilkd. 227(4):342–4. PMID:20408096
826. Mouriaux F, Vincent S, Kherrouche Z, Maurage CA, Planque N, Monté D, et al. (2003). Microphthalmia transcription factor analysis in posterior uveal melanomas. Exp Eye Res. 76(6):653–61. PMID:12742347
827. Muci-Mendoza R, Arevalo JF, Ramella M, Fuenmayor-Rivera D (2001). Optic nerve metastasis from oat cell lung adenocarcinoma: regression after radiotherapy. Ophthalmic Surg Lasers. 32(4):349–51. PMID:11475407
828. Mudhar HS, Doherty R, Salawu A, Sisley K, Rennie IG (2013). Immunohistochemical and molecular pathology of ocular uveal melanocytoma: evidence for somatic GNAQ mutations. Br J Ophthalmol. 97(7):924–8. PMID:23685997
828A. Mudhar HS, Saunders E, Rundle P, Rennie IG, Sisley K (2009). The in vivo modulatory effects of an anterior-chamber microenvironment on uveal melanoma. Br J Ophthalmol. 93(4):535–40. PMID:19019926
829. Mudhar HS, Scott I, Ul-Hassan A, Burton D, Doherty R, Cross N, et al. (2012). Bilateral diffuse uveal melanocytic hyperplasia: molecular characterization and novel association with bilateral renal papillary carcinoma. Histopathology. 61(4):751–4. PMID:22803781
830. Mudhar HS Sethuraman C, Khan MD, Jan SU (2007). Intracular, pan-uveal intravascular large B-cell lymphoma associated with choroidal infarction and choroidal tri-lineage extramedullary haemtopoiesis. Histopathology. 51(2):275–9. PMID:17593210
831. Munch-Petersen HD, Rasmussen PK, Coupland SE, Esmaeli B, Finger PT, Graue GF, et al. (2015). Ocular adnexal diffuse large B-cell lymphoma: a multicenter international study. JAMA Ophthalmol. 133(2):165–73. PMID:25393033
832. Munier FL (2014). Classification and management of seeds in retinoblastoma. Ellsworth Lecture Ghent August 24th 2013. Ophthalmic Genet. 35(4):193–207. PMID:25321846
833. Munier FL, Gaillard MC, Balmer A, Soliman S, Podilsky G, Moulin AP, et al. (2012). Intravitreal chemotherapy for vitreous disease in retinoblastoma revisited: from prohibition to conditional indications. Br J Ophthalmol. 96(8):1078–83. PMID:22694968
834. Munro S, Brownstein S, Liddy B (1993). Conjunctival keratoacanthoma. Am J Ophthalmol. 116(5):654–5. PMID:8238236
835. Muthiah S, Radhakrishnan N (2017). Management of extraocular infections. Indian J Pediatr. 84(12):945–52. PMID:28707045
836. Nabavizadeh SA, Santi M, Belasco JB, Zimmerman RA (2014). Primary atypical optic nerve sheath meningioma in a child with restricted diffusion on magnetic resonance imaging. J Neuroophthalmol. 34(2):173–6. PMID:24705258
837. Nagaishi M, Sugiura Y, Takano I, Tanaka Y, Suzuki K, Yokoo H, et al. (2015). Clinicopathological and molecular features of malignant optic pathway glioma in an adult. J Clin Neurosci. 22(1):207–9. PMID:25150758
838. Nair AG, Kaliki S, Kamal S, Mishra DK, Vemuganti GK (2015). Conjunctival leiomyosarcoma: a report of two cases. Orbit. 34(5):274–8. PMID:26214581
839. Nair AG, Pathak RS, Iyer VR, Gandhi RA (2014). Optic nerve glioma: an update. Int Ophthalmol. 34(4):999–1005. PMID:24736941
840. Nakamura Y, Mashima Y, Kameyama K (1995). Human papilloma virus DNA detected in case of inverted squamous papilloma of the lacrimal sac. Br J Ophthalmol. 79(4):392–3. PMID:7742294
841. Nakamura Y, Mashima Y, Kameyama K, Mukai M, Oguchi Y (1997). Detection of human papillomavirus infection in squamous tumours of the conjunctiva and lacrimal sac by immunohistochemistry, in situ hybridisation, and polymerase chain reaction. Br J Ophthalmol. 81(4):308–13. PMID:9215061
842. Nakashima M, Miyajima M, Sugano H, Iimura Y, Kato M, Tsurusaki Y, et al. (2014). The somatic GNAQ mutation c.548G>A (p.R183Q) is consistently found in Sturge-Weber syndrome. J Hum Genet. 59(12):691–3. PMID:25374402
843. Nakazawa T, Abe T, Sato Y, Yuda F, Omura M, Tamai M (2000). Magnetic resonance imaging of a non-pigmented adenoma of the ciliary epithelium. Acta Ophthalmol Scand. 78(4):470–3. PMID:10990055
844. Nangia V, Jonas JB, Agarwal S, Khare A, Lambat S, Panda-Jonas S (2012). Choroidal nevi in adult Indians: the Central India Eye and Medical Study. Br J Ophthalmol. 96(11):1443–4. PMID:22872672
845. Naumann G, Yanoff M, Zimmerman LE (1966). Histogenesis of malignant melanomas of the uvea. I. Histopathologic characteristics of nevi of the choroid and ciliary body. Arch Ophthalmol. 76(6):784–96. PMID:5924936
846. Nelson KD, McSoley JJ (2011). Clinical findings and management of conjunctival intraepithelial neoplasia. Optometry. 82(1):15–21. PMID:21071282
847. Neren A, Reich I, Torno R, Shinder R (2017). Minor salivary gland acinic cell carcinoma with orbital extension. Ophthal Plast Reconstr Surg. 33(3S Suppl 1):S66–8. PMID:26068556
848. National Institutes of Health (1988). Neurofibromatosis. Conference statement. National Institutes of Health Consensus Development Conference. Arch Neurol. 45(5):575–8. PMID:3128965
849. Nevares RL, Mulliken JB, Robb RM (1988). Ocular dermoids. Plast Reconstr Surg. 82(6):959–64. PMID:3200959
850. Newman NM, Smith ME, Gay AJ (1972). An unusual case of leukemia involving the eye: a clinico-pathological study. Surv Ophthalmol. 16(5):316–21. PMID:4549896
851. Newton R, Ferlay J, Reeves G, Beral V, Parkin DM (1996). Effect of ambient solar ultraviolet radiation on incidence of squamous-cell carcinoma of the eye. Lancet. 347(9013):1450–1. PMID:8676629
852. Newton R, Ziegler J, Ateenyi-Agaba C, Bousarghin L, Casabonne D, Beral V, et al. (2002). The epidemiology of conjunctival squamous cell carcinoma in Uganda. Br J Cancer. 87(3):301–8. PMID:12177799
853. Ng CH, Wang JJ, Mitchell P, Amirul Islam FM, Wong TY (2009). Prevalence and characteristics of choroidal nevi in an Asian vs white population. Arch Ophthalmol. 127(3):314–9. PMID:19273796
854. Ni C, D'Amico DJ, Fan CQ, Kuo PK (1982). Tumors of the lacrimal sac: a clinicopathological analysis of 82 cases. Int Ophthalmol Clin. 22(1):121–40. PMID:6277817
855. Ni C, Liu SL, Zhong CS (1989). Spindle cell carcinoma of cornea and conjunctiva with pseudosarcomatous metaplasia. Light microscopic, electron microscopic and immunohistochemical findings in 2 patients. Chin Med J (Engl). 102(5):387–91. PMID:2509163
856. Ni C, Wagoner MD, Wang WJ, Albert DM, Fan CO, Robinson N (1983). Mucoepidermoid carcinomas of the lacrimal sac. Arch Ophthalmol. 101(10):1572–4. PMID:6626013
857. Nickelsen MN, von Holstein S, Hansen AB, Prause JU, Heegaard S (2015). Breast carcinoma metastasis to the lacrimal gland: two case reports. Oncol Lett. 10(2):1031–5. PMID:26622620
858. Nicolò M, Nicolò G, Zingirian M (2002). Pleomorphic adenocarcinoma of the ciliary epithelium: a clinicopathological, immunohistochemical, ultrastructural, DNA-ploidy and comparative genomic hybridization analysis of an unusual case. Eur J Ophthalmol. 12(4):319–23. PMID:12220004
859. Ninane J, Taylor D, Day S (1980). The eye as a sanctuary in acute lymphoblastic leukaemia. Lancet. 1(8166):452–3. PMID:6102185
860. Niu L, Zhang C, Meng F, Cai R, Bi Y, Wang Y, et al. (2015). Ocular juvenile xanthogranuloma. Optom Vis Sci. 92(6):e126–33. PMID:25969381
861. Niu P, Zhao XX, Yan F, Zhou YM, Jian P (2014). Influence of Ginkgo biloba extract on proliferation of ACC-2 cell, survivin and TIP30 gene expression in adenoid cystic carcinoma of lacrimal gland. Zhongguo Zhong Yao Za Zhi. 39(24):4860–4. [Chinese] PMID:25898592
862. Njauw CN, Kim I, Piris A, Gabree M, Taylor M, Lane AM, et al. (2012). Germline BAP1 inactivation is preferentially associated with metastatic ocular melanoma and cutaneous-ocular melanoma families. PLoS One. 7(4):e35295. PMID:22545102
863. Nomura S, Suzuki R, Sugiyama S, Nogami K, Ito H (1999). Optic glioma with characteristic bilateral optic atrophy in a 3-year-old girl. Pediatr Neurosurg. 31(4):213–8. PMID:10705932
864. Norregaard JC, Gerner N, Jensen OA, Prause JU (1996). Malignant melanoma of the conjunctiva: occurrence and survival following surgery and radiotherapy in a Danish population. Graefes Arch Clin Exp Ophthalmol. 234(9):569–72. PMID:8880155
865. Noshiro S, Wanibuchi M, Akiyama Y, Okawa S, Ohtaki S, Sugino T, et al. (2015). IgG4-related disease initially presented as an orbital mass lesion mimicking optic nerve sheath meningioma. Brain Tumor Pathol. 32(4):286–90. PMID:26037238
866. Nusliha A, Dalpatadu U, Amarasinghe B, Chandrasinghe PC, Deen KI (2014). Congenital hypertrophy of retinal pigment epithelium (CHRPE) in patients with familial adenomatous polyposis (FAP); a polyposis registry experience. BMC Res Notes. 7:734. PMID:25326340
867. O'Neal KD, Butnor KJ, Perkinson KR, Proia AD (2003). Bilateral diffuse uveal melanocytic proliferation associated with pancreatic carcinoma: a case report and literature review of this paraneoplastic syndrome. Surv Ophthalmol. 48(6):613–25. PMID:14609707
868. O'Reilly FM, Brat DJ, McAlpine BE, Grossniklaus HE, Folpe AL, Arbiser JL (2001). Microphthalmia transcription factor immunohistochemistry: a useful diagnostic marker in the diagnosis and detection of cutaneous melanoma, sentinel lymph node metastases, and extracutaneous melanocytic neoplasms. J Am Acad Dermatol. 45(3):414–9. PMID:11511840
869. Obi EE, Drummond SR, Kemp EG, Roberts F (2013). Pleomorphic adenomas of the lower eyelid: a case series. Ophthal Plast Reconstr Surg. 29(1):e14–7. PMID:22743699
870. Oellers P, Karp CL, Shah RR, Winnick M, Matthews J, Dubovy S (2014). Conjunctival keratoacanthoma. Br J Ophthalmol. 98(2):275–6,285. PMID:24288390
871. Ohashi A, Elsayed AA, Yasuma T, Iijima T, Nakamura S (2015). Conjunctival mucoepithelial hyperplasia of the elderly. Int Ophthalmol. 35(4):611–4. PMID:25975460
872. Ohkoshi K, Tsiaras WG (1992). Prognostic importance of ophthalmic manifestations in childhood leukaemia. Br J Ophthalmol. 76(11):651–5. PMID:1477038
873. Oliver WR, Reddick RL, Gillespie GY, Siegal GP (1985). Juxtadrenal schwannoma: verification of the diagnosis by immunohistochemical and ultrastructural studies. J Surg Oncol. 30(4):259–68. PMID:2417059
874. Onken MD, Li J, Cooper JA (2014). Uveal melanoma cells utilize a novel route for transendothelial migration. PLoS One. 9(12):e115472. PMID:25506912
875. Onken MD, Worley LA, Ehlers JP, Harbour JW (2004). Gene expression profiling in uveal melanoma reveals two molecular classes and predicts metastatic death. Cancer Res. 64(20):7205–9. PMID:15492234
875A. Onken MD, Worley LA, Long MD, Duan S, Council ML, Bowcock AM, et al. (2008). Oncogenic mutations in GNAQ occur early in uveal melanoma. Invest Ophthalmol Vis Sci. 49(12):5230–4. PMID:18719078
876. Ordóñez NG (2012). Immunohistochemical endothelial markers: a review. Adv Anat Pathol. 19(5):281–95. PMID:22885378
877. Orduña-Azcona J, Gili P, De Manuel-Triantafilo S, Flores-Rodriguez P (2014). Solitary congenital hypertrophy of the retinal pigment epithelium features by high-definition optical coherence tomography. Eur J Ophthalmol. 24(4):566–9. PMID:24366775
878. Ortiz JM, Yanoff M (1979). Epipalpebral conjunctival osseous choristoma. Br J Ophthalmol. 63(3):173–6. PMID:435428
879. Østergaard J, Prause JU, Heegaard S (2011). Oncocytic lesions of the ophthalmic region: a clinicopathological study with emphasis on cytokeratin expression. Acta Ophthalmol. 89(3):263–7. PMID:19843013
880. Othmane IS, Shields CL, Shields JA, Gunduz K, Mercado G (1999). Circumscribed choroidal hemangioma managed by transpupillary thermotherapy. Arch Ophthalmol. 117(1):136–7. PMID:9930182

881. Otto MJ, Löw O, Schneider A (1991). The nominal section thickness–importance of their correction for morphometry. Exp Pathol. 42(3):129–36. PMID:1915756
882. Oworu O, Kyle P, Morton R (2004). Metastatic oesophageal carcinoma presenting as a lacrimal gland tumour. Br J Ophthalmol. 88(7):972–3. PMID:15205254
883. Paal E, Thompson LD, Heffess CS (1998). A clinicopathologic and immunohistochemical study of ten pancreatic lymphangiomas and a review of the literature. Cancer. 82(11):2150–8. PMID:9610694
884. Palma J, Sasso DF, Dufort G, Koop K, Sampor C, Diez B, et al. (2012). Successful treatment of metastatic retinoblastoma with high-dose chemotherapy and autologous stem cell rescue in South America. Bone Marrow Transplant. 47(4):522–7. PMID:21602901
885. Palme C, Bechrakis NE, Stattin M, Haas G, Zehetner C (2016). Decreased vision as initial presenting symptom of acute lymphoblastic leukemia: a case report. Case Rep Ophthalmol. 7(2):377–83. PMID:27721787
886. Pan Y, Xing Y, Wang H (2015). Expression of survivin in adenoid cystic carcinoma of the lacrimal gland and the effect of intervention with arsenic trioxide in vitro. Exp Ther Med. 10(1):330–4. PMID:26170957
887. Panagopoulos I, Gorunova L, Bjerkehagen B, Lobmaier I, Heim S (2015). LAMTOR1-PRKCD and NUMA1-SFMBT1 fusion genes identified by RNA sequencing in aneurysmal benign fibrous histiocytoma with t(3;11)(p21;q13). Cancer Genet. 208(11):545–51. PMID:26432191
888. Pang CS, Brown JD, Ganote CE, Youngberg GA (2005). A mass of the right lacrimal sac in a 53-year-old man. Arch Pathol Lab Med. 129(11):1493–4. PMID:16253035
889. Pantanowitz L, Dezube BJ (2008). Kaposi sarcoma in unusual locations. BMC Cancer. 8:190. PMID:18605999
890. Papalas JA, Manavi CK, Woodward JA, Sangueza OP, Cummings TJ (2010). Angiosarcoma of the eyelid: a clinicopathologic comparison between isolated unilateral tumors and tumors demonstrating extrapalpebral involvement. Am J Dermatopathol. 32(7):694–9. PMID:20559124
891. Pappas S, Jin K, Tse BC, Tse DT, Pelaez D, Tao W (2017). Adenoid cystic carcinoma of the lacrimal gland: clinical, genetic and molecular characteristics. In: Farooqi AA, Ismail M, editors. Molecular oncology: underlying mechanisms and translational advancements. Cham: Springer.
892. Paridaens AD, Minassian DC, McCartney AC, Hungerford JL (1994). Prognostic factors in primary malignant melanoma of the conjunctiva: a clinicopathological study of 256 cases. Br J Ophthalmol. 78(4):252–9. PMID:8199108
893. Park GC, Cho KJ, Kang J, Roh JL, Choi SH, Kim SY, et al. (2012). Relationship between histopathology of pleomorphic adenoma in the parotid gland and recurrence after superficial parotidectomy. J Surg Oncol. 106(8):942–6. PMID:22740329
894. Parmar DN, Rose GE (2003). Management of lacrimal sac tumours. Eye (Lond). 17(5):599–606. PMID:12855966
895. Parsons MA, Rennie IG, Rundle PA, Dhingra S, Mudhar H, Singh AD (2005). Congenital hypertrophy of retinal pigment epithelium: a clinico-pathological case report. Br J Ophthalmol. 89(7):920–1. PMID:15965180
896. Pasqualucci L, Zhang B (2016). Genetic drivers of NF-κB deregulation in diffuse large B-cell lymphoma. Semin Cancer Biol. 39:26–31. PMID:27546290
897. Pastora-Salvador N, Abelairas-Gómez J, Peralta-Calvo J, García-Fernández E, Morales-Bastos C, Asencio-Durán M, et al. (2012). Atypical clinical presentation and long-term survival in a patient with optic nerve medulloepithelioma: a case report. J Med Case Rep. 6:123. PMID:22571440
898. Patel AV, Miller JB, Nath R, Shih HA, Yoon MK, Freitag SK, et al. (2016). Unilateral eye findings: a rare herald of acute leukemia. Ocul Oncol Pathol. 2(3):166–70. PMID:27239459
899. Patel NR, Sanghvi S, Khan MN, Husain Q, Baredes S, Eloy JA (2014). Demographic trends and disease-specific survival in salivary acinic cell carcinoma: an analysis of 1129 cases. Laryngoscope. 124(1):172–8. PMID:23754708
900. Patrón-Bolaños C, Acosta-Torres L, Tenorio-Rocha F, Jacinto-Alemán LF, Leyva-Huerta E (2016). Immunohistochemical patterns in different stromal variants of pleomorphic adenomas: literature review. Histol Histopathol. 31(3):239–48. PMID:26507835
901. Pe'er J (2005). Ocular surface squamous neoplasia. Ophthalmol Clin North Am. 18(1):1–13,vii. PMID:15763187
902. Pe'er J, Hidayat AA (1986). Myxomas of the conjunctiva. Am J Ophthalmol. 102(1):80–6. PMID:3728629
903. Pe'er J, Hidayat AA, Ilsar M, Landau L, Stefanyszyn MA (1996). Glandular tumors of the lacrimal sac. Their histopathologic patterns and possible origins. Ophthalmology. 103(10):1601–5. PMID:8874432
904. Pe'er J, Levinger S, Ilsar M, Climenhaga H, Okon E (1990). Malignant fibrous histiocytoma of the conjunctiva. Br J Ophthalmol. 74(10):624–8. PMID:1704795
905. Pekmezci M, Reuss DE, Hirbe AC, Dahiya S, Gutmann DH, von Deimling A, et al. (2015). Morphologic and immunohistochemical features of malignant peripheral nerve sheath tumors and cellular schwannomas. Mod Pathol. 28(2):187–200. PMID:25189642
906. Pels H, Juergens A, Schirgens I, Glasmacher A, Schulz H, Engert A, et al. (2010). Early complete response during chemotherapy predicts favorable outcome in patients with primary CNS lymphoma. Neuro-oncol. 12(7):720–4. PMID:20159882
907. Penfield W, editor (1965). Cytology and cellular pathology of the nervous system. 2nd ed. New York: Hafner Publishing Company.
908. Peris K, Onorati MT, Keller G, Magrini F, Donati P, Muscardin L, et al. (1997). Widespread microsatellite instability in sebaceous tumours of patients with the Muir-Torre syndrome. Br J Dermatol. 137(3):356–60. PMID:9349329
909. Peshtani A, Kaliki S, Eagle RC, Shields CL (2014). Medulloepithelioma: a triad of clinical features. Oman J Ophthalmol. 7(2):93–5. PMID:25136238
910. Pfaffenbach DD, Green WR (1971). Ectopic lacrimal gland. Int Ophthalmol Clin. 11(3):149–59. PMID:5152651
911. Pfeiffer ML, Ozgur OK, Myers JN, Peng A, Ning J, Zafereo ME, et al. (2017). Sentinel lymph node biopsy for ocular adnexal melanoma. Acta Ophthalmol. 95(4):e323–8. PMID:27775232
912. Phelps CD (1978). The pathogenesis of glaucoma in Sturge-Weber syndrome. Ophthalmology. 85(3):276–86. PMID:662281
913. Pilarski R, Rai K, Cebulla C, Abdel-Rahman M (1993). BAP1 tumor predisposition syndrome. In: Adam MP, Ardinger HH, Pagon RA, Wallace SE, Bean LJH, Stephens K, et al., editors. GeneReviews®. Seattle: University of Washington, Seattle. PMID:27748099
914. Pineda R 2nd, Urban RC Jr, Bellows AR, Jakobiec FA (1995). Ciliary body neurilemoma. Unusual clinical findings intimating the diagnosis. Ophthalmology. 102(6):918–23. PMID:7777299
916. Płaszczyca A, Nilsson J, Magnusson L, Brosjö O, Larsson O, Vult von Steyern F, et al. (2014). Fusions involving protein kinase C and membrane-associated proteins in benign fibrous histiocytoma. Int J Biochem Cell Biol. 53:475–81. PMID:24721208
917. Plateroti AM, Scavella V, Abdolrahimzadeh B, Plateroti R, Rahimi S (2017). An update on oculodermal melanocytosis and rare associated conditions. Semin Ophthalmol. 32(4):524–8. PMID:27083007
918. Plocharczyk EF, Frankel WL, Hampel H, Peters SB (2013). Mismatch repair protein deficiency is common in sebaceous neoplasms and suggests the importance of screening for Lynch syndrome. Am J Dermatopathol. 35(2):191–5. PMID:22722469
919. Podgrabinska S, Braun P, Velasco P, Kloos B, Pepper MS, Skobe M (2002). Molecular characterization of lymphatic endothelial cells. Proc Natl Acad Sci USA. 99(25):16069–74. PMID:12446836
920. Pokhrel SM, Badu BP, Lavaju P, Shrestha BG, Pant AR, Agarwal M (2014). Unusual presentation of lacrimal gland pleomorphic adenoma. JNMA J Nepal Med Assoc. 52(195):949–51. PMID:26982673
921. Pokorny KS, Hyman BM, Jakobiec FA, Perry HD, Caputo AR, Iwamoto T (1987). Epibulbar choristomas containing lacrimal tissue. Clinical distinction from dermoids and histologic evidence of an origin from the palpebral lobe. Ophthalmology. 94(10):1249–57. PMID:3684203
922. Pollock SC, Awh CC, Dutton JJ (1991). Cutaneous melanoma metastatic to the optic disc and vitreous. Arch Ophthalmol. 109(10):1352–4. PMID:1929918
923. Polvi A, Linnankivi T, Kivelä T, Herva R, Keating JP, Mäkitie O, et al. (2012). Mutations in CTC1, encoding the CTS telomere maintenance complex component 1, cause cerebroretinal microangiopathy with calcifications and cysts. Am J Hum Genet. 90(3):540–9. PMID:22387016
924. Poole Perry LJ, Jakobiec FA, Zakka FR, Reichel E, Herwig MC, Perry A, et al. (2013). Reactive retinal astrocytic tumors (so-called vasoproliferative tumors): histopathologic, immunohistochemical, and genetic studies of four cases. Am J Ophthalmol. 155(3):593–608.e1. PMID:23219067
925. Porcelli AM, Ghelli A, Ceccarelli C, Lang M, Cenacchi G, Capristo M, et al. (2010). The genetic and metabolic signature of oncocytic transformation implicates HIF1alpha destabilization. Hum Mol Genet. 19(6):1019–32. PMID:20028790
926. Potter HD, Lee V, Hinshaw MA, Khedr SS, Albert DM, Burkat CN (2013). Lichen simplex chronicus of the conjunctiva. JAMA Ophthalmol. 131(6):816–8. PMID:23559160
927. Prabhakaran VC, Cannon PS, McNab A, Davis G, O'Donnell B, Dolman PJ, et al. (2010). Lesions mimicking lacrimal gland pleomorphic adenoma. Br J Ophthalmol. 94(11):1509–12. PMID:20962353
928. Praidou A, Jacob S, Irion L, Sivaraj R, Groenewald C, Coupland SE, et al. (2017). Retinal and vitreous metastases from hepatocholangiocarcinoma. BMC Cancer. 17(1):430. PMID:28629380
929. Prakalapakorn SG, Bernardino CR, Auclair PL, Grossniklaus HE (2008). Carcinosarcoma of the orbit: report of two cases and review of the literature. Ophthalmology. 115(11):2065–70. PMID:18562006
930. Preechawai P, Della Roccad RC, Della Rocca D, Schaefer S, McCormack S (2005). Transitional cell carcinoma of the lacrimal sac. J Med Assoc Thai. 88 Suppl 9:S138–42. PMID:16681067
931. Priest JR, Williams GM, Manera R, Jenkinson H, Bründler MA, Davis S, et al. (2011). Ciliary body medulloepithelioma: four cases associated with pleuropulmonary blastoma–a report from the International Pleuropulmonary Blastoma Registry. Br J Ophthalmol. 95(7):1001–5. PMID:21156700
932. Pujari A, Ali MJ, Mulay K, Naik MN, Honavar SG (2014). The black lacrimal sac: a clinicopathological correlation of a malignant melanoma with anterior lacrimal crest infiltration. Int Ophthalmol. 34(1):111–5. PMID:23456510
933. Pulido JS, Flotte TJ, Raja H, Miles S, Winters JL, Niles R, et al. (2013). Dermal and conjunctival melanocytic proliferations in diffuse uveal melanocytic proliferation. Eye (Lond). 27(9):1058–62. PMID:23788206
934. Punia RS, Nanda A, Mohan H, Bansal RK (2006). Clinicopathological study of dermolipoma–a report of four cases. Indian J Pathol Microbiol. 49(4):605–7. PMID:17183873
935. Purcell JJ Jr, Shields JA (1975). Hypertrophy with hyperpigmentation of the retinal pigment epithelium. Arch Ophthalmol. 93(11):1122–6. PMID:1191102
936. Pusateri A, Margo CE (2014). Intraocular astrocytoma and its differential diagnosis. Arch Pathol Lab Med. 138(9):1250–4. PMID:25171711
937. Pushker N, Kashyap S, Sen S, Bajaj MS, Hada M (2017). Cystic pleomorphic adenoma of the lacrimal gland: a clinicopathologic study. Can J Ophthalmol. 52(1):e7–9. PMID:28237174
938. Pushker N, Shrey D, Bajaj MS, Kashyap S, Yadav P, Mehta M, et al. (2010). Malignant non-teratoid medulloepithelioma of the optic nerve with intraocular extension. Clin Experiment Ophthalmol. 38(7):731–3. PMID:20497433
939. Pyo EY, Mun GH, Yoon KC (2016). The prevalence and risk factors for pterygium in South Korea: the Korea National Health and Nutrition Examination Survey (KNHANES) 2009-2010. Epidemiol Health. 38:e2016015. PMID:27156345
940. Qannam A, Bello IO (2016). Comparison of histological grading methods in mucoepidermoid carcinoma of minor salivary glands. Indian J Pathol Microbiol. 59(4):457–62. PMID:27721274
941. Qiu M, Shields CL (2015). Choroidal nevus in the United States adult population: racial disparities and associated factors in the National Health and Nutrition Examination Survey. Ophthalmology. 122(10):2071–83. PMID:26255109
942. Qualman SJ, Coffin CM, Newton WA, Hojo H, Triche TJ, Parham DM, et al. (1998). Intergroup Rhabdomyosarcoma Study: update for pathologists. Pediatr Dev Pathol. 1(6):550–61. PMID:9724344
943. Quhill H, Rennie IG, Rundle PA, Mudhar HS (2013). Three cases of intraocular mesectodermal leiomyoma expressing progesterone and androgen receptors. Eye (Lond). 27(5):669–72. PMID:23519275
944. Racher H, Soliman S, Argiropoulos B, Chan HS, Gallie BL, Perrier R, et al. (2016). Molecular analysis distinguishes metastatic disease from second cancers in patients with retinoblastoma. Cancer Genet. 209(7–8):359–63. PMID:27318443
945. Radu O, Pantanowitz L (2013). Kaposi sarcoma. Arch Pathol Lab Med. 137(2):289–94. PMID:23368874
946. Rahangdale SR, Castillo M, Shockley W (1995). MR in squamous cell carcinoma of the lacrimal sac. AJNR Am J Neuroradiol. 16(6):1262–4. PMID:7677021
947. Rahimi-Movaghar V, Karimi M (2003). Meningeal melanocytoma of the brain and

oculodermal melanocytosis (nevus of Ota): case report and literature review. Surg Neurol. 59(3):200–10. PMID:12681556
948. Rahimy E, Coffee RE, McCannel TA (2015). Bilateral diffuse uveal melanocytic proliferation as a precursor to multiple systemic malignancies. Semin Ophthalmol. 30(3):206–9. PMID:24124896
949. Rai K, Pilarski R, Cebulla CM, Abdel-Rahman MH (2016). Comprehensive review of BAP1 tumor predisposition syndrome with report of two new cases. Clin Genet. 89(3):285–94. PMID:26096145
950. Ramasubramanian A, Shields CL, Harmon SA, Shields JA (2010). Autofluorescence of choroidal hemangioma in 34 consecutive eyes. Retina. 30(1):16–22. PMID:19952988
951. Ramos A, Pozo CD, Chinchurreta A, García F, Lorenzo M, Gismero S (2016). Adenoid cystic carcinoma of the lacrimal sac: case report. Arq Bras Oftalmol. 79(5):333–5. PMID:27982216
952. Ramstead C, Buffam F, White V (2012). Caruncular alveolar rhabdomyosarcoma in a woman previously treated for breast cancer. Arch Ophthalmol. 130(8):1087–8. PMID:22893093
953. Rao NA, Font RL (1976). Mucoepidermoid carcinoma of the conjunctiva: a clinicopathologic study of five cases. Cancer. 38(4):1699–709. PMID:991088
954. Rao NA, Hidayat AA, McLean IW, Zimmerman LE (1982). Sebaceous carcinomas of the ocular adnexa: a clinicopathologic study of 104 cases, with five-year follow-up data. Hum Pathol. 13(2):113–22. PMID:7076199
955. Rao RC, Elner VM, Demirci H (2015). A red and swollen eyelid. Breast carcinoma metastasis to left lacrimal gland. JAMA Oncol. 1(4):537–8. PMID:26181264
956. Rao RS, Patil S, Amrutha N, Sanketh D, Agarwal A (2014). The ambiguous salivary myoepithelial cells. J Contemp Dent Pract. 15(4):523–8. PMID:25576124
957. Raparia K, Chang CC, Chévez-Barrios P (2009). Intraocular lymphoma: diagnostic approach and immunophenotypic findings in vitrectomy specimens. Arch Pathol Lab Med. 133(8):1233–7. PMID:19653716
958. Rashid A, Jakobiec FA (2014). Avoiding the major complication of ophthalmic pathology: misdiagnosis. A review of three common diagnostic challenges. Semin Ophthalmol. 29(5–6):468–74. PMID:25325875
959. Rasmussen P, Ralfkiaer E, Prause JU, Sjö LD, Siersma VD, Heegaard S (2011). Malignant lymphoma of the lacrimal gland: a nation-based study. Arch Ophthalmol. 129(10):1275–80. PMID:21987669
960. Rasmussen P, Sjö LD, Prause JU, Ralfkiaer E, Heegaard S (2009). Mantle cell lymphoma in the orbital and adnexal region. Br J Ophthalmol. 93(8):1047–51. PMID:19429588
961. Rasmussen PK, Ralfkiaer E, Prause JU, Sjö LD, Specht L, Rossing HH, et al. (2015). Follicular lymphoma of the ocular adnexal region: a nation-based study. Acta Ophthalmol. 93(2):184–91. PMID:25125069
962. Rath S, Connors JM, Dolman PJ, Rootman J, Rootman DB, White VA (2014). Comparison of American Joint Committee on Cancer TNM-based staging system (7th edition) and Ann Arbor classification for predicting outcome in ocular adnexal lymphoma. Orbit. 33(1):23–8. PMID:24180616
963. Rath S, Honavar SG, Reddy VA, Naik MN, Vemuganti GK, Murthy R (2009). Sebaceous carcinoma of the eyelid metastasizing to the lacrimal sac after 5 years. Orbit. 28(5):309–12. PMID:19874127
964. Reddy HS, Keene CD, Chang SH, Jian-Amadi A, Cimino PJ (2017). Immunohistochemical profiling including beta-catenin in conjunctival melanocytic lesions. Exp Mol Pathol. 102(2):198–202. PMID:28161440
965. Reddy S, Gorin MB, McCannel TA, Tsui I, Straatsma BR (2010). Novel KRIT1/CCM1 mutation in a patient with retinal cavernous hemangioma and cerebral cavernous malformation. Graefes Arch Clin Exp Ophthalmol. 248(9):1359–61. PMID:20306072
966. Reddy SC, Jackson N, Menon BS (2003). Ocular involvement in leukemia–a study of 288 cases. Ophthalmologica. 217(6):441–5. PMID:14573980
967. Reddy SC, Quah SH, Low HC, Jackson N (1998). Prognostic significance of retinopathy at presentation in adult acute leukemia. Ann Hematol. 76(1):15–8. PMID:9486919
968. Regillo CD, Eagle RC Jr, Shields JA, Shields CL, Arbizo VV (1993). Histopathologic findings in congenital grouped pigmentation of the retina. Ophthalmology. 100(3):400–5. PMID:8460012
969. Reis GF, Bloomer MM, Perry A, Phillips JJ, Grenert JP, Karnezis AN, et al. (2013). Pilocytic astrocytomas of the optic nerve and their relation to pilocytic astrocytomas elsewhere in the central nervous system. Mod Pathol. 26(10):1279–87. PMID:23702730
970. Reiser BJ, Mok A, Kukes G, Kim JW (2007). Non-AIDS-related Kaposi sarcoma involving the tarsal conjunctiva and eyelid margin. Arch Ophthalmol. 125(6):838–40. PMID:17563000
971. Ren M, Zeng JH, Luo QL, Bi F, Chen J (2014). Primary malignant melanoma of lacrimal sac. Int J Ophthalmol. 7(6):1069–70. PMID:25540768
972. Rennie IG, Parsons MA, Benson MT (1991). Neurilemoma of the caruncle: a clinicopathological report. Br J Ophthalmol. 75(12):749–51. PMID:1768668
973. Ricci M, Amadori E, Chiesa F, Bongiovanni A, Liverani C, Fabbri L, et al. (2014). Single bone metastasis from adenocarcinoma of the lacrimal gland: a case report. Future Oncol. 10(10):1735–9. PMID:25303054
974. Rickman DS, Bobek MP, Misek DE, Kuick R, Blaivas M, Kurnit DM, et al. (2001). Distinctive molecular profiles of high-grade and low-grade gliomas based on oligonucleotide microarray analysis. Cancer Res. 61(18):6885–91. PMID:11559565
975. Riemens A, Bromberg J, Touitou V, Sobolewska B, Missotten T, Baarsma S, et al. (2015). Treatment strategies in primary vitreoretinal lymphoma: a 17-center European collaborative study. JAMA Ophthalmol. 133(2):191–7. PMID:25412269
976. Rishi P, Dixit A, Verma A (2015). Bilateral optic disk metastasis from breast carcinoma. Indian J Ophthalmol. 63(5):451–2. PMID:26139809
977. Rishi P, Shields CL (2016). Intralesional and topical interferon therapy following incomplete primary excision of ocular surface squamous neoplasia. Indian J Ophthalmol. 64(6):460–1. PMID:27488156
978. Rivolta C, Royer-Bertrand B, Rimoldi D, Schalenbourg A, Zografos L, Leyvraz S, et al. (2016). UV light signature in conjunctival melanoma; not only skin should be protected from solar radiation. J Hum Genet. 61(4):361–2. PMID:26657935
979. Robertson AG, Shih J, Yau C, Gibb EA, Oba J, Mungall KL, et al. (2017). Integrative analysis identifies four molecular and clinical subsets in uveal melanoma. Cancer Cell. 32(2):204–20.e15. PMID:28810145
980. Robertson DM, Campbell RJ, Salomão DR (2002). Mushroom-shaped choroidal melanocytoma mimicking malignant melanoma. Arch Ophthalmol. 120(1):82–5. PMID:11786063
981. Robinson DR, Wu YM, Kalyana-Sundaram S, Cao X, Lonigro RJ, Sung YS, et al. (2013). Identification of recurrent NAB2-STAT6 gene fusions in solitary fibrous tumor by integrative sequencing. Nat Genet. 45(2):180–5. PMID:23313952
982. Robinson JW, Brownstein S, Jordan DR, Hodge WG (2006). Conjunctival mucoepidermoid carcinoma in a patient with ocular cicatricial pemphigoid and a review of the literature. Surv Ophthalmol. 51(5):513–9. PMID:16950250
983. Rockey JH, Donnelly JJ, Stromberg BE, Soulsby EJ (1979). Immunopathology of Toxocara canis and Ascaris suum infections of the eye: the role of the eosinophil. Invest Ophthalmol Vis Sci. 18(11):1172–84. PMID:511459
984. Rodrigues FW, Arruda JT, Silva RE, Moura KK (2008). TP53 gene expression, codon 72 polymorphism and human papillomavirus DNA associated with pterygium. Genet Mol Res. 7(4):1251–8. PMID:19065760
985. Rodrigues M, Hidayat A, Karesh J (1988). Pleomorphic adenocarcinoma of ciliary epithelium simulating an epibulbar tumor. Am J Ophthalmol. 106(5):595–600. PMID:2461084
986. Rodriguez FJ, Ligon AH, Horkayne-Szakaly I, Rushing EJ, Ligon KL, Vena N, et al. (2012). BRAF duplications and MAPK pathway activation are frequent in gliomas of the optic nerve proper. J Neuropathol Exp Neurol. 71(9):789–94. PMID:22892521
987. Rodriguez FJ, Perry A, Gutmann DH, O'Neill BP, Leonard J, Bryant S, et al. (2008). Gliomas in neurofibromatosis type 1: a clinicopathologic study of 100 patients. J Neuropathol Exp Neurol. 67(3):240–9. PMID:18344915
988. Rodríguez-Francia P, Sánchez-Tocino H, García-Cantera M, Martín-Castillo J (2005). Optic nerve pilocytic astrocytoma with retinal involvement. Arch Soc Esp Oftalmol. 80(12):733–6. [Spanish] PMID:16372218
989. Rodriguez-Galindo C, Wilson MW, Haik BG, Lipson MJ, Cain A, Merchant TE, et al. (2003). Treatment of metastatic retinoblastoma. Ophthalmology. 110(6):1237–40. PMID:12799253
990. Rodriguez-Sains RS (2002). Pigmented conjunctival neoplasms. Orbit. 21(3):231–8. PMID:12187419
991. Roh MR, Eliades P, Gupta S, Tsao H (2015). Genetics of melanocytic nevi. Pigment Cell Melanoma Res. 28(6):661–72. PMID:26300491
992. Rohrbach JM, Steuhl KP, Thanos S (1991). Monoclonal antibody HMB-45 in diagnosis of intra-ocular melanoma. Klin Monatsbl Augenheilkd. 199(4):274–7. [German] PMID:1762354
993. Rollins BJ (2015). Genomic alterations in Langerhans cell histiocytosis. Hematol Oncol Clin North Am. 29(5):839–51. PMID:26461146
994. Rolston JD, Han SJ, Cotter JA, El-Sayed IH, Aghi MK (2014). Gangliogliomas of the optic pathway. J Clin Neurosci. 21(12):2244–9. PMID:25043166
995. Rosenbaum PS, Kress Y, Slamovits TL, Font RL (1992). Phakomatous choristoma of the eyelid. Immunohistochemical and electron microscopic observations. Ophthalmology. 99(12):1779–84. PMID:1282696
996. Rosenbaum PS, Mahadevia PS, Goodman LA, Kress Y (1995). Acinic cell carcinoma of the lacrimal gland. Arch Ophthalmol. 113(6):781–5. PMID:7540387
997. Rosenthal AR (1983). Ocular manifestations of leukemia. A review. Ophthalmology. 90(8):899–905. PMID:6195573
998. Rosso R, Colombo R, Ricevuti G (1983). Neurilemmoma of the ciliary body: report of a case. Br J Ophthalmol. 67(9):585–7. PMID:6882714
999. Rotellini M, Palomba A, Baroni G, Franchi A (2014). Diagnostic utility of PLAG1 immunohistochemical determination in salivary gland tumors. Appl Immunohistochem Mol Morphol. 22(5):390–4. PMID:23958548
1000. Roth AM (1978). Solitary keratoacanthoma of the conjunctiva. Am J Ophthalmol. 85(5 Pt 1):647–50. PMID:655243
1001. Rubinstein LJ (1988). Pathological features of optic nerve and chiasmatic gliomas. Neurofibromatosis. 1(3):152–8. PMID:3152462
1002. Rummelt V, Folberg R, Woolson RF, Hwang T, Pe'er J (1995). Relation between the microcirculation architecture and the aggressive behavior of ciliary body melanomas. Ophthalmology. 102(5):844–51. PMID:7777286
1003. Ruppenstein M, Straub BK, Ach T, Völcker HE, Dithmar S (2010). Primary intrastromal iris cysts. Klin Monatsbl Augenheilkd. 227(5):425–9. [German] PMID:20490997
1004. Rush JA, Younge BR, Campbell RJ, MacCarty CS (1982). Optic glioma. Long-term follow-up of 85 histopathologically verified cases. Ophthalmology. 89(11):1213–9. PMID:6818504
1005. Rushlow DE, Mol BM, Kennett JY, Yee S, Pajovic S, Thériault BL, et al. (2013). Characterisation of retinoblastomas without RB1 mutations: genomic, gene expression, and clinical studies. Lancet Oncol. 14(4):327–34. PMID:23498719
1006. Rutzen AR, Ortega-Larrocea G, Dugel PU, Chong LP, Lopez PF, Smith RE, et al. (1995). Clinicopathologic study of retinal and choroidal biopsies in intraocular inflammation. Am J Ophthalmol. 119(5):597–611. PMID:7733185
1007. Ryan G, Glasson B, Foster A (2012). Benign fibrous histiocytoma of the conjunctiva. Case Rep Ophthalmol Med. 2012:786260. PMID:23320226
1008. Ryan SJ, Schachat AP, Wilkinson CP, Hinton DR, Sadda SR, Wiedemann P, editors (2012). Retina. 5th ed. Philadelphia: Elsevier.
1009. Ryan SJ, Font RL (1973). Primary epithelial neoplasms of the lacrimal sac. Am J Ophthalmol. 76(1):73–88. PMID:4352147
1010. Ryan SJ, Zimmerman LE, King FM (1972). Reactive lymphoid hyperplasia. An unusual form of intraocular pseudotumor. Trans Am Acad Ophthalmol Otolaryngol. 76(3):652–71. PMID:4126438
1011. Saavedra E, Singh AD, Sears JE, Ratliff NB (2006). Plexiform pigmented schwannoma of the uvea. Surv Ophthalmol. 51(2):162–8. PMID:16500216
1012. Sabatini P, Ducic Y (2009). Bilateral lacrimal gland masses: unusual case of metastatic renal cell carcinoma. J Otolaryngol Head Neck Surg. 38(1):E1–2. PMID:19344596
1013. Sadegh L, Chen PW, Brown JR, Han Z, Niederkorn JY (2015). NKT cells act through third party bone marrow-derived cells to suppress NK cell activity in the liver and exacerbate hepatic melanoma metastases. Int J Cancer. 137(5):1085–94. PMID:25683463
1015. Sadun F, Hinton DR, Sadun AA (1996). Rapid growth of an optic nerve ganglioglioma in a patient with neurofibromatosis 1. Ophthalmology. 103(5):794–9. PMID:8637690
1016. Saeed MU, Chang BY, Anand S, Chakrabarty A (2007). Diagnostic surprise in an evisceration specimen. Orbit. 26(2):129–31. PMID:17613862
1017. Saegusa M, Takano Y, Hashimura M, Okayasu I, Shiga J (1995). HPV type 16 in conjunctival and junctional papilloma, dysplasia, and squamous cell carcinoma. J Clin Pathol. 48(12):1106–10. PMID:8567996
1018. Safneck JR, Napier LB, Halliday WC (1992). Malignant astrocytoma of the optic nerve in a child. Can J Neurol Sci. 19(4):498–503. PMID:1330262
1019. Sagoo MS, Mruthyunjaya P, Cree I,

Luthert PJ, Hungerford JL (2007). Malignant transformation of iris melanocytoma to iris ring melanoma. Br J Ophthalmol. 91(11):1571–2. PMID:17947283
1020. Sahm F, Jakobiec FA, Meyer J, Schrimpf D, Eberhart CG, Hovestadt V, et al. (2016). Somatic mutations of DICER1 and KMT2D are frequent in intraocular medulloepitheliomas. Genes Chromosomes Cancer. 55(5):418–27. PMID:26841698
1021. Sakaida H, Kobayashi M, Yuta A, Imanishi Y, Majima Y (2009). Squamous cell carcinoma of the nasolacrimal duct. Eur Arch Otorhinolaryngol. 266(3):455–8. PMID:18488243
1022. Salero E, Blenkinsop TA, Corneo B, Harris A, Rabin D, Stern JH, et al. (2012). Adult human RPE can be activated into a multipotent stem cell that produces mesenchymal derivatives. Cell Stem Cell. 10(1):88–95. PMID:22226358
1023. Sali PA, Yadav KS, Bushan K, Rajpurohit V, Varty PP, Sharma S (2016). A rare case of lacrimal adenoid cystic carcinoma with large hepatic and multiple pulmonary metastases with successful surgical treatment. Int J Surg Case Rep. 20:151–4. PMID:26866882
1024. Salib RJ, Afoakwah EO (2003). De novo papillary squamous carcinoma of the lacrimal sac. Auris Nasus Larynx. 30(2):205–8. PMID:12753996
1025. Salour H, Hatami MM, Parvin M, Ferdowsi AA, Abrishami M, Bagheri A, et al. (2010). Clinicopathological study of lacrimal sac specimens obtained during DCR. Orbit. 29(5):250–3. PMID:20812824
1026. Salvanos P, Utheim TP, Moe MC, Eide N, Bragadóttir R (2015). Autofluorescence imaging in the differential diagnosis of optic disc melanocytoma. Acta Ophthalmol. 93(5):476–80. PMID:25923254
1027. Samara WA, Khoo CT, Magrath G, Shields CL (2015). Multimodal imaging for detection of clinically inapparent diffuse iris juvenile xanthogranuloma. J Pediatr Ophthalmol Strabismus. 52 Online:e30–3. PMID:25992541
1028. Samara WA, Khoo CT, Say EA, Saktanasate J, Eagle RC Jr, Shields JA, et al. (2015). Juvenile xanthogranuloma involving the eye and ocular adnexa: tumor control, visual outcomes, and globe salvage in 30 patients. Ophthalmology. 122(10):2130–8. PMID:26189188
1029. Sandboe FD, Elgjo K, Eide N, Medin W, Scott H (1994). An intraocular paraganglioma? Acta Ophthalmol (Copenh). 72(1):138–41. PMID:8017189
1030. Sandell RF, Carter JM, Folpe AL (2015). Solitary (juvenile) xanthogranuloma: a comprehensive immunohistochemical study emphasizing recently developed markers of histiocytic lineage. Hum Pathol. 46(9):1390–7. PMID:26220162
1031. Sangwan VS, Sridhar MS, Vemuganti GK (2003). Treatment of complex choristoma by excision and amniotic membrane transplantation. Arch Ophthalmol. 121(2):278–80. PMID:12583800
1032. Saornil MA, Egan KM, Gragoudas ES, Seddon JM, Walsh SM, Albert DM (1992). Histopathology of proton beam-irradiated vs enucleated uveal melanomas. Arch Ophthalmol. 110(8):1112–8. PMID:1323252
1033. Sarafzadeh S, Corrêa ZM, Dhamija A, Augsburger JJ, Trichopoulos N (2010). Intraocular lymphoma diagnosed by fine-needle aspiration biopsy. Acta Ophthalmol. 88(6):705–10. PMID:19604155
1034. Sasco AJ, Jaquet A, Boidin E, Ekouevi DK, Thouillot F, Lemabec T, et al. (2010). The challenge of AIDS-related malignancies in sub-Saharan Africa. PLoS One. 5(1):e8621. PMID:20066157
1035. Sastre X, Chantada GL, Doz F, Wilson MW, de Davila MT, Rodríguez-Galindo C, et al. (2009). Proceedings of the consensus meetings from the International Retinoblastoma Staging Working Group on the pathology guidelines for the examination of enucleated eyes and evaluation of prognostic risk factors in retinoblastoma. Arch Pathol Lab Med. 133(8):1199–202. PMID:19653709
1036. Satchi K, McKelvie P, McNab AA (2015). Malignant melanoma of the lacrimal drainage apparatus complicating conjunctival melanoma. Ophthal Plast Reconstr Surg. 31(3):207–10. PMID:25126770
1037. Saunders T, Margo CE (2012). Intraocular medulloepithelioma. Arch Pathol Lab Med. 136(2):212–6. PMID:22288972
1038. Savagner F, Franc B, Guyetant S, Rodien P, Reynier P, Malthiery Y (2001). Defective mitochondrial ATP synthesis in oxyphilic thyroid tumors. J Clin Endocrinol Metab. 86(10):4920–5. PMID:11600563
1039. Schachat AP, Shields JA, Fine SL, Sanborn GE, Weingeist TA, Valenzuela RE, et al. (1984). Combined hamartomas of the retina and retinal pigment epithelium. Ophthalmology. 91(12):1609–15. PMID:6521994
1040. Schalenbourg A, Coupland S, Kacperek A, Damato B (2008). Iridocyclectomy for neovascular glaucoma caused by proton-beam radiotherapy of pigmented ciliary adenocarcinoma. Graefes Arch Clin Exp Ophthalmol. 246(10):1499–501. PMID:18581131
1041. Schalenbourg A, Moulin A, Guillou L, Zografos L (2011). Metastatic choroidal paraganglioma. Ophthalmology. 118(11):2238–41. PMID:21906814
1042. Schefler AC, Abramson DH (2008). Retinoblastoma: what is new in 2007-2008. Curr Opin Ophthalmol. 19(6):526–34. PMID:18854698
1043. Scheithauer BW, Silva AI, Ketterling RP, Pula JH, Lininger JF, Krinock MJ (2009). Rosette-forming glioneuronal tumor: report of a chiasmal-optic nerve example in neurofibromatosis type 1: special pathology report. Neurosurgery. 64(4):E771–2. PMID:19349806
1044. Schellini SA, Marques ME, Milanezi MF, Bacchi CE (1997). Conjunctival keratoacanthoma. Acta Ophthalmol Scand. 75(3):335–7. PMID:9253992
1045. Scheuermann JC, de Ayala Alonso AG, Oktaba K, Ly-Hartig N, McGinty RK, Fraterman S, et al. (2010). Histone H2A deubiquitinase activity of the Polycomb repressive complex PR-DUB. Nature. 465(7295):243–7. PMID:20436459
1046. Schlesinger T, Appukuttan B, Hwang T, Atchaneeyakasul LO, Chan CC, Zhuang Z, et al. (2007). Internal en bloc resection and genetic analysis of retinal capillary hemangioblastoma. Arch Ophthalmol. 125(9):1189–93. PMID:17846357
1047. Schmitz EJ, Herwig-Carl MC, Holz FG, Loeffler KU (2017). Sebaceous gland carcinoma of the ocular adnexa - variability in clinical and histological appearance with analysis of immunohistochemical staining patterns. Graefes Arch Clin Exp Ophthalmol. 255(11):2277–85. PMID:28741159
1048. Scholz SL, Möller I, Reis H, Süßkind D, van de Nes JAP, Leonardelli S, et al. (2017). Frequent GNAQ, GNA11, and EIF1AX mutations in iris melanoma. Invest Ophthalmol Vis Sci. 58(9):3464–70. PMID:28700778
1049. Scholz SL, Thomasen H, Reis H, Möller I, Darawsha R, Müller B, et al. (2015). Frequent TERT promoter mutations in ocular surface squamous neoplasia. Invest Ophthalmol Vis Sci. 56(10):5854–61. PMID:26348634
1050. Schroeder B, Hesse L, Brück W, Gal A (1997). Histopathological and immunohistochemical findings associated with a null mutation in the Norrie disease gene. Ophthalmic Genet. 18(2):71–7. PMID:9228243
1051. Schwab C, Mayer C, Zalaudek I, Riedl R, Richtig M, Wackernagel W, et al. (2017). Iris freckles a potential biomarker for chronic sun damage. Invest Ophthalmol Vis Sci. 58(6):BIO174–9. PMID:28715582
1052. Schwab C, Wackernagel W, Grinninger P, Mayer C, Schwab K, Langmann G, et al. (2016). A unifying concept of uveal pigment cell distribution and dissemination based on an animal model: insights into ocular melanogenesis. Cells Tissues Organs. 201(3):232–8. PMID:27002320
1053. Schwab C, Zalaudek I, Mayer C, Riedl R, Wackernagel W, Juch H, et al. (2015). New insights into oculodermal nevogenesis and proposal for a new iris nevus classification. Br J Ophthalmol. 99(5):644–9. PMID:25359901
1054. Schweizer L, Koelsche C, Sahm F, Piro RM, Capper D, Reuss DE, et al. (2013). Meningeal hemangiopericytoma and solitary fibrous tumors carry the NAB2-STAT6 fusion and can be diagnosed by nuclear expression of STAT6 protein. Acta Neuropathol. 125(5):651–8. PMID:23575898
1055. Schwent BJ, Wojno TH, Grossniklaus HE (2007). Hemangiopericytoma of the optic nerve sheath. Am J Ophthalmol. 143(5):904–6. PMID:17452190
1056. Searl SS, Krigstein HJ, Albert DM, Grove AS Jr (1982). Invasive squamous cell carcinoma with intraocular mucoepidermoid features. Conjunctival carcinoma with intraocular invasion and diphasic morphology. Arch Ophthalmol. 100(1):109–11. PMID:7055460
1057. Seca M, Borges P, Reimão P, Gomes M, Meireles A (2012). Conjunctival lymphangioma: a case report and brief review of the literature. Case Rep Ophthalmol Med. 2012:836573. PMID:22666617
1058. Seddon JM, Gragoudas ES, Glynn RJ, Egan KM, Albert DM, Blitzer PH (1990). Host factors, UV radiation, and risk of uveal melanoma. A case-control study. Arch Ophthalmol. 108(9):1274–80. PMID:2400347
1059. Seethala RR (2017). Salivary gland tumors: current concepts and controversies. Surg Pathol Clin. 10(1):155–76. PMID:28153132
1060. Seethala RR, Barnes EL (2011). Rare malignant and benign salivary gland epithelial tumors. Surg Pathol Clin. 4(4):1217–72. PMID:26837791
1061. Seethala RR, Griffith CC (2016). Molecular pathology: predictive, prognostic, and diagnostic markers in salivary gland tumors. Surg Pathol Clin. 9(3):339–52. PMID:27523965
1062. Seethala RR, Stenman G (2017). Update from the 4th edition of the World Health Organization classification of head and neck tumours: tumors of the salivary gland. Head Neck Pathol. 11(1):55–67. PMID:28247227
1063. Seregard S (1999). Phakomatous choristoma may be located in the eyelid or orbit or both. Acta Ophthalmol Scand. 77(3):343–6. PMID:10406159
1064. Seregard S, Kock E (1992). Conjunctival malignant melanoma in Sweden 1969-91. Acta Ophthalmol (Copenh). 70(3):289–96. PMID:1636385
1065. Shah SU, Mashayekhi A, Shields CL, Walia HS, Hubbard GB 3rd, Zhang J, et al. (2014). Uveal metastasis from lung cancer: clinical features, treatment, and outcome in 194 patients. Ophthalmology. 121(1):352–7. PMID:23988200
1066. Shammas HF, Blodi FC (1977). Orbital extension of choroidal and ciliary body melanomas. Arch Ophthalmol. 95(11):2002–5. PMID:921579
1067. Shao L, Newell B, Quintanilla N (2007). Atypical fibroxanthoma and squamous cell carcinoma of the conjunctiva in xeroderma pigmentosum. Pediatr Dev Pathol. 10(2):149–52. PMID:17378688
1068. Shapey J, Sabin HI, Danesh-Meyer HV, Kaye AH (2013). Diagnosis and management of optic nerve sheath meningiomas. J Clin Neurosci. 20(8):1045–56. PMID:23809100
1069. Sharara NA, Alexander RA, Luthert PJ, Hungerford JL, Cree IA (2001). Differential immunoreactivity of melanocytic lesions of the conjunctiva. Histopathology. 39(4):426–31. PMID:11683945
1070. Sharma N, O'Hagan S, Phillips G (2016). Conjunctival myxoma - atypical presentation of a rare tumour: case report and review of literature. BMC Ophthalmol. 16(1):54. PMID:27177589
1071. Sharma P, Shields CL, Turaka K, Eagle RC Jr, Shields JA (2011). Ciliary body medulloepithelioma with neoplastic cyclitic membrane imaging with fluorescein angiography and ultrasound biomicroscopy. Graefes Arch Clin Exp Ophthalmol. 249(8):1259–61. PMID:21505878
1072. Sharma T, Grewal J, Gupta S, Murray PI (2004). Ophthalmic manifestations of acute leukaemias: the ophthalmologist's role. Eye (Lond). 18(7):663–72. PMID:15002029
1073. Sharma V, Finger PT, Sidoti PA, Semenova E, Iacob CE (2016). Rapidly growing iris melanocytoma with secondary glaucoma in a 6-year-old child. Eur J Ophthalmol. 26(4):e71–3. PMID:26692065
1074. Shehri M, Bouhenni R, Ghazi NG, Abu Safieh L, Edward DP (2014). Retinal reactive astrocytic tumor: gene expression profiling. JAMA Ophthalmol. 132(6):773–5. PMID:24921169
1075. Shenoy SB, Karam T, Udupa K, Nayal B (2016). Leukaemic infiltration of the optic nerve head: a rare site of initial relapse. BMJ Case Rep. 2016. PMID:27797802
1076. Shields CL, Alset AE, Boal NS, Casey MG, Knapp AN, Sugarman JA, et al. (2017). Conjunctival tumors in 5002 cases. Comparative analysis of benign versus malignant counterparts. The 2016 James D. Allen Lecture. Am J Ophthalmol. 173:106–33. PMID:27725148
1077. Shields CL, Arepalli S, Atalay HT, Ferenczy SR, Fulco E, Shields JA (2015). Choroidal osteoma shows bone lamella and vascular channels on enhanced depth imaging optical coherence tomography in 15 eyes. Retina. 35(4):750–7. PMID:25296127
1078. Shields CL, Benevides R, Materin MA, Shields JA (2006). Optical coherence tomography of retinal astrocytic hamartoma in 15 cases. Ophthalmology. 113(9):1553–7. PMID:16949441
1079. Shields CL, Chien JL, Surakiatchanukul T, Sioufi K, Lally SE, Shields JA (2017). Conjunctival tumors: review of clinical features, risks, biomarkers, and outcomes–the 2017 J. Donald M. Gass Lecture. Asia Pac J Ophthalmol (Phila). 6(2):109–20. PMID:28399347
1080. Shields CL, Demirci H, Karatza E, Shields JA (2004). Clinical survey of 1643 melanocytic and nonmelanocytic conjunctival tumors. Ophthalmology. 111(9):1747–54. PMID:15350332
1081. Shields CL, Douglass AM, Beggache M, Say EA, Shields JA (2016). Intravitreous chemotherapy for active vitreous seeding from retinoblastoma: outcomes after 192 consecutive injections. The 2015 Howard Naquin Lecture. Retina. 36(6):1184–90. PMID:26630319
1082. Shields CL, Fasiuddin AF, Mashayekhi A, Shields JA (2004). Conjunctival nevi: clinical features and natural course in 410 consecutive patients. Arch Ophthalmol. 122(2):167–75. PMID:14769591
1083. Shields CL, Furuta M, Mashayekhi A,

Berman EL, Zahler JD, Hoberman DM, et al. (2008). Clinical spectrum of choroidal nevi based on age at presentation in 3422 consecutive eyes. Ophthalmology. 115(3):546–52.e2. PMID:18067966
1084. Shields CL, Furuta M, Thangappan A, Nagori S, Mashayekhi A, Lally DR, et al. (2009). Metastasis of uveal melanoma millimeter-by-millimeter in 8033 consecutive eyes. Arch Ophthalmol. 127(8):989–98. PMID:19667335
1085. Shields CL, Hasanreisoglu M, Saktanasate J, Shields PW, Seibel I, Shields JA (2015). Sclerochoroidal calcification: clinical features, outcomes, and relationship with hypercalcemia and parathyroid adenoma in 179 eyes. Retina. 35(3):547–54. PMID:25574788
1086. Shields CL, Hogarty MD, Kligman BE, Christian C, Ehya H, Shields JA (2010). Langerhans cell histiocytosis of the uvea with neovascular glaucoma: diagnosis by fine-needle aspiration biopsy and management with intraocular bevacizumab and brachytherapy. J AAPOS. 14(6):534–7. PMID:21168078
1087. Shields CL, Honavar SG, Shields JA, Cater J, Demirci H (2001). Circumscribed choroidal hemangioma: clinical manifestations and factors predictive of visual outcome in 200 consecutive cases. Ophthalmology. 108(12):2237–48. PMID:11733265
1088. Shields CL, Kaliki S, Arepalli S, Atalay HT, Manjandavida FP, Pieretti G, et al. (2013). Uveal melanoma in children and teenagers. Saudi J Ophthalmol. 27(3):197–201. PMID:24227986
1089. Shields CL, Kaliki S, Furuta M, Mashayekhi A, Shields JA (2012). Clinical spectrum and prognosis of uveal melanoma based on age at presentation in 8,033 cases. Retina. 32(7):1363–72. PMID:22466491
1090. Shields CL, Kaliki S, Hutchinson A, Nickerson S, Patel J, Kancherla S, et al. (2013). Iris nevus growth into melanoma: analysis of 1611 consecutive eyes: the ABCDEF guide. Ophthalmology. 120(4):766–72. PMID:23290981
1091. Shields CL, Kaliki S, Livesey M, Walker B, Garoon R, Bucci M, et al. (2013). Association of ocular and oculodermal melanocytosis with the rate of uveal melanoma metastasis: analysis of 7872 consecutive eyes. JAMA Ophthalmol. 131(8):993–1003. PMID:23681424
1092. Shields CL, Kancherla S, Patel J, Vijayvargiya P, Suriano MM, Kolbus E, et al. (2012). Clinical survey of 3680 iris tumors based on patient age at presentation. Ophthalmology. 119(2):407–14. PMID:22035581
1093. Shields CL, Kels JG, Shields JA (2015). Melanoma of the eye: revealing hidden secrets, one at a time. Clin Dermatol. 33(2):183–96. PMID:25704938
1094. Shields CL, Manalac J, Das C, Ferguson K, Shields JA (2014). Choroidal melanoma: clinical features, classification, and top 10 pseudomelanomas. Curr Opin Ophthalmol. 25(3):177–85. PMID:24614143
1095. Shields CL, Manchandia A, Subbiah R, Eagle RC Jr, Shields JA (2008). Pigmented squamous cell carcinoma in situ of the conjunctiva in 5 cases. Ophthalmology. 115(10):1673–8. PMID:18378314
1096. Shields CL, Markowitz JS, Belinsky I, Schwartzstein H, George NS, Lally SE, et al. (2011). Conjunctival melanoma: outcomes based on tumor origin in 382 consecutive cases. Ophthalmology. 118(2):389–95.e1–2. PMID:20723990
1097. Shields CL, Mashayekhi A, Cater J, Shelil A, Meadows AT, Shields JA (2004). Chemoreduction for retinoblastoma: analysis of tumor control and risks for recurrence in 457 tumors. Trans Am Ophthalmol Soc. 102:35–45. PMID:15747743
1098. Shields CL, Mashayekhi A, Ho T, Cater J, Shields JA (2003). Solitary congenital hypertrophy of the retinal pigment epithelium: clinical features and frequency of enlargement in 330 patients. Ophthalmology. 110(10):1968–76. PMID:14522773
1099. Shields CL, Materin MA, Walker C, Marr BP, Shields JA (2006). Photoreceptor loss overlying congenital hypertrophy of the retinal pigment epithelium by optical coherence tomography. Ophthalmology. 113(4):661–5. PMID:16581426
1100. Shields CL, McMahon JF, Atalay HT, Hasanreisoglu M, Shields JA (2014). Retinal metastasis from systemic cancer in 8 cases. JAMA Ophthalmol. 132(11):1303–8. PMID:25033168
1101. Shields CL, Pellegrini M, Ferenczy SR, Shields JA (2014). Enhanced depth imaging optical coherence tomography of intraocular tumors: from placid to seasick to rock and rolling topography–the 2013 Francesco Orzalesi Lecture. Retina. 34(8):1495–512. PMID:25014847
1102. Shields CL, Perez B, Benavides R, Materin MA, Shields JA (2008). Optical coherence tomography of optic disk melanocytoma in 15 cases. Retina. 28(3):441–6. PMID:18327136
1103. Shields CL, Pirondini C, Bianciotto C, Harmon SA, Shields JA (2007). Autofluorescence of congenital hypertrophy of the retinal pigment epithelium. Retina. 27(8):1097–100. PMID:18040252
1104. Shields CL, Qureshi A, Eagle RC Jr, Lally SE, Shields JA (2012). Epibulbar osseous choristoma in 8 patients. Cornea. 31(7):756–60. PMID:22516954
1105. Shields CL, Ramasubramanian A, Ganguly A, Mohan D, Shields JA (2011). Cytogenetic testing of iris melanoma using fine needle aspiration biopsy in 17 patients. Retina. 31(3):574–80. PMID:21336070
1106. Shields CL, Ramasubramanian A, Rosenwasser R, Shields JA (2009). Superselective catheterization of the ophthalmic artery for intraarterial chemotherapy for retinoblastoma. Retina. 29(8):1207–9. PMID:19734768
1107. Shields CL, Schoenberg E, Kocher K, Shukla SY, Kaliki S, Shields JA (2013). Lesions simulating retinoblastoma (pseudoretinoblastoma) in 604 cases: results based on age at presentation. Ophthalmology. 120(2):311–6. PMID:23107579
1108. Shields CL, Shields JA (2004). Tumors of the conjunctiva and cornea. Surv Ophthalmol. 49(1):3–24. PMID:14711437
1109. Shields CL, Shields JA (2015). Ocular surface squamous neoplasia: from blue skies to blue dyes–we still need our ophthalmic pathologists. JAMA Ophthalmol. 133(11):1321–2. PMID:26378883
1110. Shields CL, Shields JA, Augsburger JJ (1988). Choroidal osteoma. Surv Ophthalmol. 33(1):17–27. PMID:3051466
1111. Shields CL, Shields JA, Barrett J, De Potter P (1995). Vasoproliferative tumors of the ocular fundus. Classification and clinical manifestations in 103 patients. Arch Ophthalmol. 113(5):615–23. PMID:7748132
1112. Shields CL, Shields JA, De Potter P, Minelli S, Hernandez C, Brady LW, et al. (1993). Plaque radiotherapy in the management of retinoblastoma. Use as a primary and secondary treatment. Ophthalmology. 100(2):216–24. PMID:8437830
1113. Shields CL, Shields JA, Gross NE, Schwartz GP, Lally SE (1997). Survey of 520 eyes with uveal metastases. Ophthalmology. 104(8):1265–76. PMID:9261313
1114. Shields CL, Shields JA, Honavar SG, Demirci H (2001). Clinical spectrum of primary ophthalmic rhabdomyosarcoma. Ophthalmology. 108(12):2284–92. PMID:11733272
1115. Shields CL, Shields JA, Marr BP, Sperber DE, Gass JD (2003). Congenital simple hamartoma of the retinal pigment epithelium: a study of five cases. Ophthalmology. 110(5):1005–11. PMID:12750104
1116. Shields CL, Shields JA, Materin M, Gershenbaum E, Singh AD, Smith A (2001). Iris melanoma: risk factors for metastasis in 169 consecutive patients. Ophthalmology. 108(1):172–8. PMID:11150284
1117. Shields CL, Shields JA, Shields MB, Augsburger JJ (1987). Prevalence and mechanisms of secondary intraocular pressure elevation in eyes with intraocular tumors. Ophthalmology. 94(7):839–46. PMID:3658352
1118. Shields CL, Shields JA, White D, Augsburger JJ (1986). Types and frequency of lesions of the caruncle. Am J Ophthalmol. 102(6):771–8. PMID:3789057
1119. Shields CL, Sioufi K, Alset AE, Boal NS, Casey MG, Knapp AN, et al. (2017). Clinical features differentiating benign from malignant conjunctival tumors in children. JAMA Ophthalmol. 135(3):215–24. PMID:28125759
1120. Shields CL, Sun H, Demirci H, Shields JA (2005). Factors predictive of tumor growth, tumor decalcification, choroidal neovascularization, and visual outcome in 74 eyes with choroidal osteoma. Arch Ophthalmol. 123(12):1658–66. PMID:16344436
1121. Shields CL, Zahler J, Falk N, Furuta M, Eagle RC Jr, Espinosa LE, et al. (2007). Neovascular glaucoma from advanced Coats disease as the initial manifestation of facioscapulohumeral dystrophy in a 2-year-old child. Arch Ophthalmol. 125(6):840–2. PMID:17563001
1122. Shields JA (1984). Ocular toxocariasis. A review. Surv Ophthalmol. 28(5):361–81. PMID:6719335
1123. Shields JA (2006). Photodynamic therapy for choroidal hemangioma. Graefes Arch Clin Exp Ophthalmol. 244(9):1071–2. PMID:16506073
1124. Shields JA, Decker WL, Sanborn GE, Augsburger JJ, Goldberg RE (1983). Presumed acquired retinal hemangiomas. Ophthalmology. 90(11):1292–300. PMID:6664668
1125. Shields JA, Demirci H, Marr BP, Eagle RC Jr, Shields CL (2005). Sebaceous carcinoma of the ocular region: a review. Surv Ophthalmol. 50(2):103–22. PMID:15749305
1126. Shields JA, Demirci H, Mashayekhi A, Eagle RC Jr, Shields CL (2006). Melanocytoma of the optic disk: a review. Surv Ophthalmol. 51(2):93–104. PMID:16500211
1127. Shields JA, Demirci H, Mashayekhi A, Shields CL (2004). Melanocytoma of optic disc in 115 cases: the 2004 Samuel Johnson Memorial Lecture, part 1. Ophthalmology. 111(9):1739–46. PMID:15350331
1128. Shields JA, Eagle RC Jr, Dutton J, Ehya H, Shields CL (2014). Adenocarcinoma of the retinal pigment epithelium: clinicopathologic correlation with paradoxical immunohistochemical findings. JAMA Ophthalmol. 132(10):1249–52. PMID:24993572
1129. Shields JA, Eagle RC Jr, Ferguson K, Shields CL (2015). Tumours of the nonpigmented epithelium of the ciliary body: the Lorenz E. Zimmerman Tribute Lecture. Retina. 35(5):957–65. PMID:25545484
1130. Shields JA, Eagle RC, Marr BP, Shields CL, Grossniklaus HE, Stulting RD (2007). Invasive spindle cell carcinoma of the conjunctiva managed by full-thickness eye wall resection. Cornea. 26(8):1014–6. PMID:17721310
1131. Shields JA, Eagle RC Jr, Shields CL (1999). Adenoma of nonpigmented ciliary epithelium with smooth muscle differentiation. Arch Ophthalmol. 117(1):117–9. PMID:9930173
1132. Shields JA, Eagle RC Jr, Shields CL, Brown GC, Lally SE (2009). Malignant transformation of congenital hypertrophy of the retinal pigment epithelium. Ophthalmology. 116(11):2213–6. PMID:19744732
1133. Shields JA, Eagle RC Jr, Shields CL, De Potter P (1996). Acquired neoplasms of the nonpigmented ciliary epithelium (adenoma and adenocarcinoma). Ophthalmology. 103(12):2007–16. PMID:9003334
1134. Shields JA, Eagle RC Jr, Shields CL, De Potter P, Poliak JG (1995). Natural course and histopathologic findings of lacrimal gland choristoma of the iris and ciliary body. Am J Ophthalmol. 119(2):219–24. PMID:7832229
1135. Shields JA, Eagle RC Jr, Shields CL, Marr BP (2005). Aggressive retinal astrocytomas in 4 patients with tuberous sclerosis complex. Arch Ophthalmol. 123(6):856–63. PMID:15955990
1136. Shields JA, Eagle RC Jr, Shields CL, Potter PD (1996). Congenital neoplasms of the nonpigmented ciliary epithelium (medulloepithelioma). Ophthalmology. 103(12):1998–2006. PMID:9003333
1137. Shields JA, Eagle RC Jr, Shields CL, Singh AD, Robitaille J (2002). Pigmented medulloepithelioma of the ciliary body. Arch Ophthalmol. 120(2):207–10. PMID:11831926
1138. Shields JA, Eagle RC Jr, Shields CL, Singh AD, Torrisi PF (2001). Clinicopathologic reports, case reports, and small case series: progressive growth of benign adenoma of the pigment epithelium of the ciliary body. Arch Ophthalmol. 119(12):1859–61. PMID:11735805
1139. Shields JA, Font RL, Eagle RC Jr, Shields CL, Gass JD (1994). Melanotic schwannoma of the choroid. Immunohistochemistry and electron microscopic observations. Ophthalmology. 101(5):843–9. PMID:8190469
1140. Shields JA, Hogan RN, Shields CL, Eagle RC Jr, Weakley DR Jr (2000). Intraocular lacrimal gland choristoma involving iris and ciliary body. Am J Ophthalmol. 129(5):673–5. PMID:10844067
1141. Shields JA, Kligman BE, Mashayekhi A, Shields CL (2011). Acquired sessile hemangioma of the conjunctiva: a report of 10 cases. Am J Ophthalmol. 152(1):55–59.e1. PMID:21529766
1142. Shields JA, Magrath GN, Shields C, Mackool R, Eagle RC Jr, Grossniklaus HE (2016). Dissecting aortic aneurysm 55 years after diagnosis of iris flocculi. Ocul Oncol Pathol. 2(4):222–5. PMID:27843899
1143. Shields JA, Mashayekhi A, Kligman BE, Kunz WB, Criss J, Eagle RC Jr, et al. (2011). Vascular tumors of the conjunctiva in 140 cases. Ophthalmology. 118(9):1747–53. PMID:21788081
1144. Shields JA, Mashayekhi A, Ra S, Shields CL (2005). Pseudomelanomas of the posterior uveal tract: the 2006 Taylor R. Smith Lecture. Retina. 25(6):767–71. PMID:16141866
1145. Shields JA, Sanborn GE, Augsburger JJ (1983). The differential diagnosis of malignant melanoma of the iris. A clinical study of 200 patients. Ophthalmology. 90(6):716–20. PMID:6888862
1146. Shields JA, Sanborn GE, Kurz GH, Augsburger JJ (1981). Benign peripheral nerve tumor of the choroid: a clinicopathologic correlation and review of the literature. Ophthalmology. 88(12):1322–9. PMID:7322483
1147. Shields JA, Shields CL (2001). Differentiation of Coats' disease and retinoblastoma. J Pediatr Ophthalmol Strabismus. 38(5):262–6. PMID:11587173
1148. Shields JA, Shields CL (2002). Review: Coats disease: the 2001 LuEsther T. Mertz Lecture. Retina. 22(1):80–91. PMID:11884883
1149. Shields JA, Shields CL (2009). Glial tumors of the retina. The 2009 King Khaled Memorial Lecture. Saudi J Ophthalmol. 23(3–4):197–201. PMID:23960860
1150. Shields JA, Shields CL (2009).

Sebaceous adenocarcinoma of the eyelid. Int Ophthalmol Clin. 49(4):45–61. PMID:20348857
1151. Shields JA, Shields CL, editors (2015). Eyelid, conjunctival, and orbital tumors: an atlas and textbook. 3rd ed. Philadelphia: Wolters Kluwer.
1152. Shields JA, Shields CL (2017). Cysts of the iris pigment epithelium. What is new and interesting? The 2016 Jose Rizal International Medal Lecture. Asia Pac J Ophthalmol (Phila). 6(1):64–9. PMID:28161919
1153. Shields JA, Shields CL (2017). Tumors and related lesions of the pigmented epithelium. Asia Pac J Ophthalmol (Phila). 6(2):215–23. PMID:28399346
1154. Shields JA, Shields CL, Brotman HK, Carvalho C, Perez N, Eagle RC Jr (2001). Cancer metastatic to the orbit: the 2000 Robert M. Curts Lecture. Ophthal Plast Reconstr Surg. 17(5):346–54. PMID:11642491
1155. Shields JA, Shields CL, Eagle RC Jr (2007). Melanocytoma (hyperpigmented magnocellular nevus) of the uveal tract: the 34th G. Victor Simpson Lecture. Retina. 27(6):730–9. PMID:17621182
1156. Shields JA, Shields CL, Eagle RC Jr, Arevalo JF, DePotter P (1997). Ocular manifestations of the organoid nevus syndrome. Ophthalmology. 104(3):549–57. PMID:9082288
1157. Shields JA, Shields CL, Eagle RC Jr, De Potter P (1994). Observations on seven cases of intraocular leiomyoma. The 1993 Byron Demorest Lecture. Arch Ophthalmol. 112(4):521–8. PMID:8155052
1158. Shields JA, Shields CL, Eagle RC Jr, Friedman ES, Wheatley HM (2009). Age-related hyperplasia of the nonpigmented ciliary body epithelium (Fuchs adenoma) simulating a ciliary body malignant neoplasm. Arch Ophthalmol. 127(9):1224–5. PMID:19752438
1159. Shields JA, Shields CL, Eagle RC Jr, Singh AD (2001). Adenocarcinoma arising from congenital hypertrophy of retinal pigment epithelium. Arch Ophthalmol. 119(4):597–602. PMID:11296028
1160. Shields JA, Shields CL, Eagle RC Jr, Singh AD, Armstrong T (2001). Metastatic renal cell carcinoma to the palpebral lobe of the lacrimal gland. Ophthal Plast Reconstr Surg. 17(3):191–4. PMID:11388385
1161. Shields JA, Shields CL, Gündüz K, Eagle RC Jr (1999). Neoplasms of the retinal pigment epithelium: the 1998 Albert Ruedemann, Sr, Memorial Lecture, Part 2. Arch Ophthalmol. 117(5):601–8. PMID:10326956
1162. Shields JA, Shields CL, Lois N, Mercado G (1999). Iris cysts in children: classification, incidence, and management. The 1998 Torrence A Makley Jr Lecture. Br J Ophthalmol. 83(3):334–8. PMID:10365043
1163. Shields JA, Shields CL, Mashayekhi A, Marr BP, Benavides R, Thangappan A, et al. (2008). Primary acquired melanosis of the conjunctiva: risks for progression to melanoma in 311 eyes. The 2006 Lorenz E. Zimmerman Lecture. Ophthalmology. 115(3):511–9.e2. PMID:17884168
1164. Shields JA, Shields CL, Shah PG, Pastore DJ, Imperiale SM Jr (1992). Lack of association among typical congenital hypertrophy of the retinal pigment epithelium, adenomatous polyposis, and Gardner syndrome. Ophthalmology. 99(11):1709–13. PMID:1333580
1165. Shields JA, Shields CL, Singh AD (2000). Acquired tumors arising from congenital hypertrophy of the retinal pigment epithelium. Arch Ophthalmol. 118(5):637–41. PMID:10815155
1166. Shields JA, Shields CL, Singh AD (2000). Metastatic neoplasms in the optic disc: the 1999 Bjerrum Lecture: Part 2. Arch Ophthalmol. 118(2):217–24. PMID:10676787
1167. Shields JA, Shields CL, Suvarnamani C, Schroeder RP, DePotter P (1991). Retinoblastoma manifesting as orbital cellulitis. Am J Ophthalmol. 112(4):442–9. PMID:1928248
1168. Shields JA, Stephens RF, Eagle RC Jr, Shields CL, De Potter P (1992). Progressive enlargement of a circumscribed choroidal hemangioma. A clinicopathologic correlation. Arch Ophthalmol. 110(9):1276–8. PMID:1520116
1169. Shields JA, Tso MO (1975). Congenital grouped pigmentation of the retina. Histopathologic description and report of a case. Arch Ophthalmol. 93(11):1153. PMID:1191104
1170. Shneor E, Millodot M, Barnard S, Gantz L, Koslowe K, Gordon-Shaag A (2014). Prevalence of congenital hypertrophy of the retinal pigment epithelium (CHRPE) in Israel. Ophthalmic Physiol Opt. 34(3):385. PMID:24750466
1171. Shofty B, Ben-Sira L, Kesler A, Constantini S (2015). Optic pathway gliomas. Adv Tech Stand Neurosurg. 42:123–46. PMID:25411148
1172. Shoji J, Inada N, Sawa M (2006). Antibody array-generated cytokine profiles of tears of patients with vernal keratoconjunctivitis or giant papillary conjunctivitis. Jpn J Ophthalmol. 50(3):195–204. PMID:16767372
1173. Shukla SY, Shields JA, Eagle RC, Shields CL (2012). Transformation of optic disc melanocytoma into melanoma over 33 years. Arch Ophthalmol. 130(10):1344–7. PMID:23044959
1174. Shuler JD, Holland GN, Miles SA, Miller BJ, Grossman I (1989). Kaposi sarcoma of the conjunctiva and eyelids associated with the acquired immunodeficiency syndrome. Arch Ophthalmol. 107(6):858–62. PMID:2471496
1175. Ashur-Fabian O, Blumenthal DT, Bakon M, Nass D, Davis PJ, Hercbergs A (2013). Long-term response in high-grade optic glioma treated with medically induced hypothyroidism and carboplatin: a case report and review of the literature. Anticancer Drugs. 24(3):315–23. PMID:23348245
1176. Sia KJ, Tang IP, Kong CK, Tan TY (2012). Nasolacrimal relapse of nasopharyngeal carcinoma. J Laryngol Otol. 126(8):847–50. PMID:22804860
1177. Siddens JD, Fishman JR, Jackson IT, Nesi FA, Tsao K (1999). Primary orbital angiosarcoma: a case report. Ophthal Plast Reconstr Surg. 15(6):454–9. PMID:10588260
1178. Simunovic MP, Thaung C, da Cruz L, Sagoo MS, Egan C (2015). Small cell carcinoma of the lung metastatic to the retina: a clinicopathologic case report. Can J Ophthalmol. 50(6):e119–21. PMID:26651321
1179. Singh AD, Bergman L, Seregard S (2005). Uveal melanoma: epidemiologic aspects. Ophthalmol Clin North Am. 18(1):75–84,viii. PMID:15763193
1180. Singh AD, De Potter P, Fijal BA, Shields CL, Shields JA, Elston RC (1998). Lifetime prevalence of uveal melanoma in white patients with oculo(dermal) melanocytosis. Ophthalmology. 105(1):195–8. PMID:9442799
1181. Singh AD, Kalyani P, Topham A (2005). Estimating the risk of malignant transformation of a choroidal nevus. Ophthalmology. 112(10):1784–9. PMID:16154197
1182. Singh AD, Nouri M, Shields CL, Shields JA, Perez N (2002). Treatment of retinal capillary hemangioma. Ophthalmology. 109(10):1799–806. PMID:12359597
1183. Singh AD, Santos CM, Shields CL, Shields JA, Eagle RC Jr (2000). Observations on 17 patients with retinocytoma. Arch Ophthalmol. 118(2):199–205. PMID:10676785
1184. Singh AD, Shields CL, Shields JA, Sato T (2000). Uveal melanoma in young patients. Arch Ophthalmol. 118(7):918–23. PMID:10900104
1185. Singh AD, Topham A (2003). Incidence of uveal melanoma in the United States: 1973-1997. Ophthalmology. 110(5):956–61. PMID:12750097
1186. Singh AD, Turell ME, Topham AK (2011). Uveal melanoma: trends in incidence, treatment, and survival. Ophthalmology. 118(9):1881–5. PMID:21704381
1187. Singh AD (2007). Tumors of the uvea: benign melanocytic tumors. In: Singh AD, Damato BE, Pe'er J, Murphree AL, Perry J, editors. Clinical ophthalmic oncology. Philadelphia: Elsevier; pp. 185–97.
1189. Singh G, Sharma MC, Agarwal S, Prasad GL, Mishra S, Singh MM, et al. (2012). Epithelial-myoepithelial carcinoma of the lacrimal gland: a rare case. Ann Diagn Pathol. 16(4):292–7. PMID:21546298
1190. Singh P, Mathur SK, Singh S, Marwah N, Kalra R, Arora B (2005). Cystic lymphangioma of the spleen–a case report. Indian J Pathol Microbiol. 48(2):202–3. PMID:16758665
1191. Sisley K, Rennie IG, Parsons MA, Jacques R, Hammond DW, Bell SM, et al. (1997). Abnormalities of chromosomes 3 and 8 in posterior uveal melanoma correlate with prognosis. Genes Chromosomes Cancer. 19(1):22–8. PMID:9135991
1192. Sjö LD (2009). Ophthalmic lymphoma: epidemiology and pathogenesis. Acta Ophthalmol. 87 Thesis 1:1–20. PMID:19178392
1193. Sjö LD, Ralfkiaer E, Juhl BR, Prause JU, Kivelä T, Auw-Haedrich C, et al. (2006). Primary lymphoma of the lacrimal sac: an EORTC Ophthalmic Oncology Task Force study. Br J Ophthalmol. 90(8):1004–9. PMID:16672329
1194. Sjö N, Heegaard S, Prause JU (2000). Conjunctival papilloma. A histopathologically based retrospective study. Acta Ophthalmol Scand. 78(6):663–6. PMID:11167228
1195. Sjö NC, Heegaard S, Prause JU, von Buchwald C, Lindeberg H (2001). Human papillomavirus in conjunctival papilloma. Br J Ophthalmol. 85(7):785–7. PMID:11423448
1196. Sjö NC, von Buchwald C, Cassonnet P, Flamant P, Heegaard S, Norrild B, et al. (2007). Human papillomavirus: cause of epithelial lacrimal sac neoplasia? Acta Ophthalmol Scand. 85(5):551–6. PMID:17362365
1197. Skálová A, Gnepp DR, Lewis JS Jr, Hunt JL, Bishop JA, Hellquist H, et al. (2017). Newly described entities in salivary gland pathology. Am J Surg Pathol. 41(8):e33–47. PMID:28614209
1198. Skálová A, Weinreb I, Hyrcza M, Simpson RH, Laco J, Agaimy A, et al. (2015). Clear cell myoepithelial carcinoma of salivary glands showing EWSR1 rearrangement: molecular analysis of 94 salivary gland carcinomas with prominent clear cell component. Am J Surg Pathol. 39(3):338–48. PMID:25581728
1199. Skippen B, Lane CM, Hourihan M, Morris DS (2017). A case of mistaken identity: the role of lacrimal gland pleomorphic adenoma tissue diagnosis. Int Ophthalmol. 38(1):381–4. PMID:28108899
1200. Smedby KE, Hjalgrim H, Askling J, Chang ET, Gregersen H, Porwit-MacDonald A, et al. (2006). Autoimmune and chronic inflammatory disorders and risk of non-Hodgkin lymphoma by subtype. J Natl Cancer Inst. 98(1):51–60. PMID:16391371
1201. Smith PA, Damato BE, Ko MK, Lyness RW (1987). Anterior uveal neurilemmoma–a rare neoplasm simulating malignant melanoma. Br J Ophthalmol. 71(1):34–40. PMID:3545285
1202. Soler VJ, Tran-Viet KN, Galiacy SD, Limviphuvadh V, Klemm TP, St Germain E, et al. (2013). Whole exome sequencing identifies a mutation for a novel form of corneal intraepithelial dyskeratosis. J Med Genet. 50(4):246–54. PMID:23349227
1203. Soliman SE, Racher H, Zhang C, MacDonald H, Gallie BL (2017). Genetics and molecular diagnostics in retinoblastoma–an update. Asia Pac J Ophthalmol (Phila). 6(2):197–207. PMID:28399338
1204. Sommacal A, Campbell RJ, Helbig H (2003). Adenocarcinoma of the retinal pigment epithelium. Arch Ophthalmol. 121(10):1481–3. PMID:14557190
1205. Soon AK, Brownstein S, O'Connor M, Iordanous Y (2017). Fibrous histiocytoma of the conjunctiva. Ophthal Plast Reconstr Surg. 33(5):e133. PMID:27636240
1206. Sousa DC, Leal I (2016). Bilateral optic nerve metastases. Ophthalmology. 123(2):360. PMID:26802708
1207. Spaide RF (2016). Unilateral diffuse uveal melanocytic proliferation. Retin Cases Brief Rep. [EPUB ahead of print] PMID:28005580
1208. Spencer WH, Jesberg DO (1973). Glioneuroma (choristomatous malformation of the optic cup margin). A report of two cases. Arch Ophthalmol. 89(5):387–91. PMID:4697215
1209. Spitznas M, Koch F, Pohl S (1990). Ultrastructural pathology of anterior persistent hyperplastic primary vitreous. Graefes Arch Clin Exp Ophthalmol. 228(5):487–96. PMID:2227497
1210. Srikanth D, Devi V, Polishetty N, Singh D (2016). Subcutaneous benign fibrous histiocytoma: rare presentation on cheek-case report and review of literature. J Maxillofac Oral Surg. 15(Suppl 2):282–6. PMID:27408454
1211. Stacy RC, Kenyon KR, Jakobiec FA, Colby KA (2010). Conjunctival melanoma arising from primary acquired melanosis in a patient with neurofibromatosis type I. Cornea. 29(2):232–4. PMID:20023582
1212. Stadigh A, Puska P, Vesti E, Ristimäki A, Turunen JA, Kivelä TT (2017). Ring melanoma of the anterior chamber angle as a mimicker of pigmentary glaucoma. Surv Ophthalmol. 62(5):670–6. PMID:28159633
1213. Stagner AM, Jakobiec FA (2016). Updates on the molecular pathology of selected ocular and ocular adnexal tumors: potential targets for future therapy. Semin Ophthalmol. 31(1–2):188–96. PMID:26959146
1214. Stefanyszyn MA, Hidayat AA, Pe'er JJ, Flanagan JC (1994). Lacrimal sac tumors. Ophthal Plast Reconstr Surg. 10(3):169–84. PMID:7947444
1215. Stemmer-Rachamimov AO, Xu L, Gonzalez-Agosti C, Burwick JA, Pinney D, Beauchamp R, et al. (1997). Universal absence of merlin, but not other ERM family members, in schwannomas. Am J Pathol. 151(6):1649–54. PMID:9403715
1216. Stenman G (2013). Fusion oncogenes in salivary gland tumors: molecular and clinical consequences. Head Neck Pathol. 7 Suppl 1:S12–9. PMID:23821214
1217. Stephenson JA, Mayland DM, Ingall G, Frank TW (1988). Squamous cell carcinoma of the lacrimal sac. Otolaryngol Head Neck Surg. 99(5):524–7. PMID:3147447
1218. Stergiopoulos P, Link B, Naumann GO, Seitz B (2009). Solid corneal dermoids and subconjunctival lipodermoids: impact of differentiated surgical therapy on the functional long-term outcome. Cornea. 28(6):644–51. PMID:19512907
1219. Stern J, Jakobiec FA, Housepian EM (1980). The architecture of optic nerve gliomas with and without neurofibromatosis. Arch Ophthalmol. 98(3):505–11. PMID:6767467
1220. Stiller CA, Parkin DM (1996). Geographic and ethnic variations in the incidence of childhood cancer. Br Med Bull. 52(4):682–703. PMID:9039726
1221. Streeten BW, McGraw JL (1972). Tumor of the ciliary pigment epithelium. Am J Ophthalmol. 74(3):420–9. PMID:4115451
1222. Strominger MB, Schatz NJ, Glaser JS

(1993). Lymphomatous optic neuropathy. Am J Ophthalmol. 116(6):774–6. PMID:8250089
1223. Sturm V, Richard G (2007). The prevalence of bilateral malignant uveal melanoma. Klin Monatsbl Augenheilkd. 224(10):770–4. [German] PMID:17952820
1224. Subramaniam SS, Anand R, Mellor TK, Brennan PA (2017). Primary lacrimal sac melanoma with metastatic cervical disease: a review of the literature and case report. J Oral Maxillofac Surg. 75(7):1438–41. PMID:28215853
1225. Sugiura M, Colby KA, Mihm MC Jr, Zembowicz A (2007). Low-risk and high-risk histologic features in conjunctival primary acquired melanosis with atypia: clinicopathologic analysis of 29 cases. Am J Surg Pathol. 31(2):185–92. PMID:17255762
1226. Sukeda A, Mori T, Suzuki S, Ochiai A (2014). Adenocarcinoma of the pigmented ciliary epithelium. BMJ Case Rep. 2014. PMID:25015166
1227. Sultan I, Qaddoumi I, Yaser S, Rodriguez-Galindo C, Ferrari A (2009). Comparing adult and pediatric rhabdomyosarcoma in the Surveillance, Epidemiology and End Results program, 1973 to 2005: an analysis of 2,600 patients. J Clin Oncol. 27(20):3391–7. PMID:19398574
1228. Sumich P, Mitchell P, Wang JJ (1998). Choroidal nevi in a white population: the Blue Mountains Eye Study. Arch Ophthalmol. 116(5):645–50. PMID:9596501
1229. Sun EC, Fears TR, Goedert JJ (1997). Epidemiology of squamous cell conjunctival cancer. Cancer Epidemiol Biomarkers Prev. 6(2):73–7. PMID:9037556
1230. Sung KS, Kim DC, Ahn HB, Song YJ (2015). Pleomorphic adenoma with sarcomatous change in a lacrimal gland. J Korean Neurosurg Soc. 57(6):473–7. PMID:26180619
1231. Swerdlow SH, Campo E, Harris NL, Jaffe ES, Pileri SA, Stein H, et al., editors (2017). WHO classification of tumours of haematopoietic and lymphoid tissues. Revised 4th ed. Lyon: International Agency for Research on Cancer. Available from: http://publications.iarc.fr/556.
1232. Syed ZA, Chen TC (2016). New ultrasound biomicroscopy iris findings in juvenile xanthogranuloma. J Glaucoma. 25(8):e759–60. PMID:27483333
1233. Szalai E, Wells JR, Grossniklaus HE (2017). Mechanisms of optic nerve invasion in primary choroidal melanoma. Ocul Oncol Pathol. 3(4):267–75. PMID:29344479
1234. Szanto PA, Luna MA, Tortoledo ME, White RA (1984). Histologic grading of adenoid cystic carcinoma of the salivary glands. Cancer. 54(6):1062–9. PMID:6088017
1235. Szudek J, Joe H, Friedman JM (2002). Analysis of intrafamilial phenotypic variation in neurofibromatosis 1 (NF1). Genet Epidemiol. 23(2):150–64. PMID:12214308
1236. Tabin G, Levin S, Snibson G, Loughnan M, Taylor H (1997). Late recurrences and the necessity for long-term follow-up in corneal and conjunctival intraepithelial neoplasia. Ophthalmology. 104(3):485–92. PMID:9082277
1237. Tagawa Y, Namba K, Ogasawara R, Kanno H, Ishida S (2015). A case of mature natural killer-cell neoplasm manifesting multiple choroidal lesions: primary intraocular natural killer-cell lymphoma. Case Rep Ophthalmol. 6(3):380–4. PMID:26668579
1238. Takahashi BS, Bruè C, Spaide RF (2008). Autofluorescence characteristics of congenital hypertrophy of the retinal pigment epithelium. Retin Cases Brief Rep. 2(4):259–61. PMID:25390583
1239. Takahashi Y, Takahashi E, Nakakura S, Kitaguchi Y, Mupas-Uy J, Kakizaki H (2016). Risk factors for local recurrence or metastasis of eyelid sebaceous gland carcinoma after wide excision with paraffin section control. Am J Ophthalmol. 171:67–74. PMID:27590119
1240. Takahashi Y, Takahashi E, Nishimura K, Kakizaki H (2017). Immunoglobulin G4-related dacryocystitis. Can J Ophthalmol. 52(5):e188–90. PMID:28985831
1241. Takahira M, Nakamura Y, Shimizu S, Minato H, Katori N, Kobayashi H, et al. (2005). Carcinosarcoma of the lacrimal gland arising from a pleomorphic adenoma. Am J Ophthalmol. 140(2):337–40. PMID:16086968
1242. Talcott KE, Garg RJ, Garg SJ (2016). Ophthalmic manifestations of leukemia. Curr Opin Ophthalmol. 27(6):545–51. PMID:27585213
1243. Tan ACS, Yzer S, Atebara N, Marr BP, Verdijk RM, Dalm VASH, et al. (2017). Three cases of Erdheim-Chester disease with intraocular manifestations: imaging and histopathology findings of a rare entity. Am J Ophthalmol. 176:141–7. PMID:28153505
1244. Altan-Yaycioglu R, Bolat F, Akova YA (2007). Basosquamous carcinoma of the lacrimal sac: a case report. Orbit. 26(4):267–9. PMID:18097965
1245. Tang W, Hei Y, Xiao L (2013). Recurrent orbital space-occupying lesions: a clinicopathologic study of 253 cases. Chin J Cancer Res. 25(4):423–9. PMID:23997529
1246. Tay A, Scheithauer BW, Cameron JD, Myhre MJ, Boerner MJ (2009). Retinal ependymoma: an immunohistologic and ultrastructural study. Hum Pathol. 40(4):578–83. PMID:18835620
1247. Taylor BS, Barretina J, Maki RG, Antonescu CR, Singer S, Ladanyi M (2011). Advances in sarcoma genomics and new therapeutic targets. Nat Rev Cancer. 11(8):541–57. PMID:21753790
1248. Taylor HR, Burton MJ, Haddad D, West S, Wright H (2014). Trachoma. Lancet. 384(9960):2142–52. PMID:25043452
1249. Teixeira AI, Neno M, Badura R, Borges-Costa J, Filipe PL (2016). Kaposi sarcoma of the eyelid as an initial manifestation of AIDS. Dermatol Online J. 22(7). PMID:27617725
1250. Teo L, Seah LL, Choo CT, Chee SP, Chee E, Looi A (2013). A survey of the histopathology of lacrimal gland lesions in a tertiary referral centre. Orbit. 32(1):1–7. PMID:23387446
1251. Tetzlaff MT, Curry JL, Yin V, Pattanaprichakul P, Manonukul J, Uiprasertkul M, et al. (2015). Distinct pathways in the pathogenesis of sebaceous carcinomas implicated by differentially expressed microRNAs. JAMA Ophthalmol. 133(10):1109–16. PMID:26203913
1252. Thareja S, Rashid A, Grossniklaus HE (2014). Spontaneous necrosis of choroidal melanoma. Ocul Oncol Pathol. 1(1):63–9. PMID:27175363
1253. Thaung C, Bonshek RE, Leatherbarrow B (2006). Phakomatous choristoma of the eyelid: a case with associated eye abnormalities. Br J Ophthalmol. 90(2):245–6. PMID:16424545
1254. Collaborative Ocular Melanoma Study Group (1998). The Collaborative Ocular Melanoma Study (COMS) randomized trial of pre-enucleation radiation of large choroidal melanoma I: characteristics of patients enrolled and not enrolled. COMS report no. 9. Am J Ophthalmol. 125(6):767–78. PMID:9645715
1255. Thériault BL, Dimaras H, Gallie BL, Corson TW (2014). The genomic landscape of retinoblastoma: a review. Clin Experiment Ophthalmol. 42(1):33–52. PMID:24433356
1256. Thiagalingam S, Johnson MM, Colby KA, Zembowicz A (2008). Juvenile conjunctival nevus: clinicopathologic analysis of 33 cases. Am J Surg Pathol. 32(3):399–406. PMID:18300811
1257. Thomas AC, Zeng Z, Rivière JB, O'Shaughnessy R, Al-Olabi L, St-Onge J, et al. (2016). Mosaic activating mutations in GNA11 and GNAQ are associated with phakomatosis pigmentovascularis and extensive dermal melanocytosis. J Invest Dermatol. 136(4):770–8. PMID:26778290
1258. Thomas AJ, Erickson CA (2008). The making of a melanocyte: the specification of melanoblasts from the neural crest. Pigment Cell Melanoma Res. 21(6):598–610. PMID:19067969
1259. Thong BY (2017). Allergic conjunctivitis in Asia. Asia Pac Allergy. 7(2):57–64. PMID:28487836
1260. Thuro BA, Ning J, Peng SA, Pace ST, Dudeja G, Ozgur O, et al. (2017). Rates of positive findings on positron emission tomography and bone marrow biopsy in patients with ocular adnexal lymphoma. Ophthal Plast Reconstr Surg. 33(5):355–60. PMID:27636243
1261. Tibolt RE, Meyer DR, Wobig JL (1991). Small-cell carcinoma metastatic to the lacrimal gland. Arch Ophthalmol. 109(7):921–2. PMID:1648346
1262. Tijl J, Koornneef L, Eijpe A, Thomas L, Gonzalez DG, Veenhof C (1992). Metastatic tumors to the orbit–management and prognosis. Graefes Arch Clin Exp Ophthalmol. 230(6):527–30. PMID:1427135
1263. Timoney PJ, Bradley M, Cowen DE (2011). A rare case of progressive ptosis caused by lacrimal gland oncocytoma. Ophthal Plast Reconstr Surg. 27(4):e85–7. PMID:21283034
1264. Tiong T, Borooah S, Msosa J, Dean W, Smith C, Kambewa E, et al. (2013). Clinicopathological review of ocular surface squamous neoplasia in Malawi. Br J Ophthalmol. 97(8):961–4. PMID:23613511
1265. Torbidoni AV, Laurent VE, Sampor C, Ottaviani D, Vazquez V, Gabri MR, et al. (2015). Association of cone-rod homeobox transcription factor messenger RNA with pediatric metastatic retinoblastoma. JAMA Ophthalmol. 133(7):805–12. PMID:25928893
1266. Toth J, Karcioglu ZA, Moshfeghi AA, Issa TM, Al-Ma'ani JR, Patel KV (2000). The relationship between human papillomavirus and p53 gene in conjunctival squamous cell carcinoma. Cornea. 19(2):159–62. PMID:10746446
1267. Traber GL, Pangalu A, Neumann M, Costa J, Weller M, Huna-Baron R, et al. (2015). Malignant optic glioma - the spectrum of disease in a case series. Graefes Arch Clin Exp Ophthalmol. 253(7):1187–94. PMID:26004076
1268. Traboulsi EI, Krush AJ, Gardner EJ, Booker SV, Offerhaus GJ, Yardley JH, et al. (1987). Prevalence and importance of pigmented ocular fundus lesions in Gardner's syndrome. N Engl J Med. 316(11):661–7. PMID:3821797
1269. Traboulsi EI, Maumenee IH, Krush AJ, Giardiello FM, Levin LS, Hamilton SR (1988). Pigmented ocular fundus lesions in the inherited gastrointestinal polyposis syndromes and in hereditary nonpolyposis colorectal cancer. Ophthalmology. 95(7):964–9. PMID:2845322
1270. Traboulsi EI, Murphy SF, de la Cruz ZC, Maumenee IH, Green WR (1990). A clinicopathologic study of the eyes in familial adenomatous polyposis with extracolonic manifestations (Gardner's syndrome). Am J Ophthalmol. 110(5):550–61. PMID:2173407
1271. Traynis I, Singer S, Winterkorn J, Rosenblum M, Dinkin M (2014). Infiltration of the optic chiasm, nerve, and disc by gliomatosis cerebri. J Neuroophthalmol. 34(1):44–6. PMID:23287703
1272. Triay E, Bergman L, Nilsson B, All-Ericsson C, Seregard S (2009). Time trends in the incidence of conjunctival melanoma in Sweden. Br J Ophthalmol. 93(11):1524–8. PMID:19628487
1273. Trichopoulos N, Augsburger JJ, Schneider S (2006). Adenocarcinoma arising from congenital hypertrophy of the retinal pigment epithelium. Graefes Arch Clin Exp Ophthalmol. 244(1):125–8. PMID:15983818
1274. Tripathi RC, Tripathi BJ, Ringus J (1981). Phakomatous choristoma of the lower eyelid with psammoma body formation: a light and electron microscopic study. Ophthalmology. 88(12):1198–206. PMID:7322468
1275. Tripathy D, Mittal R (2014). Dermolipoma of the lower eyelid. Orbit. 33(3):193–5. PMID:24409831
1276. Trubnik V, Conley R, Ritterband DC, Udell I, Thompson G, Shih C, et al. (2011). Progressive growth in epibulbar complex choristomas: report of 2 cases and review of literature. Cornea. 30(11):1267–9. PMID:21885965
1277. Ts'o MO, Fine BS, Zimmerman LE (1969). The Flexner-Wintersteiner rosettes in retinoblastoma. Arch Pathol. 88(6):664–71. PMID:5357720
1278. Ts'o MO, Fine BS, Zimmerman LE (1970). The nature of retinoblastoma. II. Photoreceptor differentiation: an electron microscopic study. Am J Ophthalmol. 69(3):350–9. PMID:5418851
1279. Ts'o MO, Zimmerman LE, Fine BS (1970). The nature of retinoblastoma. I. Photoreceptor differentiation: a clinical and histopathologic study. Am J Ophthalmol. 69(3):339–49. PMID:4190798
1280. Tsai AS, Lee KY, Al Jajeh I, Sittampalam K, Fong KS (2008). Epibulbar osseous choristoma: a report of two cases. Orbit. 27(3):231–3. PMID:18569837
1281. Tsai JH, Galaydh F, Ching SS (2005). Anterior uveitis and iris nodules that are associated with Langerhans cell histiocytosis. Am J Ophthalmol. 140(6):1143–5. PMID:16376670
1282. Tso MO (1980). Clues to the cells of origin in retinoblastoma. Int Ophthalmol Clin. 20(2):191–210. PMID:6995387
1283. Tso MO, Albert DM (1972). Pathological condition of the retinal pigment epithelium. Neoplasms and nodular non-neoplastic lesions. Arch Ophthalmol. 88(1):27–38. PMID:5049451
1284. Tsuchihashi T, Murayama K, Saito T, Ebisawa N, Yoneya S (2005). Midperipheral mottling pigmentation with familial choroidal osteoma. Retina. 25(1):63–8. PMID:15655443
1285. Tucker N, Chow D, Stockl F, Codère F, Burnier M (1997). Clinically suspected primary acquired nasolacrimal duct obstruction: clinicopathologic review of 150 patients. Ophthalmology. 104(11):1882–6. PMID:9373121
1286. Tuncer S, Cebeci Z (2014). Dramatic regression of presumed acquired retinal astrocytoma with photodynamic therapy. Middle East Afr J Ophthalmol. 21(3):283–6. PMID:25100919
1287. Tuomaala S, Eskelin S, Tarkkanen A, Kivelä T (2002). Population-based assessment of clinical characteristics predicting outcome of conjunctival melanoma in whites. Invest Ophthalmol Vis Sci. 43(11):3399–408. PMID:12407149
1288. Tuomaala S, Kivelä T (2004). Metastatic pattern and survival in disseminated conjunctival melanoma: implications for sentinel lymph node biopsy. Ophthalmology. 111(4):816–21. PMID:15051218
1289. Turner HC, Budak MT, Akinci MA, Wolosin JM (2007). Comparative analysis of human conjunctival and corneal epithelial gene expression with oligonucleotide microarrays. Invest Ophthalmol Vis Sci. 48(5):2050–61. PMID:17460260
1290. Turunen JA, Markkinen S, Wilska R, Saarinen S, Raivio V, Täll M, et al. (2016). BAP1 germline mutations in Finnish patients with uveal melanoma. Ophthalmology. 123(5):1112–7. PMID:26876698
1291. Tzu JH, Cavuoto KM, Villegas VM,

Dubovy SR, Capo H (2014). Optical coherence tomography findings of pigmented fundus lesions in familial adenomatous polyposis. Ophthalmic Surg Lasers Imaging Retina. 45(1):69–70. PMID:24266367
1292. Ulbright TM, Fulling KH, Helveston EM (1984). Astrocytic tumors of the retina. Differentiation of sporadic tumors from phakomatosis-associated tumors. Arch Pathol Lab Med. 108(2):160–3. PMID:6421263
1293. Ustaalioglu BB, Bilici A, Seker M, Gumus M, Ozdemir N, Salman T, et al. (2009). Bilateral primary small lymphocytic lymphoma of the lacrimal sac and review of the literature. Leuk Res. 33(11):e184–5. PMID:19493568
1293A. Usui M, Ishii S, Yamawaki S, Hirayama T (1984). The occurrence of soft tissue sarcomas in three siblings with Werner's syndrome. Cancer. 54(11):2580–6. PMID:6498750
1294. Uusitalo E, Leppävirta J, Koffert A, Suominen S, Vahtera J, Vahlberg T, et al. (2015). Incidence and mortality of neurofibromatosis: a total population study in Finland. J Invest Dermatol. 135(3):904–6. PMID:25354145
1295. Auw-Haedrich C, Danielewicz KD, Mendoza PR, Reinhard T, Grossniklaus HE (2016). Conjunctival stromal tumor: expansion of findings in a newly described entity. Ophthalmology. 123(5):1166–7. PMID:26778331
1296. Vachette M, Moulin A, Zografos L, Schalenbourg A (2012). Epibulbar osseous choristoma: a clinicopathological case series and review of the literature. Klin Monatsbl Augenheilkd. 229(4):420–3. PMID:22496017
1297. Vader MJC, Madigan MC, Versluis M, Suleiman HM, Gezgin G, Gruis NA, et al. (2017). GNAQ and GNA11 mutations and downstream YAP activation in choroidal nevi. Br J Cancer. 117(6):884–7. PMID:28809862
1298. Vagge A, Camicione P, Capris C, Sburlati C, Panarello S, Calevo MG, et al. (2015). Choroidal abnormalities in neurofibromatosis type 1 detected by near-infrared reflectance imaging in paediatric population. Acta Ophthalmol. 93(8):e667–71. PMID:25990002
1299. Vagia E, Economopoulou P, Oikonomopoulos N, Athanasiadis I, Dimitriadis G, Psyrri A (2015). Androgen-receptor positive lacrimal sac adenocarcinoma demonstrating long-lasting response to LHRH analog plus abiraterone treatment. Front Oncol. 5:10. PMID:25699235
1300. Vajdic CM, van Leeuwen MT, McDonald SP, McCredie MR, Law M, Chapman JR, et al. (2007). Increased incidence of squamous cell carcinoma of eye after kidney transplantation. J Natl Cancer Inst. 99(17):1340–2. PMID:17698951
1301. Valenzuela AA, McNab AA, Selva D, O'Donnell BA, Whitehead KJ, Sullivan TJ (2006). Clinical features and management of tumors affecting the lacrimal drainage apparatus. Ophthal Plast Reconstr Surg. 22(2):96–101. PMID:16550051
1302. van de Nes JA, Nelles J, Kreis S, Metz CH, Hager T, Lohmann DR, et al. (2016). Comparing the prognostic value of BAP1 mutation pattern, chromosome 3 status, and BAP1 immunohistochemistry in uveal melanoma. Am J Surg Pathol. 40(6):796–805. PMID:27015033
1303. van Essen TH, van Pelt SI, Versluis M, Bronkhorst IH, van Duinen SG, Marinkovic M, et al. (2014). Prognostic parameters in uveal melanoma and their association with BAP1 expression. Br J Ophthalmol. 98(12):1738–43. PMID:25147369
1304. van Poppelen NM, Vaarwater J, Mudhar HS, Sisley K, Rennie IG, Rundle P, et al. (2018). Genetic background of iris melanomas and iris melanocytic tumors of uncertain malignant potential. Ophthalmology. 125(6):904–12. PMID:29371009
1305. Van Raamsdonk CD, Bezrookove V, Green G, Bauer J, Gaugler L, O'Brien JM, et al. (2009). Frequent somatic mutations of GNAQ in uveal melanoma and blue naevi. Nature. 457(7229):599–602. PMID:19078957
1306. Van Raamsdonk CD, Griewank KG, Crosby MB, Garrido MC, Vemula S, Wiesner T, et al. (2010). Mutations in GNA11 in uveal melanoma. N Engl J Med. 363(23):2191–9. PMID:21083380
1307. van Klink F, de Keizer RJ, Jager MJ, Kakebeeke-Kemme HM (1992). Iris nevi and melanomas: a clinical follow-up study. Doc Ophthalmol. 82(1–2):49–55. PMID:1305027
1308. Vander Poorten V, Triantafyllou A, Thompson LD, Bishop J, Hauben E, Hunt J, et al. (2016). Salivary acinic cell carcinoma: reappraisal and update. Eur Arch Otorhinolaryngol. 273(11):3511–31. PMID:26685679
1309. Vangveeravong S, Katz SE, Rootman J, White V (1996). Tumors arising in the palpebral lobe of the lacrimal gland. Ophthalmology. 103(10):1606–12. PMID:8874433
1310. Vannas S, Raitta C, Tarkkanen A (1974). Neurilemmoma of the choroid in Recklinghausen's disease. Acta Ophthalmol Suppl. 123:126–33. PMID:4368953
1311. Vatansever M, Bozkurt FM, Dinç E, Yılmaz EB, Nayir E, Sarı AA, et al. (2016). Orbital metastasis of multiple myeloma: case report. Turk J Ophthalmol. 46(3):148–50. PMID:27800278
1312. Vékony H, Leemans CR, Ylstra B, Meijer GA, van der Waal I, Bloemena E (2009). Salivary gland carcinosarcoma: oligonucleotide array CGH reveals similar genomic profiles in epithelial and mesenchymal components. Oral Oncol. 45(3):259–65. PMID:18693132
1313. Vékony H, Röser K, Löning T, Raaphorst FM, Leemans CR, Van der Waal I, et al. (2008). Deregulated expression of p16INK4a and p53 pathway members in benign and malignant myoepithelial tumours of the salivary glands. Histopathology. 53(6):658–66. PMID:19076682
1314. Velazquez-Martin JP, Krema H, Fulda E, Yücel YH, Simpson ER, Pavlin CJ (2013). Ultrasound biomicroscopy of the ciliary body in ocular/oculodermal melanocytosis. Am J Ophthalmol. 155(4):681–7.e1-2. PMID:23219068
1315. Vemuganti GK, Honavar SG, Jalali S (2002). Intraocular osseous metaplasia. A clinico-pathological study. Indian J Ophthalmol. 50(3):183–8. PMID:12355691
1316. Venkatesulu BP, Pathy S, Vallonthaiel AG, Chawla B (2015). Epithelial-myoepithelial carcinoma of lacrimal gland from an ex pleomorphic adenoma. BMJ Case Rep. 2015. PMID:26231189
1317. Venturini G, Moulin AP, Deprez M, Uffer S, Bottani A, Zografos L, et al. (2012). Clinicopathologic and molecular analysis of a choroidal pigmented schwannoma in the context of a PTEN hamartoma tumor syndrome. Ophthalmology. 119(4):857–64. PMID:22281088
1318. Verdijk RM (2016). On the classification and grading of medulloepithelioma of the eye. Ocul Oncol Pathol. 2(3):190–3. PMID:27239464
1319. Verdijk RM, Pecorella I, Mooy CM (2015). The orbit, including the lacrimal gland and lacrimal drainage system. In: Heegaard S, Grossniklaus H, editors. Eye pathology: an illustrated guide. Berlin: Springer-Verlag; pp. 547–731.
1323. Verma V, Shen D, Sieving PC, Chan CC (2008). The role of infectious agents in the etiology of ocular adnexal neoplasia. Surv Ophthalmol. 53(4):312–31. PMID:18572051
1324. Vermeulen TL, Isaacs TW, Spagnolo D, Amanuel B (2013). Rosai-Dorfman disease presenting as choroidal melanoma: a case report and review of the literature. Graefes Arch Clin Exp Ophthalmol. 251(1):295–9. PMID:23090417
1325. Vervaet N, Van Ginderdeuren R, Van Den Oord JJ, Foets B (2007). A rare conjunctival Spitz nevus: a case report and literature review. Bull Soc Belge Ophtalmol. (303):63–7. PMID:17894290
1326. Vickers JL, Matherne RJ, Allison AW, Wilkerson MG, Tyring SK, Bartlett BL, et al. (2010). Transitional cell neoplasm of the nasolacrimal duct associated with human papillomavirus type 11. J Cutan Pathol. 37(7):793–6. PMID:19615034
1327. Villegas VM, Hess DJ, Wildner A, Gold AS, Murray TG (2013). Retinoblastoma. Curr Opin Ophthalmol. 24(6):581–8. PMID:24100372
1328. Viola F, Villani E, Natacci F, Selicorni A, Melloni G, Vezzola D, et al. (2012). Choroidal abnormalities detected by near-infrared reflectance imaging as a new diagnostic criterion for neurofibromatosis 1. Ophthalmology. 119(2):369–75. PMID:21963267
1329. Virgili G, Gatta G, Ciccolallo L, Capocaccia R, Biggeri A, Crocetti E, et al. (2007). Incidence of uveal melanoma in Europe. Ophthalmology. 114(12):2309–15. PMID:17498805
1330. Vizcaíno MA, Bishop J, Sharma R, Refaey K, Quiñones-Hinojosa A, Rodriguez FJ (2016). Intracranial solitary fibrous tumor/hemangiopericytoma with osteoclast-like multinucleated giant cells: comparison with giant cell-rich solitary fibrous tumor. Clin Neuropathol. 35(4):171–7. PMID:27049065
1331. von Holstein SL (2013). Tumours of the lacrimal gland. Epidemiological, clinical and genetic characteristics. Acta Ophthalmol. 91 Thesis 6:1–28. PMID:24893972
1332. von Holstein SL, Coupland SE, Briscoe D, Le Tourneau C, Heegaard S (2013). Epithelial tumours of the lacrimal gland: a clinical, histopathological, surgical and oncological survey. Acta Ophthalmol. 91(3):195–206. PMID:22471335
1333. Von Holstein SL, Fehr A, Heegaard S, Therkildsen MH, Stenman G (2012). CRTC1-MAML2 gene fusion in mucoepidermoid carcinoma of the lacrimal gland. Oncol Rep. 27(5):1413–6. PMID:22323114
1334. von Holstein SL, Fehr A, Persson M, Nickelsen M, Therkildsen MH, Prause JU, et al. (2014). Lacrimal gland pleomorphic adenoma and carcinoma ex pleomorphic adenoma: genomic profiles, gene fusions, and clinical characteristics. Ophthalmology. 121(5):1125–33. PMID:24468654
1335. von Holstein SL, Rasmussen PK, Heegaard S (2016). Tumors of the lacrimal gland. Semin Diagn Pathol. 33(3):156–63. PMID:26849904
1336. von Holstein SL, Therkildsen MH, Prause JU, Stenman G, Siersma VD, Heegaard S (2013). Lacrimal gland lesions in Denmark between 1974 and 2007. Acta Ophthalmol. 91(4):349–54. PMID:22471375
1337. von Goscinski C, Koch KR, Cursiefen C, Heindl LM (2016). Tumors of the lacrimal drainage system. HNO. 64(6):386–93. [German] PMID:27222017
1338. Vora GK, Demirci H, Marr B, Mruthyunjaya P (2017). Advances in the management of conjunctival melanoma. Surv Ophthalmol. 62(1):26–42. PMID:27321895
1339. Vortmeyer AO, Frank S, Jeong SY, Yuan K, Ikejiri B, Lee YS, et al. (2003). Developmental arrest of angioblastic lineage initiates tumorigenesis in von Hippel-Lindau disease. Cancer Res. 63(21):7051–5. PMID:14612494
1340. Vozmediano-Serrano MT, Toledano-Fernández N, Fdez-Aceñero MJ, Gil-Díez JL, García-Saenz S (2006). Lacrimal sac metastases from renal cell carcinoma. Orbit. 25(3):249–51. PMID:16987775
1341. Wachtel JG, Caplan CW, Makley TA Jr (1967). Juvenile melanoma (mixed spindle cell and epithelioid cell nevus) of the conjunctiva. Surv Ophthalmol. 12(1):12–6. PMID:6040928
1342. Wada K, Arai C, Suda T, Nagaoka M, Shimura E, Yanagisawa S, et al. (2015). Primary adenoid cystic carcinoma of the nasolacrimal duct treated with proton beam therapy. Auris Nasus Larynx. 42(6):496–500. PMID:25998851
1343. Walijee HZ, Berry S, Quine S, Lane C, Morris DS, Bowman B (2015). Inverted papilloma originating primarily from the nasolacrimal duct: a case report and review of the pertinent literature. Case Rep Otolaryngol. 2015:123694. PMID:26649215
1344. Walker BA, Saltzman BS, Herlihy EP, Luquetti DV (2017). Phenotypic characterization of epibulbar dermoids. Int Ophthalmol. 37(3):499–505. PMID:27405313
1345. Walter JW, Blei F, Anderson JL, Orlow SJ, Speer MC, Marchuk DA (1999). Genetic mapping of a novel familial form of infantile hemangioma. Am J Med Genet. 82(1):77–83. PMID:9916848
1346. Walter JW, North PE, Waner M, Mizeracki A, Blei F, Walker JW, et al. (2002). Somatic mutation of vascular endothelial growth factor receptors in juvenile hemangioma. Genes Chromosomes Cancer. 33(3):295–303. PMID:11807987
1347. Walter SD, Chao DL, Feuer W, Schiffman J, Char DH, Harbour JW (2016). Prognostic implications of tumor diameter in association with gene expression profile for uveal melanoma. JAMA Ophthalmol. 134(7):734–40. PMID:27123792
1348. Walther C, Hofvander J, Nilsson J, Magnusson L, Domanski HA, Gisselsson D, et al. (2015). Gene fusion detection in formalin-fixed paraffin-embedded benign fibrous histiocytomas using fluorescence in situ hybridization and RNA sequencing. Lab Invest. 95(9):1071–6. PMID:26121314
1349. Wan WL, Geller JL, Feldon SE, Sadun AA (1990). Visual loss caused by rapidly progressive intracranial meningiomas during pregnancy. Ophthalmology. 97(1):18–21. PMID:2314836
1350. Wang W, Chen L (2017). Cavernous hemangioma of the retina: a comprehensive review of the literature (1934-2015). Retina. 37(4):611–21. PMID:27820777
1351. Wang XN, Qian J, Yuan YF, Zhang R, Zhang YQ (2012). Space-occupying lesions of the lacrimal gland at one tertiary eye center in China: a retrospective clinical study of 95 patients. Int J Ophthalmol. 5(2):208–11. PMID:22762051
1352. Watanabe A, Andrew NH, Ueda K, Kinoshita S, Katori N, Reid M, et al. (2016). Clinico-radiological features of primary lacrimal gland pleomorphic adenoma: an analysis of 37 cases. Jpn J Ophthalmol. 60(4):286–93. PMID:27184391
1353. Webster AR, Anderson JR, Richards EM, Moore AT (1995). Ischaemic retinopathy occurring in patients receiving bone marrow allografts and campath-1G: a clinicopathological study. Br J Ophthalmol. 79(7):687–91. PMID:7662637
1354. Weinreb I, Tabanda-Lichauco R, Van der Kwast T, Perez-Ordoñez B (2006). Low-grade intraductal carcinoma of salivary gland: report of 3 cases with marked apocrine differentiation. Am J Surg Pathol. 30(8):1014–21. PMID:16861974
1355. Weis E, Rootman J, Joly TJ, Berean KW, Al-Katan HM, Pasternak S, et al. (2009). Epithelial lacrimal gland tumors: pathologic classification and current understanding. Arch Ophthalmol. 127(8):1016–28. PMID:19667339

1356. Weisbrod DJ, Pavlin CJ, Xu W, Simpson ER (2010). Long-term follow-up of 42 patients with small ciliary body tumors with ultrasound biomicroscopy. Am J Ophthalmol. 149(4):616–22. PMID:20346778
1357. Weiss SW, Langloss JM, Enzinger FM (1983). Value of S-100 protein in the diagnosis of soft tissue tumors with particular reference to benign and malignant Schwann cell tumors. Lab Invest. 49(3):299–308. PMID:6310227
1358. Weiss SW, Goldblum JR, editors (2008). Malignant vascular tumors. In: Enzinger and Weiss's soft tissue tumors. Philadelphia: Elsevier; pp. 703–30.
1360. Wemmert S, Willnecker V, Brunner C, Wenzel GI, Sauter B, Meinelt H, et al. (2013). New genetic findings in parotid gland pleomorphic adenomas. Head Neck. 35(10):1431–8. PMID:22987447
1361. Werner JU, Lang GK, Enders C (2017). Free-floating intraocular cysts. Klin Monbl Augenheilkd. [German] [EPUB ahead of print] PMID:28470658
1362. Werner RL, Castle JT (2014). Recurrent pleomorphic adenoma. Head Neck Pathol. 8(3):303–6. PMID:24197723
1363. Whalen KE, Eagle RC Jr, Vrabec TR (2018). A case of metastatic urothelial carcinoma of the retina and vitreous. Retin Cases Brief Rep. 12(3):177–180. PMID:27930437
1364. White VA (2012). Update on lacrimal gland neoplasms: molecular pathology of interest. Saudi J Ophthalmol. 26(2):133–5. PMID:23960983
1365. White VA, Chambers JD, Courtright PD, Chang WY, Horsman DE (1998). Correlation of cytogenetic abnormalities with the outcome of patients with uveal melanoma. Cancer. 83(2):354–9. PMID:9669819
1366. White VA, Damji KF, Richards JS, Rootman J (1991). Leiomyosarcoma of the conjunctiva. Ophthalmology. 98(10):1560–4. PMID:1961645
1367. Wiesner T, Obenauf AC, Murali R, Fried I, Griewank KG, Ulz P, et al. (2011). Germline mutations in BAP1 predispose to melanocytic tumors. Nat Genet. 43(10):1018–21. PMID:21874003
1368. Wilkes SR, Campbell RJ, Waller RR (1981). Ocular malformation in association with ipsilateral facial nevus of Jadassohn. Am J Ophthalmol. 92(3):344–52. PMID:7294093
1369. Williams AT, Font RL, Van Dyk HJ, Riekhof FT (1978). Osseous choristoma of the choroid simulating a choroidal melanoma. Association with a positive 32P test. Arch Ophthalmol. 96(10):1874–7. PMID:697626
1370. Wilson DJ, Braziel R, Rosenbaum JT (1992). Intraocular lymphoma. Immunopathologic analysis of vitreous biopsy specimens. Arch Ophthalmol. 110(10):1455–8. PMID:1417546
1371. Wimmer K, Eckart M, Meyer-Puttlitz B, Fonatsch C, Pietsch T (2002). Mutational and expression analysis of the NF1 gene argues against a role as tumor suppressor in sporadic pilocytic astrocytomas. J Neuropathol Exp Neurol. 61(10):896–902. PMID:12387455
1372. Wirz K, Lee WR, Coaker T (1982). Progressive changes in congenital hypertrophy of the retinal pigment epithelium. Graefes Arch Clin Exp Ophthalmol. 219(5):214–21. PMID:7160628
1373. Witschel H, Font RL (1976). Hemangioma of the choroid. A clinicopathologic study of 71 cases and a review of the literature. Surv Ophthalmol. 20(6):415–31. PMID:820013
1374. Witt RL, Eisele DW, Morton RP, Nicolai P, Poorten VV, Zbären P (2015). Etiology and management of recurrent parotid pleomorphic adenoma. Laryngoscope. 125(4):888–93. PMID:25289881
1375. Wittekindt C, Streubel K, Arnold G, Stennert E, Guntinas-Lichius O (2007). Recurrent pleomorphic adenoma of the parotid gland: analysis of 108 consecutive patients. Head Neck. 29(9):822–8. PMID:17563905
1376. Wiwatwongwana D, Berean KW, Dolman PJ, Rootman J, White VA (2009). Unusual carcinomas of the lacrimal gland: epithelial-myoepithelial carcinoma and myoepithelial carcinoma. Arch Ophthalmol. 127(8):1054–6. PMID:19667347
1377. Wiwatwongwana D, White VA, Dolman PJ (2010). Two cases of periocular cutaneous angiosarcoma. Ophthal Plast Reconstr Surg. 26(5):365–6. PMID:20856078
1378. Wladis EJ, Frempong T, Gausas R (2007). Nasolacrimal metastasis from heptocellular carcinoma masquerading as dacryocystitis. Ophthal Plast Reconstr Surg. 23(4):333–5. PMID:17667118
1379. Wolber RA, Talerman A, Wilkinson EJ, Clement PB (1991). Vulvar granular cell tumors with pseudocarcinomatous hyperplasia: a comparative analysis with well-differentiated squamous carcinoma. Int J Gynecol Pathol. 10(1):59–66. PMID:1848836
1380. Wolf EJ, Wessel MM, Hirsch MD, Leib ML (2007). Reactive lymphoid hyperplasia of the nasolacrimal duct presenting as bloody epiphora. Ophthal Plast Reconstr Surg. 23(3):242–3. PMID:17519671
1381. Wong AJ, Planck SR, Choi D, Harrington CA, Troxell ML, Houghton DC, et al. (2014). IgG4 immunostaining and its implications in orbital inflammatory disease. PLoS One. 9(10):e109847. PMID:25303270
1382. Wong JY, Uhl V, Wara WM, Sheline GE (1987). Optic gliomas. A reanalysis of the University of California, San Francisco experience. Cancer. 60(8):1847–55. PMID:3652011
1383. Woo KI, Yeom A, Esmaeli B (2016). Management of lacrimal gland carcinoma: lessons from the literature in the past 40 years. Ophthal Plast Reconstr Surg. 32(1):1–10. PMID:26291539
1384. Wright JE, McNab AA, McDonald WI (1989). Primary optic nerve sheath meningioma. Br J Ophthalmol. 73(12):960–6. PMID:2611192
1385. Xian J, Xu Q, Wang Z, Yang B, Wei W, Yan Z, et al. (2010). MR imaging of adenomas of the nonpigmented ciliary epithelium of the eye. AJNR Am J Neuroradiol. 31(5):886–90. PMID:20044507
1386. Xiong MJ, Dim DC (2015). Conjunctival myxoma: a synopsis of a rare ocular tumor. Arch Pathol Lab Med. 139(5):693–7. PMID:25927154
1387. Xu XL, Fang Y, Lee TC, Forrest D, Gregory-Evans C, Almeida D, et al. (2009). Retinoblastoma has properties of a cone precursor tumor and depends upon cone-specific MDM2 signaling. Cell. 137(6):1018–31. PMID:19524506
1388. Yalcinbayir O, Gelisken O, Sen F, Yasar S, Alizadegan F (2017). Retinal metastasis from squamous cell carcinoma of the lung: a case presentation. Retin Cases Brief Rep. [EPUB ahead of print] PMID:28221259
1389. Yamamoto N, Kiyosawa M, Kawasaki T, Miki T, Fujino T, Tokoro T (1994). Successfully treated optic nerve infiltration with adult T-cell lymphoma. J Neuroophthalmol. 14(2):81–3. PMID:7951932
1390. Yan J, Liu X, Zhang P, Li Y (2015). Acquired adenoma of the nonpigmented ciliary epithelium: analysis of five cases. Graefes Arch Clin Exp Ophthalmol. 253(4):637–44. PMID:25605545
1391. Yang BT, Wang YZ, Wang XY, Wang ZC (2012). Mesenchymal chondrosarcoma of the orbit: CT and MRI findings. Clin Radiol. 67(4):346–51. PMID:22177886
1392. Yang HS, Jeong HR, Kim CW, Yoon YH, Kim JG (2013). Histological heterogeneity between primary and metastatic cancer in a pathologic confirmed case of isolated optic disc metastasis of prostate adenocarcinoma. Graefes Arch Clin Exp Ophthalmol. 251(1):375–8. PMID:23188520
1393. Yang J, Foster CS (1997). Squamous cell carcinoma of the conjunctiva. Int Ophthalmol Clin. 37(4):73–85. PMID:9429933
1394. Yanoff M, Zimmerman LE (1967). Histogenesis of malignant melanomas of the uvea. 3. The relationship of congenital ocular melanocytosis and neurofibromatosis in uveal melanomas. Arch Ophthalmol. 77(3):331–6. PMID:6019552
1395. Yasunari T, Shiraki K, Hattori H, Miki T (2000). Frequency of choroidal abnormalities in neurofibromatosis type 1. Lancet. 356(9234):988–92. PMID:11041400
1396. Yeh S, Wilson DJ (2010). Pars plana vitrectomy and endoresection of a retinal vasoproliferative tumor. Arch Ophthalmol. 128(9):1196–9. PMID:20837805
1397. Yen MT, Bilyk JR, Wladis EJ, Bradley EA, Mawn LA (2018). Treatments for ocular adnexal lymphoma: a report by the American Academy of Ophthalmology. Ophthalmology. 125(1):127–36. PMID:28712656
1398. Yildiz I, Sen F, Tuncer S, Kilic L, Basaran M, Bavbek S (2011). Optic disc and choroidal metastasis from sporadic medullary thyroid carcinoma: case report and review of the literature. Onkologie. 34(11):630–3. PMID:22104161
1399. Yilmaz I, Gamsizkan M, Sari SO, Yaman B, Demirkesen C, Heper A, et al. (2015). Molecular alterations in malignant blue nevi and related blue lesions. Virchows Arch. 467(6):723–32. PMID:26403583
1400. Yip CC, Au EK, Choo CT (2002). Lacrimal sac tumour presenting with blood-stained ocular discharge. Singapore Med J. 43(3):156–8. PMID:12005344
1401. Yip CC, Bartley GB, Habermann TM, Garrity JA (2002). Involvement of the lacrimal drainage system by leukemia or lymphoma. Ophthal Plast Reconstr Surg. 18(4):242–6. PMID:12142754
1402. Yonekawa Y, Kim IK (2012). Epidemiology and management of uveal melanoma. Hematol Oncol Clin North Am. 26(6):1169–84. PMID:23116575
1403. You JY, Finger PT, Iacob C, McCormick SA, Milman T (2013). Intraocular schwannoma. Surv Ophthalmol. 58(1):77–85. PMID:22981398
1404. Yousef YA, Finger PT (2012). Squamous carcinoma and dysplasia of the conjunctiva and cornea: an analysis of 101 cases. Ophthalmology. 119(2):233–40. PMID:22189448
1405. Yu FX, Luo J, Mo JS, Liu G, Kim YC, Meng Z, et al. (2014). Mutant Gq/11 promote uveal melanoma tumorigenesis by activating YAP. Cancer Cell. 25(6):822–30. PMID:24882516
1406. Yu GP, Hu DN, McCormick S, Finger PT (2003). Conjunctival melanoma: is it increasing in the United States? Am J Ophthalmol. 135(6):800–6. PMID:12788119
1407. Zako M, Takeyama M, Naito E, Mizumoto K, Iwaki M (2012). Choroidal and optic disc metastases from breast cancer and their response to combination pharmacotherapy with tamoxifen, cyclophosphamide hydrate, letrozole, and bevacizumab. J Ocul Pharmacol Ther. 28(1):89–93. PMID:22011078
1408. Zamir E, Mechoulam H, Micera A, Levi-Schaffer F, Pe'er J (2002). Inflamed juvenile conjunctival naevus: clinicopathological characterisation. Br J Ophthalmol. 86(1):28–30. PMID:11801498
1409. Zelefsky JR, Revercomb CH, Lantos G, Warren FA (2008). Isolated lymphoma of the anterior visual pathway diagnosed by optic nerve biopsy. J Neuroophthalmol. 28(1):36–40. PMID:18347457
1410. Zemba M, Stamate AC, Papadatu CA, Avram CI, Malciolu R, Ochinciuc U, et al. (2014). The significance of imaging in a case of intraorbital cystic tumor. Oftalmologia. 58(2):18–24. [Romanian] PMID:25300124
1411. Zembowicz A, Mandal RV, Choopong P (2010). Melanocytic lesions of the conjunctiva. Arch Pathol Lab Med. 134(12):1785–92. PMID:21128776
1412. Zhan KY, Khaja SF, Flack AB, Day TA (2016). Benign parotid tumors. Otolaryngol Clin North Am. 49(2):327–42. PMID:27040584
1413. Zhang J, Jianmin, Wang N, Shi J, Ge X (2009). A case of primary oncocytic adenocarcinoma of the lacrimal sac. BMJ Case Rep. 2009. PMID:21747898
1414. Zhang R, Qian J, Yuan Y, Bi Y (2015). Atypical clinical presentation of orbital adenoid cystic carcinoma. J Cancer Res Ther. 11(4):1035. PMID:26881639
1415. Zhao M, Mu Y, Dang Y, Zhu Y (2014). Secondary glaucoma as initial manifestation of ring melanoma: a case report and review of literature. Int J Clin Exp Pathol. 7(11):8163–9. PMID:25550867
1416. Zhong FL, Mamaï O, Sborgi L, Boussofara L, Hopkins R, Robinson K, et al. (2016). Germline NLRP1 mutations cause skin inflammatory and cancer susceptibility syndromes via inflammasome activation. Cell. 167(1):187–202.e17. PMID:27662089
1417. Zhou M, Shen D, Head JE, Chew EY, Chévez-Barrios P, Green WR, et al. (2007). Ocular clusterin expression in von Hippel-Lindau disease. Mol Vis. 13:2129–36. PMID:18079682
1418. Zhou Q, Chang H, Zhang H, Han Y, Liu H (2012). Increased numbers of p63-positive/CD117-positive cells in advanced adenoid cystic carcinoma give a poorer prognosis. Diagn Pathol. 7:119. PMID:22963430
1419. Zhu MM, Cui HG, Teng XD (2015). GCDFP-15, AR, and Her-2 as biomarkers for primary ductal adenocarcinoma of the lacrimal gland: a Chinese case and literature review. Onco Targets Ther. 8:1017–24. PMID:25999735
1420. Zimmer-Galler I, Lie JT (1994). Choroidal infiltrates as the initial manifestation of lymphoma in rheumatoid arthritis after treatment with low-dose methotrexate. Mayo Clin Proc. 69(3):258–61. PMID:7510810
1421. Zimmerman LE (1965). Melanocytes, melanocytic nevi, and melanocytomas. Invest Ophthalmol. 4:11–41. PMID:14271285
1422. Zimmerman LE (1970). The remarkable polymorphism of tumours of the ciliary epithelium. Trans Aust Coll Ophthalmol. 2:114–25. PMID:5525160
1423. Zimmerman LE (1971). Phakomatous choristoma of the eyelid. A tumor of lenticular anlage. Am J Ophthalmol. 71(1 Pt 2):169–77. PMID:5542122
1424. Zimmerman LE, Thoreson HT (1964). Sudden loss of vision in acute leukemia. A clinicopathologic report of two unusual cases. Surv Ophthalmol. 9:467–73. PMID:14199728
1425. Zimmermann-Paiz MA, García de la Riva JC (2015). Conjunctival tumors in children: histopathologic diagnosis in 165 cases. Arq Bras Oftalmol. 78(6):337–9. PMID:26677032
1426. Zinkham WH (1978). Visceral larva migrans. A review and reassessment indicating two forms of clinical expression: visceral and ocular. Am J Dis Child. 132(6):627–33. PMID:350038
1427. Zoeller GK, Brathwaite CD, Sandberg

DI (2010). Malignant transformation of an optic pathway glioma without prior radiation therapy. J Neurosurg Pediatr. 5(5):507–10. PMID:20433265

Subject index

Numbers

A

B

C

D

E

F

G

Q

R

S

List of abbreviations

AIDS	acquired immunodeficiency syndrome
APAAP	alkaline phosphatase–antialkaline phosphatase
A-scan	amplitude scan (ultrasonography)
ATP	adenosine triphosphate
B-scan	brightness scan (ultrasonography)
CNS	central nervous system
DAB	3,3′-diaminobenzidine
DNA	deoxyribonucleic acid
EBV	Epstein–Barr virus
FISH	fluorescence in situ hybridization
H&E	haematoxylin and eosin
HHV8	human herpesvirus 8
HIV	human immunodeficiency virus
HPV	human papillomavirus
HTLV-1	human T-lymphotropic virus type 1
IARC	International Agency for Research on Cancer
ICD-O	International Classification of Diseases for Oncology
ICRB	International Classification of Retinoblastoma
Ig	immunoglobulin
MALT lymphoma	extranodal marginal zone lymphoma of mucosa-associated lymphoid tissue
MIM number	Mendelian Inheritance in Man number
MRI	magnetic resonance imaging
mRNA	messenger ribonucleic acid
N:C ratio	nuclear-to-cytoplasmic ratio
NK cell	natural killer cell
NOS	not otherwise specified
PCR	polymerase chain reaction
PET-CT	positron emission tomography–computed tomography
RNA	ribonucleic acid
RPE	retinal pigment epithelium
TNM	tumour, node, metastasis
UV	ultraviolet
VEGF	vascular endothelial growth factor